Emergency Medicine

Second Edition

Emergency Medicine

Second Edition

S.N. Chugh
MD, MNAMS, FICP, FIACM, FICN, FISC, FIMSA

Professor of Medicine and Head
Endocrine and Metabolism
Pt. B.D. Sharma PGIMS
Rohtak

PEEPEE
PUBLISHERS AND DISTRIBUTORS (P) LTD.

Emergency Medicine

Published by
Pawaninder P. Vij

Peepee Publishers and Distributors (P) Ltd.
Head Office: 160, Shakti Vihar, Pitam Pura, Delhi-110 034 (India)

Corporate Office: 7/31, Ansari Road, Daryaganj, Post Box-7243
New Delhi-110 002 (India)
Ph: 55195868, 9811156083
e-mail: peepee160@yahoo.co.in
e-mail: peepee160@rediffmail.com
e-mail: peepee160@gmail.com
www.peepeepub.com

© 2006 Dr. S.N. Chugh

All rights reserved

No part of this publication may be reproduced or transmitted in any form or by any means, electronic, mechanical, photocopy, recording, translated, or any information storage and retrieval system, without permission in writing from the editor and the publisher.

This book has been published in good faith that the material provided by authors/contributors is original. Every effort is made to ensure accuracy of material, but publisher and printer will not be held responsible for any inadvertent errors. In case of any dispute, all legal matters to be settled under Delhi jurisdiction only.

First Edition: **2004**

Second Edition: **2006**

ISBN: 81-88867-79-9

Printed at
Lordson, C-5/19, Rana Pratap Bagh, Delhi-110 007

To
My Parents
WIFE
Dr. Kiran Chugh
SON
Dr. Anshul Chugh
DAUGHTER
Dr. Ashima Chugh

A Request

Dear Students/Physicians

This second edition of my book "Emergency Medicine" is colourful mega edition, containing the comprehensive text in the coloured boxes and tables that soothe one's eyes. The text has been revised and updated after consultations with my colleagues and resident staff. I have added few new emergencies on the request of students and practitioners. The success of this edition depends entirely on the students and readers. I have made every effort to provide detailed informations to the readers on each and every emergency, still, if there is any lapse on my part, I may be excused. Comments and suggestions from the readers will be appreciated if sent to the publisher directly.

S.N. Chugh

Preface to the Second Edition

The success of the first edition of "Emergency Medicine", has encouraged me to bring out this second multi-coloured and mega edition of this book. I have enjoyed the opportunity to enlarge this edition as well as to alter the previous text in the light of new literature. The illustrations and colour pictures in this book themselves speak the status and standard of the book. Certain new topics have been added according to the demands of the students and the practitioners. Few topics have been fully revised and updated.

I hereby stress that the basic aim of this book remains unchanged. Each emergency discussed in the book is according to international standard. I have tried my maximum to explain the text with the help of figures and the diagrams. The coloured boxes and tables further beautify the book.

The book is intended for the students of medicine and the clinicians dealing with these emergencies. This book will also help those students who intend to pursue further study in medicine.

I am thankful to Mr. Pawaninder P. Vij, Director, Peepee Publishers and Distributors (P) Ltd., New Delhi, who has put sincere efforts to bring this colourful mega edition of the book. This book itself speaks the efficiency and proficiency of the publisher. I congratulate him for this new edition.

S.N. Chugh

Preface to the First Edition

Most of the clinical conditions present acutely as an emergency and patient lands in the casualty and accidental department of a hospital or an institution. Every physician has to deal with the emergency situations in clinical practice, while resident staff deal them in a hospital. The clinical efficiency and capabilities of the doctor/physician depends on the up-date knowledge and acquaintance with recent advances in medicine. For every physician, it is must to be well versed with these emergencies and equipment/procedure required for that. Every physician is duty-bound to refer the patient to an institution if the necessary facility/equipment/expertise is not available.

To write a book on emergency as a single handed physician is a formidable and challenging task. No body will accept the challenge of writing a book unless or until he/she possesses the knowledge to deal with the acute medical conditions. To write a book by multiple authors has become not only customary but is essential because it is not possible for one author to deal with such a fast-changing subject of medicine.

Having a very long experience of teaching undergraduates and postgraduates, I decided to write this book on the request of my resident staff and students. I have the blessings of my teachers as well as my colleagues, Dr Harpreet Singh, Dr. H.K. Aggarwal, Associate Professor of Medicine to write the necessary book. They assured me necessary help and even helped me whenever I needed.

My sole purpose of writing this book was to teach the undergraduates and postgraduates the necessary management of emergencies through this book which is handy, concise and updated. I think it will be useful to students and practising physicians and will make them acquainted with necessary decisions to be taken in emergency situations.

S.N. Chugh

Contents

Part I: Pulmonary Medicine

1. Severe or Massive Haemoptysis 3
2. Community-Acquired Pneumonia 7
3. Acute Severe Bronchial Asthma 12
4. Acute Respiratory Distress Syndrome (ARDS) 16
5. Pulmonary Embolism 20
6. Pneumothorax 29
7. Asphyxia 34
8. Respiratory Failure 39
9. Acute Empyema Thoracis 45

Part II: Gastroenterology

10. Acute Vomiting 53
11. Acute Diarrhoea 57
12. Upper Gastrointestinal Bleed 61
13. Lower Gastrointestinal Bleed 65
14. Acute Pancreatitis 68
15. Amoebic Liver Abscess 75
16. Hepatic Encephalopathy 79
17. Biliary Colic 85

Part III: Infections

18. Septic Shock 91
19. Dengue Fever 96
20. Typhoid Fever and its Complications 99
21. Rabies 102
22. Tetanus 106
23. Myonecrosis (Gas Gangrene) 110
24. Cholera 112
25. Bacterial Food Poisoning 115

26. Acute Dysentery *119*
27. Cerebral Malaria *121*

Part IV: Cardiology

28. Acute ST-Elevation Myocardial Infarction (STEMI) *127*
29. Cardiogenic Shock *134*
30. Shock (Acute Circulatory Failure) *140*
31. Heart Failure *147*
32. Left Ventricular Failure (Pulmonary Oedema) *153*
33. Management of Tachyarrhythmias *159*
34. Management of Bradyarrhythmias and Stokes-Adam Attacks *169*
35. Acute Coronary Syndrome *177*
36. Cardiac Tamponade *182*
37. Acute Chest Pain *187*
38. Cardiac Arrest and Sudden Cardiac Death *191*
39. Hypertensive Emergencies/Urgencies *197*

Part V: Neurology

40. Acute Confusional State (Delirium) *207*
41. The Unconsciousness or Coma *213*
42. Acute Headache *219*
43. Acute Syncope *225*
44. Acute Vertigo *230*
45. Acute Ischaemic Stroke *235*
46. Subarachnoid Haemorrhage *246*
47. Status Epilepticus` *251*
48. Acute Meningitis *255*
49. Acute Viral Encephalitis *265*
50. Acute Transverse Myelitis *269*
51. Acute Spinal Cord Compression *273*
52. Acute Inflammatory Demyelinating Polyradiculoneuropathy *280*
53. Cortical Venous and Dual Sinus Thrombosis *286*
54. Raised Intracranial Pressure *289*

Part VI: Haematology

55. Acute Haemolytic Anaemia *295*
56. Thrombocytopenia *301*
57. Thrombotic Thrombocytopenic Purpura (TTP) *306*

58. Haemophilia 309
59. Disseminated Intravascular Coagulation (DIC) 314
60. Agranulocytosis or Severe Neutropenia 319
61. Aplastic Anaemia 323
62. Acute Leukaemias 328
63. Blood Transfusion Related Complications 336

Part VII: Endocrinology and Metabolism

64. Diabetic Ketoacidosis (Diabetic Coma) 345
65. Hyperosmolar Hyperglycaemic Non-Ketotic Coma (HHNKC) 352
66. Hypoglycaemia 356
67. Thyroid Crisis or Storm 361
68. Myxoedema Coma 365
69. Acute Adrenal Crisis/Insufficiency 368
70. Pituitary Apoplexy 372
71. Hypocalcaemia 375
72. Hypercalcaemia (Hypercalcaemic Crisis) 379

Part VIII: Nephrology

73. Acute Nephritic Syndrome 385
74. Acute Renal Failure 390

Part IX: Poisonings

75. Management of a Case with Poisoning 401
76. Corrosive (Acid and Alkali) Poisoning 409
77. Methylalcohol (Methanol) Poisoning 414
78. Carbon Monoxide Poisoning 418
79. Copper Sulphate Poisoning 421
80. Epidemic Dropsy 424
81. Organophosphates (Organophosphorus) 427
82. Aluminium and Zinc Phosphide Poisoning 432
83. Organochlorines 437
84. Plant Poison 439
85. Snake and Lizard Bites 442
86. Scorpion Sting 450
87. Sedative and Hypnotic Poisoning 454

Part X: Internal Medicine

88. Systemic Anaphylaxis *461*
89. Heat Hyperpyrexia *464*
90. Hypothermia *468*
91. High Altitude Related Emergencies *472*
92. Electrical and Lightning Injuries *476*
93. Drowning and Near Drowning *479*
94. Hanging and Strangulation *483*

Part XI: Acid-base and Electrolyte Disturbance

95. Acid-base Disturbance *489*
96. Disorders of Sodium Balance *502*
97. Acute Disturbance of Potassium Balance (Dyskalaemia) *510*

Part XII: Skin Emergencies

98. Acute Urticaria and Angioedema *521*
99. Erythroderma and Exfoliative Dermatitis *524*
100. Pemphigus *526*
101. Skin Infections *528*
102. Stevens-Johnson Syndrome *530*

Index *533*

Part One

Pulmonary Medicine

Chapter 1

Severe or Massive Haemoptysis

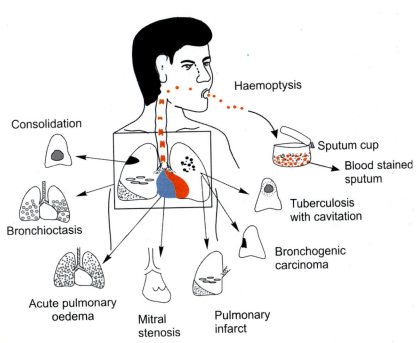

Fig. 1.1: Some common causes of haemoptysis

MASSIVE HAEMOPTYSIS

Definition

Massive haemoptysis is defined as expectoration of more than 200 ml of blood in 24 hours. Massive haemoptysis can represent acute life-threatening emergency, should be subjected to appropriate diagnostic tests to find out the specific cause. Expectoration of even small amount of blood is a frightening symptom. Large amounts of blood can fill the airways and alveolar spaces, not only seriously disturbing the alveolar gas exchange but also causing choking or suffocation.

Pseudo-haemoptysis means the blood expectorated is not coming from the lungs; is actually coming from upper respiratory tract (sinus, nares, pharynx or mouth) initiating the coughing with blood.

4 Pulmonary Medicine

Box 1.1: Causes of haemoptysis

1. **Diseases of bronchi**
   - Bronchial adenoma
   - Bronchial carcinoma
   - Acute bronchitis
   - Bronchiectasis
   - Foreign body
2. **Diseases of lung parenchyma**
   - Tuberculosis
   - Suppurative pneumonia
   - Lung abscess
   - Trauma
   - Parasitic, e.g. lung flukes
   - Fungal, e.g. aspergilloma, actinomycosis
3. **Lung vascular disease**
   - Pulmonary embolism
   - Goodpasture's syndrome
   - Polyarteritis nodosa
   - Wegner's granulomatosis
4. **Cardiovascular diseases**
   - Acute left ventricular failure
   - Mitral stenosis
   - Aortic aneurysm
5. **Haematological diseases**
   - Anticoagulants therapy
   - Thrombocytopenia
   - Leukaemia
   - Haemophilia
6. **Iatrogenic**
   - Bronchoscopy
   - Pulmonary artery rupture during catheterisation

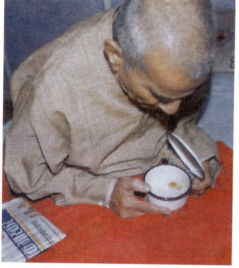

Fig. 1.2: Haemoptysis in a patient with pneumonic consolidation. Note the blood stained sputum

Causes

Although there are a large number of causes of haemoptysis (see the Box 1.1 and Fig. 1.1), but common causes encountered in clinical practice are bronchitis, bronchiectasis, pneumonia, tuberculosis, lung abscess and bronchogenic carcinoma, etc.

Clinical Work-up

It includes:
1. History.
2. Physical examination.
3. Laboratory investigations.

History

The duration, character and precipitating factors of haemoptysis provide helpful diagnostic clues:
- The purulent sputum streaked with blood suggests an infection as the cause (Fig. 1.2).
- Haemoptysis lasting more than 24 hours despite appropriate treatment of infection suggests an endobronchial lesion such as tuberculosis or cancer as the causes of bleeding.
- Expectoration of frank blood in smokers over the age of 40 years suggests a bronchogenic carcinoma.
- Recurrent haemoptysis of small amounts of blood over a period of years suggest underlying bronchial adenoma.
- Fever, recurrent pneumonias with haemoptysis indicate bronchiectasis as the underlying cause.
- If haemoptysis is due to cardiovascular cause, then associated symptoms such as dyspnoea

orthopnoea, PND help in the diagnosis.
- If haemoptysis is associated with pain chest and wheezing in a patient with deep vein thrombosis, then possibility of acute pulmonary embolism is most likely.
- History of drugs such as anticoagulants should also be taken.
- History of any procedure.

Physical Examination

A thorough physical examination should be done to find out the underlying cause (listed in the Box 1.1). Finger clubbing is common in bronchiectasis, lung cancer, lung abscess. Look for signs of malignancy, i.e. cachexia, hepatomegaly, lymphadenopathy. Signs of consolidation and pleurisy indicate pneumonia or a pulmonary infarct. Look for systemic signs such as rash, purpura, haematuria, splinter haemorrhage for systemic vascular diseases. Look for signs of mitral valve disease and signs of left heart failure.

Laboratory Investigations

- *Blood count:* Total leucocytes count and differential leucocyte count to be done for any evidence of infection. Haemoglobin estimation to be done for severity of blood loss and anaemia. Blood count is also important for haematological malignancy.
- *Urine examination* for systemic diseases such as polyarteritis nodosa, Goodpasture's syndrome or vasculitis.
- *Coagulation studies* to identify the correctable haematological abnormalities.
- *Chest X-ray* provides valuable informations of pulmonary congestion (oedema), pneumonia (consolidation), tuberculosis (a cavity), lung abscess (a cavity with fluid and air), pulmonary infarcts (multiple peripheral triangular shadows), lung cancer (a big solid lesion with atelectasis), etc. The chest X-ray has its limitations. It has been reported that 30% of chest X-ray of the patients with haemoptysis may be normal. In addition, when abnormalities are detected on the X-ray, the bronchoscopy frequently reveals another location of haemorrhage.
- *Sputum examination* by Gram and acid-fast stains (along with corresponding culture) is indicated. In suspected mass lesion, sputum may be examined for malignant cells.
- *Fibreoptic bronchoscopy* is particularly useful for localising the site of bleeding and for visualisation of endobronchial lesions. When bleeding is massive, rigid bronchoscopy is often preferable than fibreoptic because of better airways control and efficient suction capabilities.

Bronchoscopy has the highest diagnostic yield when performed during bleeding.

Bronchoscopy may not be necessary when other tests have pinpointed the bleeding site and is also not recommended in mild haemoptysis which is likely to be due to acute respiratory infection (tracheobronchitis, pneumonia). In patients suspected of bronchiectasis, HRCT (high resolution computed tomography) is now the procedure of choice instead of bronchography.

Bronchoscopy has little role in haemoptysis with normal chest X-ray.

Angiography: It is most helpful when vascular lesions are suspected. It is helpful in diagnosis of pulmonary embolism. CT pulmonary angiography may be necessary in patients with pre-existing lung disease where ventilation perfusion scan is difficult to interpret.

Ventilation-perfusion (V/Q) lung scan: It is useful in establishing the diagnosis of suspected thromboembolic disease.

CT scan: It is particularly useful in investigating peripheral lesions seen on chest X-ray which may not be accessible to bronchoscopy and facilitates accurate *percutaneous* needle biopsy, if indicated.

Management

The rapidity of bleeding and its effect on gas exchange determine the urgency of management. Establish the diagnosis first, and find out the cause if bleeding is mild and gas exchange is preserved; but if there is massive haemoptysis, then to maintain adequate gas exchange, following steps may be taken:

1. Bed-rest, mild sedation and cough suppression may help the bleeding to subside.
2. If origin of the blood is known and is limited to one lung, the bleeding lung should be placed in the dependent position so that blood is not aspirated into unaffected lung.
3. Oxygen supplementation is guided by blood gas analysis. With massive haemoptysis, the need to control the airway and maintain adequate gas exchange, endotracheal intubation and mechanical ventilation may be necessary.
4. Blood volume should be replaced by blood transfusions, if necessary. Coagulopathies should be treated with transfusion of the appropriate coagulation factors and platelets.
5. Resuscitation of shock by fluids, blood transfusions and drugs, if necessary.
6. Chest physiotherapy, spirometry and postural drainage should be avoided.
7. In massive haemoptysis, if there is danger of flooding of the lung with blood contralateral to the side of haemorrhage despite the proper positioning, isolation of right and left bronchi from each other can be achieved with specially designed double lumen endotracheal tube.
8. Endoscopic balloon tamponade is done to occlude the bronchus having the bleeding site by inserting a balloon catheter through a bronchoscope after direct visualisation of bleeding site, and by inflating the balloon. This technique not only prevents the aspiration of blood into unaffected areas but also may promote tamponade (compression) the bleeding site and stoppage of bleeding.
9. Other available techniques to control the bleeding in massive haemoptysis include laser photocoagulation, embolotherapy and surgical resection of the involved area of lung. Haemoptysis due to bleeding from an endobronchial tumour can be stopped temporarily by coagulating the bleeding site by laser therapy (neodymium-Yttrium-aluminium-garnet—Nd:YAG). Embolotherapy, is an angiographic procedure in which a vessel proximal to the bleeding site is cannulated and *gel foam* is injected to occlude the vessel like an embolus.

Chapter 2

Community-Acquired Pneumonia

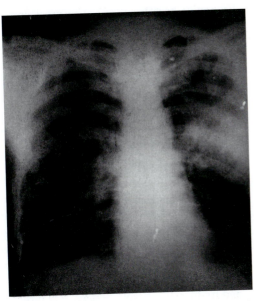

Fig. 2.1: Chest X-ray showing consolidation left mid-zone. Note the homogenous opacity

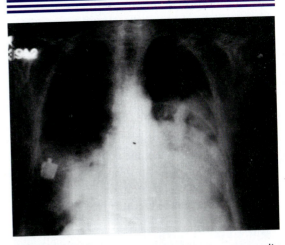

Fig. 2.2: Bilateral consolidation due to community acquired pneumonia. Note the homogenous opacities in the mid and lower zones of both the lungs

COMMUNITY-ACQUIRED PNEUMONIA

Definition

Pneumonia is an acute inflammation of the lung parenchyma by infective or noninfective process presenting with features of consolidation on clinical and radiological examination. It is a leading cause of death and morbidity in the developing as well as in developed countries. It is one of the most common cause for hospital admission in adults and children.

Community-acquired pneumonia refers to pneumonia occurring in young healthy adults. Infection is usually spread by droplets inhalation and, most patients affected are previously well. Cigarette smoking, alcoholism, and corticosteroid or immunosuppressive therapy all impair mucociliary clearance and immune defense and predispose to it.

Community-acquired pneumonia may present as *lobar pneumonia* which is a radiological and pathological term referring to a homogenous consolidation (clinical term) of one or more lobes (Figs 2.1 and 2.2) often associated with pleural inflammation. *Bronchopneumonia* refers to a more patchy alveolar consolidation associated with bronchial and bronchiolar inflammation often affecting both the lower lobes.

Causative Pathogens

Identification of the aetiological micro-organism is of prime importance, since, this is key to start the antimicrobial therapy. However, despite intensive investigations the causative organism is not isolated in a large number of cases and, therefore, the initial antimicrobial therapy is empirical and is based on (i) the setting in which infection was acquired, (ii) the clinical presentation, (iii) pattern of radiological findings, (iv) result of Gram-staining of the sputum, and (v) current trend of susceptibility of the suspected pathogens to antimicrobial agents. When the causative organism is found, then specific antibiotic therapy can be chosen. The common pathogens causing community-acquired pneumonia are given in the Box 2.1.

Box 2.1: Causative pathogens responsible for community-acquired pneumonia

Common	Uncommon
• Streptococcus pneumoniae	• Legionella species
• Mycoplasma pneumoniae	• Staphylococcus aureus
• H. influenzae	• Coxiella burnetci/ Chlamydia
	• Oral anaerobes
	• Viruses, e.g. influenza, parainfluenza
	• Fungal

The *predisposing factors* to community-acquired pneumonia are:
1. Alcoholism.
2. Chronic obstructive pulmonary disease.
3. Recent attack of influenza.
4. Old age.
5. Contact with sick bird (*chlamydia* species) and from environment (*coxiella burneti*).
6. Poor orodental hygiene (oral anaerobes).
7. Travelling (endemic mycosis).

Clinical Features

1. *Typical presentation:* The 'typical' pneumonia syndrome presents with sudden onset of fever, productive cough with purulent sputum, haemoptysis, and in some cases, pleuritic chest pain and physical signs of consolidation (dullness on percussion, increased vocal fremitus and bronchial breath sound). The most common pathogen is *S. pneumoniae*.

2. *Atypical presentation:* It is characterised by a gradual onset, dry cough, extrapulmonary symptoms (headache, myalgia, fatigue, sore throat, nausea, vomiting and diarrhoea) and minimal findings on chest examination despite abnormal chest X-ray (no correlation between physical and radiological findings). The causative organisms include *Mycoplasma pneumoniae, L. pneumophila, P. carinii, anaerobes,* etc. Certain viruses (influenza), and tuberculosis also produce atypical manifestations of pneumonia. In immunocompromised host, *Pneumocystis carinii* is the most common pathogen. These patients have concurrent infections with other opportunistic pathogens such pulmonary and frequently extrapulmonary, oral thrush due to candida or extensive perineal ulcers due to herpes simplex virus.

Sudden onset of fever, productive cough, haemoptysis and pleuritic chest pain are classical manifestations of pneumonia. Physical findings are consistent with consolidation of lung seen on chest X-ray.

Investigations

1. *Chest X-ray is useful:*
   i. To confirm the presence and location of pulmonary infiltrates. Most pulmonary

pathogens produce focal lesions. Multiple areas of involvement suggest hematogenous spread. Diffuse lesions in immunocompromised host suggest infection by *P. carinii* and viral infections.

ii. To assess the extent of lung involvement.
iii. To detect pleural and lymph node (hilar lymphadenopathy) involvement and pulmonary cavitation.
iv. To assess the response to antimicrobial therapy.
v. To rule out other conditions that simulate pneumonia on X-ray.

Usually X-ray chest shows reticular pattern in *Mycoplasma* infection, homogenous localised opacity and air bronchogram is seen in *S. pneumoniae* infection.

2. ***Sputum examination:*** It remains the mainstay of the diagnosis but its specificity is decreased because it gets contaminated during expectoration with bacteria that colonise the upper respiratory tract. It has low sensitivity also. However, an acceptable sample should have less than 10 epithelial cells and more than 25 leucocytes per low power field. Sputum should be examined by Gram staining which may show gram-positive diplococci in pneumococcal pneumonia. Ziehl-Neelsen stain for *Mycobacterium tuberculosis* (AFB) must be done, as well as Giemsa staining for *P. carinii*. Sputum culture should also be done.

Expectorated sputum is easily collected from patients with a vigorous cough but may be scanty in patients with atypical pneumonia, in elderly and in patients with disturbed sensorium. In such a situation, sputum can be induced with ultrasonic nebulization of 3% saline.

3. ***Blood culture:*** It is useful if pneumonia is associated with bacteremia.
4. ***Blood test:*** Total and differential leucocyte count and ***ESR*** may suggest an evidence of infection.
5. ***Serological tests:*** *These* tests are sometimes helpful. They depend on the host immune response and usually become positive later in the course of the disease. They are:
   - Indirect immunofluorescence test: (IgA, IgM 4-6 fold rise in antibody titre suggests. *M. pneumoniae* infection).
   - Indirect fluorescent antibody test for legionella.
   - Microimmunofluorescence for *C. psittaci*.
6. ***ECG:*** It shows myocarditis in *C. burnetti* infection.
7. **Invasive procedures:** These may be required to obtain the pulmonary material sometimes to establish the diagnosis when other investigations are non-contributory and patient has failed to respond to antimicrobial therapy. These are:
   - Transtracheal aspiration.
   - Percutaneous transthoracic lung puncture and aspiration.
   - Fibreoptic bronchoscopy. Either bronchoalveolar lavage of aspirated material after brushing or transbronchial lung biopsy specimens may be obtained.
   - Open lung biopsy.
8. ***Other tests:*** If empyema is a clinical consideration, then diagnostic thoracentesis is indicated. Pleural fluid culture is generally considered diagnostic of the aetiology of pneumonia.
9. Arterial blood gas or oxygen saturation.

Assessment of Severity and Decision to Hospitalise

Unnecessary admission of a patient to a hospital not only burden the hospital resources, but also poses the patient to risk of nosocomial infections. Therefore, utmost care to be exercised to admit the patient because most of the patients with pneumonia can be treated on out-patient basis. The criteria for hospital admission include:

1. Elderly patients > 65 years of age.
2. Significant comorbidity (e.g., kidney, heart or lung disease, immunocompromised state).
3. Leucopenia (WBC < 5000 cells/µL) not attributed to a known cause.
4. *S. aureus,* gram-negative organism or anaerobes as the suspected cause of pneumonia.
5. Severe pneumonia, e.g. multilobar involvement, hypoxia, tachypnoea (> 30/min), tachycardia (> 140/min), hypotension (systolic BP < 90 mm).
6. Presence of complications, e.g. empyema thoracis, meningitis, endocarditis.
7. Inability to take oral medication or altered mental status.
8. Failure of out-patient management, e.g. treatment compliance is poor.

Management

The plan of management of community-acquired pneumonia includes:
1. To decide whether patient needs out of hospital or in-hospital treatment (read the criteria).
2. To determine the most likely organism depending on the age and choice of empirical therapy.
3. To determine the prevalence of antibiotic resistance pattern in the community.
4. Associated illness or comorbidity.

Outpatient Management

Pneumonia in an otherwise healthy adult is most likely to be due to *Mycoplasma pneumoniae, S. pneumoniae* or *Chlamydia pneumoniae*, hence, empirical therapy with penicillin, ampicillin or amoxycillin (500 mg 8 hourly for 7-10 days) remains the treatment of choice. Erythromycin (500 mg every 6 hourly) or doxycycline (100 mg every 12 hourly) is another option. Fluoroquinolones can also be used but has borderline activity against pneumococci *in vitro*.

In older patients with underlying chronic respiratory disease, *Legionella pneumophilia, H. influenzae* organisms should be considered in addition to abovementioned organisms. In older patients or adult outpatients with pre-existing respiratory disease with typical presentation of pneumonia, either *amoxycillin plus* the β-lactamase inhibitor clavulanic acid or doxycycline can be used. The new macrolides (azithromycin—a single dose of 500 mg on first day and 250 mg once daily for next 4 days or clarithromycin—500 mg twice daily for 7 to 10 days) are other options. For *Mycoplasma* and *Legionella pneumoniae*, a macrolide is the drug of choice but doxycycline, cotrimoxazole and ciprofloxacin have also been used successfully. The duration of therapy for such pneumonia is 2-3 weeks; the long duration is frequently recommended to prevent relapse.

Pneumonia due to anaerobes is treated with clindamycin (300 mg 6 hourly or 450 mg 8 hourly for 7 to 10 days) with amoxycillin (500 mg 8 hourly) plus metronidazole (500 mg 6 hourly) or with amoxycillin/clavulanic acid combination.

The outpatient treatment is summarised in the Box 2.2.

Box 2.2: Outpatient empirical treatment for community-acquired pneumonia

Without cardiopulmonary and/or comorbid condition	With cardiopulmonary and/or comorbid condition
• Newer macrolide (azithromycin or clarithromycin) or	• Beta-lactam plus macrolide or
• Antipneumococcal quinolone (e.g. levofloxacin, sparfloxacin, gatfloxacin or High dose amoxycillin/ doxycycline	• Antipneumococcal fluoroquinolone

In-hospital Management

1. ***Antibiotic therapy***
   The hospitalised patients must undergo prompt microbial evaluation and receive empirical antimicrobial therapy based on Gram's staining of the sputum and knowledge of the current

antimicrobial sensitivity. Parenteral antibiotic therapy is mandatory. The empirical therapy for hospitalised patient depends on the presence or absence of comorbid conditions (see Box 2.3). On improvement, therapy can be switched from intravenous to oral agents to complete 7-10 days course of antibiotics.

Box 2.3: Empirical antibiotic therapy for hospitalised patients

No cardiopulmonary or comorbid condition	With cardiopulmonary or comorbid condition
• Parenteral azithromycin or clarithromycin or • Beta-lactam and doxycycline or • Antipneumococcal fluoroquinolones	• I.V Beta-lactam plus I.V or oral macrolide or • I.V antipneumococcal fluoroquinolone

The antibiotic therapy to be modified after culture and sensitivity report of sputum. If sputum production is scanty and patient's condition is critical, invasive methods may be used to procure the pulmonary specimen for isolation of pathogens.

2. *Oxygen therapy:* Oxygen should be administered to all the hypoxaemic patients and high concentration (> 35%) should be used in all patients who do not exhibit hypercapnia associated with COPD. Assisted ventilation may be considered if patient remains hypoxaemic despite O_2 therapy.
3. *Treatment of hypotension* with I.V fluids and inotropic support if needed.
4. *Treatment of pleural pain:* It is important to relieve pleural pain in order to allow the patient to feel better and to breath properly and cough effectively. Parenteral pethidine (50-100 mg) or morphine (5-10 mg) may be used with utmost caution in patient's with poor respiratory function.
5. *Physiotherapy:* With relief of pleural pain, patient should be encouraged to cough efficiently to help in mucus clearance and to improve gas exchange and to assist in resolution of pneumonia.

Chapter 3

Acute Severe Bronchial Asthma

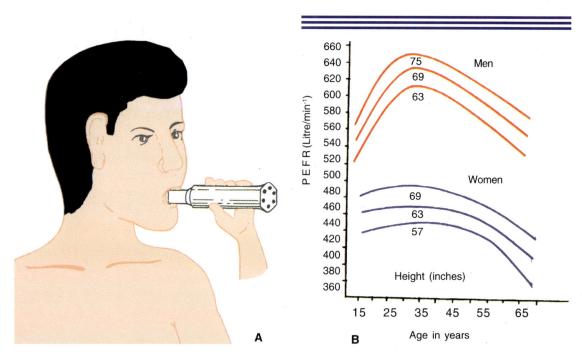

Fig. 3.1: Peak flow measurement (A) Peak flowmeter (B) Graph of normal recording for men and women. Note: In asthmatic patients recordings of < 200 L/min indicate severe disease and values of < 100 L/min indicate life-threatening asthma

ACUTE SEVERE BRONCHIAL ASTHMA

Definition

Acute severe bronchial asthma (previously called status asthmaticus) is used to describe life-threatening episodes of asthma during which the patient is distressed by severe breathlessness, cough, wheeze and other symptoms of asthma due to severe airway obstruction resulting in pulsus paradoxus and use of accessory muscles of respiration; and response to maintenance therapy fails and aggressive therapy becomes necessary.

Acute episodes of severe bronchial asthma are one of the most common respiratory emergencies

Acute Severe Bronchial Asthma

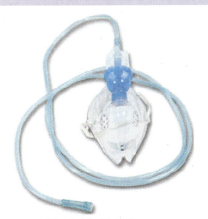

Fig. 3.2A: Nebuliser

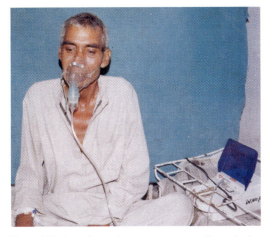

Fig. 3.2B: A patient of acute severe asthma being nebulised at the bed-side

seen in clinical practice, hence, it is essential to recognise them early with early institution of therapy.

Precipitating Factors

A stable patient of asthma develops an acute severe attack either due to omission or inadequacy of the maintenance drug treatment. Other factors that push the patient into acute attack are:
1. Infection (upper respiratory infection or pneumonia).
2. Pollutants (e.g., exposure to pollen, smoke).
3. Smoking.
4. Change of local environment such as seasonal change, shifting into a new house, a new pet, white-washing or painting in house, taking out old shelved books or clothes.
5. Drugs (β-blockers and NSAIDs)
6. Acute anxiety or stress.

Clinical Features

The clinical features result due to acute severe reversible airway obstruction resulting in hyper-inflated lungs, use of extra-respiratory muscles for respiration and fall in pulse pressure on inspiration (pulsus paradoxus). There is loss of adventitial breath sounds and wheezing becomes high-pitched and may become absent. The clinical features are given in the Box 3.1.

In extreme situations, wheezing may lessen markedly or even disappear, cough may become ineffective and patient may develop gasping type of respiration. These findings indicate excessive mucus plugging and impending suffocation. Central cyanosis develops and chest becomes silent and bradycardia may occur. All these are ominous signs.

Life-threatening features include:
- Inability to speak.
- Central cyanosis.
- Reduced or altered consciousness.
- Silent chest.
- Bradycardia.
- PEF < 100 L/min.

Investigations

Investigations are done to grade the severity and to identify the complications (e.g., atelectasis, spontaneous pneumothorax, etc.). These are:
1. **Chest X-ray:** It is done to see any evidence of infection, e.g. pneumonia or complications such as atelectasis or pneumothorax.
2. **Peak expiratory flow rate (PEFR):** It is useful to assess the severity. PEFR < 50% of predicted value or his/her personal best suggests severe obstruction (Fig. 3.1). Majority of patients with

Pulmonary Medicine

Box 3.1: Clinical features of acute severe asthma

Symptoms	Signs
• Severe respiratory distress, cough and wheezing	• Tachypnoea (respiratory rate > 25/min) and tachycardia (HR > 100/min)
• Feeling of heaviness/tightness of chest due to increase in anteroposterior diameter of chest	• Use of accessory muscles and indrawing of intercostal spaces
• Inability to complete the sentences without becoming breathless	• Wheezing become extensive and high-pitched (may become absent in severe attack)
• Inability to get out of bed or get proper sleep	• Silent chest—breath sounds may be inaudible
	• Pulsus paradoxus due to reduced cardiac return as a result of hyperinflated lungs. This sign may become absent if the patient's breathing is shallow as it requires a large negative intrathoracic pressure to produce it

acute severe asthma have PEFR less than 100 L/min and find difficulty in blowing into peak flowmeter.

3. *Arterial gas analysis:*
   - Presence of hypoxaemia (PaO_2 < 60 mmHg) indicates a very serious state.
   - Acidosis (pH < 7.38) and hypercapnia ($PaCO_2$ > 40 mmHg) indicate fear of impending death. In fact, $PaCO_2$ is generally low during an acute attack (hypocapnia), hence, rise in $PaCO_2$ even to normal or above is an ominous sign.
4. *Other tests:*
   - TLC and DLC for an evidence of infection.
   - Blood biochemistry and serum electrolytes to assess the effect of an acute attack.
   - ECG to look for ischaemic changes as a result of hypoxaemia, right heart strain and arrhythmias.

Differential Diagnosis

Acute attack of bronchial asthma must be differentiated from cardiac asthma (acute left ventricular failure). Other conditions that simulate an acute attack of asthma are:
- Pulmonary embolism.
- Acute upper respiratory obstruction (suffocation by tumour or laryngeal oedema).
- Hypersensitivity pneumonia (eosinophilic pneumonias).
- Vocal cord dysfunction presenting with severe laryngospasm or laryngotracheal hyper-reactivity.
- Endobronchial disease such as foreign body aspiration, a neoplasm or bronchial stenosis. These conditions produce localised persistent wheezing with paroxysmal attacks of coughing.

Management

Aims and Objectives

- Early recognition and early institution of therapy so as to prevent death.
- Correction of hypoxaemia.
- To overcome airflow obstruction as early as possible.
- To reduce recurrences or early relapse.
- Removal of the precipitating factor.

One of the most important cause of mortality in asthma is delayed institution of treatment or worsening episodes of asthma, therefore, for early diagnosis and assessment of severity, peak expiratory flow rate (PEFR) should be measured in all patients presenting with asthma; less than 50% of predicted value or patient best value or < 200L/min indicates severe asthma; the value < 30% of the predicted value or < 100 L/min indicates life-threatening situation necessitating hospital admission. Treatment of acute severe asthma is divided into:

1. ***Treatment at home:***
   - The patient is assessed. Tachycardia (HR> 110 min), tachypnoea (> 25/min), pulsus paradoxus, inability to speak, PEFR < 50% of predicted value indicate severe asthma.
   - If PEFR is < 150 L/min in an adult, patient should be shifted to a hospital.
   - Nebulised salbutamol 5 mg or terbutaline 2.5 mg is administered 2-4 hourly or as required (Figs 3.2A and 3.2B).
   - Prednisolone 40 mg orally or hydrocortisone 200 mg I.V.
   - Oxygen—high flow (40-60%).
   - Maintain I.V. access and take chest X-ray.
   - Sedatives should be avoided.
2. ***Treatment in hospital:***
   - Proper hydration of the patient with I.V. fluids
   - The patient is reassessed after admission to the hospital for severity and life-threatening situation.
   - Oxygen therapy 40-60% is continued.
   - The PEFR is measured and if asthma is under control, then continue nebulised salbutamol or terbutaline 4 hourly, prednisolone 40-60 mg/day for 2 days or hydrocortisone I.V.

   If features of severity persist:
   - Add ipratropium bromide 0.5 mg to the nebulised salbutamol/terbutaline.
   - Continue nebulised salbutamol/terbutaline treatment every 15-30 min if necessary, reduce to 4 hourly once clear response to treatment occurs.
   - Magnesium sulphate (25 mg/kg I.V. or max 2.0 g).
   - Arterial blood gases are measured; the PaCO$_2$ greater than 6 kPa and PaO$_2$ less than 8 kPa alongwith deteriorating consciousness (confusion, drowsiness, coma) are indications for assisted ventilation.
   - *Antibiotics:* They are indicated in the presence of infection (purulent sputum, leucocytosis). Amoxycillin or one of the macrolides is adequate.
   - *Intravenous aminophylline:* Recent trials have shown that addition of I.V. aminophylline to initial standard therapy with nebulised beta 2-agonists and systemic steroids in acute asthma fail to demonstrate any beneficial effect, hence, aminophylline has no role in acute severe asthma but certain physicians still persist to it.

   Monitoring of treatment
   - PEFR recordings should be made every 15-30 minutes to assess the early response and as and when required basis. In hospital, PEFR values should be charted 4-6 hourly, before and after inhaled bronchodilator treatment throughout the period of hospital stay.
   - Repeated measurement of arterial blood gas tensions and pH within 1-2 hours is necessary in all patients if first arterial sample shows features of life-threatening situation (PaO$_2$ < 8kPa and PaCO$_2$ > 6kPa and rising).
   - Oxygen saturation by pulse oximetry is valuable in all patients to assess response.
3. ***Recovery phase of asthma***: Aggressive treatment should continue for 7 to 10 days; thereafter, it may be stepped down. Physiotherapy and expectorants to assist expectoration may be useful at this stage. Oral corticosteroids should be continued for 2 weeks then substituted by steroids inhalers for maintenance.
4. ***Correction of precipitating factor:*** Triggering or provoking agents must be avoided.

Prevention

Along with avoidance of triggering agents/factors, maintenance therapy with inhaled bronchodilators should continue to prevent early relapse. Those who develop an acute severe worsening asthma are likely to have similar episodes in future; therefore, early recognition and initiation of treatment is necessary.

Chapter 4
Acute Respiratory Distress Syndrome (ARDS)

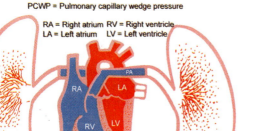

A

Diagnostic Criteria
1. Inspired oxygenation < 200 mmHg.
2. PCWP < 18 mm with normal left atrial pressure.
3. Bilateral diffuse pulmonary infiltrates.

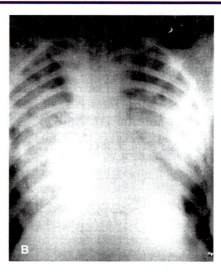

X-ray Chest AP view: Non-cardiogenic pulmonary oedema (Adult respiratory distress syndrome)

Figs 4.1A and B: Acute respiratory distress syndrome (ARDS) (A) Diagnostic criteria (B) Radiological appearance—pulmonary oedema with normal cardiac shadow

ACUTE RESPIRATORY DISTRESS SYNDROME (ARDS)

Definition

Acute respiratory distress syndrome is defined as an acute hypoxic lung injury resulting in extensive bilateral pulmonary infiltrates, refractory hypoxaemia, stiff lung (decreased compliance) and respiratory distress. It is an emergency and carries a high mortality rate (40-60%).

Recently European-American consensus conference defined ARDS as a condition of acute onset with following features:
i. Impaired oxygenation (it is defined as a ratio of PaO_2 to the fraction of inspired O_2 (FiO_2) that is < 200 mmHg.
ii. Chest X-ray showing diffuse bilateral infiltrates.
iii. Pulmonary capillary wedge pressure (PCWP) less than or equal to 18 mmHg when measured

Acute Respiratory Distress Syndrome (ARDS)

Box 4.1: Causes of acute respiratory distress syndrome

Common	Uncommon

1. Infection
   • Sepsis
   • Pneumonia, e.g., bacterial, viral, mycoplasma, *Pneumocystis carinii*
2. Acute pancreatitis
3. Severe burns
4. Aspiration of gastric contents
5. Blunt chest trauma (bilateral lung contusion)
6. Inhalation of toxic gases or fumes
7. Near-drowning
	1. Multiple blood transfusions reactions.
	2. Cardiopulmonary bypass
	3. Inhalational injury
	4. Fat or amniotic fluid embolism
	5. Goodpasture's syndrome
	6. Raised intracranial pressure
	7. Anaphylaxis (wasp, bee, snake venom)
	8. Falciparum malaria
	9. Tuberculosis
	10. Drugs, e.g., heroin, barbiturates, thiazides
	11. Carcinomatosis

and no clinical evidence of left atrial hypertension to exclude cardiogenic pulmonary oedema.

Causes

ARDS can occur as a nonspecific reaction of the lungs to a wide variety of insults, including shock, sepsis, embolism, trauma, inhalation of toxic gases and smoke, etc. (see the Box 4.1). Pneumonia is a common complication of ARDS.

Pathophysiology

ARDS can be considered as the earliest manifestation of a generalised inflammatory reaction and irrespective of its cause evolves through the following phases:

1. ***Exudative phase (noncardiogenic pulmonary oedema):*** This is the early phase of ARDS; occurs within 24-96 hours following a precipitating event. It is characterised by endothelial injury, denudation of type I epithelial cells, increase in vascular permeability caused by microcirculatory changes, release of inflammatory mediators, hyaline membrane formation and interstitial neutrophilic infiltrates. There is decreased surfactant production. It usually lasts for 3-7 days. The clinical hallmarks of this phase are; bilateral pulmonary infiltrates (noncardiogenic pulmonary oedema), dyspnoea and marked hypoxaemia.

2. ***Proliferative phase (stage of development of pulmonary hypertension):*** By 3-7 days, patient who survives the initial phase progresses to proliferative stage. Necrotic type I cells are replaced by type II epithelial cells which proliferate and form new alveolar epithelium. Interstitial and alveolar oedema starts decreasing and these spaces are filled with RBCs, inflammatory cells and cellular debris. This phase is characterised by worsening hypoxaemia as a result of pulmonary shunting of blood and development of pulmonary hypertension as a result of hypoxic vasoconstrictive response (hypoxia is vasoconstrictor of pulmonary vasculature), precipitated by microthrombi formation, platelets aggregation and vasoactive substances.

3. ***Fibrotic phase:*** After about 7-10 days of onset of ARDS, formation of a new epithelial lining is underway and activated fibroblasts accumulate in the interstitial spaces. Subsequently fibrosis sets in with loss of elastic tissue and obliteration of the lung vasculature. This may slowly resolve or may result in lung destruction which may be irreversible.

4. ***Phase of repair and recovery:*** Very little is known about this phase. During this phase mechanical properties and gas exchange functions of the lungs return towards normal. This phase may continue for as long as 6-12 months after discontinuation of mechanical ventilation.

Clinical Features

In addition to the clinical manifestations of the provoking condition, the patients usually develop unexplained dyspnoea, dry cough, labored breathing, and may become agitated and disoriented usually after 24-72 hours of precipitating event. Tachypnoea, tachycardia and cyanosis appear later. Fine crackles are heard throughout both lung fields.

Investigations

Investigations are done to find out the treatable underlying cause such as infections and to assess the progress of the disease.

1. **Chest X-ray:** The radiological features become evident by about 12 hours after the clinical onset of type I respiratory failure. Initially, patchy ill-defined opacities may become apparent throughout the lungs. They rapidly coalesce and massive air-space or alveolar consolidation become evident. Later, the chest X-ray shows bilateral, diffuse shadowing with an alveolar pattern and air bronchogram is frequently visible which distinguishes it from cardiogenic pulmonary oedema, and last of all it may progress to the picture of complete "white out". After about a week, the lungs remain diffusely abnormal but the pattern changes to reticular or bubbly shadowing suggestive of interstitial and air-space fibrosis.
2. **Arterial blood gas analysis:** It shows characteristic of type I respiratory failure, i.e.
   - Refractory hypoxaemia (PaO_2 < 60 mmHg/ or < 8.0 kPa).
   - Hypocapnia ($PaCO_2$ < 6.6 kPa).
   - Alkalosis (pH > 7.39).
3. **CT scan:** CT scan of the chest reveals diffusely distributed non-uniform ground glass opacification or consolidation, which may not conform to the gravity distribution. Later, the opacification becomes more homogenous and gravity dependent. As the disease progresses, reticular appearance becomes evident indicating interstitial fibrosis. Complications of ARDS such as small pneumothorax, pneumomediastinum and interstitial emphysema become evident.
4. **Measurement of pulmonary capillary wedge pressure (PCWP)** by Swan-Ganz catheter is less than 18 mmHg. The cardiac index is > 2.1 L/min.
5. **Broncho-alveolar lavage** may reveal increased number of polymorph leucocytes. This is nonspecific finding.

Differential Diagnosis

Several conditions stimulate clinical and radiological findings of ARDS, hence, have to be differentiated. These are:

1. **Cardiogenic pulmonary oedema** (acute left ventricular failure). The PCWP is elevated (> 18 mmHg).
2. **Diffuse alveolar haemorrhage:** There is haemoptysis, fall in haemoglobin, frothy red fluid on bronchoscopy and haemosiderin laden macrophages—a characteristic finding, may be seen in the bronchoalveolar lavage fluid.
3. **Metastatic carcinomatosis.**

Management

Attempts should be made to establish the cause of ARDS and institute the specific therapy to treat it, if treatable. The other steps of management are:

1. **General measures:**
   - Procure pulmonary and systemic I.V. access for haemodynamic monitoring and fluid therapy.
   - Arterial O_2 saturation and arterial blood gas analysis must be monitored for progress.
   - Adequate nutrition should be ensured through enteral feeding.
   - If sepsis is the cause, empirical antibiotic therapy may be begun followed by specific therapy depending on the culture and sensitivity reports.
2. **Fluid therapy:** Adequate circulation and BP must be maintained for adequate oxygenation

by using fluids (crystalloid or colloids) and/or vasopressors, taking the PCWP as the guide for therapy. Transfusion of blood or packed red cells is indicated if the patient is anaemic.

3. *Oxygen therapy:* The simplest method and the lowest inspired fraction of O_2 (FiO_2) should be used to achieve a PaO_2 of 60 mmHg (O_2 saturation of about 90%). Initially spontaneous ventilation using a facemask with high flow rate can be used to improve PaO_2 without increasing FiO_2. If a FiO_2 more than 0.6 and CPAP more than 10 cm H_2O are needed to achieve PaO_2 > 60 mmHg, then endotracheal intubation and mechanical ventilation must be considered.

4. *Mechanical ventilation (assisted ventilatory support):* In the presence of ARDS, adequate oxygenation is usually not achieved with these less invasive measures listed above. Mechanical ventilatory support after endotracheal intubation is initially started with volume cycled mechanical ventilators. To begin with, the initial ventilator setting could be FiO_2 as 1.0 (or a lower value that can achieve a PaO_2 > 60 mmHg and oxygen saturation > 90%), tidal volume 6-10 ml/kg body weight, PEEP less than or equal to 5 cm of water and inspiratory flow 760 L/min. PEEP may be applied to increase the lung volume and keep the alveoli open. PEEP is applied in small increments of 3-5 cm H_2O upto a maximum of 15 cm of H_2O to achieve oxygen saturation of > 90% with non-toxic FiO_2 levels (< 0.6). Ventilatory rate of 20-25 breaths/minute is needed to keep $PaCO_2$ and pH normal.

5. *Other ventilatory strategies:* Controlled hypoventilation with permissive hypercapnia or pressure targeted ventilation may be useful in patients of ARDS who have peak airway resistance > 40-45 cm H_2O despite conventional ventilatory support.

Airway-pressure release ventilation and high frequency ventilation are other newer methods of ventilation.

6. *Prone position:* In situations where maximal PEEP with FiO_2 of 1.0 does not supply sufficient oxygen, placing the patient in the prone position has been found helpful.

7. *Pharmacological treatment:* Though various pharmacological therapy have been tried in ARDS, but none of them have been found effective.

   i. *Corticosteroids therapy:* It has been established that steroid therapy has no role in ARDS except in special setting such as patients of ARDS with high eosinophil count in blood and lungs. In this setting, corticosteroids therapy should be started early in course of the disease. In a desperate situation such as severe ARDS which does not show signs of improvement 7-14 days after its onset, a trial of 1-2 weeks of corticosteroids is worth attempting.

   ii. *Recent reports using nitric oxide* (NO) inhalation (5-80 parts per million) or prostacycline (PGI_2) as a selective pulmonary vasodilator showed promising results on initial evaluation.

   iii. *Certain antioxidants* (N-acetylcysteine, glutathione, vitamin E) have been tried to overcome free radical-mediated injury without much success.

Chapter 5

Pulmonary Embolism

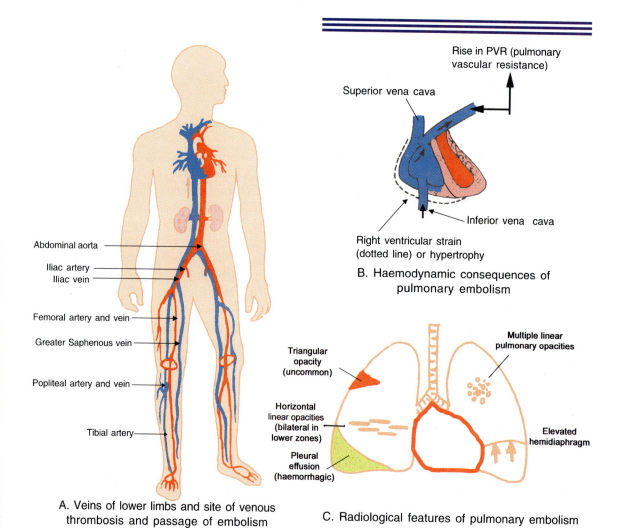

Figs 5.1A to C: Pulmonary embolism

PULMONARY EMBOLISM

Definition

Lungs are connected to the venous side of circulation, hence, act as a first filter for a variety of diverse materials gaining access to venous circulation, thus, is a common site for embolism. In strict sense, pulmonary embolism represents formation of a clot or thrombus in the venous circulation, its dislodgement and propagation through venous circulation and ultimately its lodgement in pulmonary circulation. Clinically, it is defined as acute haemodynamic disturbance due to occlusion of pulmonary vasculature due to an embolus or emboli.

It is a very common condition complicating deep vein thrombosis. It is very difficult to predict its incidence because of disparity between clinical detection and autopsy diagnosis. A great majority of patients die within first few hours of the embolic episode due to inadequate therapy because the diagnosis is either missed or delayed.

Causes

The causes of pulmonary embolism are given in the Table 5.1. The common sites of venous thrombosis are represented in Figure 5.1A.

The most common cause of pulmonary embolisation is deep vein thrombosis (DVT) which constitutes 90-95% of patients, out of which 70-80% originate from the veins of the legs (Fig. 5.2)

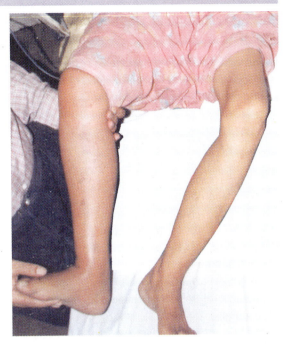

Fig. 5.2: Deep vein thrombosis (DVT) of right leg. Note the swelling of the leg and positive Homan's sign (the sign is now-a-days not elicited). The patient presented with pain chest and haemoptysis. CT angiogram confirmed the diagnosis of pulmonary embolism

and 10-15% from pelvic veins. The mechanism of thrombus formation in the veins is similar to thrombus formation anywhere, and involves three factors, i.e., stasis of blood, hypercoagulability of the blood and abnormalities of the vessel wall.

The clinical risk factors that predispose to DVT and embolism are:

1. Surgery, trauma (in-plastic injuries or fracture of lower limb bones).
2. Prolonged immobilisation (stroke, or intensive care unit patients).
3. Oral contraceptives, pregnancy, postpartum.
4. Cancer and cancer chemotherapy.
5. Varicosity of the veins.
6. Congestive heart failure (stasis of blood).
7. Obesity.
8. Hypercoagulable state.

Table 5.1: Causes of pulmonary embolism

1. *Thrombotic*
   - Deep vein thrombosis
   - Congestive heart failure
   - Right sided endocarditis
   - Atrial fibrillation
2. *Nonthrombotic*
   - Fat embolism following bone trauma or a fracture
   - Amniotic fluid embolism following delivery and caesarean section
   - Tumour embolism (choriocarcinoma)
   - Parasitic embolism (schistosomiasis)
   - Air embolism (pulmonary barotrauma in drivers)

Pathophysiological Consequences
(Fig. 5.1B)

1. ***Increased pulmonary vascular resistance*** due to vascular obstruction and release of serotonin.
2. ***Impaired gas exchange due to:***
   - Increased alveolar dead space from vascular obstruction leading to wasted ventilation. There will be large areas of the lungs which are ventilated but not perfused.
   - Hypoxaemia from alveolar hypoventilation in the non-obstructed lung.
   - Right to left shunting (patent foramen ovale).
   - Loss of gas exchange surface.
3. ***Increased airway resistance*** due to bronchoconstriction.
4. ***Reduced pulmonary compliance*** due to lung oedema, lung haemorrhage and loss of surfactants.
5. ***Right ventricular dysfunction:*** Progressive right heart failure is the usual immediate cause of death. As pulmonary vasculature resistance increases, it puts strain on the right ventricle and causes right ventricular dilatation and dysfunction. Consequently the interventricular septum bulges into normal left ventricle reducing left ventricular cavity and its filling (Bernheim effect). Increased right ventricular wall tension also compresses the right coronary artery and precipitates myocardial ischaemia and right ventricular infarction. Underfilling of left ventricle may lead to fall in left ventricular output causing hypotension thereby provoking myocardial ischaemia due to compromised coronary artery perfusion. Eventually, circulatory collapse and death may occur.

Clinical Features

The clinical picture is highly variable from asymptomatic disease to catastrophic acute illness. The massive pulmonary embolism produces features of acute cor pulmonale; while multiple microembolisation leads to features of chronic cor pulmonale. The triad of a pulmonary infarct is *haemoptysis, pleuritic chest pain* and *wheeze* that occurs due to embolisation of small peripheral blood vessels near the pleura. The clinical features of pulmonary embolism are given in the Table 5.2.

Dyspnoea, syncope, hypotension or shock indicate massive embolisation; while pleuritic pain, cough, haemoptysis, wheeze indicate a small embolisation located distally near the pleura. The physical signs depend on the severity of embolism, type of vessel/vessels involved and development of an infarct.

Investigations

1. ***Blood examination:*** It may show leucocytosis and raised ESR if patient develops a pulmonary infarct.
2. ***Chest X-ray:*** It may be normal even in severe embolism. However, the most frequent radiological findings are (Fig 5.1C):
   - Atelectasis.
   - Elevated hemidiaphragm.
   - Enlargement of cardiac shadow.
   - Enlarged pulmonary conus.
   - Pleural effusion.
   - Consolidation.
   - Avascular lung zone (*Westermark's sign*), wedge-shaped opacity above hemidiaphragm (*Hampton's hump*) and an enlarged right descending pulmonary artery (*Palla's sign*).

   Note: All these signs are nonspecific. The chest X-ray is done to exclude the other possibilities that mimic pulmonary embolism such as pneumonia, pneumothorax, etc. and to provide information that could help in the interpretation of radionuclide scans.
3. ***The ECG:*** The 12 lead ECG may be normal (70-80% of cases just show tachycardia). In severe cases, the ECG changes represent acute right ventricular strain or myocardial ischaemia or both. Right axis deviation and clockwise rotation is common. The S_1, Q_{111}, T_{111} syndrome in which there is S wave in lead I and Q wave in lead III with T inversion, if present is highly suggestive of acute

Table 5.2: Clinical features of pulmonary embolism

Size of vessel involved	Severity	Clinical syndrome	Haemodynamic consequences	Symptoms	Signs
Large vessel embolisation	Massive	Acute cor pulmonale (primary pulmonary hypertension)	• > 50% ↓ in PV bed • ↑↑ PVR • ↑↑ RV afterload • RV failure • ↓ CO and shock	• Acute dyspnoea • Tachypnoea • Tachycardia • Sweating • Haemoptysis • Chest pain • Syncope	• Hypotension or shock • Raised JVP • Cyanosis • Loud P_2 with wide splitting • An ejection systolic murmur at P_2 area • Signs of RV hypertrophy
Multiple or recurrent embolism (Chronic pulmonary embolism)	Moderate to severe	Primary pulmonary hypertension or chronic cor pulmonale	• > 50% ↓ in PV bed • ↑ PVR • ↑ RV afterload • RV dysfunction • No shock	• Dyspnoea • Fatigue • Weakness • Syncope	• Raised JVP • Cyanosis • Oedema • Hepatomegaly • Loud P_2 with narrow splitting • Parasternal heave and RV hypertrophy
Small or medium sized vessels	Mild to moderate	Pulmonary infarct(s) or asymptomatic	• < 50 ↓ in PV bed • PVR—Normal • No RV dysfunction • No shock	• Pleuritic chest pain • Haemoptysis • Wheeze • Jaundice, mild, occasional • Fever	• Pleural rub • Tachycardia • Either signs of pleural effusion or atelectasis • Crackles

Abbreviations: ↓ means decrease; ↑ means increase; ↑↑ means marked increase; RV means right ventricle; PVR means pulmonary vascular resistance; PV bed means pulmonary vascular bed, CO means cardiac output

pulmonary embolism. There may be ST segment depression in leads I and II with T wave inversion in leads V_1-V_4 indicating right ventricular strain.

In appropriate clinical setting, transient development of incomplete RBBB is indicative of acute pulmonary embolism. Recurrent episodes of arrhythmias, e.g. sinus tachycardia, atrial flutter or fibrillation may also occur.

Tip: ECG changes are transient in nature, hence, appearance and disappearance of above mentioned changes on serial ECGs is highly diagnostic. It must be born in mind that normal ECG does not rule out pulmonary embolism

4. ***Arterial blood gas (ABG) abnormalities:*** It shows hypoxaemia with respiratory alkalosis.
5. ***Echocardiogram:*** The two-dimensional-echocardiography is particularly helpful as it may reveal right ventricular dilatation/dysfunction, hypokinesia, septal flattening and tricuspid regurgitation. These echocardiographic findings in right clinical setting (positive findings of venous thrombosis on USG of the legs) is virtually pathognomonic. Transthoracic echocardiography is particularly helpful in critically ill patients as it may show a clot in right heart or the main pulmonary arteries.
6. ***Plasma D-dimers:*** D-dimer; a specific degradation product of fibrin is released into

circulation after fibrinolysis of the clot. Its elevated levels in blood (ELISA method) suggest active thrombosis. It has not much diagnostic value as it may be raised in other conditions such as myocardial infarction, pneumonia, heart failure, cancer, etc. On the other hand, it is an excellent tool to exclude the pulmonary embolism, i.e. low levels of D-dimers (< 500 mg/ml) exclude pulmonary embolism, hence, is most useful initial screening investigation (Fig. 5.3). A positive D-dimer is not diagnostic of PE since it may be raised in inflammatory conditions such as pneumonia.

7. ***Noninvasive tests for deep vein thrombosis:*** Any objective evidence confirming DVT (Doppler ultrasound, impedances plethysmography, ascending venography, etc.) definitely raises the possibility of thromboembolism in an appropriate setting (echocardiographic evidence of right ventricular dysfunction, dilatation, etc.)

8. ***Radioisotopic ventilation perfusion (V/Q) scan:*** It includes two scans done simultaneously, i.e. lung perfusion scan (^{99m}technetium) and ventilation scan (by radioactive ^{133}Xenon). Lung perfusion scan is a simple procedure in which particles of macroaggregated tumour albumin labelled with ^{99m}technetium are injected intravenously. These particles act as microemboli and get lodged in small pulmonary vessels and cause an occlusion of only a small fraction of pulmonary vasculature temporarily. The under perfused area(s) of the lung is shown as '*cold area/spot*' or '*avascular zone*' in the scan.

   A perfusion scan can demonstrate area/areas of hypoperfusion but cannot identify the cause of perfusion defect.

   A perfusion defect/defects can occur with any parenchymal or pleural lesion such as COPD, asthma, atelectasis, pneumonia and pleural effusion.

   A normal perfusion scan in a patient with suspected pulmonary embolism virtually excludes it.

   In a ventilation scan, radioactive ^{133}Xenon is inhaled and exhaled by the patient, while the gamma camera records its distribution throughout the alveolar gas exchange units. The test is based on the assumption that ventilation is preserved in areas of reduced perfusion due to pulmonary embolism and is abnormal when perfusion defects are due to pulmonary disease. The sensitivity and specificity of V/Q scans were established in general representative US Population by Prospective Investigation of Pulmonary Embolism Diagnosis (PIOPED) study and is used as a criteria for interpretation of V/Q scan (i.e., *high probable*, *intermediate* and *low probable*). A high probable scan indicates pulmonary embolism. A low probability scan and a strong clinical impression that pulmonary embolism is unlikely make the possibility of pulmonary embolism remote.

9. ***Spiral CT angiography:*** It is an alternate if facility of V/Q scan is not available. This approach is best suited for identifying emboli that are situated in the proximal pulmonary vasculature but may not pick up emboli in distal vascular bed.

   CT pulmonary angiography is now-a-days investigation of choice than V/Q scan in PE.

10. ***Pulmonary angiography:*** It is accepted as a *gold standard* for the diagnosis of pulmonary embolism. Contrast material is injected in the main pulmonary artery which provides direct visualisation of the filling defects caused by pulmonary embolism. It is hazardous in patients with pulmonary hypertension, right heart failure or respiratory failure. It is strongly indicated in establishing the diagnosis of life-threatening embolism where thrombolytic therapy or mechanical intervention or surgery are being considered.

Diagnosis

Well's Diagnostic scoring system for clinical likelihood is depicted in the Box 5.1.

Box 5.1: Well's diagnostic scoring system

Feature	Points
• Clinical symptoms/signs of DVT	3.0
• An alternative diagnosis is less likely i.e. other conditions have been excluded	3.0
• Heart rate > 100/min	1.5
• Immobilisation or surgery during past 4 weeks	1.5
• Previous episode of DVT/ pulmonary embolism	1.5
• Haemptosis	1.0
• Malignancy (on treatment/treated in past 6 month)	1.0

Note: Total score is 12.5. If score is ≤ 4.0, then clinical diagnosis is less likely

The recommendations for the diagnosis on V/Q scan are depicted in Figures 5.3 and 5.4.

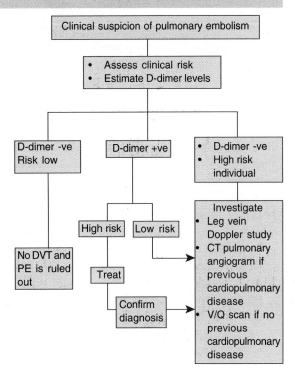

Fig. 5.3: Initial screening of the patients with suspicion of pulmonary embolism (PE)

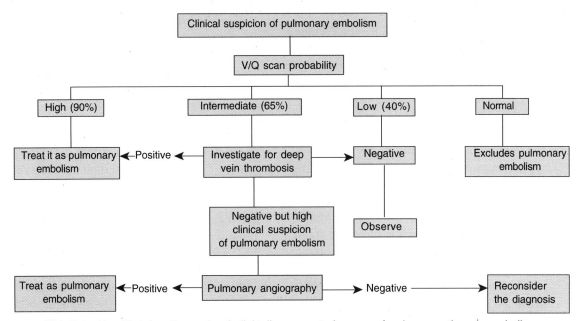

Fig. 5.4: Algorithm for diagnosis of clinically suspected cases of pulmonary thromboembolism

Management

Massive pulmonary thromboembolism is a life-threatening emergency, carries a mortality of 43-80% in first two hours following the event, hence, appropriate preventive measures in high-risk patients are most useful. However, once massive pulmonary thromboembolism has occurred, immediate recognition and institution of treatment are mandatory. Diagnosis mainly rests on the clinical suspicion together with V/Q scan (as discussed in algorithm). The steps of management are:

1. **Initial supportive measures:** Opiates may be necessary to relieve pain and distress but should be used with caution in hypotensive patients. Resuscitation by external cardiac massage may be sometimes successful in moribund patient by dislodging and breaking up a large central thrombus. Other measures include"
   i. Oxygen administration through mask to restore arterial oxygen saturation over 90%.
   ii. Fluid therapy for hypotensive and shocked patients. It should be given continuously because these patients have increase in pulmonary vascular resistance and right ventricular failure.
   iii. Vasoactive drugs such as norepinephrine and dobutamine to raise the BP in hypotensive or shocked patients in acute massive pulmonary embolism.
   iv. Diuretics and vasodilators should be avoided during acute setting.

2. **Prompt anticoagulation:** If the patient remains haemodynamically stable with or without supportive treatment, anticoagulation with heparin should be given to all patients with a high clinical suspicion of pulmonary embolism whilst confirmatory test results are awaited. Heparin accelerates the action of antithrombin III, thereby preventing the further formation and extension of thrombosis and permitting endogenous fibrinolysis to dissolve some of the clots. Initial therapy for 3 months to one year is the treatment of choice for most patients with pulmonary embolism. Heparin without oral anticoagulation is the treatment used throughout pregnancy to manage pulmonary embolism in high-risk pregnant patients. Heparin is used in the dose which prolongs the activated PTT to 1.5 to 2 times over control.

   Different modes of anticoagulation are:
   i. *Aggressive heparin therapy:* Heparin is started in the dose of 5000-7500 units as a bolus dose, followed by 1000 U/hr as an infusion monitoring the PTT and the dose is adjusted to maintain the PTT at 1.5 to 3 times that of control.
   ii. *Short course of heparin* (5 days) and simultaneous administration of warfarin. Early discharge of the patient from hospital is possible with this treatment.
   Note: International normalisation ratio (INR) is the PT ratio that would be obtained if the WHO standard thromboplastin was used in performing a given PT test. An INR of 2.0 to 3 is equal to a PT ratio of 1.3 to 1.5 approx, Warfarin monitoring should ideally be done with INR.
   iii. *A low molecular heparin* given subcutaneously in a weight adjusted dosage is equally effective in the treatment of pulmonary thromboembolism.

3. **Thrombolysis:** Patient with an acute massive pulmonary embolism with haemodynamically compromised state, i.e. evidence of right ventricular dysfunction on ECHO or of hypotension, should be considered for urgent thrombolytic therapy when the diagnosis is confirmed. Streptokinase is given as a loading dose of 250,000 I.V. over 20 to 30 minutes, after pretreatment with 100 mg of I.V. hydrocortisone. This is followed by continuous I.V. infusion of streptokinase 100,00. I.V. per hour for 24 hours. The lysis can be confirmed by measuring either PTT, FT, TT, fibrin split products or whole blood euglobin lysis time. Treatment with urokinase (a loading dose of 4400 IU/kg over 10 minutes followed by 4400 IU/Kg/hr for 12 to 24 hours) is equally effective. Before initiation of thrombolytic therapy, heparin is administered.

Alteplase (human tissue plasminogen activator-tPA) can be used. It is more expensive but less likely to lead systemic side-effects and hypotension. A dose of 60 mg I.V. administered over 15 minutes is sufficient. Heparin should be given subsequently.

Surgery

The advent of thrombolytic treatment has reduced the need for surgical procedures (embolectomy, percutaneous transvenous catheter fragmentation and distal dissipation of proximal pulmonary embolism). However, contraindications (see Box 5.2) to thrombolytic therapy or refractory hypotension despite thrombolytic therapy have kept embolectomy a viable option (Box 5.3).

Prophylaxis

The incidence of pulmonary embolism and deaths due to pulmonary embolism can be reduced by applying prophylactic strategies given in the Table 5.3. Prevention of DVT in lower limbs will reduce the frequency of embolism. Patients with a high risk for developing pulmonary embolism should be given prophylactic therapy. Prophylactic therapy may be medical or surgical. The medical therapy in high risk patients is given in Table 5.3.

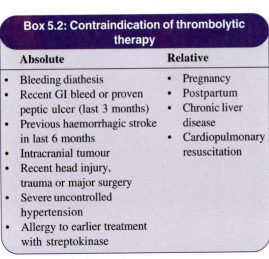

Box 5.2: Contraindication of thrombolytic therapy

Absolute	Relative
• Bleeding diathesis	• Pregnancy
• Recent GI bleed or proven peptic ulcer (last 3 months)	• Postpartum
	• Chronic liver disease
• Previous haemorrhagic stroke in last 6 months	• Cardiopulmonary resuscitation
• Intracranial tumour	
• Recent head injury, trauma or major surgery	
• Severe uncontrolled hypertension	
• Allergy to earlier treatment with streptokinase	

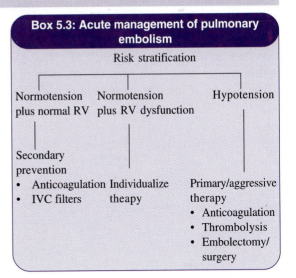

Box 5.3: Acute management of pulmonary embolism

Risk stratification

- Normotension plus normal RV → Secondary prevention
  - Anticoagulation
  - IVC filters
- Normotension plus RV dysfunction → Individualize theapy
- Hypotension → Primary/aggressive therapy
  - Anticoagulation
  - Thrombolysis
  - Embolectomy/surgery

Table 5.3: Prophylaxis of DVT and pulmonary thromboembolism

Risk factors	*Preventive measures/treatments*
1. High to moderate risk general surgery patients	• Low dose heparin, or • Low molecular weight heparin (LMWH) • Intermittent pneumatic compression devices. These devices apply pressure to calf, enhance venous return and fibrinolytic activity
2. Neurosurgery, urosurgery, major knee surgery	• Intermittent pneumatic compression
3. Effective hip surgery, surgery for fracture hip	• Low molecular weight heparin, or • Adjusted dose heparin to keep PTT at upper half of normal control value
4. Very high-risk general surgery patients	• Low molecular weight heparin or low dose heparin started preoperatively • Intermittent pneumatic compression
5. Medical patients with clinical risk factors for venous thromboembolism	• Low molecular weight heparin or low dose heparin

Surgical Methods (Caval Filters)

Patients with recurrent pulmonary embolism despite adequate anticoagulation or failure of anticoagulation control get benefit from the insertion of a filter placed in inferior vena cava (caval filter obstruction) below the origin of the renal vessels. Such filters can be placed in patients in whom anticoagulants are contraindicated. These have occlusion rate of 5%, are safe and effective in preventing embolisation.

Chapter 6

Pneumothorax

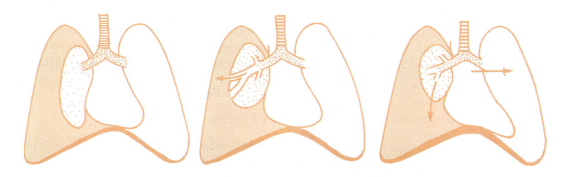

Fig. 6.1: Various types of pneumothorax

PNEUMOTHORAX

Definition

Pneumothorax is defined as the entry of air into the pleural space. The incidence is higher in males aged 15-30 years.

Classification

The pneumothorax is divided into two main categories, i.e. spontaneous and traumatic (see Box 6.1). The spontaneous pneumothorax may be primary (underlying lung is healthy) or secondary (occurs as a complication of some lung disease).

The traumatic pneumothorax results either from a chest injury or from a clinical procedure (iatrogenic).

> **Box 6.1: Classification of pneumothorax**
>
> **A. Spontaneous:**
> i. *Primary:* There is no evidence of overt lung disease. Air enters into the pleural space either through rupture of a small subpleural emphysematous bulla or a pleural bleb at the pulmonary end of pleural adhesion.
> ii. *Secondary:* There is an overt underlying lung disease, most commonly COPD or tuberculosis. It is also seen in bronchial asthma, pulmonary infarct, lung abscess, bronchogenic carcinoma and all forms of fibrotic and cystic lung lesions. In tuberculosis or lung abscess, there is usually hydropneumothorax because these lesions lead to exudative pleural fluid.
>
> **B. Traumatic:**
> It occurs following chest trauma/injury or may result following thoracic surgery or biopsy-called *iatrogenic*.

Causes

1. *Primary spontaneous pneumothorax:* It is caused by rupture of subpleural emphysematous blebs or a pleural bleb which may be congenital or acquired (pulmonary end of a pleural adhesion). Now, it has been established that 80% of patients with primary spontaneous pneumothorax have some emphysematous changes on CT scan. The *risk factors* identified for primary pneumothorax are:
   - Thin as well as tall body habitus.
   - Heavy smoking (> 20 cigarettes/day).
   - Marfan's syndrome.
   - Mitral valve prolapse.
   - Going to high altitude.
   - Bronchial anatomical abnormalities.
2. *Secondary spontaneous pneumothorax:* It is most commonly seen in patients of COPD and pulmonary tuberculosis. Almost every lung disease may be associated with pneumothorax. *Pneumocystis carinii pneumonia* is an emerging cause of pneumothorax in patients of AIDS. The other lung diseases associated with pneumothorax are:
   - Infections, e.g. necrotising pneumonia, lung abscess. These commonly cause hydropneumothorax or pyopneumothorax.
   - Interstitial lung diseases.
   - Occupational lung disease, e.g. silicosis, coal-workers pneumoconiosis.
   - Malignancy lung, e.g. bronchogenic carcinoma.
   - Miscellaneous rare causes such as pulmonary infarct, asthma, cystic fibrosis, eosinophilic granuloma, post-irradiation, tuberous sclerosis, catamenial pneumothorax (endometriosis).
3. *Traumatic pneumothorax:* It results from:
   - Blunt injury to thorax or abdomen.
   - Penetrating thoracic injury.
   - Procedural (iatrogenic), e.g. pleural tap, pleural biopsy, bronchoscopy, lung biopsy, endoscopy and sclerotherapy.

Pathological Types
(see Figure 6.1 on front page)

1. *Closed:* The rupture site closes and lung is deflated. The air in the pleural space is absorbed slowly and lung expands to its original position over few weeks. The mean pleural pressure is negative (less than atmospheric pressure).
2. *Open:* The rupture site does not close but forms a communication between the pleural cavity and the bronchus (*bronchopleural fistula*). The mean pleural pressure is atmospheric, hence, the lung cannot re-expand. Infection such as pyopneumothorax is a common complication of bronchopleural fistula. Open pneumothorax also can result from penetrating chest wall injury.
3. *Tension (valvular):* The communication between the pleura and the lung persists, and acts as a check valve (discussed on next page).

Clinical Features

Symptoms

Primary spontaneous pneumothorax develops suddenly without any provocation. Symptoms of pneumothorax depend on the amount of air in the pleural cavity. A small pneumothorax is usually asymptomatic and detected by chance on routine chest X-ray. Moderate amount of air in pleural space produces chest pain and dyspnoea. Chest pain is sharp, pleuritic and localised to the side of pneumothorax. Dyspnoea is proportional to the amount of pneumothorax.

Secondary pneumothorax is usually more symptomatic because of pre-existing lung disease.

Signs

The clinical signs of pneumothorax are localised to the side involved. These are:
1. Fullness of intercostal spaces.
2. Decreased movement of chest wall.
3. Hyper-resonant percussion note.
4. In closed pneumothorax, breath sounds, vocal fremitus and vocal resonance are diminished.

In open pneumothorax, an *amphoric bronchial breathing* with increased vocal fremitus and vocal resonance and presence of whispering pectoriloquy if a large broncho-pleural fistula develops. In tension pneumothorax, one may hear amphoric breath sounds at a localised place; otherwise breath sounds are diminished.

5. If associated with infection, e.g. open pneumothorax (commonly associated with infection) or pneumothorax due to tuberculosis, there will be accumulation of fluid or pus in the pleural cavity (hydro or pyopneumothorax), then there will be physical signs like horizontal shifting level of dullness and succussion splash, and in addition there will be signs of toxaemia.
6. *Recurrent spontaneous pneumothorax occur* in patients with emphysema due to rupture of bullae and these invariably occur on the same side.
7. Very rarely, one may get bilateral small spontaneous pneumothorax; it may be difficult to diagnose such a case clinically as there will be hyper-resonant note and diminished breath sounds on both the sides and there will be no shift of trachea. All these signs are also present in emphysema from which it will be differentiated only on X-ray chest.

Tension Pneumothorax

As the name suggests, the air in pleural cavity (pneumothorax) is under tension, i.e. mean pleural pressure is positive, hence, causes compression collapse of the lung. It is a medical emergency. It develops due to persistent air leak into the pleural cavity by a communication which opens during inspiration allowing the air to enter, and closes during expiration, preventing the air to escape, thus, acts as check valve. In this way, air accumulates with each successive breath and causes rise in intrapleural pressure thereby shifting the mediastinum to the opposite side and puts pressure on the great vessels. There is decreased venous return to the heart and cardiac output falls leading to hypotension (cardiac tamponade) and cyanosis.

It can occur with any sort of pneumothorax. The clinical features include:

- Patients may present with acute onset of dyspnoea and cough or there may be sudden increase in symptoms in a patient of pneumothorax.
- Prominent chest (hyperinflated chest) with diminished or absent movement on the side involved.
- Trachea and mediastinum are shifted to the opposite side due to push of air pressure.
- Decreased or absent breath sounds on the side affected. Occasionally, there may amphoric breathing at a localised place.
- Tachypnoea, tachycardia, hypotension, cyanosis and pulsus paradoxus are usually present.

Investigations

1. **Chest X-ray:** A high degree of suspicion is required to diagnose pneumothorax clinically, which is confirmed on X-ray chest. Air in the pleural cavity gives hypertranslucent area devoid of lung markings in the periphery with a thin pleural line indicating the outer border of the collapsed lung (Fig. 6.2). In a doubtful case of small pneumothorax, a lateral decubitus or an end-expiratory film may help to delineate the free air in the pleural cavity. The diagnosis of pneumothorax on a film taken in supine position is more difficult and may be suggested by *"deep sulcus sign"*, i.e. the presence of rim of air on the superior border of the diaphragm, making the diaphragmatic outline very sharp on the affected side.

The amount of air can be calculated by the following formula on chest X-ray:

$$\text{Pneumothorax (\%)} = \frac{(d_L)^3}{(d_T)^3} \times 100$$

It is represented as percentage (%) of hemithorax volume occupied by air, roughly derived by measuring the average diameter of the collapsed lung (d_L) and hemithorax (d_T).

Tension pneumothorax on chest X-ray produces typical signs of increased volume of the affected hemithorax i.e. shift of the trachea and mediastinum to the opposite side. Lung on the affected side is markedly collapsed and pasted along the hilum;

32 Pulmonary Medicine

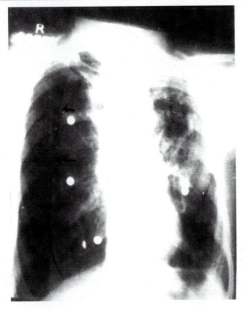

Fig. 6.2: Pneumothorax. X-ray chest (PA view) shows hyperinflated right lung with hyperlucency in the periphery devoid of markings. The underlying lung is collapsed indicated by a thin line (darkened) indicated by arrows

but may not collapse if it is already diseased and fibrosed and fixed. Similarly, mediastinum may not be shifted and yet the hemodynamic compromise of tension pneumothorax may be evident.

In addition to pneumothorax, the chest X-ray may show signs of underlying disease (COPD or tuberculosis) or pleural fluid with horizontal level (hydropneumothorax).

Differential Diagnosis

It has to be differentiated from a large emphysematous bulla, which at times, may be difficult. The distinguishing feature is the outline or pleural margins of the collapse or deflated lung, but if pneumothorax is also loculated, then **CT** scan is helpful for differentiation.

Management

Aims

- To remove the air from the pleural space and to allow the lung to expand.
- To prevent recurrence.

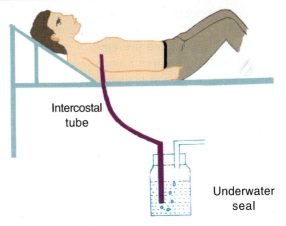

Fig. 6.3: Intercostal tube drainage of pneumothorax

Steps of Treatment

A. ***Removing air from pleural space:***
   i. *Conservative approach:* A small pneumothorax (< 20%) is usually asymptomatic and should be left as such for spontaneous reabsorption and resolution with re-expansion of the lung which may take four weeks. This process can be hastened by oxygen inhalation at high concentration.
   ii. *Aspiration of air:* Any pneumothorax which is > 20% and symptomatic needs to be aspirated by the methods described below:
   1. *Simple needle aspiration:* Simple needle (16/18G) or catheter (I.V. cannula) is used for aspiration. A small pneumothorax can easily be drained with a 50 CC syringe and a three-way valve attached to it. Air is continuously drained till no air comes out and then catheter is left *in situ* for 4 to 6 hours keeping it well closed. Repeat chest X-ray is taken and compared with original one. If X-ray chest shows no recurrence or a small amount of air (< 20%), catheter is removed. If recurrence is seen, then alternative procedure given below is required.
   2. *Intercostal tube drainage:* It is required for all patients with moderate to large pneumothorax who fail on simple needle aspiration or who present with tension

pneumothorax. Even a small pneumothorax can cause severe respiratory distress/failure in patients with underlying chronic lung disease, hence, all such patients require intercostal tube drainage and in-hospital observation.

If required, an intercostal drain should be inserted in the 3rd or 4th intercostal space in mid-axillary line following blunt dissection through to the parietal pleura. The tube is advanced in the apical direction and connected to underwater seal (Fig. 6.3). Once the lung expands, chest X-ray should be repeated to exclude the recurrence before removing the tube. Clamping of the tube before removal is potentially dangerous, should not be attempted. The drain should be removed 24 hours after the lung has fully reinflated and bubbling stopped. If bubbling in the underwater seal stops prior to full reinflation of the lung, then the tube is either blocked, kinked or displaced.

3. All patients should receive supplement O_2 as this accelerates the rate at which air is reabsorbed by the pleura.

> *Note: Tension pneumothorax needs immediate relief of tension. It can be accomplished by just simply inserting the needle (16G) into the second intercostal space and removing 2-2.5 litre of air or till the patient gets relief in dyspnoea even without any underwater seal. This arrangement is prior to insertion of intercostal drainage.*

4. Patients should not fly or dive for 3 months after full expansion of the lung. They should stop smoking to reduce the risk of a further attack.

B. *Prevention of spontaneous pneumothorax:* About 25% patients with primary pneumothorax have recurrence during the first year. Risks for further recurrences are still higher reaching upto 80% after the third episode. The recurrence rate in secondary pneumothorax is low.

Due to seriousness of this condition, pleurodhesis (chemical or surgical) is recommended in all such patients with primary spontaneous pneumothorax following a second episode (even if ipsilateral) or in patients following their first pneumothorax where there is persistent air leak (> 7 days). Surgical pleurodhesis is recommended in all patients with secondary pneumothorax.

In chemical pleurodhesis, the drug of choice is injectable tetracycline, doxycycline or minocycline which is instilled into pleural space in doses of 20 to 25 mg/kg. Alternative is talc insufflation. Currently, pleurodhesis is limited due to non-availability of these drugs in our country, hence, surgical pleurodhesis is done wherever indicated. This can be achieved by pleural abrasion, or parietal pleurectomy at thoracotomy or thoracoscopy.

Patients who plan to continue activities that increase the risk of complications (e.g., flying or diving) should also undergo preventive treatment after the first episode of spontaneous pneumothorax.

Re-expansion Pulmonary Oedema

This is a rare complication that can occur with sudden withdrawal of air or fluid from the pleural space. This is unilateral pulmonary oedema that occurs more frequently if the lung has remained collapsed for longer period and if negative pressure is applied for drainage. The pathogenesis is not well understood. Loss of surfactants from the collapsed lung is the presumed hypothesis. Unilateral pulmonary oedema can lead to variable degree of hypoxia and cardiovascular compromise, and rarely, can be fatal. It is recognised by sudden onset of cough and dyspnoea soon after or during thoracocentesis or ICTD. Chest X-ray shows unilateral pulmonary oedema.

Treatment is supportive once it occurs. It can be prevented by slow removal of air/fluid, avoidance of negative pressure during drainage and monitoring of intrapleural pressure during such procedures.

Chapter 7

Asphyxia

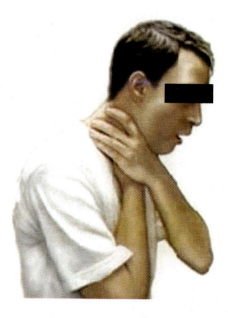

Fig. 7.1: Asphyxia due to foreign body airway obstruction

DEFINITION

Asphyxia literally (GK. asphuxia; **A** means without **sphuxia** means heart beat) means stoppage of the heart beat. Clinically it refers to airway obstruction leading to less or non-delivery of atmospheric O_2 to the lungs resulting in CO_2 retention. Asphyxia can be *mechanical* (obstruction extrinsic to airways) or *nonmechanical* (obstruction intrinsic to airways).

Causes

I. *Mechanical*
- Closing of face (e.g. plastic bag).
- Gag or pad smothering (closing of the external respiratory orifice by hand or by other means such as closing of nose and mouth with cloth, pad etc).
- Gagging.
- Food or foreign body obstruction (choking).
- Throttling (compression of the neck manually).
- Hanging and strangulation.
- Drowning
- Traumatic asphyxia.

II. *Nonmechanical*
Suffocation may occur from diseases such as:
- Diphtheria, infectious mononucleosis, H influenzae in children.
- Rupture of aortic aneurysm in air passages.
- Haemoptysis in pulmonary tuberculosis.
- Erosion of bronchus by a tubercular gland.

- Laryngeal oedema due to any cause (e.g. steam inhalation, ingestion of irritant substances, drug allergies and poisons).
- Pharyngeal abscess.
- Laryngeal or bronchial growths.
- Nonpenetrating injury to front of the neck.

FOREIGN BODY AIRWAY OBSTRUCTION (CHOKING)

Choking is a form of asphyxia caused by an obstruction within air-passages.

Choking is almost always accidental. It results from the objects being lodged in the throat, is commonly seen in the children, elderly persons, psychiatric patients and in the infirms particularly where the ability to swallow or masticate is severely impaired.

Causes

1. It commonly occurs during a meal when the food is accidentally inhaled especially when victim is laughing or crying.
2. Vomitus may be inhaled by a person under the influence of liquor, during anaesthesia or an epileptic fit.
3. Infants usually regurgitate clotted milk after a meal and this mayb fall into the larynx.
4. Choking may occur due to inhalation of blood from facial injury, dislodged teeth, impaction of solid object, i.e. piece of meat, fruitstone, corn, button, coin, tag and rubber teat, gauge piece.
5. *Cafe coronary* (obstruction by a bolus of food or meat results in heart attack).

The choking or obstruction may be partial or complete. In complete obstruction, the victim becomes severely asphyxiated and may die suddenly or may develop severe brain damage or complication if obstruction is not relieved immediately.

If obstruction is partial, the resultant hypoxia may result in complications involving various organs.

Clinical Manifestations

The clinical feature varies according to severity of obstruction.

I. In partial obstruction due to a foreign body, the patient may struggle with the obstruction and tries to *'cough it out'* or *tries to swallow or wash it down with water*. The victim is responsive and can cough forcibly. If air entry is poor, then signs of poor air exchange will appear such as weak ineffective cough, high-pitched noise while inspiration (stridor), increased respiratory difficulty and cyanosis.

II. With complete airway obstruction, the patient may clutch the neck with the thumb and fingers (universal distress sign for choking Fig. 7.1 on front page) and following signs may appear:
- Inability to speak, breath and cough.
- Pallor followed by cyanosis.
- Loss of consciousness and collapse.

If obstruction is not relieved immediately patient may develop cardiac arrest and die.

Diagnosis

The diagnosis is based on the circumstances and the clinical features. To find out the cause of obstruction, ask the following points in the history:
- Age of the patient.
- History of epilepsy, recent surgery or anaesthesia or psychiatric illness.
- History of recent intake of food or milk. If the obstructing agent is a fragment of food, the victim will be invariably the infant/child and the mother will tell the history of milk feed.
- Any history of trauma or facial injury.

Examination

- Examine the patient for signs of injury, loosening or missing of any teeth or wearing of artificial denture especially in old persons.
- Examine the mouth for sticking of food or any other material that can choke the throat.
- *Vital signs:* Examine the pulse, BP, temperature and respiratory rate. Look for cyanosis.

36 Pulmonary Medicine

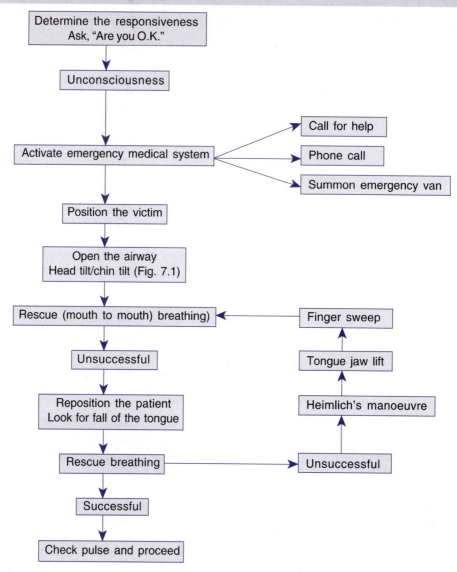

Fig. 7.2: Action plan for foreign body airway obstruction

Management

The basic aim of management is to relieve the obstruction either by expelling the foreign body by artificial coughing (Heimlich's manoeuvre or subdiaphragmatic abdominal thrusts) or its removal by sweeping the middle and index finger into the mouth cavity or with forceps. The plan of action in suspected foreign body airway obstruction is depicted in the Figure 7.2.

A. AIRWAY

Clearing the airway is critical step in preparation of the victim for cardiac resuscitation. If tilting the head and lifting the chin (Fig. 7.3) do not clear

Asphyxia

the airway, then it seems that a foreign body might be obstructing the airway. First try to remove it by sweeping the fingers in the mouth. If desired result is not achieved, give five firm blows between the scapulae (Fig. 7.4), this may dislodge a foreign body by compressing the air that remains in the lungs, thereby producing an upward thrust of force behind the obstructing material and dislodging it and leading to its subsequent expulsion.

If both fingers sweep and back blows are not able to clear the airway, then try five abdominal thrust (Fig. 7.5A). If person is unconscious, then kneel over the victim, make a fist of one of your hand (place one hand over the other) and place it immediately below the victim's xiphisternum (Fig. 7.5B) and discharge the thrusts.

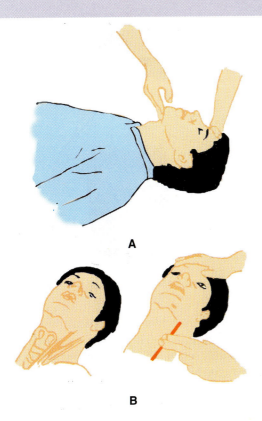

Fig. 7.3: (A) Head tilt and chin lift (B) Checking the pulse

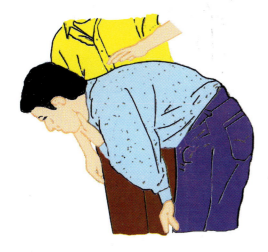

Fig. 7.4: Discharge the back blows to dislodge a foreign body

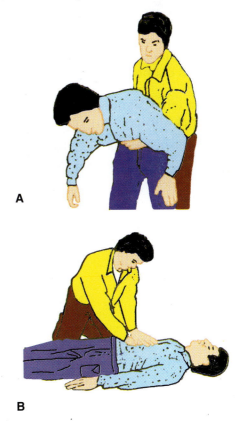

Fig. 7.5A and B: Abdominal thrust (A) Conscious patient (B) In unconscious patient

38 Pulmonary Medicine

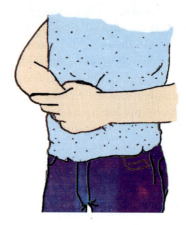

Fig. 7.6: Heimlich's manoeuver in conscious patient

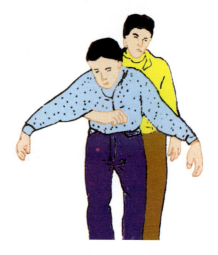

Fig. 7.7: Alternate abdominal thrust with back slaps

In conscious patient, one can use. Heimlich's manoeuvre or discharge abdominal thrusts with back slaps as described below.

The Heimlich's Manoeuvre (Abdominal Thrust)

Grasp your fist with your other hand and push firmly and suddenly upward and backwards (Fig. 7.6). Discharge alternative abdominal thrust with back slaps (Fig. 7.7). The Heimlich's manoeuvre is not entirely benign. Rupture of abdominal viscera in the victim have been reported.

Note: It there is strong suspicion that respiratory arrest precipitates cardiac arrest, particularly in the presence of mechanical airway obstruction, a second precordial thump should be delivered after the airway is cleared.

Chapter 8

Respiratory Failure

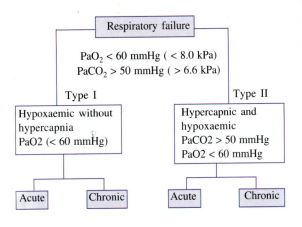

Fig. 8.1: Classification of respiratory failure

RESPIRATORY FAILURE

Definition

The primary function of the lungs is to supply the body with adequate O_2 and to remove CO_2. Normally the respiratory system maintains partial pressure of oxygen ($PaO_2 > 95$ mmHg) and CO_2 ($PaCO_2$ 36-45 mmHg) with a narrow margin of variation. When the respiratory system can no longer function to keep the gas exchange within normal range, respiratory failure is said to be present. The condition is suspected on the clinical ground, but confirmation is done by arterial blood

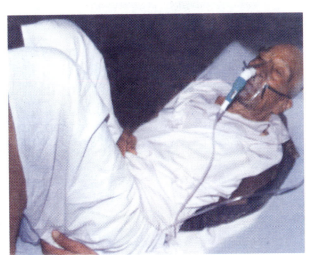

Fig. 8.2: A patient of type II respiratory failure with venture mask for O_2 therapy. The patient is not much distressed in spite of being critically ill

gas analysis. For all practical purposes, PaO_2 less than 60 mmHg or $PaCO_2$ more than 50 mmHg indicates respiratory failure.

Classification (Fig. 8.1)

In respiratory failure, hypoxaemia (low PaO_2) is always present but partial pressure of CO_2 in the blood varies from low, normal to high. The retention of CO_2 in blood more than normal is called *hypercapnia*. Depending on the arterial blood gas analysis, respiratory failure is divided into hypoxaemic (type I) and hypercapnic (type II); each of which is further subdivided into acute and chronic depending on the acute and chronic alterations in arterial blood gases.

1. *Hypoxaemic (type I) respiratory failure:* It is defined as the failure of the lungs to maintain adequate oxygenation leading to significant fall in partial pressure of O_2 ($PaO_2 < 60$ mmHg) while breathing room air. There is no hypercapnia.
2. *Hypercapnic (type II) respiratory failure:* It is defined as the failure of the lungs to maintain an adequate alveolar ventilation as evidenced by rise in $PaCO_2 > 50$ mmHg. There is always hypoxaemia. Therer is always hypoxaemia.

Note: Respiratory failure is a dynamic process, it is not uncommon for a patient presenting with type I respiratory failure to progress to type II failure as fatigue of respiratory muscles develops.

Type I Respiratory Failure

A. *Acute:* There is an acute alteration in blood gases concentration with hypoxaemia and normo or hypocapnia due to tachypnoea or hyperventilation.
B. *Chronic:* Chronic alteration in blood gases occurs because of slow diffusion of CO_2 through lungs, hence hypoxaemia and normocapnia occur. The pH and HCO_3 levels remain normal and maintained through kidneys.

The various pathophysiological mechanisms involved in type I respiratory failure are:
1. *A low fraction of inspired oxygen (FiO_2):* It is generally seen at high altitude.
2. *Hypoventilation:* It is a decrease in alveolar ventilation for a given level of CO_2 production.
3. *Ventilation/perfusion (V/Q) mismatch:* It represents areas with inadequate ventilation for a given level of perfusion (low V/Q mismatch).
4. *Shunt:* It refers to areas with normal perfusion with no ventilation (wasted perfusion).

A variety of diseases that result in this type of respiratory failure through mechanisms described above are depicted in the Box 8.1.

Hypercapnic (type II) Respiratory Failure

A. *Acute:* This is called asphyxia. There is hypercapnia with acidosis.
B. *Chronic:* There is slow and insidious rise in CO_2 in the blood.
C. *Acute on chronic type of respiratory failure* (acute exacerbation of stable type II respiratory failure).

The pathophysiological mechanisms involved are:
1. Alveolar hypoventilation

Box 8.1: Causes of type I respiratory failure

Acute	Chronic
$PaO_2 \downarrow\downarrow$	$PaO_2 \downarrow$
$PaCO_2$: N or $\downarrow$	$PaCO_2$: N or $\uparrow$
pH: N or $\downarrow$	pH: N
HCO_3: N	HCO_3: N
• Acute asthma	• Interstitial lung disease
• Pulmonary embolism	• Pulmonary fibrosis
• Pulmonary oedema (LVF)	• Emphysema
• ARDS	• Right to left shunt (Eisenmenger's syndrome)
• Pneumothorax	
• Pneumonia	• Anaemia
• CO poisoning	• High altitude
• Aspiration	• Pulmonary AV fistula
• Lung contusion	

N = Normal, $\downarrow$ = decrease $\downarrow\downarrow$ markedly decreased

Respiratory Failure

2. Severe low ventilation/perfusion (V/Q) mismatch.
3. Increased CO_2 production.
   The causes of type II respiratory failure are given in the Box 8.2.

Diagnosis

The diagnosis is based on the clinical features (listed in the Box 8.3). The symptoms and signs of hypoxia and hypercapnia are nonspecific and overlapping. Dyspnoea is the presenting feature irrespective of the type of respiratory failure. The confirmation of the diagnosis is done by arterial blood gas analysis which also judge the type and severity of respiratory failure.

Once the diagnosis of respiratory failure is confirmed, the cause of respiratory failure should be established by history, detailed physical examination and specific investigations.

- A history of wheezing, cough, mucoid expectoration, shortness of breath and seasonal variations indicate asthma as the cause.
- History of cough with or without expectoration on most of the days for consecutive three months in a year for two consecutive years in a person indicates COPD (chronic bronchitis).

Box 8.3: Symptoms and signs of respiratory failure

Hypoxia	Hypercapnia
• Mental confusion	• Disorientation
• Agitation	• Somnolence
• Tachypnoea	• CO_2 narcosis
• Tachycardia	• Flapping tremors
• Restlessness	• Headache
• Cyanosis	• Papilloedema
	• Bounding pulses

- A short history of fever, pain chest with rusty sputum indicates pneumonia.
- A history of exertional dyspnoea and dry cough indicates an interstitial lung disease.
- A history of sudden onset of dyspnoea and chest discomfort indicates pneumothorax.
- A detailed neurological examination may reveal neuropathy, myopathy or CNS disease as the underlying cause.

Management

A. *Treatment of acute type I (hypoxaemic) respiratory failure:*
   - To improve oxygenation and ventilation.
   - To remove or correct the underlying cause.
   1. *To improve oxygen and ventilation:*

Box 8.2: Causes of type II respiratory failure

Acute	Chronic
1. Respiratory	• Chronic bronchitis (COPD)
• Severe acute asthma	• Terminally ill patients
• Pulmonary embolism	• Any progressive respiratory disease
• An inhaled foreign body	• Kyphoscoliosis (severe chest deformity)
• Laryngeal oedema	• Obesity (Pickwickian syndrome)
• Multiple fractured ribs (flail chest)	• Sleep-apnoea syndrome
2. Extrarespiratory	*Acute on chronic*
• Drug overdose (narcotics)	• Infections
• Brain-stem infarction	• Retention of secretions (sputum retention syndrome)
• Respiratory muscles paralysis	• Pulmonary embolism
• GB syndrome	• Bronchospasm
• Myxoedema	• Heart failure
• Metabolic alkalosis	• Ribs fracture
• Myasthenia gravis and Eaton-Lambert syndrome	• Pneumothorax
	• Drug overdose (narcotics)

i. These patients are hospitalised and treated in RICU.
ii. *Correction of hypoxaemia:* The supportive treatment includes; administration of O_2, endotracheal intubation, mechanical ventilation and nutrition. The goal is to ensure adequate O_2 delivery to the tissues generally to achieve a PaO_2 of more than 60 mmHg. The administration of O_2 is guided by pathological mechanisms underlying the respiratory failure. For example:
- If hypoxaemia is due to V/Q mismatch, supplemental oxygen with the help of nasal cannula or venture mask may be sufficient.
- If shunt is the underlying cause of hypoxia, then patient may require mechanical ventilation and use of PEEP along with O_2.

All patients with type I respiratory failure may be treated with high concentration (> 35%) of O_2 delivered by an oronasal mask. Young patients may need to be treated in oxygen tents. Very critically ill patients may require ventilatory support often involving endotracheal intubation and mechanical ventilation.

2. *Specific treatment of underlying disorders:*
- Effective management requires prompt diagnosis and treatment of underlying cause given in the Box 8.4.
- The treatment of infection, removal of secretions may help to reverse the airflow resistance in COPD and bronchial asthma and improve oxygenation.
- No sedative or CNS depressants are employed for agitation or insomnia. For pain, non-narcotic analgesic may be employed.
- Intravenous fluids and electrolytes therapy is started and monitored by CVP and serum electrolytes. Intravenous H_2 blockers are administered in the drip to prevent GI bleed in stressed patients.

3. *Monitoring:* Close monitoring is essential and arterial blood gases taken on presentation should be repeated after 20 minutes to establish that treatment has achieved acceptable PaO_2 levels. If there is no improvement despite the treatment of underlying cause, an early decision about mechanical ventilation is necessary.

B. *Treatment of type II respiratory failure: Acute:*

In acute type II respiratory failure—also called *asphyxia*, CO_2 retention occurs suddenly and causes severe acute respiratory acidosis. The main aim of treatment is immediate or very rapid reversal of the precipitating factor and ventilatory support, if necessary. The steps of treatment are:
i. Dislodgement of a laryngeal foreign body (if being the cause) or tracheostomy.
ii. Fixation of ribs in flail chest injury.
iii. Removal of narcotic drugs
iv. Treatment of acute severe asthma
v. Temporary ventilatory support by means of noninvasive ventilation (noninvasive intermittent positive pressure ventilation—NIPPV) or invasive mechanical ventilation (following intubation) if the condition caus-

Box 8.4: Specific treatment of underlying cause of type I respiratory failure

Condition	Principles of treatment
Bronchial asthma	Aggressive bronchodilation, systemic corticosteroids
COPD	Effective bronchodilatation, antibiotic and steroids
Bronchiectasis	Antibiotics, bronchodilators,
Pneumonia	Antibiotics
LVF	Diuretic, digitalis, treatment of hypertension if present
Pneumothorax	Intercostal tube drainage if bronchopleural fistula present
Pulmonary embolism	Low molecular weight heparin, thrombolytic therapy if indicated

ing respiratory failure cannot immediately be reversed.

Chronic:
The most common cause of chronic type II respiratory failure is COPD. In this condition, CO_2 is retained slowly and is potential for acidaemia being corrected by renal conservation of bicarbonate which results in normal plasma pH. The *status quo* is usually maintained until there is a further respiratory insult in the form of infection, retention of secretions, bronchospasm, chest injury (ribs fracture), drug overdose (CNS depression) or pneumothorax which precipitates an episode of acute on chronic respiratory failure (see the causes in the Box 8.2) or acute exacerbation of COPD.

The principal aims of treatment are:
- To achieve a safe PaO_2 (> 7.0 kPa) without inducing extremes of $PaCO_2$ or pH.
- To identify and treat the precipitating cause. These patients of type II respiratory failure may not be overtly distressed despite being critically ill (Fig. 8.2 on front page).

Although relief of hypoxaemia is the first priority in management of type II respiratory failure, the hypercapnia and respiratory acidosis also must be addressed. Therefore, in initial assessment, it is important to evaluate the conscious level of the patient, his/her ability to respond to commands and ability to cough effectively. This will give an idea whether patient needs intubation and tracheal suction or mechanical support.

If the hypercapnia with physical signs of CO_2 nacrosis (confusion, flapping tremors, bounding pulses, etc.) is secondary to depressed CNS drive due to sedatives overdose or poisoning, the patient should be intubated and put on mechanical ventilation straightway.

Prompt intervention may occasionally be necessary for some precipitating conditions, e.g. intercostal tube drainage for pneumothorax or injection of local anaesthetic for fractured ribs and torn muscles. Such interventions can result in dramatic improvement of respiratory functions.

Acute on chronic:
Generally, the treatment of type II respiratory failure is treatment of 'acute on chronic' respiratory failure rather than chronic type II. The steps of management of acute on chronic or acute exacerbation of chronic respiratory failure are:

1. ***Initial assessment:***
   - Consciousness level (response to command, ability to cough).
   - Signs of CO_2 narcosis (confusion, warm extremities, flapping tremors, bounding pulses, etc.).
   - Signs of airway obstruction, e.g. wheeze, intercostal indrawing, pursed lips, tracheal tug,
   - Signs of right heart failure or cor pulmonale, e.g. raised JVP, oedema, hepatomegaly, ascites, etc.).
   - Signs of precipitating events or underlying cause (See Box 8.2).

2. ***Investigations:***
   - Arterial blood gas analysis for severity of hypoxaemia, hypercapnia and acidosis.
   - Chest X-ray for underlying disease or precipitating factor.

3. ***Treatment:***
   - Maintenance of airway.
   - Treatment of specific conditions as discussed above.
   - Controlled O_2 therapy. Start with 24% controlled flow mask and increase it slowly to achieve $PaO_2 \geq 7$ kPa.
   - Pharyngeal suction and physiotherapy.
   - Antibiotics for treatment of infection.
   - Nebulised bronchodilators.
   - Diuretics for right heart failure.

4. ***Progress:***
   - If $PaCO_2$ continues to rise or patient cannot achieve a safe PaO_2 without severe hypercapnia and acidosis, respiratory stimulant (e.g. doxapram 1.5 to 5 mg/min I.V infusion) or mechanical ventilation (NIPPV or invasive)

may be required. In case of COPD with acute exacerbation, if the patient is alert and the pH is > 7.25, patient can be managed on non-invasive intermittent positive pressure ventilation (NIPPV) therapy through nasal or venture masks. If patient is visibly fatigued and has pH < 7.25, then early mechanical ventilation will be ideal.

5. *Monitoring:*
   - Level of consciousness
   - CVP
   - Arterial blood gases
   - ECG, TLC, DLC.
   - Urine output
   - Pulse, BP, temperature, respiration
   - Urea, creatinine, electrolytes

Chapter 9

Acute Empyema Thoracis

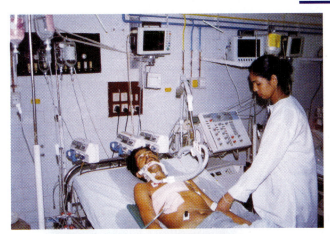

Fig. 9.1: Empyema thoracis. Intercostal tube drainage by self-retaining catheter in a patient with empyema thoracis

ACUTE EMPYEMA THORACIS

Definition

Empyema thoracis is defined as collection of pus in the pleural cavity or grossly purulent effusion (Fig. 9.1). The most common cause of empyema is the bacterial pneumonia. About 30-40% hospitalised cases of bacterial pneumonia have an associated pleural effusion. A small percentage (10%) of these parapneumonic effusions require drainage for their resolution and are called *complicated parapneumonic effusion*. Therefore, recently, the term empyema has been broadened to include all these cases of complicated parapneumonic effusions. The characteristic feature of these effusions is exudative pleural effusion which contains significant number of WBCs (but less than empyema)

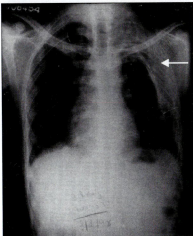

Fig. 9.2: Chronic empyema thoracis. X-ray chest shows thickened pleura on the left side(←). The shifted mediastinum has not returned to its original position

and contains organisms as demonstrated by Gram's stain and/or culture.

Parapneumonic effusions are exudative pleural effusion with low WBC count as compared to empyema but contain organisms as demonstrated on Gram's stain and/or culture, are included in the designated term 'empyema' which was previously used for frank pus in the pleural space.

Pathology

In acute empyema, there is accumulation of large amount of pleural fluid with many polymorphs, bacteria and cellular debris. Fibrin gets deposited on both the layers of pleura (visceral and parietal) and there is tendency towards loculation. Later, as the empyema becomes chronic, fibroblasts grow from both the layers into the exudate resulting in adhesions of both the surfaces of pleura and form an inelastic membrane called *thickened pleura* or *pleural peel* (Fig. 9.2).

Causes

The empyema results from infection of pleura which may travel from the lungs, abdominal viscera or mediastinum. It may result from blood born infection (septicaemia) or iatrogenic infection (following procedures). There may be secondary pleural infection following chest injuries or postoperative. The causes are given in the Table 9.1.

Pathogenic Organisms

1. Gram-positive aerobic organisms, e.g. *S. aureus, S. pneumonia, S. pyogenes.*
2. Gram-negative aerobic organisms, e.g. *E. coli, B. proteus, H. influenza, Klebsiella, pseudomonas* and *Enterobacter* species.
3. Anaerobic bacteria, e.g., *bacteriodes, fusobacterium, pepto-streptococci.*
4. *M. Tuberculosis.*
5. Parasites. *E. histolytica, T. echinococcus.*
6. Fungi, e.g. *Aspergillus, cryptococcus, blastomycosis,* etc.

Table 9.1: Cause of empyema thoracis

1. **Diseases of lung:** Infection travels from the lung to pleura
   - Lung abscess
   - Pneumonia
   - Fungal infection
   - Bronchiectasis
   - Tuberculosis
   - Bronchopleural fistula
2. **Diseases of abdominal viscera** (infection travels from abdominal viscera to pleura)
   - Liver abscess (unruptured or ruptured)
   - Subphrenic abscess
   - Perforated peptic ulcer
3. **Diseases of mediastinum:** There may be infective focus in the mediastinum from which it travels to pleura
   - Cold abscess
   - Oesophageal perforation
   - Osteomyelitis e.g. vertebrae, sternum
4. **Trauma with superadded infection**
   - Chest wall injuries (gunshot wound, stab wound)
   - Postoperative.
5. **Iatrogenic:** Infection introduced during procedure
   - Chest aspiration
   - Liver biopsy
6. **Blood-borne infection**
   - Septicaemia

Clinical Features

The empyema can occur in any age group but commoner in elderly and debilitated persons. The common predisposing conditions include; cardiopulmonary disorders, diabetes, alcoholism, drug abuse, malnutrition, presence of neoplasm, neurological disorders and immunocompromised state (e.g. HIV, use of corticosteroids or cytotoxic drugs). Mortality is high in immunocompromised patients.

Patients with aerobic infections present with acute onset of symptoms such as fever with chills, cough with purulent expectoration (bronchopleural fistula), dyspnoea and chest discomfort. In many patients, empyema develops as a complication of pneumonia and pleural effusion. Patients with anaerobic infections present with subacute illness with nonspecific symptom and signs such as weight loss, leucocytosis, mild anaemia and history/evidence of predisposing factor for aspiration from oral cavity. Tubercular empyema presents with low grade fever of weeks and months duration with weakness and cough.

Physical signs: Physical examination reveals signs of toxaemia (fever, tachypnoea, tachycardia) and pleural effusion during acute phase. Presence of tenderness on percussion with some oedema of chest wall provides a clue to empyema. Clubbing of fingers and toes is usually seen. Rarely, empyema may track into subcutaneous tissue of chest wall and presents as a localised swelling with positive cough impulse. This is termed as *empyema necessitans* and is mostly seen with actinomycotic infections.

Chronic cases with pleural thickening (thickened pleura Fig. 9.2) and loculation of pus will show significant deformity with retraction of chest on the same side of empyema and even scoliosis. The signs will be dull percussion note with diminished breath sounds. Extensive pleural calcification may occur. Tubercular empyema is often chronic and present with thickened pleura.

Investigations

The possibility of a parapneumonic effusion and empyema should be considered in each and every case of pneumonia if patients develops signs of pleural effusion. Investigations to be done include:

1. **Leucocyte count:** There is leucocytosis with raised ESR in acute empyema.
2. *Chest X-ray:* All the three views (PA, lateral and decubitus) of chest X-ray are helpful. The X-ray picture of empyema initially is same as pleural effusion (Fig. 9.3A). Later on loculation of empyema which occurs posterolaterally is better seen on a lateral film. An air and fluid level if present, indicates pyopneumothorax which may be due to bronchopleural fistula. A large lung abscess with thin walls may have to be differentiated from a loculated pyopneumothorax.
3. *Ultrasonography:* It is most helpful investigations and guides the site of aspiration of loculated empyema. Fibrin strands and loculations (pockets) of empyema may be seen on USG and may be aspirated under ultrasound guidance to confirm the diagnosis. All loculations should be aspirated as character of pleural fluid may vary from one loculation to other.
4. *CT scan:* It is most useful to distinguish pleural fluid loculations from peripheral parenchymal infiltrates, pleural thickening or lung abscess. It is particularly useful in identifying multiple small loculations.
5. *Aspiration of pus (thoracentesis Fig. 9.1):* Initial aspiration of pus (thoracentesis) should be therapeutic *cum* diagnostic. The fluid (pus) aspirated should be examined for colour (anchovy source pus in ruptured amoebic liver abscess), turbidity (thick pus is pyogenic) and odour (foul putrid smell is due to anaerobic infections) and discharge of sulphur granules (actinomycosis). Alquots are sent for cytology and biochemical analysis (i.e., glucose, proteins, pH, LDH, amylase level and TLC and DLC). Acidic effusion tends to loculate rapidly than alkaline.

Pleural fluid should be subjected to Gram-staining and culture for pyogenic organisms and AFB. The pleural fluid pH is usually less than 7.2, the LDH level is more than 1000 IU/L and glucose content is < 60 mg/dl. Low pH of parapneumonic pleural effusion indicates impending empyema.

Complications

1. Thickening of pleura with calcification (Fig. 9.2).
2. Empyema necessitans and chronic discharging sinus.
3. Bronchopleural fistula.
4. Fibrosis with bronchiectasis in the underlying lung.
5. Metastatic infection, e.g. brain abscess, meningitis, suppurative pericarditis.

6. Amyloidosis.
7. Gross deformity of thoracic cage.
8. Septicaemia.

Management

Aims

- To sterilize the pleural space by antibiotics and pus drainage.
- To achieve expansion of lung by early drainage of pus and chest physiotherapy.
- To control septicaemia or systemic infection with appropriate antibiotic therapy.

1. **Antibiotic therapy based on culture and sensitivity:** In gram-negative infection, a 3rd generation cephalosporins along with an aminoglycoside is used. In community-acquired infection, β-lactam (oral cefpodoxime, cefuroxime, amoxycillin and clavulanic acid combination) *plus* an oral macrolide may be used. If staphylococcal infection is suspected, then *targocid* or vancomycin is preferred. For anaerobes, a combination of clindamycin or metronidazole and amoxycillin *plus* clavulanic acid is used.

   In the absence of culture and sensitivity report, a combination of penicillin (amoxycillin), an aminoglycoside (gentamicin, amikacin) and metronidazole may be used to cover both aerobic and anaerobic infections. In severe infections, systemic antibiotics in standard doses should be used. The duration of treatment is 6 weeks. Empyema due to tuberculosis or other organisms such as *Entamoeba histolytica* and *Actinomyces* should be treated accordingly.

2. **Drainage of the pus or empyema fluid:** The aim is to evacuate the pus rapidly to allow the underlying lung to re-expand. Drainage of pus may be closed or open. The closed drainage may be either intermittent via a wide-bore needle aspirations (thoracentesis) or continuous intercostal tube drainage.

   A. *Intermittent needle aspiration (thoracentesis):* The first needle aspiration is indicated in all cases of empyema to classify the nature of fluid (pus). During initial aspiration, the fluid or pus should be removed as much as possible and sent for diagnostic evaluation, hence, it is therapeutic cum diagnostic aspiration. If fluid recurs, serial thoracenteses (aspirations) are to be done provided patient is clinically better and there is no formation of loculations. Before each aspiration, chest X-ray is to be repeated (Figs 9.3A and B) or USG done to decide the site of aspiration. After each aspiration, fluid should be sent for cytology and biochemistry along with Gram-stain and culture. During aspiration, a three-way cannula should be used to prevent air entry into pleural cavity. If response to antibiotic treatment is good, then fluid will become more serous (thin) at each aspiration and will become sterile after 3-4 aspirations. Chest X-ray repeated after each aspiration will demonstrate lung expansion (Fig. 9.3B) provided there is no underlying cause for nonexpansion (underlying lung disease).

   > *During aspiration, if patient develops, respiratory distress, pain and tachycardia, aspiration should be stopped immediately as uncommonly pleural shock and air embolism can occur.*

   Failure to needle aspiration: Needle aspiration will fail if:
   1. Wrong site is selected.
   2. Needle is too narrow and syringe is small sized.
   3. Thick clot and fibrin tags block the aspirating needle, which should be made thin with use of fibrinolytic agents or proteolytic enzyme (hylase).

   B. *Closed intercostal tube drainage:* The decision to institute chest tube drainage is mainly based on the pleural fluid examination. Any of the following is an indication for intercostal tube drainage:

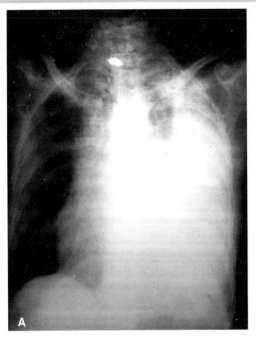 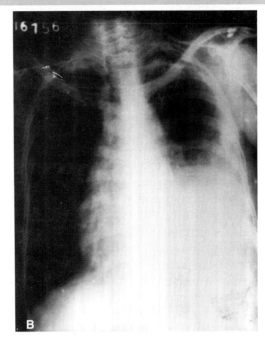

Figs 9.3A and B: Empyema thoracis. Chest X-rays are displayed showing: (A) Empyema thoracis before needle aspiration. (B) After needle aspiration and removal of 400 ml of pus

- The presence of thick pus in the pleural space which is difficult to aspirate through needle.
- Organisms visible on Gram-stain of pleural fluid.
- Glucose level of the fluid is < 50 mg/dl.
- Pleural fluid pH < 7.2 or 0.15 units lower than the arterial pH. This is because acidic pleural fluid is likely to loculate rapidly, at times, within hours.
- Marked elevated WBC count in the pleural fluid.
- Bronchopleural fistula.
- Failure of serial thoracentesis.
- Bilateral acute empyema.
- Severe toxaemia.

The chest tube, traditionally, a large bore (28 to 32 French) catheter or any self-retaining catheter is put in the most dependent part of the empyema cavity and connected to underwater seal (Fig. 9.1). Recently, it has been advocated that in complicated parepneumonic effusions, smaller catheters (8 to 16 French) can be used percutaneously, especially for satellite pleural pockets formed due to pleural adhesions. These are easier to put and less painful but require ultrasonic guidance.

Success of tube drainage: If drainage is successful, then there will be clinical and radiological improvement within 24 hours.

Duration of drainage: Chest tube should be left in place until the volume of pleural drainage is less than 50 ml/24 hours for 2 consecutive days and the drainage fluid becomes clearly yellow.

Failure of tube drainage: It occurs if:
- Tube is in wrong place.
- Multiple loculations.
- Bronchopleural fistula.
- Failure of the pleural cavity to collapse and obliterate due to thickened pleural (pleural peel).
- Undiagnosed or unsuspected tuberculosis.

A CT scan will be helpful to distinguish these possibilities.

Note: If the purulent drainage continues through the chest tube for more than a week in spite of proper method of drainage and after proper selection of an antibiotic, then an aggressive method should be used for evacuation of pus.

Use of Intrapleural Thrombolytic Agents

These agents have a role to break the loculations in multiloculated empyema. Intrapleural instillation of streptokinase (usual dose is 250,000 U in 100 ml saline) or urokinase (100, 000 U diluted in 100 ml of saline) through chest tube is helpful if drainage stops because of loculations and opacities on chest X-ray persist. After each instillation, the chest tube is clamped for 2 hours to allow the thrombolytic agents to attack the fibrin membranes responsible for loculations. Thrombolytic agents can be daily instilled for upto 14 days. This is a costly treatment. The intrapleural injection of thrombolytic agents does not affect the systemic coagulation system as these do not diffuse through the pleura.

Contraindications

Thrombolytic therapy is contraindicated:
- Presence of bronchopleural fistula.
- Recent trauma.
- Recent bronchial suturing.

If the closed chest tube drainage and thrombolytic agents are unsuccessful, then surgical intervention either by rib resection, thoracoscopy with breakdown of adhesions, decortication, lung resection, thoracoplasty may be required. These are aggressive approaches of drainage of pus.

Rib resection is indicated when closed chest tube drainage has not helped the patient because now the drainage is gravity dependent or fibrin clots block the tube. Complete cure may take 6 to 8 weeks by tube drainage following rib resection. It will also fail if pus is too thick or a bronchopleural fistula has developed or pockets of pus become loculated and inaccessible. This will require major surgical interventions.

Surgical Interventions/Procedures

A. ***Thoracoscopy with manual breakdown of adhesions and chest tube drainage:*** In this, chest tube is positioned optimally with the help of thoracoscope. In addition, pleural surface can be inspected to determine the necessity for decortication. If this procedure is successful, lung expands and drainage stops and after 2 to 3 days, the tube can be removed.

B. ***Decortication:*** It is procedure of choice if:
   1. The fluid is too thick to drain.
   2. There is an evidence of pleural adhesions.
   3. The lung is not expanding on serial chest X-rays.

   In this procedure, all the fibrous tissue is removed from the visceral pleura, and all pus is evacuated from the pleural space.

Note: Decortication is not possible in heavily thickened pleura which is usually seen in tuberculosis.

C. ***Lung resection:*** If the underlying lung is diseased, or the lung does not expand after decortication and there are chances of reactivation of the disease such as tuberculosis; in such patients, pleuropneumonectomy or pleurolobectomy is indicated.

D. ***Open drainage:*** If patient is not fit for major surgical procedures described above and empyema has become completely walled off, then open drainage by flap procedure (*Floesser flap*) can be done. In this procedure, the pleural space is exposed to the surface (i.e. to atmospheric pressure), hence, there is danger of developing pneumothorax if the empyema cavity is not walled off, therefore, it should not be done too early. Open drainage should be continued till the pleural cavity is completely evacuated and obliterated. It requires regular irrigation of the cavity with antibiotics and antiseptic dressings. The cavity will become obliterated within few months.

Part Two

Gastroenterology

Chapter 10

Acute Vomiting

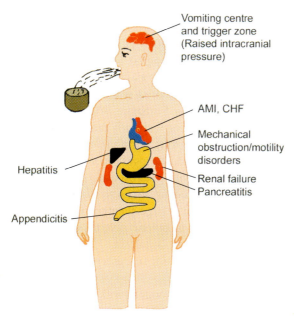

Fig. 10.1: Possible causes of vomiting

ACUTE VOMITING

Definition

Vomiting refers to forceful expulsion of gastric contents through the mouth by sustained contractions of abdominal muscles. Nausea refers to feeling of an imminent desire to vomit. Nausea often precedes or accompanies vomiting. Retching refers to laboured rhythmic contractions of respiratory and abdominal muscles. It also frequently precedes or accompanies vomiting.

Reflex Pathway of Vomiting

1. *Central control:* Vomiting is controlled by two centres located in the medulla, i.e. *vomiting centre* in lateral reticular formation and *chemoreceptor trigger zone* in the floor of 4th ventricle.
2. *Afferent pathway:* The vomiting centre receives afferent impulses from the GI tract, from the brainstem and cortical centres especially labyrinthine apparatus and from the chemoreceptor trigger zone. The chemoreceptor trigger zone by itself is incapable of mediating the act of vomiting. The activation of this zone results in efferent impulses to the medullary vomiting centre, which in turn initiates the vomiting.
3. *The efferent pathway:* The important efferent pathways in vomiting are phrenic nerves (to the diaphragm), spinal nerves (to intercostal and abdominal muscles) and visceral efferent fibers in the vagus nerve (to the larynx, pharynx, oesophagus and stomach).

The causes of vomiting are given in the Table 10.1.

Clinical Consequences of Vomiting

1. Repeated vomiting, if forceful may lead to pressure rupture of oesophagus (*Boerhave's syndrome*).

54 Gastroenterology

Table 10.1: Causes of vomiting

1. **Gastrointestinal**
   i. *Mechanical obstruction*
      - Gastric outlet obstruction following peptic ulcer or malignancy
      - Small intestinal obstruction, e.g. volvolus, adhesions, malignancy
   ii. *Motility disorders*
      - Gastroparesis due to diabetes, drugs, post-vagotomy and idiopathic
   iii. *Inflammation*
      - Bacterial food poisoning
      - Appendicitis
      - Acute pancreatitis
   iv. *Gastrointestinal irritants*
      - Alcohol
      - Drugs, e.g. NSAIDs
      - Oral antibiotics
2. **Hepatobiliary**
   - Hepatitis A and B
   - Acute cholecystitis
   - Portal hypertension
   - Gallstones
3. **CNS disorders**
   i. *Vestibular causes*
      - Labyrinthitis
      - Meniere's disease
      - Motion sickness
   ii. *Raised intracranial pressure*
      - CNS tumours
      - Subdural/subarachnoid haemorrhage
      - Hydrocephalus
      - Meningitis, encephalitis
4. **Cardiovascular**
   - Acute MI
   - Congestive heart failure
5. **Renal**
   - Renal failure
6. **Endocrinal**
   - Diabetes mellitus
   - Hypo and hyperthyroidism
   - Thyrotoxic crisis
   - Adrenal crisis
7. **Systemic causes**
   - Infection
   - Pregnancy
8. **Psychogenic**
9. **Radiation therapy**
10. **Bulmia**
    - Psychiatric disorders
11. **Postoperative**

2. It may cause a linear mucosal tear at or near the cardioesophageal junction leading to haematemesis (*Mallory-Weiss syndrome*).
3. Prolonged vomiting may lead to fluid loss (dehydration), loss of HCl (metabolic alkalosis), loss of K^+ (hypokalaemia) and loss of nutrients (malnutrition).
4. Vomiting in an unconscious patient or in patient with depressed consciousness may result in aspiration pneumonia.

Clinical Evaluation

History

The history is an important step in clinical evaluation of a case with vomiting because temporal relationship of vomiting to eating may be helpful in diagnosis as detailed below:

- Early morning vomiting without retching is seen in pregnancy and uraemia. Alcoholic gastritis produces retching with early morning vomiting.
- Vomiting occurring during or immediate after eating may indicate psychogenic vomiting or peptic ulcer with pylorospasm.
- Vomiting occurring after 4 to 6 hours of eating with expulsion of large quantities of gastric contents, is seen in pyloric obstruction or gastroparesis, or cardia achalasia.
- A projectile vomiting suggests raised intracranial pressure.
- A long history of vomiting with little or no weight loss indicates psychogenic basis.
- Associated symptoms such as tinnitus, vertigo indicate vestibular involvement (Meniere's disease).
- Relief of abdominal pain with vomiting is typical of peptic ulcer.
- A large amount of gastric contents in vomiting indicates gastric outlet obstruction or hypersecretory state such as *Zollinger-Ellison syndrome*.
- The presence of blood in the gastric contents usually denotes bleeding from the oesophagus, stomach or duodenum.

- Fever indicates inflammation or infection as the cause of vomiting.
- History of drug intake may indicate drug-induced vomiting.

Physical Examination

Every effort should be made to find out the cause of vomiting and also to assess the status of hydration.
1. Status of hydration is assessed by pulse, BP, skin turgor, moistness of mucous membrane and other vital signs.
2. Abdominal examination provides clues to the diagnosis and the cause of vomiting:
   - Abdominal distension with sluggish bowel sounds indicates either an appendicitis or cholecystitis.
   - Abdominal distension with tenderness and visible peristalsis suggest acute intestinal obstruction.
   - Abdominal distension with board-like rigidity may suggest peritonitis.
   - Presence of jaundice, hepatomegaly and subcostal tenderness (thumping sign) indicates hepatobiliary disease.
   - Altered sensorium, signs of meningeal irritation, focal neurological deficit, seizures, papilloedema indicate intracranial pathology with raised intracranial tension.
   - Nystagmus, ear discharge, deafness suggest either otogenic or cerebellar disease.

Investigations

A battery of tests to cover all the causes of vomiting, is given below out of which one has to select investigations depending on the presumptive cause.
- Complete blood count.
- Urine analysis.
- Renal profile, e.g., blood urea, creatinine.
- Serum electrolytes, e.g. K+.
- Hepatic profile, e.g. serum bilirubin, hepatic enzymes.
- Serum amylase for pancreatic disease.
- USG of abdomen for liver and pancreatic disease.
- CSF analysis and CT scan of the head for any neurological cause.
- Pregnancy test should be done in all potentially pregnant women.
- Serum drug levels of certain drugs.
- Supine and erect X-ray to be done in a case suspected of intestinal obstruction or perforation.
- Upper GI endoscopy for peptic ulcer and/or gastric outlet obstruction.
- EKG for myocardial infarction.

Management

1. The initial step of managements is to find out the cause and treat/correct it appropriately. Electrolyte imbalance, gastric outlet obstruction, systemic infections, metabolic disorders, e.g. diabetes, uraemia and CNS disorders must be identified and treated accordingly.
2. Most cases of vomiting are mild and self-limited, require no specific treatment.
3. Patients with severe vomiting should be hospitalised and intravenous fluids started to prevent or correct dehydration. Electrolyte balance is corrected by infusing saline and potassium supplementation to correct metabolic alkalosis and hypokalaemia.
4. Gastric decompression by Ryle's tube aspiration may be needed for gastric outlet obstruction, gastroparesis and acute intestinal obstruction, etc.
5. Drug therapy: Antimetics drugs vary in their usefulness, hence, choice of drug depends on the availability and extent of control of emesis. The antiemetics are given in the Table 10.2 with their action, indications and side effects.

Substance P antagonists are being tried for control of vomiting in patients receiving cancer chemotherapy. Initial trials show promising results with no side effects.

56 Gastroenterology

Table 10.2: Antiemetic drugs

Agent	Dose and route	Indications	Side effects
1. **Antihistaminics and anticholinergics**			
Diphenhydramine	25-50 mg, 4 to 6 hourly orally or parenterally	• Vomiting due to motion sickness, pregnancy, inner ear disease, uraemia and post-operative vomiting	Sedation, dizziness, dry mouth, blurred vision, epigastric discomfort, constipation, urinary retention
Meclozine	25-50 mg orally/day		
Promethazine	25 mg 4-6 hours/orally or parenterally		
Scopolamine	1.5 mg/3rd day patch		
2. **Dopamine receptors inhibitors**			
• Phenothiazine (prochlorperazine)	25 mg suppository/per rectum q 6 hours/oral, or parenteral	• All types of vomiting except motion sickness and labrinthine disease	Hypotension, extrapyramidal side-effects, akathisia, drowsiness, anxiety, sedation
• Droperidol	1-2.5 mg q 3-6 hours I.V.	• Gastroparesis	
• Metoclopramide	10-20 mg oral or I.V. 6 hourly		
• Domperidone	20-40 mg orally 3-4 times a day		
3. **Sedative**			
• Diazepam	2 to 5 mg q 4-6 hours orally or I.V.	• Psychogenic vomiting	Sedation
• Lorazepam	1 to 2 mg q 4-6 hours/ orally or I.V.	• Added to metoclopramide or steroids to control vomiting in cancer patients	
4. **Serotonin receptors antagonists**			
• Dolasetran	100 mg or 1.8 mg/kg/I.V. or 200 mg oral	• Chemotherapy induced vomiting in combination with corticosteroids	Mild headache, diarrhoea or constipation, transient rise in transaminases
• Ondansetron	8 mg or 0.15 mg/kg infusion or 8 mg tds orally		
• Granisetran	10 µg/kg infusion or 9 mg oral		
5. **Corticosteroids**			
• Dexamethasone	8-20 mg I.V. 4-20 mg oral	They are combined with metocloplamide to control vomiting due to cancer chemotherapy	Side effects are of corticosteroids
• Methylprednisolone	40-100 mg I.V.		
6. **Antibiotic**			
• Erythromycin	125 mg q 6 hours orally	• Gastroparesis	• Abdominal cramps, bloating, nausea

Vomiting due to chemotherapy in cancer patients a special problem and can pose as an emergency as these patients go into dehydration easily. The drugs used to control vomiting in such cases include a combination of metoclopramide, steroids and serotinin receptor antagonists e.g. dolasetran.

Chapter 11

Acute Diarrhoea

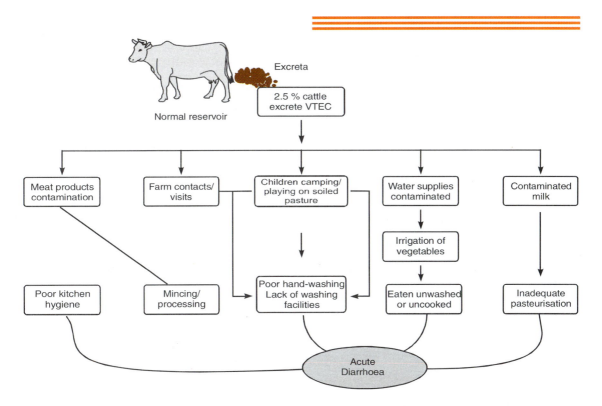

Fig. 11.1: Enterohaemorrhagic E. coli—Verocytotoxigenic E. coli (VTEC). The reservoir of infection is the gut of herbivores. Contaminated meat products are recognised source of this infection

ACUTE DIARRHOEA

Definition

Normal stool content is < 200g/day and stool is well formed. Normal bowel frequency varies from three times a week to three times a day.

Diarrhoea is defined as an increase in daily stool content > 200 g/day associated with increased stool frequency (> 3/day). In diarrhoea, stool is usually liquid due to increase in water content. Diarrhoea is said to be *acute* if its duration is less than 3 weeks.

Gastroenterology

Table 11.1: Classification of acute diarrhoea

Small bowel diarrhoea	Large bowel diarrhoea
1. Infective • Viral, e.g. rota, norwalk, adeno, corona • Bacterial, e.g. *E. coli, vibrio cholerae, yersinia* • Parasitic e.g. *Giardia* • Fungal, e.g. *Candida* 2. Drugs, e.g. laxative, digitalis, ampicillin, etc. 3. Traveller's diarrhoea	1. Infective • Bacterial, e.g., *Shigella, Salmonella, E. coli, Campylobacter* • Parasitic, e.g. *E. histolytica* • Fungal 2. Pseudomembranous colitis (antibiotic-induced diarrhoea) 3. Food poisoning 4. Spurious diarrhoea (fecal impaction) 5. Traveller's diarrhoea 6. Pelvic inflammatory disease

Diarrhoea must be distinguished from *pseudodiarrhoea* or hyperdefecation (increased frequency of defecation without increase in stool weight above normal) and *incontinence* (involuntary discharge of rectal contents).

Causes

The acute diarrhoea can be classified depending on the *aetiology*, *site of involvement* (small bowel vs large bowel) or *pathophysiology* (i.e., whether secretory, osmotic, exudative or disordered motility) and *type of involvement* (invasive vs noninvasive). Based on the aetiology and site of involvement, classification of acute diarrhoea is depicted in the Table 11.1. Contaminated food articles (water, milk, meat) or contact with farm animals (Fig. 11.1) are common reservoir of infection.

Box 11.1: Symptoms and signs of acute diarrhoea

Symptoms	Signs of dehydration may be present
• Nausea, vomiting • Abdominal pain • Fever • Watery loose stools • Blood in the stool • Excessive thirst	• Patient irritable • Weak pulse, low BP • Depressed fontanelle • Dry pinched facies • Sunken eye balls • Dryness of mouth, tongue, mucous membrane • Loss of skin turgor

Table 11.2: Characteristics of small bowel vs large bowel diarrhoea

Characteristic	Small bowel	Large bowel
Pathogens	• *V. cholerae* • *E. coli* • Rota virus • Norwalk virus • *Giardia*	• *Shigella* • *E coli* • *Campylobacter* • *E. histolytica*
Stool content	Large	Small
Type of stool	Loose, watery	Viscus, mucoid
Presence of blood	Rare	Common
Presence of pus cells	Rare	Common
Pain	Central (periumbilical)	Quadrantic (commonly left lower abdominal)
Proctoscopy	Normal	Abnormal

Clinical Features

Patients with acute infectious diarrhoea present with nausea, vomiting (common with toxins or toxigenic infection), abdominal pain which is mild, diffuse, crampy due to stimulation of peristalsis by hypervoluminous stool content, fever (e.g. infections) and loose watery, malabsorptive or bloody stool depending on the specific pathogen.

The presence of systemic symptoms may provide important clues to the basic underlying cause, e.g., both *shigellosis* and *E. coli* (enterohaemorrhagic strain) may be accompanied by haemolytic-uraemic syndrome particularly in very young and old persons. *Yersinia* infection and occasionally other enteric bacterial infections may be accompanied by *Reiter's syndrome* (arthritis, uveitis, urethritis), thyroiditis, pericarditis and glomerulonephritis.

The signs of dehydration may be present depending the severity of diarrhoea (see the Box 11.1). The clinical features of small bowel and large bowel diarrhoea are given in the Table 11.2. It is important from the aetiological and therapeutic point of view.

Investigations

1. Stool examination for leucocytes, ova, parasites, blood and pus cells, etc.
2. Stool culture for isolation of the infective agent.
3. Complete haemogram.
4. Blood biochemistry e.g., urea, creatinine, electrolytes.
5. Blood culture.
6. Sigmoidoscopy.
7. Abdominal X-ray.

Management

The mainstay of treatment of acute diarrhoea is rest and prevention and treatment of dehydration by fluid replacement.

1. **Correction of fluid and electrolyte deficit:** Most deaths in acute diarrhoea result from fluid and electrolyte deficit, hence, must be corrected by fluid and electrolyte replacement. Intravenous fluid therapy may be necessary in severely dehydrated individuals, especially the infants and elderly. The key to effective management of diarrhoea is early replacement of fluid losses starting from home with available fluid administration early in the illness to prevent dehydration. As long as renal function is preserved, profound disturbances of electrolytes and pH do not occur.

   Depending on the degree of dehydration, the oral rehydration solutions (ORS) used in the treatment of cholera can also be considered in patients of acute diarrhoea.

   A. *Mild dehydration* (i.e. just irritable and weak pulse). Mild dehydration is treated by home-available solution (plan A of WHO) such as coconut water, lemon sugar beverage (shikanjvi), weak tea, rice, etc. The fluid should be given as much as the patient can tolerate orally. This fluid therapy may be given in small sips or with teaspoon. If situation does not come under control, then home made oral rehydration solution (mixing of 6-8 TSF of sugar, one TSF of salt with or without lemon squeeze in one litre of water) should be started.

   B. *Moderate dehydration* (dry tongue, depressed fontanella, irritability, reduced urine output, feeble pulse, excessive thirst, loss of skin turgor), requires WHO recommended ORS (i.e. glucose 20 g, NaCl 3.5 g, trisodium citrate 2.9 g and KCl 1.5 g dissolved in one litre of safe drinking water). It is administered in small sips or with a teaspoon freely as much as person can tolerate without vomiting. It should be continued till dehydration is corrected.

   ORS provides 90 mEq/L of Na^+, 20 mEq/L of K^+; 80 mEq/L of Cl^+ and 30 mEq/L of HCO_3^- which is usually sufficient for all types of diarrhoea at all ages.

   C. *Severe dehydration* with signs of acute peripheral circulatory failure requires intravenous fluid replacement starting with Ringer's lactate or glucose saline solution at a rate of 20 ml/kg/hr in the next 2 hours. An adult should receive about 2 L of fluids within 2-3 hours.

   A child who starts passing urine within two hours should receive 40 ml/kg of Ringer's lactate solution I.V. over next two hours as well. Concurrently, oral rehydration therapy should also be started as described above. Oral rehydration therapy should be continued till losses have been corrected and patient is on maintenance requirement of fluids.

2. ***Antibiotics:*** Antibiotic therapy in bacterial diarrhoea is controversial and generally not required in patients with mild or resolving disease but should be considered in patients with shigellosis, traveller's diarrhoea, pseudomembranous colitis, cholera, food poisoning, etc. Only 5-10% of patients with diarrhoea require antibiotic therapy; the choice of which depends on the causative agent (see Box 11.2).

3. ***Antidiarrhoeal drugs:*** Most of these drugs have little beneficial effect and can have potential side effects. These are not recommended in children. Loperamide and bismuth subsalicylate have been shown to be safe in patients with traveller's diarrhoea who have neither fever nor blood or pus in the stool. Loperamide is also a widely used drug for social convenience to decrease the frequency of stools in profuse diarrhoea.

4. ***Symptomatic treatment of vomiting and distention of abdomen:*** Occasional vomiting does not require treatment except the adjustment of oral rehydration therapy. Persistent vomiting may require antiemetic therapy.

Box 11.2: Antibiotic treatment of acute diarrhoea

Organism	Choice of antibiotic
Shigella	Quinolones (Norfloxacin 400 mg bid or ciprofloxacin 500 mg bid for 5 days)
E. coli and traveller's diarrhoea	
Cholera (*Vibrio cholerae*)	Tetracycline (see the treatment of cholera)
C. difficile	Vancomycin orally (250-500 mg qid for 7-10 days)
Campylobacter	Erythromycin 250-500 mg qid for 5 days
Yersinia	Tetracycline 1-2 g/day for 7 days
Giardia	Metronidazole 200-400 mg tid for 7 days
E. histolytica	Metronidazole (400-800 mg tid for 5-7 days) or tinidazole 600 mg bid for 5-7 days or ornidazole 500 mg bid.

Abdominal distention due to hypokalaemia may be treated by withholding oral feeding and its replacement with parenteral fluids with potassium supplementation.

5. ***Monitoring:*** Patient with acute diarrhoea should be monitored for vitals, electrolytes, pH, urea and creatinine.

Chapter 12

Upper Gastrointestinal Bleed

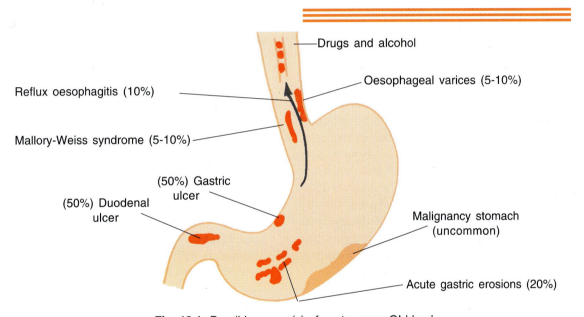

Fig. 12.1: Possible source(s) of acute upper GI bleed

ACUTE UPPER GASTROINTESTINAL BLEED

Definition

Bleeding occurring from upper gastrointestinal tract upto the ligament of *Treitz* is called as upper GI (UGI) bleed. It is most common gastrointestinal emergency presenting as haemetemesis, malena or both. For malena to result, there must be at least 50-100 ml of blood loss in upper GI tract.

Causes

The causes according to frequency are given in the Box 12.1 and Fig. 12.1.

Clinical Features

Patients with upper GI bleed invariably present with haemetemesis (blood in the vomit) which may be red with clots when bleeding is profuse, or malena (black, tarry stool) in case of less severe bleeding.

Gastroenterology

> **Box 12.1: Causes of acute upper GI bleed frequency-wise**
>
> 1. Peptic ulcer (35-50%) associated with NSAIDs and H. pylori.
> 2. Acute gastric erosion (about 20%) e.g. NSAIDs, alcohol induced.
> 3. Oesophageal varices (5-10%) i.e., liver disease, portal hypertension.
> 4. Reflux oesophagitis (5-10%) usually associated with hiatus hernia.
> 5. Mallory-Weiss tear (5%)
> 6. Vascular (angiomatous) malformations (5%)
> 7. Cancer of oesophagus or stomach (2%)
> 8. Aortic graft (aorto-duodenal fistula - 0.2%)
> 9. Miscellaneous (rare) i.e., bleeding disorders, corrosive injury, post-sclerotherapy or ligation ulcers.

Blood loss of less than 500 ml is rarely associated with systemic signs. A postural fall in systolic BP > 10 mm usually indicates a 20% or more reduction in blood volume. There may be syncope, dizziness, tachycardia, tachypnoea due to hypotension resulting from intravascular volume depletion. Shock frequently ensues when blood loss is 25 to 40% of blood volume. Patients may occasionally experience vasovagal reaction with bradycardia during bleeding episodes. There may be symptoms and signs of anaemia if there has been a chronic blood loss due to repeated bleeding.

History and clinical examination may provide important clues to the possible cause:

1. A history or symptoms suggestive of peptic ulcer disease, liver disease (portal hypertension), intake of NSAIDs (erosive gastropathy), bleeding from other sites (patient on anticoagulants), cutaneous malformations (telangiectatic lesion of Osler-Rendu-Weber disease) point towards the possible cause of UGI bleed. History of retching preceding haemetemesis suggests Mallory—Weiss tear.
2. Clinical examination also yields important informations. Stigmata of alcoholic liver disease (spider angiomata, gynaecomastia, jaundice, ascites, testicular atrophy, hepatosplenomegaly) suggest portal hypertension with bleeding from the varices (oesophageal or gastric).

Investigations

1. Initial studies include *hematocrit* and *haemoglobin* which may be falsely high due to hemoconcentration, come to normal following fluid repletion.
2. *Prothrombin time and partial thromboplastin studies* are needed to exclude clotting defects (primary or secondary).
3. *Blood urea* and *serum creatinine* may be high due to pre-renal or renal azotaemia.
4. *Upper GI endoscopy:* It is the most preferred method of examination to find out the cause of upper GI bleeding. When there is history of haemetemesis or malena, a nasogastric tube should be passed to empty the stomach and to determine whether the bleeding is proximal to the ligament of Treitz.

If the initial nasogastric aspirate is clear, current active bleeding is unlikely and the tube may be removed. If **blood or "coffee ground"** material is aspirated from the nasogastric tube, water or saline lavage should be initiated. Stomach should be irrigated to have better view during emergency upper GI endoscopy.

Endoscopy should be done once the patient is hemodynamically stable. A diagnosis will be achieved in 80% of cases. Lesions located in certain blind areas may be missed on endoscopy such as fundus of the stomach, high lesser curvature and just inside the rim of pyloric opening. Oesophageal varices may not be apparent soon after UGI bleed. In case of multiple lesions, endoscopy can pinpoint the lesion responsible for bleed due to collapse. In torrential bleeding, endoscopic visualisation is impossible. Upper GI endoscopy also provides information about the risk of rebleed in patients with peptic ulcer. Patients who are found to have major endoscopic stigmata of recent haemorrhage in peptic ulcer (i.e., active spurting haemorrhage, a visible vessel) have 50-80% chances of rebleed. Similarly, varices, which are large and have stigmata of recent bleed, are likely to rebleed.

Endoscopy provides diagnosis, prognosis and a chance of treatment in upper GI bleed.

5. *Angiography:* It is useful where endoscopic examination fails to reveal the bleeding lesion or the bleeding is severe enough to obscure the endoscopic visualisation. Selective mesenteric angiography usually localises the site of bleeding in about 75% of such cases.
6. *Upper GI barium study:* In acute upper GI bleed, barium studies are rather contraindicated as the barium may obscure the proper visualisation during subsequent endoscopy.
7. *Ultrasound of abdomen:* It can provide evidence of portal hypertension especially when the patient is unfit for endoscopy.

Management

1. *Immediate management and general measures*
   - *Intravenous access:* The first step is to gain intravenous access using at least two large-bore cannula.
   - *Restoration of airway and O_2 administration:* Blood and blood clots should be removed from the mouth cavity to have patent and clear airway. Administer oxygen by facemask, if necessary.
   - *Restoration of intravascular volume:* Intravenous fluids and blood may be administered to replace lost volume. Patients with shock and patients with haemoglobin less than 10.0g should receive blood transfusions to replace the intravascular volume. Always maintain two I.V. lines in patients with shock. Saline or Ringer's lactate solution should be infused to stabilise the vital signs. The haemoglobin should be kept above 8 g %. Periodic monitoring of PCV, haemoglobin and CVP (to avoid overtransfusion) is mandatory.
   - *Vasopressors* are generally avoided because shock is hypovolaemic, needs fluid/blood replacement as early as possible.
   - *Coagulopathy* is corrected by administration of platelets, fresh frozen plasma or whole blood and vitamin K.
   - *H_2 receptors antagonists* are used on empirical basis by physicians but have no proven value. Use of antacid is also not advised as it makes the endoscopic visualisation difficult.
   - *Monitoring:* Patients are monitored carefully for heart rate, BP, CVP and urine output.
2. **Specific therapy for underlying lesions**
   A. *Peptic ulcer:*
   i. *Therapeutic endoscopy:* Endoscopic haemostasis should be attempted as soon as patient is fit for endoscopy. It is safe and effective procedure, decreases the rate of rebleeding, duration of hospital stay, need for blood transfusions and also the mortality rates. The methods employed are:
      - Injection sclerotherapy (with epinephrine, absolute alcohol, poridocanol etc.).
      - Laser photocoagulation (it is costly, not affordable, is available in specialised centres).
      - Electrocoagulation.
      - Heater probe.
      - Use of hemoclips.

      The efficacy of all the methods is almost similar but injection sclerotherapy is commonly employed because it is safe, effective and economical.
   ii. *Surgery:* An urgent surgical operation is undertaken when:
      - Endoscopic haemostasis fails to stop active bleeding.
      - Rebleeding occurs on one occasion in an elderly or frail patient, or twice in younger patients.
      - Significant number of blood transfusions (> 5 units in 24 hours) are needed.

      The choice of operation depends on the site and diagnosis of bleeding lesion.
   iii. *Angiography and arterial embolisation:* Patients with massive haemorrhage, who are not fit for surgery or endoscopic therapy, can be considered for arterial angiography (selective catheterisation of the

bleeding artery) and then either a continuous infusion of vasopressin or arterial embolisation may be attempted.

B. **Oesophageal/gastric varices (portal hypertension):**
   i. *Endoscopic haemostasis:* The endoscopic measures used to control acute variceal bleeding include *sclerotherapy* and *banding*. Both sclerotherapy and variceal band ligation are effective in upto 90% of cases. In experienced hands, they are safe and effective. Sclerotherapy carries a higher risk of complications such as oesophageal ulceration, perforation and stricture; whereas variceal ligation is equally effective and has low rate of complications.
   ii. *Reduction of portal venous pressure by vasopressin, or somatostatin/octreotide:*
   - *Vasopressin* can be given as 20 units in 100 ml of 5% dextrose as I.V. infusion over a period of 10 minutes or may be given as continuous I.V. infusion. Though therapy lowers portal venous pressure but is highly risky and should not be used in patients of IHD, hypertension or other vascular diseases.
   - *Somatostatin/octreotide:* Intravenous use of somatostatin (250 µg as a bolus dose followed by an infusion of 250 µg/hour) or octreotide (50 µg as a bolus dose followed by I.V. infusion of 50 µg/hour) can be tried. The success rate of this therapy is comparable to endoscopic treatment. The treatment is safe with minimal side-effects.
   - Terlipressin is another alternative.
   iii. *Balloon tamponade (variceal decompression):* It is quite effective in controlling the bleeding from oesophageal or gastric varices. Several tubes are available (Sengstaken-Blakemore tube, Minnesota tube, Linton tube) for decompression. Use of balloon tamponade is associated with high risk of complications, some of which may be fatal, hence, this procedure should be reserved if therapeutic endoscopy and pharmacotherapy are not available immediately.
   iv. *Surgery:* It can be done if endoscopic and pharmacotherapy fail to stop the variceal bleeding. The success of surgery depends on the status of liver functions and the surgical expertise.
   v. *Transjugular intrahepatic portosystemic shunt (TIPS):* It has been used increasingly in the recent past for control of bleeding from the gastric/oesophageal varices not responding to other therapeutic procedures. A metal stent is placed between hepatic vein and the portal vein (portosystemic shunt) to reduce the portal vein pressure by decompressing the portal vein.

C. **Erosive gastritis (acute gastric erosion):** The steps of management include:
   i. Stop NSAIDs promptly if these are the cause.
   ii. Judicious use of antacids or I.V. proton pump inhibitor (pentaprazole I.V).
   iii. Treatment of associated stress and organ dysfunction.

D. **Mallory-Weiss tear:**
   i. Most patients stop bleeding spontaneously.
   ii. Endoscopic haemostasis (injection sclerotherapy) may be tried and has been found effective.

E. **Stress ulceration:** It is a frequent cause of GI bleeding in seriously ill patients admitted in ICU with head injuries, fulminant hepatic failure, multiple organ system failure, shock etc. Prophylactic therapy in such patients with I.V. H_2 antagonists, proton pump inhibitors (PPIs) or high doses of antacids orally or through ryle's tube are very effective in preventing stress ulceration and bleed.

F. **Angiodysplasias:** These lesions are frequently multiple and may be present in other parts of the body. Gastric mucosal bleeding in this condition is treated by endoscopic means as discussed earlier. Combined use of oestrogen and progestrone is also helpful in controlling the bleeding from these lesions.

Chapter 13

Lower Gastrointestinal Bleed

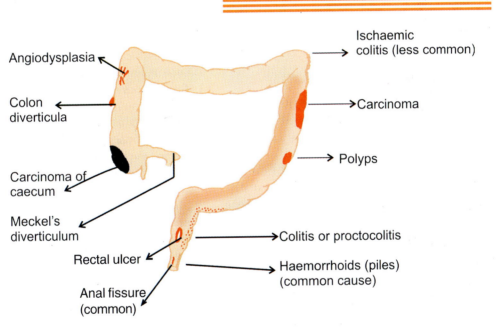

Fig. 13.1. Causes of lower GI bleed (diagrammatic representation)

LOWER GASTROINTESTINAL BLEED

Definition

Lower gastrointestinal bleeding is defined as bleed distal to ligament of *Treitz* or duodeno-jejunal flexure. It may present with fresh red blood in stool (hematochezia), maroon blood or occult blood. It must be remembered that melana (black tarry stool) is a sign of upper GI bleed, but rarely can occur in lower GI bleed such as bleeding lesion of right side of colon.

Causes

The causes of lower GI bleed are diagrammatically represented in the Fig 13.1 and summarised in the Box 13.1.

Gastroenterology

Box 13.1: Causes of lower GI bleeding

Severe acute	Moderate chronic/subacute
• Diverticular disease	• Anal disease (e.g. fissure, haemorrhoids)
• Ischaemic colitis	• Inflammatory bowel disease (e.g. crohn's disease, ulcerative colitis)
• Angiodysplasias or AV malformations	• Infections (e.g. bacillary dysentery, tuberculosis, HIV colopathy etc).
• Meckel's diverticulum	• Large polyps • Carcinoma • Angiodysplasia • Radiation enteritis, solitary rectal ulcer

Clinical Features

The clinical features depend on the site, type and severity of the bleeding from lower GI tract. The clinical features with their important causes are given in the table 13.1. The causes of acute, subacute and chronic lower GI bleed (see Box 13.1). Patients with profuse bleeding have underlying enteric or nonspecific ulcers, arteriovenous malformations (angiodysplasias) in elderly (> 55 years) or diverticular disease (erosion of an artery within mouth of a diverticulum) in the young. Ischaemic or inflammatory bowel disease or tumour results in subacute or chronic blood loss.

Investigation

1. ***Anoproctoscopy:*** It is done to detect underlying lesions (e.g. haemorrhoids, rectal ulcer or cancer, proctitis etc.).
2. ***Colonoscopy:*** It is the investigation of choice in all patients with lower GI bleeding unless massive bleeding precludes this procedure. It is done both for diagnostic (visual examination of the lesion, biopsy) and therapeutic purposes (an application of sclerotherapy/heater probe/ thermal ablation). Colonoscopy can detect many lesions that are often missed on barium enema studies. Colonoscopy also helps in localisation of the lesion (right or left colon) and to determine its possible aetiology (characteristic vascular spots in angiodysplasia).
3. ***Barium enema study:*** It is inferior than colonoscopy. Air contrast barium enema is performed to detect lesions such as benign tumour of the small intestine (an area which is beyond the reach of endoscope). Even presence of a lesion (e.g. diverticulum) on barium enema does not mean that it is actually responsible for bleeding. Barium studies should not be performed before colonoscopy as it will hinder in visual assessment on colonoscopy. Barium studies may be helpful in recurrent GI bleeding.
4. ***Angiography:*** Angiography is a tool in expert hands to localise the lesion. Angiography may also disclose lesions like angiodysplasia (vascular

Table 13.1: Clinical features with their possible causes in lower GI bleed

Features	*Possible cause(s)*
Bleeding occurring as drops or ooz at the end of defecation associated with constipation	Haemorrhoids (piles)
Bleeding per rectum with pain and tenesmus	Fissure, proctitis
Painless frequent bleeding occurring in a child	Polyposis, Meckel's diverticulum
Painful rectal bleeding with constipation	Diverticular disease
Blood mixed with mucus and diarrhoea	Inflammatory bowel disease
Bleed with a palpable abdominal lump, obstruction, weight loss, change in bowel habits, old age.	Malignancy colon
Perianal skin lesions,	Crohn's disease
Occult GI bleed (blood or blood products are present in the stool but cannot be seen) with anaemia	Colorectal cancer particularly carcinoma of right side of colon or of caecum

Box 13.2: Treatment of commonly encountered lesions in lower GI bleeding

Lesion	Treatment
Haemorrhoids/piles	Injection sclerotherpay/banding/laser photocoagulation
Polyp(s)	Polypectomy
Amoebic colitis	Metronidazole/tinidazole
Bacillary dysentery	Appropriate antibiotics
Typhoid ulcers	Ciprofloxacin or ceftriaxone; if conservative treatment fails, then surgery
Malignancy	Endoscopic hemostasis, surgery
Nonspecific/ulcerative colitis	Steroids/5-ASA enemas
Angiodysplasias	Laser/heater probe/surgery
Rectocolonic varices	Somatostatin/surgery

spots as reminiscent of spider naevi) and diverticulosis even when active bleeding has stopped. During this procedure, vasopressin can be given intraarterially. *Gelfoam* or *steel coils* can be injected into a bleeding vessel to stop the bleeding. This procedure is available only at specialised centres.

5. **Radionuclide scanning:** It is useful to detect lesions with low rates of bleeding but can be normal in upto 30% of cases with bleeding from colonic site. Tc^{99m} pertechnetate scans are useful to detect ectopic gastric epithelium in Meckel's diverticulum in children and adolescents. In the presence of massive GI bleed (an emergency), angiography is preferred over scan.

6. **Upper GI endoscopy:** It should be done if no lesion is found on investigations in lower GI bleed. About 5 to 10% of patients with bleeding per rectum may have a lesion found on upper GI endoscopy. It is advisable to perform upper GI endoscopy in each and every case of lower GI bleed to rule out upper GI lesion even when nasogastric aspirate is negative for blood.

Management

1. *General treatment:* The primary consideration in the case of bleeding patient is:
   - To maintain intravascular volume by fluids and blood transfusions.
   - Resuscitation of shock and to maintain haemodynamic stability. These measures have already been discussed in management of upper GI bleed.

2. *Specific treatment:* It depends on the cause (see Box 13.2). Specific treatment can be endoscopic (e.g. polypectomy, injection sclerotherapy, laser/thermal ablation), angiographic (arterial embolisation) or pharmacological (vasopressin, somatostatin in case of UGI bleed). Surgery is indicated for inaccessible lesions e.g. small bowel tumours or when source of bleeding remains unknown. In case of nonlocalisation of lesion with continued bleeding, hemicolectomy/colectomy may be performed as a life-saving measure.

Chapter 14

Acute Pancreatitis

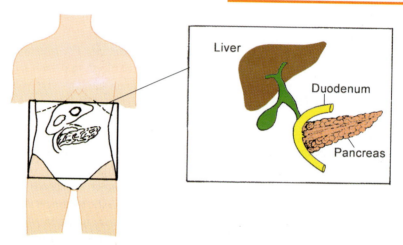

Fig. 14.1A: Structures in relation to pancreas, likely to be involved

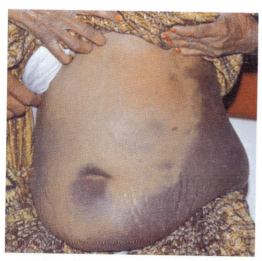

Fig. 14.1B: Acute pancreatitis. A patient of pancreatitis showing haemorrhagic manifestations e.g. brownish discolouration in periumbilical region (Cullen's sign) and in the flanks (Grey-Turner sign). Both the signs indicate acute necrotising haemorrhagic pancreatitis

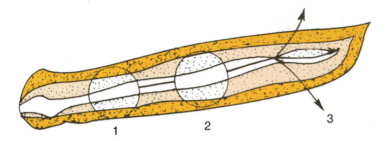

1. Initial insult
Zymogen activation
due to Ischaemia or
obstruction
2. Release of
activated enzymes,
vasoactive substances,
cytokines (IL-1, TNF-α)
3. Pancreatic/extrapancreatic
inflammation, ischaemia,
tissue damage

Fig. 14.2: Pathophysiology of pancreatitis

ACUTE PANCREATITIS

Definition

Acute pancreatitis is defined as an acute inflammation of the pancreas with variable involvement of regional tissues (Fig. 14.1) and remote organ system. It results from premature activation of zymogen granules which activate and release pancreatic enzymes (proteases), vasoactive substances and toxic material that digest the pancreas and the surrounding tissues leading to local and systemic complications.

Classification

The currently used terminology based on Atlanta system of classification is tabulated (Table 14.1).

Pathogenesis and Pathophysiology (Fig. 14.2)

The most accepted pathogenesis of pancreatitis is its autodigestion by its enzymes. It occurs as a result of:
1. Premature activation of zymogen granules.
2. Release of activated proteolytic enzymes e.g. proteases.
3. Autodigestion (inflammation) of the pancreas and surrounding tissue.

Table 14.1: Terminologies used in acute pancreatitis

1. *Severe acute pancreatitis:*
   Associated with multisystem organ failure (MSOF) and/or local complications such as necrosis, abscess or pseudocyst.
2. *Mild acute pancreatitis:*
   Uneventful recovery takes place within 3-5 days without organ dysfunction.
3. *Acute fluid collections:* Occurs in severe acute pancreatitis and detected on CT scan.
4. *Acute pseudocyst:* Collection of pancreatic juice and inflammatory exudate in lesser omentum enclosed by a wall of fibrous or granulation tissue.
5. *Pancreatic necrosis:*
   Widespread focal areas of non-viable parenchyma that may be infected or sterile.
6. *Pancreatic abscess:*
   Collection of pus within pancreas.
7. *Pancreatic ascites:*
   Exudative fluid in peritoneal cavity rich in amylase and lipase

The normal pancreas has only a poorly developed capsule, and adjacent structures including the common bile duct, duodenum, splenic vein and transverse colon are commonly involved in the inflammatory process (Fig. 14.1A). The severity of pancreatitis depends on the balance between

> **Box 14.1: Causes of acute pancreatitis**
>
> | Common (90%) | Uncommon/rare |
> |---|---|
> | • Gallstones | • Trauma |
> | • Alcohol abuse | • Hyperlipidaemia |
> | • Idiopathic | • Infections e.g. viral (mumps, coxsackie), bacterial (salmonella) fungal and parasitic (round worm) |
> | • Post-ERCP | • Drugs (azathioprine, thiazides, sodium valproate) |
> | • Post-surgical (abdominal/ extraabdominal) | • Perforating peptic ulcer |
> | | • End-stage renal disease |
> | | • Congenital anomaly (pancreas divisium) |
> | | • Pancreatic outflow obstruction. |
> | | • Severe hypothermia, shock, bites etc |
> | | • Organ transplantation (kidney, liver) |

proteolytic enzymes injury and anti-proteolytic defence.

Causes

The gall stones, alcohol, post-ERCP (endoscopic retrograde cholangiopancreatography) and idiopathic constitute 90% of cases of pancreatitis. Rest 10% are due to many other conditions given in the Box 14.1.

Clinical Features

Symptoms

1. Upper abdominal pain localised to the epigastrium, which is severe and commonly radiates to the back is the presenting symptom. Radiation of pain to the left upper quadrant or periumbilical region is also seen. Pain may be dull or boring in character and is deep-seated. The patient may feel relief of pain by sitting forward with bent-knees against the chest or lying on one side with knees flexed.
2. Associated nausea and vomiting.
3. Distention of abdomen.
4. Symptoms of other organ systems involvement e.g. dyspnoea, GI bleed.

Signs

1. In severe cases, the patient looks acutely ill, restless with low grade fever and tachycardia. Later, they become hypoxic, develop hypovolaemic shock and oliguria due to retroperitoneal sequetration of fluid.
2. *Abdominal signs* are absent initially, but develop gradually. These are:
   - Abdominal tenderness, guarding and rigidity due to peritoneal involvement.
   - Abdominal distension and absent bowel sounds due to development of paralytic ileus.
   - Mild jaundice may be seen. This is due to compression of intrapancreatic portion of common bile duct by inflammatory exudate.
   - *Grey-Turner's sign* (brown discolouration of the flanks-Fig. 14.1B) may be seen in acute haemorrhagic pancreatitis.
   - *Cullen's sign* (bluish-brown discolouration of the periumbilical region Fig. 14.1B) is also seen in haemorrhagic pancreatitis due to blood dissecting along the tissue planes giving this discolouration.
3. *Chest signs:* Chest examination may reveal pleural effusion, commonly on the left, is usually small, haemorrhagic and has high amylase content. Sometimes, there may be pneumonitis or development of ARDS (hypoxic respiratory failure).
4. *A palpable mass* two or more weeks after the onset may represent inflammatory mass/ necrosis or pseudocyst. Ascites may be present if pancreatitis is complicated.

Diagnosis

Diagnosis initially rests on the clinical picture. Acute pancreatitis should be suspected in any patient with severe upper abdominal pain or unexplained hypovolaemic shock. Ultimately, diagnosis is made on the basis of symptoms, signs, compatible biochemical and radiological investigations and exclusion of the other causes.

Investigations

i. **Serum enzyme levels:** A number of enzymes i.e. amylase, lipase, elastase, phospholipase A etc. are released into circulation during acute pancreatitis, hence, their estimation form an important diagnostic clue.

Serum *amylase* is elevated in 75% of cases, starts rising within few hours and persists for 3 to 5 days. It is not specific for pancreatitis because many extra-pancreatic conditions (e.g. perforated bowel, intestinal obstruction, mesenteric infarction, peritonitis, acute appendicitis, renal failure, diabetic keto acidosis, salpingitis, diagnostic and therapeutic GI tract procedures etc.) can raise it 2 to 3 times than normal. Therefore, higher levels more than 3 times than normal are suggestive of pancreatitis in a patient with upper abdominal pain. Persistence of high levels beyond first week indicates presence of extensive necrosis or pseudocyst formation. Separation of serum amylase into pancreatic and salivary fractions is more diagnostic than total amylase.

Serum lipase levels are raised by two to three times than normal in about 80% cases of acute pancreatitis. Its elevation is more specific than serum amylase. Its estimation is helpful in conditions where hyperamylasemia is due to non-pancreatic causes. Therefore, combined measurement of serum amylase and lipase increases the sensitivity as well as specificity to about 90% in acute pancreatitis.

> *An elevated serum amylase or lipase at least 3 times than normal in a patient with recent onset of upper abdominal pain with or without shock is diagnostic of acute pancreatitis.*

ii. **Inflammatory markers:** Certain inflammatory markers such as IL-6 released by macrophages increase during acute pancreatitis. C-reactive protein also increases, indicates an acute inflammatory response, is not specific for pancreatitis. However these markers have prognostic rather than diagnostic value in follow-up of cases.

iii. **Blood tests:** There may be leucocytosis (10,000-20,000 cells/mm^3) and hematocrit may be high.

iv. **Liver function tests:** Raised serum bilirubin, alkaline phosphatase and aminotransferases may occur.

v. **Serum calcium:** Hypocalcaemia may be seen in 25% of cases of severe pancreatitis. It results from sequestration of Ca^{++} in saponification of fats, increased glucagon and calcitonin levels. It is associated with bad prognosis.

vi. **Blood sugar:** There may hyperglycaemia.

vii. **Methemoglobinemia** may be seen in haemorrhagic pancreatitis due to entry of haematin into the circulation.

Radiological Studies

The radiological findings which may be seen on plain X-ray abdomen and X-ray chest are given in the Box 14.2.

X-ray abdomen is also useful to rule out other causes of acute abdominal pain such as ruptured viscus and bowel infarction.

Imaging Studies

i. **Abdominal ultrasound:** It is very useful in diagnosis and management of acute pancreatitis and its local complications. It is useful in detection of gall stones, helps in identification of pseudocyst and ascites. In the early stage, it may show the swollen gland with periglandular fluid collections.

ii. **CT scan/MRI scan:** CT scan shows swollen, oedematous gland with obliteration of peripancreatic fat. Inflammation and necrosis of surrounding organs may also be seen. MRI has no added advantages over CT scan, to be

Gastroenterology

> **Box 14.2: Radiological findings in acute pancreatitis**
>
> **Plain X-ray abdomen**
> - Ill defined tissue planes, dilated bowel loops and hazy renal and psoas shadows.
> - Isolated small bowel dilated loops near the pancreas due to isolated ileus *(sentinal loop)*
> - *Colon cut-off sign:* It is a nonspecific finding. There is spasm in the transverse colon with absence of colonic gas beyond it.
> - Hazziness due to ascites
> - Extraluminal gas bubbles indicating pancreatic abscess
>
> **X-ray chest (PA view)**
> - Raised domes of diaphragm
> - Pleural effusion (left)
> - Atelectasis
> - Pneumonitis
> - Cardiomegaly or CHF
> - Interstitial fluffy shadows

done if CT scan cannot be done. A contrast enhanced CT scan provides valuable information or the estimation of the presence and extent of pancreatic necrosis.

iii. **Barium studies:** These have been largely replaced by ultrasonography and CT scan. However, if done, may show widened 'C' loop of the duodenum, swollen mucosal folds and lobulated filling defect due to swollen papilla.

Complications

They are given the Table 14.1 with there pathogenesis.

Management

There is no specific therapy which can arrest or interrupt the process of autodigestion, hence, the treatment is mainly supportive and symptomatic.

Steps of Treatment

- To establish the diagnosis and to assess its severity.
- Early institution of treatment whether disease is mild or severe.
- Resuscitation of shock or maintenance of intravascular volume.
- Relief of pain.
- Detection and treatment of complications.
- Nutritional support and rest to the gland.
- Treatment of underlying cause, if found, specifically gallstones.

A. **Mild pancreatitis:** Mild pancreatitis is treated by:
  i. *Relief of pain* by meperidine hydrochloride I.M. or I.V. Morphine is not preferred as it may cause spasm of *sphincter of oddi* and may exacerbate the disease.
  ii. *Fluid replacement:* The fluid deficit must be corrected immediately so as to correct hypotension. The fluid therapy must be monitored by pulse, BP, skin turgor and urine output.
  iii. *Rest to the gland:* Patient is kept on nil orally. A nasogastric aspiration should be done to keep the stomach empty in an attempt to prevent gastric acid from entering into the duodenum and stimulating the pancreatic secretions.
  There is no use of administering H_2 receptors antagonists or proton pump inhibitor in order to reduce pancreatic secretions.
  iv. *Antibiotics:* Prophylactic use of antibiotics in mild pancreatitis is not recommended.
  v. *Nutrition:* Current evidence indicates that intrajejunal tube feeding is idcal than total parenteral nutrition (TPN) since it bypasses the duodenum avoiding the stimulation of pancreas and provides adequate nutrition.

Acute Pancreatitis

Table 14.1: Complications of acute pancreatitis

I. Local
- Pancreatic necrosis
- Pancreatic fluid collection e.g. abscess, pseudocyst
- Pancreatic ascites
- Involvement of adjoining organs and vessels.
- Obstructive jaundice

II. Systemic
- *Pulmonary*
  Pleural effusion
  Atelectasis
  Mediastinal abscess
  Pneumonitis
  ARDS
- *Renal*
  Oliguria
  Azotemia
  ATN (acute tubular necrosis)
  Renal artery/vein thrombosis
- *Cardiovascular*
  Hypotension
  Sudden death
  Non specific ST-T Changes
  Pericardial effusion
- *Haematological*
  Disseminated
  Intravascular coagulation
- *GI haemorrhage*
  Peptic ulcer disease
  Hemorrhagic pancreatic necrosis portal vein thrombosis
- *Metabolic*
  Hyperglycemia
  Hpertriglyceridemia
  Hypocalcemia
  Encephalopathy
  Purtscher's retinopathy
- *CNS*—Psychosis, fat emboli.

Nasojejunal tube is double lumen tube, provides simultaneous gastric aspiration and jejunal feeding. Enteral feeding is less expensive and avoids complications of parenteral feeding.

B. *Severe pancreatitis:* Patients with severe pancreatitis are best managed in ICU. Management include:
1. *Relief of pain* by analgesic.
2. *Nasogastric aspiration* to keep the stomach empty and to provide rest to the gland.
3. *Parenteral nutrition:* After 3-4 days of I.V. fluids, if pain continues, there are a number of options to provide continuous nutrition including total parenteral nutrition with intralipids. Lipid infusion does not stimulate pancreatic secretions but it can produce hyperlipidaemia that can trigger further pancreatitis. As soon as pain is relieved, enteral feeding may be started with a low fat diet.
4. *Antibiotics:* Antibiotic therapy is indicated in severe pancreatitis with or without complications. Antibiotics having good diffusion capacity into pancreas (e.g. imipenem, ofloxacin, metronidazole, and mezlocillin) may be started in severe pancreatitis. Those with necrotising pancreatitis should preferably receive imipenem 500 mg I.V. every 12 hourly for 2 weeks.
5. *Resuscitation of shock* by I.V. fluids and pressor agents like dopamine.
6. *Severe hypocalcaemia* is corrected by giving 10 ml of calcium gluconate I.V. slowly.
7. *Patient with ARDS or respiratory distress* require O_2 therapy and respiratory support.
8. *Renal failure* is treated on the same lines as acute renal failure (Read acute renal failure).
9. Patients who present with cholangitis or jaundice in association with acute severe pancreatitis should undergo urgent ERCP to diagnose and treat gallstones. Otherwise, ERCP has to be done once acute phase is over.

Management of Complications

Patients who have developed *necrotising pancreatitis* or *pancreatic abscess* require urgent surgical debridement of the pancreas, followed by drainage of the pancreatic bed.

Pancreatic pseudocysts are treated by drainage into the stomach or duodenum. This is usually done after at least 6 weeks, once a pseudocapsule is formed, using open surgery or endoscopic method.

Pancreatic abscess is treated by antibiotics and fine needle aspiration. Surgical drainage is

Box 14.3: Bad prognostic indicators in acute pancreatitis

Ranson's criteria	Glasgow criteria
1. At admission	• Age > 55 years
• Age > 55 years	• PO_2 < 8 kPa
• TLC > 16000/mm^3	• WBC > 15 × 10^9/L
• Blood sugar > 200 mg %	• Albumin < 32 g/L (3.2g%)
• LDH > 350 IU/L	• Serum calcium < 2 mmol/L (corrected)
• Base deficit > 4 mEq/L	
• Fluid sequestration > 6L	
2. Initial 48 hours	• Glucose > 10 mmol/L
• Haematocrit decrease by > 10%	• Urea > 16 mmol/L (after rehydration)
• BUN increase by > 5 mg%	• ALT > 200 U/L
• Serum calcium < 8 mg%	• LDH > 800 U/L
• PaO2 < 60 mmHg	
• AST > 250 U/L	

required when percutaneous drainage of pus is not helpful.

Pancreatic ascites is exudative (protein > 2.5 g/L) and has high serum amylase levels (> 1000 U/dl). Medical treatment include nasogastric aspiration, total parenteral nutrition and octreotide therapy. As it occurs due to leakage from the cyst or duct, hence, surgery may be needed to correct this leakage.

Prognosis

Despite recent advances in management, the mortality remains unchanged (10-15%) in acute pancreatitis. The adverse prognostic factors (Ranson's criteria and Glasgow criteria) are given in the Box 14.3. Contrast-enhanced CT provides valuable information on the grade and severity of pancreatic necrosis which influence the prognosis of patients with pancreatitis (Box. 14.4).

Three or more risk factors imply severe disease, worsen the prognosis in both the criteria, hence these patients should be treated in ICU.

Box 14.4: CECT severity index (scoring system) in acute pancreatitis

Finding	Points
A. Degree of pancreatic necrosis	
• No necrosis	0
• Necrosis of 1/3rd of pancreas	2
• Necrosis of ½ (one half) of pancreas	4
• Necrosis more than one-half of pancreas	6
B. Grade of acute pancreatitis	
• Normal pancreas	0
• Pancreatic enlargement alone	1
• Inflammation of pancreas and peripancreatic fat	2
• One peripancreatic fluid collection	3
• Two or more fluid collections	4

Severity index = CT grade + necrosis score (0-10)

Note:
1. Complications and mortality rates are negligible when severity index is 1 or 2; and low when score is 3 to 6.
2. High morbidity (92%) and significant mortality (17%) is reported when the severity score is >7.

Chapter 15

Amoebic Liver Abscess

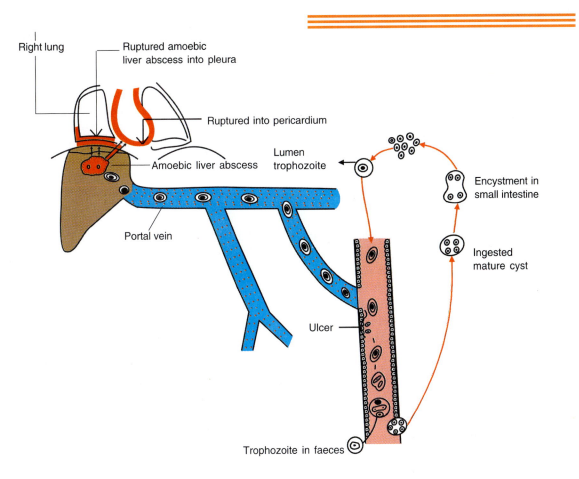

Fig. 15.1: Amoebic liver abscess-pathogenesis and its rupture into pleural space

AMOEBIC LIVER ABSCESS

Definition

Amoebic liver abscess is an inflammatory space occupying lesion of the liver caused by *Entamoeba histolytica*. It is the most common form of liver abscess encountered in clinical practice as an emergency. It is endemic in India, and is the most common presentation of extraintestinal invasive amoebiasis.

Pathogenesis

Liver abscess is always preceded by amoebic intestinal involvement which may be symptomatic or asymptomatic. Trophozoites invade the veins in the intestine by lysis of the wall and reach the liver through portal circulation (Fig. 15.1). Pathogenic strains are resistant to complement-mediated lysis—a property which makes them survive in the blood stream. In contrast, *nonpathogenic* strains are rapidly lysed by complement and are thus restricted to the bowel lumen. The active trophozoites in the liver incite inflammatory reaction consisting predominantly of neutrophils. Later, the neutrophils are lysed by contact with amoebae and release of neutrophil toxin that may contribute to necrosis of hepatocytes. The liver parenchyma is replaced by necrotic material that is surrounded by a thin margin of congested liver tissue i.e. there is formation of liver abscess demarcated by inflamed congested liver tissue. The oozing of blood from the vessel into necrotic tissue makes the liver abscess—a classical anchovy paste—called *anchovy sauce like pus* but the colour of fluid is variable with treatment and is composed of bacteriologically sterile granular debris with few or no pus cells. Trophozoites, if seen, tend to be found only near the walls of the abscess.

Clinical Features

Of traveller's who develop amoebic liver abscess after leaving an endemic area, 95% do so within 4-5 months. Young patients with abscess are more likely to present in the acute phase with prominent symptoms of less than 10 days duration. The presenting symptom is fever with right upper quadrantic pain which may be dull or pleuritic in nature and radiates to shoulders. Point tenderness over the liver and left sided pleural effusion (sympathetic effusion) are common. Although the parasites reach the liver from the intestine, concomitant diarrhoea is common. In older patients, unexplained weight loss without fever or pain may be seen as a presenting complaint.

Hepatomegaly with intercostal tenderness (thumping sign) is a characteristic finding but may be absent in deep or centrally located lesion. Jaundice is not a common finding but a large abscess can cause compression of bile ducts and produce obstructive jaundice at a later stage.

Persistent or increase in local signs of inflammation on the skin suggest impending rupture. Complications occur due to rupture of the abscess into subdiaphragmatic, pleural, pericardial, intraperitoneal or intrabiliary space. Compression of inferior vena cava (IVC) or hepatic veins may cause an outflow obstruction (Budd-Chiari syndrome).

Fever, tender hepatomegaly with intercostal tenderness of less than 10 days duration in a young person suggest an amoebic liver abscess.

Since 10-15% of patients present only with fever, therefore, amoebic liver abscess should be considered in the differential diagnosis of PUO (pyrexia of unknown origin).

Diagnosis

The diagnosis of amoebic liver abscess is made on history of fever, right hypochondrial pain with tender hepatomegaly. It is confirmed on ultrasound and other tests.

Investigations

1. **Stool examination** for trophozoites is usually negative.
2. **WBC count** may show leucocytosis (> 10,000 cells/mm^3). There may be anaemia.

Amoebic Liver Abscess

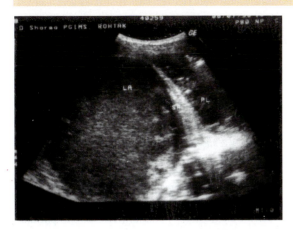

Fig. 15.2: Amoebic liver abscess-USG of liver showing a large abscess (LA) in right lobe of the liver (12 × 8 cm)

3. *Ultrasonography of liver:* It is useful non-invasive test to identify an abscess as a hypoechoic cyst or cavity with irregular shaggy walls. The abscess is more common in right than left lobe on its posterosuperior surface (Fig. 15.2). Multiple abscesses are likely to be pyogenic. Satellite lesions (microabscesses) may be present around the main lesion. However, multiple lesions spread all over the liver in amoebic liver abscess should make one to suspect an immunocompromised state which should be investigated. The USG findings change with the duration of the illness from a solid lesion, abscess-in-evolution to abscess formation. It is made clear that size usually increases with treatment and does not warrant aspiration unless associated with a no response to treatment or impending rupture.
4. *CT scan/MRI.* These investigations do not have any advantage over USG which is gold standard for diagnosis of an amoebic liver abscess.
5. *Serological tests:* Indirect haemagglutination (IHA) and ELISA tests for amoebiasis have been the most extensively employed confirmatory tests. Low titres are not diagnostic of recent infection. Titres > 1:1024 are diagnostic of amoebic liver abscess. A negative IHA rules out amoebic liver abscess and should warrant further investigations to look for other aetiologies like pyogenic abscess, primary or secondary heptocellular carcinoma or an infected cyst.
6. When diagnosis is uncertain and there is high possibility of the abscess to be pyogenic, *a diagnostic aspiration* may be done. Demonstration of trophozoites in the aspirated fluid is not easy and their absence does not help in the differentiation of amoebic from pyogenic abscess. Aspiration for gram-staining and culture will help when diagnosis is in doubt.
7. *Other routine tests* such as liver function tests are normal. However with large liver abscess, the alkaline phosphatase, bilirubin and aminotransferases may be elevated slightly.
8. *Fluoroscopy* may show limitation of movement of right dome of the diaphragm.
9. *X-ray chest (PA views):* It is done to detect the complications such as pleural or pericardial effusion. Right dome of the diaphragm may be raised in amoebic liver abscess.

Treatment

1. *Relief of pain and fever* with analgesics.
2. *Drug treatment:* Single drug therapy with *metronidazole* (800 mg tid or 40 mg/kg/day) is treatment of choice for amoebic liver abscess. *Tinidazole, secnidazole* and *ornidazole* are other nitromidazoles derivatives found to be effective in amoebic liver abscess. The second line therapeutic drugs i.e., emetine and chloroquine should be avoided because of cardiovascular and GI side-effects of the former and high relapse rates with the latter. These drugs should be reserved for nonresponders. South African studies done on liver abscesses have recommended an addition of luminal agent (diloxanide furoate) to metronidazole to eradicate cysts and prevent further transmission even if there is no evidence or past history of invasive amoebiasis.

Response to anti-amoebic therapy is seen usually within 48-72 hours with prompt resolution of fever, pain, toxaemia, tender hepatomegaly; and therapy must be continued for 10 days. Relapses

78 Gastroenterology

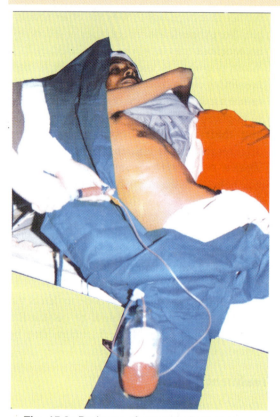

Fig. 15.3: Drainage of amoebic liver abscess

> **Box 15.1: Indications for aspiration of amoebic liver abscess**
> - No response to medical treatment
> - Impending rupture. Thin rim (< 1 cm) between abscess wall and liver capsule on USG
> - Abscess in the left lobe of the liver
> - Abscess size > 10 cm
> - When distinction between pyogenic and amoebic liver abscess is uncertain

after adequate therapy are uncommon when a luminicidal agent has been added. Routine administration of antibiotics is not indicated as superadded bacterial infection is not common.

3. *Aspiration of the abscess (Fig. 15.3):* Routine aspiration of the abscess is not indicated because it has been shown clearly that aspiration does not change the course of the disease as compared to medical therapy alone. Most of the patients responds to medical therapy. Aspiration is indicated in certain situations given in the Box 15.1. Its distinction from pyogenic abscess is not easy. Patients with pyogenic liver abscess typically are older and have history of underlying bowel disease or recent surgery. There will be symptoms and sign of toxaemia. In pyogenic abscess sometimes, repeated aspiration of the amoebic liver abscess may lead to its conversion into pyogenic abscess, hence, repeated aspirations are to be avoided. Serial ultrasonographic follow up should be done to detect resolution of the abscess, which takes 3-6 months.

4. *Catheter drainage*: Along with medical therapy, aspiration with catheter may be required to treat abscess with complications (e.g. rupture).

5. *Surgical exploration* may become necessary in certain situations like bowel perforation or rupture into the pericardium.

Chapter 16

Hepatic Encephalopathy

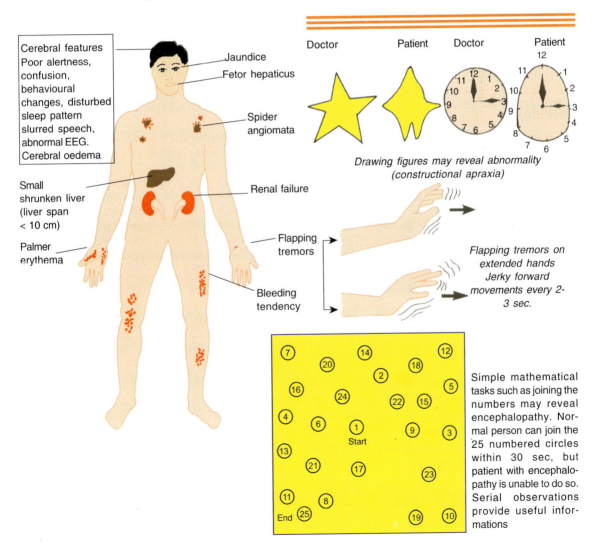

Fig. 16.1: Clinical spectrum of acute hepatic encephalopathy

Gastroenterology

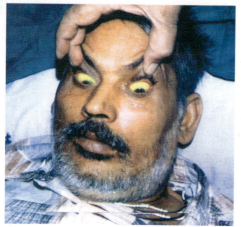

Fig. 16.2: A patient of hepatic coma. There was severe jaundice and unconsciousness

ACUTE HEPATIC ENCEPHALOPATHY

Definition

Acute hepatic encephalopathy is a clinical syndrome of neuropsychiatric manifestations developing within a period of 8 weeks in a patient with acute fulminant hepatitis as a result of massive acute hepatocellular necrosis without any evidence of previous liver disease. This is due to entry of nitrogenous products in the circulation and the brain. These nitrogenous products normally originate in the intestine and are inactivated and metabolised in the liver. In hepatic failure, they bypass the diseased liver and reach the CNS through circulation leading to encephalopathy.

Causes

It is primarily seen in hepatitis B and D, as well as in E but is rare in hepatitis A and C. Hepatitis B accounts for more than 50% of cases; one third of which are associated with Hepatitis D virus (HDV) infection. It is a life-threatening syndrome. The causes are given in the Box 16.1.

Clinical Features (Fig. 16.1)

It consists of features of:
  i. Encephalopathy (cerebral features).
  ii. Liver cell failure.

1. *Cerebral features:* These include poor alertness, disturbed concentration, behavioural changes, drowsiness, confusion, disorientation, disturbed sleep pattern, slurred speech, convulsions and coma. These cerebral features are divided into 4 grades depending on severity of liver disease (see Box 16.2).
2. *Features of acute hepatocellular failure:* These include:
   - *Jaundice:* It is moderate to severe. Bilirubin > 20 mg% carries poor prognosis.
   - *Fetor hepaticus:* It is an ammonical smell in patients's breath due to excretion of methylmercaptans.

Box. 16.1: Causes of acute hepatic encephalopathy

1. **Infection:** Viral hepatitis (B and D), yellow fever leptospirosis.
2. **Hepatotoxic drugs:** e.g. anaesthetics (halothane), NSAIDs, acetaminophen overdose, antitubercular drugs.
3. **Vascular:** Hepatic vein thrombosis (*Budd-chiari syndrome*), veno-occlusive disease.
4. **Poisons:** e.g. carbon tetrachloride, poisonous fungi (*amanita phalloides*), phosphorous.
5. **Miscellanous:** Wilson's disease, Reye's syndrome, fatty liver of pregnancy, autoimmune hepatitis etc.

Box. 16.2: Clinical features of acute hepatic encephalopathy

Stage	Cerebral features	Asterixis (tremors)	EEG
I	Confusion, mood changes, slurred speech, disordered sleep	+/–	Tri phasic slow waves
II	Lethargy, drowsy but arousable, confusion, behavioural disturbances	+	–do–
III	Marked confusion, incoherent speech, sleepy but arousable	+	–do–
IV	Coma, initially responsive to noxious stimuli, later non-responsive	–	Delta waves

(+) means present (–) means absent

- *Flapping tremors:* A flap on extended hands is visible in grade II and III coma but is lost in grade IV coma.
- *Bleeding diathesis:* In some patients, purpura or severe gastrointestinal bleeding may occur due to lowered coagulation factors. Bleeding can occur from any site, may be evident in the form of epistaxis, black coloured gastric aspirate, purpura, ecchymosis or from a punctured site.
- *Liver dullness:* The liver span is reduced to < 10 cm (normal > 14 cm) due to shrinkage.
- *Neurological manifestations* e.g. hypertonia, decerebration may develop but are less common. Cerebral oedema and brainstem compression are terminal event.

Note: Patient may develop **acute on chronic hepatic encephalopathy** in patient with pre-existing liver disease such as cirrhosis. In such cases, features of chronic liver disease (clubbing, white nails, spider naevi, palmer erythema, gynaecomastia testicular atrophy, parotid enlargement and symptoms and signs of portal hypertension) will be present.

> Tip: Recent onset of encephalopathic features in a patient of hepatitis (within 8 weeks of onset) with small strunken liver on clinical examination (reduced liver span) as well as on USG suggest acute hepatic encephalopathy in a young person without any evidence of pre-existing liver disease.

Investigations

1. *Complete haemogram* may reveal anaemia and leucocytosis.
2. *Serum bilirubin* is raised. Both conjugated and unconjugated fractions are increased. Serum bilirubin > 30 mg% is a bad prognostic sign.
3. *Serum transaminases:* They are raised initially, may fall progressively with progression of the disease, hence, fall of SGOT/SGPT in acute hepatic coma is not a healthy sign but constitutes a bad prognostic parameter. The alkaline phosphatase levels are normal.
4. *Virological studies:* This includes estimation of IgM anti-HBc, IgM anti-HAV, anti HEV, HCV, CMV, herpes simplex and EBV.
5. *Serology:* Serum autoantibodies, ANA, anti-mitochondrial antibodies must be assessed.
6. *Serum albumin* level is usually normal to low.
7. *Coagulation profile*: Prothrombin time (PT) and PTT are prolonged in severe form of the disease. PT > 50 sec is also a bad prognostic sign in acute hepatic coma.
8. *EEG:* It is done to grade the hepatic coma. A characteristic symmetric high voltage triphasic slow waves pattern (2-5/sec) on ECG seen in grade 1 to 3 while delta wave activity appears in grade IV coma.
9. *Serum ammonia* levels are high.
10. *Ultrasonography (USG)* of the liver shows reduced liver size (usually < 10 cm) with normal echotexture.
11. Toxicology screen of blood and urine. Ceruloplasmin, serum and urinary copper may be done.

Management

Patient should be treated in intensive care unit under the direct supervision of specialists. Early diagnosis and early institution of therapy is essential to prevent its further progression.

Steps of Treatment

General measures:
- Patient should be isolated.
- Barrier nursing care.
- All medical personnel and attendants looking after the patient must be vaccinated against hepatitis B.
- A large bore central venous line should be put in for fluids, CVP measurements, drug administration and sample collection.

- A nasogastric tube and condom urinary drainage or catheter are also put. Maintain intake and output chart. Measure urine output.
- Monitor pulse, BP, temperature, respiration, size of pupils, ocular fundus, plantar response and grade of coma. Liver size on percussion or ultrasound be monitored periodically.
- Check the blood counts, urine, LFT, coagulation profile, blood urea, creatinine, arterial blood gases, electrolytes and blood sugar almost every day/alternate day.
- The cause of acute hepatic encephalopathy if known should be treated simultaneously. Infections surveillance by culture of blood, urine, cannulasites, sputum, chest X-ray and TLC and DLC must be done.

Specific measures:

1. *Sedation:* No sedation is to be given until the patient is violent or irritable. However, if necessary, a small dose of phenobarbitone or 5 mg I.V. diazepam may be given. Phenothiazines being hepatotoxic should not be used either as an antiemetic or as a sedative.
2. *Nutrition:* Withdraw oral protein intake from all sources. Hypoglycaemia is an important cause of death, hence, 10-20% glucose drip is given continuously with potassium supplements. In early stages of coma, glucose can be given through nasogastric tube. Blood glucose is to be monitored frequently with a glucometer and should be kept above 100 mg%. Oral feeds including proteins are to be substituted once the patient starts recovering.
3. *Sterilisation of the gut and its emptying:*
   - Sterlisation of gut by neomycin 1 gm through nasogastric tube after every 6 hours. To avoid nephrotoxicity, one can use metronidazole or broad spectrum antibiotic.
   - Increase the nitrogen content of stool by changing the bacterial flora with lactulose (30-60 ml through nasogastric tube after every 2-3 hours) till one or two loose stools are passed. Lactilol 30 g powder per day is also effective.
   - Repeated bowel/colonic wash to evacuate the bowel (colon) off its contents so as to reduce the ammonia formation from breakdown of proteins by coliform bacteria.
4. *Treatment of infection:* Sputum, urine, intravenous catheter tip/site and blood culture should be obtained periodically. Antibiotic should be given at the evidence of infection. Prophylactic antibiotics have no role. Non hepatotoxic antibiotics (amoxycillin, gentamicin, third generation cephalosporin) and metronidazole may be used.
5. *Treatment of bleeding:* Patients may develop mucocutaneous bleeding, GI bleed or frank DIC. Often the haemorrhage is fatal. Bleeding is treated with fresh blood/packed RBCs infusion, fresh frozen plasma and vit K intravenously. Intravenous H_2 blockers (ranitidine) or proton pump inhibitors can be given through nasogastric tube. Prothrombin time, BT, CT and platelet count are done daily. Active suction through nasogastric tube should be avoided as it can produce gastric erosions.
6. *Treatment of renal failure:* Progressive azotaemia is a dangerous situation in acute hepatic encephalopathy, can be worsened by haemorrhage and sepsis. It should be corrected by volume repletion and monitored by CVP. Nitrogenous matter is removed by gastric lavage. Renal failure is managed by low dose dopamine, hemodialysis or continuous arterio-venous haemofiltration (CAVH) or continuous venovenous haemofiltration. The only satisfactory treatment is liver transplantation.
7. *Cerebral oedema:* It is the most important cause of death. The diagnostic clues to cerebral oedema include; poorly reacting pupils, fluctuating BP, hypertonia and decerebrate posture. It is treated by rapid infusion of mannitol (20%) at a dose of 100 ml and can be repeated after 4-6 hours if patient passes adequate amount of

urine. In the absence of diuresis, mannitol can produce hyponatraemia and water retention.
8. *Liver transplantation:* If available, is the treatment of choice in patients with grade III-IV coma.
9. *Other recent therapies:* Acetyl-cysteine in paracetamol overdoses and role of prostaglandin E1 intravenously; penicillin and silymarin infusion for amanita (mushroom) poisoning, appear to be effective. Flumazenil-a benzodiazepine antagonist may have a role in hepatic encephalopahty precipitated by use of benzodiazepine (diazepam, lorazepam).

Complications of Acute Hepatic Failure

- Hypoglycaemia, hypokalemia, hypocalcaemia, hypomagnesaemia metabolic acidosis.
- Cerebral oedema.
- Hypothermia.
- Hypotension.
- Respiratory failure.
- Pancreatitis.
- Progressive azotemia (renal failure).
- Bleeding tendencies.
- Sepsis.

ACUTE ON CHRONIC HEPATIC ENCEPHALOPATHY

Definition

This is a syndrome of mental and neurological features that occur acutely in patients with long-standing cirrhosis with or without portal hypertension. It is intermittent and reversible in nature if treated early and properly. Rarely irreversible CNS changes occur producing paraplegia, parkinsonism and epileptic fits.

Precipitating Factors

Chronic hepatic disease i.e. cirrhosis due to any cause is the underlying cause of chronic hepatic encephalopathy which is precipitated acutely by certain precipitating factors i.e.:

1. High protein diet.
2. Infections.
3. Trauma.
4. Surgery (portosystemic shunts)
5. GI bleed.
6. Hypokalaemia.
7. Constipation.
8. Rapid removal of ascitic fluid.
9. Uraemia (spontaneous or diuretic-induced).
10. Drugs e.g. sedative, hypnotics, antidepressants.

Clinical Features

Apart from encephalopathy, clinical features include stigmata of cirrhosis and liver cell failure.
1. Feature of encephalopathy—read acute hepatic encephalopathy.
2. Stigmata of cirrhosis of liver and liver cell failure These include:
   - *Mild to moderate jaundice* due to hepatic decompensation.
   - *Ascites* It is due to combined effect of portal hypertension and liver cell failure.
   - *Circulatory changes* e.g. palmar erythema, spider angiomata, cyanosis (AV shunting in the lungs).
   - *Endocrinial changes* e.g. loss of axillary and pubic hair, loss of libido.
     - *Men:* Gynaecomastia, impotence, testicular atrophy.
     - *Women:* Menstrual irregularity, ammenorrhoea, breast atrophy.
   - *Haematological* e.g. anaemia, pancytopenia (hypersplenism), bruises, purpura, menorrhagia.
   - *Symptoms and sign of portal hypertension* e.g. caput medusae (collaterals around the umbilicus), variceal bleed (hemetemesis) and fetor hepaticus.
   - *Others* e.g. pigmentation and Dupuytren's contractures, clubbing of fingers, white nails etc.

Investigations

They have been discussed in acute hepatic encephalopathy. In addition, the following investigations may be done:

1. *Ascitic fluid examination for biochemistry and cytology*. The fluid is transudate in cirrhosis of the liver with encephalopahty. An ascitic fluid with total leucocyte count > 500 cells/mm^3 or > 250 polymorphonuclear leucocytes suggests spontaneous bacterial peritonitis which is treated with antibiotics (amoxycillin and gentamicin or cefotaxime).
2. *USG of liver* will show evidence of chronic liver disease (disturbed shape, size and echotexture), presence of ascites, splenomegaly, increased portal vein diameter (> 14 mm).

Treatment

It is same as discussed under the heading of acute hepatic encephalopathy. In addition to it, the management include:

1. Treatment of ascites by salt restriction and diuretics (potassium sparing or a combination of loop diuretic with potassium sparing). Hypokalaemia must be avoided. Ascites should not be tapped routinely except for diagnostic purpose. If ascites is tense and causing respiratory embarrassment, then it should be tapped keeping in mind that sudden withdrawal of large amount of fluid can precipitate coma. Ascitic fluid can be shunted by a *Leveen shunt* to the central veins in patients, who fail to respond to medical treatment.
2. Treatment of complications, if and when develop.
3. Once the acute phase is over and patient has regained consciousness, then chronic encephalopathy can be managed on out-patient basis with dietary protein restrictions (< 60 g/day) in combination with low doses of lactulose or neomycin.

Complications

- Severe GI bleed (fatal bleeding).
- Hepatorenal syndrome. It is rare in acute hepatic encephalopathy. It occurs in chronic or acute on chronic hepatic encephalopathy.
- Fulminant septicaemia
- Spontaneous bacterial peritonitis.
- Cerebral oedema.

Chapter 17

Biliary Colic

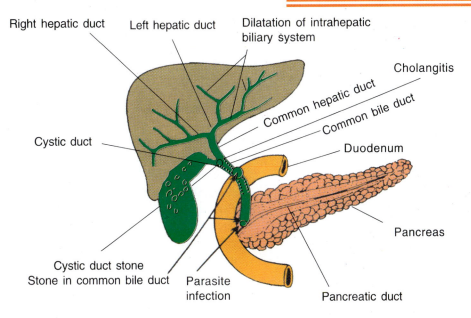

Fig. 17.1: Functional anatomy of biliary tract and aetiology of biliary colic

BILIARY COLIC

Definition

It is an acute intermittent abdominal colic resulting from an obstruction in the biliary tract leading to increased intraluminal pressure and acute distension of biliary system (Fig. 17.1) followed by intermittent repeated biliary contractions to overcome this obstruction. Intermittent biliary contractions are responsible for pain. Infection usually supervenes producing acute cholangitis and/or acute cholecystitis and then the two conditions i.e. obstruction and infection co-exist.

Pathogenesis

Two important factors in pathogenesis of acute biliary colic are: obstruction with superadded or concomittant infection. Obstruction leads to dilatation of the biliary system distal to obstruction resulting in rise in intraluminal pressure followed by or concomittent infection of the stagnant bile (Fig. 17.2). Infection or acute cholangitis causing

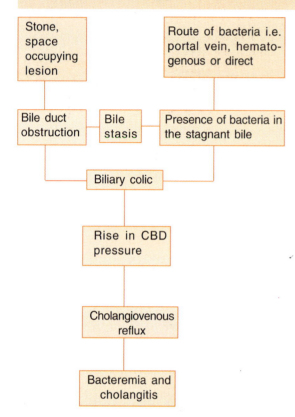

Fig. 17.2: Pathogenesis of acute biliary colic and its consequences

3. Malignant obstruction of biliary tract.
4. Parasitic infection (ascariasis, clonorchis sinensis).
5. Ductal compression by lymphadenopathy.
6. Primary sclerosing cholangitis.
7. Congenital anomalies of bile ducts such as choledochal cyst.
8. Chronic pancreatitis.

Clinical Features

1. *Acute abdominal pain*, colicky in nature, intermittent or continuous, is felt in the epigastrium or right upper quadrant of abdomen. It may radiate to interscapular region, right scapula or shoulder. There is no guarding or rigidity of abdomen.
2. *Associated features:*
   - Vomiting nearly always accompany pain, at times, may be severe.
   - *Jaundice:* There may be intermittent jaundice, i.e. during an attack of pain, slight jaundice may appear and when present is helpful in diagnosis of biliary obstruction. In some cases, frank jaundice (obstructive) develops.
   - *Pyrexia and chills:* Moderate pyrexia is not uncommon. The *Charcot's triad* (fever with chills and rigors, jaundice and right upper quadrantic pain) indicates obstructive cholangitis, is found in 70% of cases.

Investigations

- *Plain X-ray abdomen* will demonstrate calcified stones in less than 20% of cases.
- *USG* is the method of choice to diagnose gall stones, cystic duct stone and stone in the common bile duct. This investigation has replaced other radiological studies such as oral cholecystography or CT scan.
- *MRI* is becoming increasingly available which can demonstrate gall stones and their complications such as cholangitis.
- *ERCP* (endoscopic retrograde cholangiopancreatography) can be used to diagnose obstruc-

acute biliary colic can occur in the absence of obstruction. Portal vein is the most significant pathway of bacterial colonisation of biliary system. Another route is invasion of biliary system directly from the gut through the sphincter of oddi or through the biliary enteric communications.

The fever and chills accompanying acute biliary colic indicate acute cholangitis due to bacteremia. As a result of obstruction, there may be regurgitation of bacteria from the bile into hepatic venous system and is directly proportional to biliary pressure.

Causes of Biliary Colic

1. Choledocholithiasis (70-75%).
2. Biliary stricture.

tion and its cause, and to remove bile duct stones. If ERCP fails, percutaneous transhepatic cholangiography may be undertaken.
- **Routine investigation** such as total leucocyte count (TLC) and differential leucocyte count (DLC) may reveal leucocytosis with neutrophilia if there is an evidence of infection i.e. cholecystitis, cholangitis etc. Serum bilirubin may some time be raised slightly with raised alkaline phosphatase and transaminases. Blood culture is usually sterile, but if there is an evidence of infection, it may yield the causative organism.

Treatment

1. *Relief of pain:* Several analgesics can be used to control pain but pethidine I.M. or pentazocine I.M. are commonly employed. Morphine is best avoided as it increases intrabiliary pressure.

2. *Treatment of gall stones:*
    i. Medical dissolution of gall stones can be achieved by oral administration of the bile acid—chenodeoxycholic acid or its congener ursodeoxycholic acid. Radiolucent stones, stones < 15 mm in diameter, extreme obesity and mild symptomatic disease are indications of medical therapy.
    ii. Direct contact dissolution therapy is attempted via percutaneous catheters or catheters placed at ERCP.
    iii. Extracorporeal shock-wave lithotripsy is expensive and is not widely available.

3. *Treatment of infections:* Effective antibiotics include amoxycillin, cephalosporins and aminoglycoside either alone or in combinations. A combination of amoxycillin with an aminoglycoside or a third generation cephalosporin is a preferred regimen.

Part Three

Infections

Chapter 18

Septic Shock

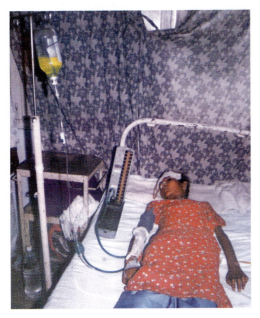

Fig. 18.1: A patient of septic shock being treated in a hospital

SEPTIC SHOCK (Fig. 18.1)

Definitions Used in Relation to Septic Patients

1. *Sepsis or systemic inflammatory response syndrome (SIRS):* In a patient with proven or suspected microbial infection, the presence of two of the following 4 conditions constitute sepsis or SIRS.
   - Oral temperature of > 38 °C or < 36 °C.
   - Respiratory rate > 20/min or $PaCO_2$ < 32 mmHg.
   - Heart rate > 90/min.
   - Leucocyte count > 12,000/μL or < 4000/μL or > 10% bands forms.
2. *Septicaemia:* Systemic illness produced as a result of spread of microbial infection or entry of their toxins into the blood stream.
3. *Bacteraemia:* Presence of viable bacteria in the blood as evidenced by positive blood culture.
4. *Hypotension:* Systolic blood pressure < 90 mm Hg or 40 mm fall of systolic BP from the baseline in a patient without any other reason for hypotension.
5. *Septic shock:* It is defined as sepsis with hypotension unresponsive to fluid resuscitation *plus* signs of organ dysfunction or hypoperfusion such as mental obtundation, oliguria, metabolic acidosis, cold extremities or adult respiratory distress syndrome. It is called refractory if it lasts > 1 hour and does not respond to fluids and pressor agents.
6. *Severe sepsis:* It is defined as sepsis with one or more signs of organ dysfunction, hypotension or hypoperfusion such as (i) metabolic acidosis, (ii) acute alteration in mental status, oliguria or adult respiratory distress syndrome.
7. *Multiple-organ dysfunction syndrome (MODS):* Dysfunction or failure of more than two organs/systems requiring intervention to maintain homeostasis.

Infections

Causes

Septic shock can result from gram-positive and gram-negative organisms and due to fungal sepsis. The most common cause is gram-negative sepsis, and common organisms involved are *E. coli, Klebsiella, pseudomonas* and *enterobacter*. The gram-positive organisms are *staphylococcus* and *meningococcus*. The portal of entry is via blood, GI tract, genitourinary tract, respiratory tract and the skin. The causes of increased incidence of severe infection are given in the Box 18.1.

Box 18.1: Sites of infection causing septic shock

Major	Others
• Intravenous lines (particularly central)	• Heart valves (prostheses)
• Respiratory tract (nosocomial infection)	• Meninges (pyogenic meningitis)
• Abdomen (intra-abdominal organ infection e.g. abscess, necrotic gut, pancreatitis, cholecystitis etc).	• Joints and bones (septic arthritis, osteomyelitis)
	• Nasal sinuses, ears, retropharyngeal space infection
	• Genitourinary tract (e.g postpartum)
• Urinary tract (e.g. infection)	• Gastrointestinal tract e.g. infection

The conditions that predispose to sepsis are tabulated (Table 18.1).

The patient may be admitted with infection from home *(community acquired)* or develop it after hospitalisation *(nosocomial)*. The risk factors for hospital-acquired infections are:
1. Mechanical ventilation.
2. Trauma.
3. Catheters (intravenous or urinary) or tubes (nasogastric).
4. Prolonged hospital stay.
5. Stress ulcer prophylaxis with H_2-antagonists.

Diagnosis and Clinical Features

The diagnosis of septic shock or sepsis syndrome rests on a high degree of suspicion in a patient with suspected or proven infection. The septic response can be quite variable especially in patients at extremes of age, those on immunosuppressive therapy (e.g. steroids, cytotoxic drugs), in patients with indwelling catheters or with co existing illness such as diabetes, malnutrition, cancer or transplantation. The clinical features are given in the Table 18.2.

Initially, patient has a stage of *warm shock* (e.g. hot body, diaphoresis, warm extremities due to vasodilatation) followed by stage of *cold shock* (cold clammy skin, vasoconstriction). The patient may recover with treatment, otherwise, there may be development of multiple organ dysfunction syndrome involving the lungs, heart, kidneys, brain, liver, etc.

Investigations

They are given in the Box 18.2.

Table 18.1: Predisposing conditions/factors to sepsis or septic shock

1. *Immunocompromised state* e.g. diabetes mellitus, AIDS, cytotoxic and steroids use.
2. *Malignancies* e.g. leukaemia, lymphoma.
3. Cirrhosis of the liver (portosystemic infection).
4. Extensive burns.
5. Neutropenia.
6. Implants, prostheses, intravenous drug abuse.
7. Antibiotic abuse.
8. Invasive procedures.
9. Malnutrition.
10. Rupture of hollow viscus.

Box 18.2: Investigations for a patient with septic shock

- Leucocytosis or leucopenia, neutrophilia with toxic granules
- Thrombocytopenia
- Rise in serum bilirubin and hepatic enzymes
- Features suggestive of DIC (prolonged thrombin time, low fibrinogen level, presence of D-dimers)
- Metabolic acidosis (lactic acidosis)
- Proteinuria
- Arterial blood gas analysis reveals hypoxia
- Chest X-ray may show infiltrates or ARDS

Table 18.2: Pathophysiology and clinical features of septic shock

Pathophysiology	Symptoms and signs
Stage I (warm shock) There is vasodilatation, opening of arteriovenous shunts and increase in cardiac output	• The skin is flushed and warm with perspiration (diaphoresis) • Impaired consciousness, irritability and mental confusion • Tachypnoea and tachycardia • Blood pressure is normal or may be decreased • Urine output is normal or slightly decreased
Stage II (cold shock) This is stage of vasoconstriction and leakage of circulating volume into interstitial spaces with decrease in cardiac output	• Cold, clammy skin and cold extremities • Seven hypotension BP < 80 mmHg • Weak, thready pulses tachycardia, tachypnoea and oliguria • Restlessness, listlessness, confusion, disorientation, stupor, coma • Arrhythmias
Stage III (multi-organ failure) There is poor tissue perfusion, microthemobi in leaking capillaries, disseminated intravascular coagulation, metabolic acidosis, circulatory collapse and respiratory and renal failure	• Cold extremities • Weak, thready pulse with severe hypotension, arrhythmias • Oliguria or anuria • Shallow respiration (acidotic breathing), worsening hypoxaemia, tachypnoea etc. • Disorientation, stupor and coma • Bleeding tendencies

Management

Aims

1. To find out the underlying cause and to treat it properly.
2. To treat local and/or systemic infection.
3. To sustain life by hemodynamic and respiratory support.
4. Symptomatic treatment, of pain, fever etc.
5. Other measures.

1. **To remove the source of infection wherever possible:** It includes: *surgical drainage of abscesses, debridement of necrotic tissue,* to relieve obstruction of hollow viscus or to exclude pelvic or soft tissue pus collection by CT scan.
2. **Antimicrobial therapy:** The indwelling I.V. catheter should be removed; culture should be taken from the tip and a new catheter should be inserted at a different site. The best way to treat septic shock is to initiate empiricial antibiotic therapy as soon as possible.
   Samples of blood and other relevant sites should be taken for culture. The choice of initial therapy is based on the knowledge of the likely organisms at specific sites of local infections and predisposing factors operating in the patient and the location (community or a hospital). Pending culture reports, it is reasonable to start an antibiotic which is effective against both gram-positive and gram-negative organisms such as a combination of third generation cephalosporin (cefotaxime 2 g I.V. 6 hourly or ceftriaxone 2 g I.V. 12 hourly) and a aminoglycoside (amikacin I g bid); if anaerobes are being suspected then add penicillin, metronidazole or clindamycin. If methicillin resistant *S. aureus* (MRSA) is suspected, then add vancomycin. For respiratory infections, a macrolide is added. Similarly a quinolone (ciprofloxacin) may be added for urogenital sepsis.
   When culture results become available, then antibiotic regimen be simplified using specific antibiotic effective against specific organism. Most patients require antibiotic therapy for one week, but can be extended depending on the underlying cause/disease.
   Antibiotic therapy is to be given intravenously in shocked patients

3. *Supportive therapy:*
   A. *Resuscitation of shock (hemodynamic support):*
      i. **Fluids therapy:** Patients of septic shock are dehydrated and need a large amount of volume replacement by fluids. Both cystalloids and colloids can be administered. Initially 1-2 L of saline is infused over a period of 1-2 hours, followed by infusion of fluids to maintain systolic BP > 90 mm and cardiac index $\geq$ 4 L/min/m^2. If these guidelines are not met by fluid replacement, then vasoactive agents are indicated.

      Adrenal insufficiency should be considered if severe, refractory hypotension is present in patients with sepsis. Supplemental hydrocortisone 50 mg I.V. after every 6 hour is recommended prior to ACTH stimulation test.

      ii. **Vasopressor agents:** Patients with low mean arterial pressure, low cardiac output and low or normal pulmonary capillary wedge pressure need inotropic support with dopamine (2-10 µg/kg/min). While those with high pulmonary capillary wedge pressure (PCWP) respond best to dobutamine.

   Fluid therapy is to be monitored by CVP (to be kept at 8-12 cm H_2O) and PCWP (to be kept 12 to 16 mmHg) and urine output (to be kept above 30 ml/hr).

   B. *Respiratory support (ventilatory support):*
      i. **Oxygenation:** Ventilatory support is needed in about 85% of patients with progressive hypoxaemia, hypercapnia, neurological deterioration and respiratory muscle failure. Intubation is often undertaken for adequate oxygenation. If respiratory drive and muscle power is adequate, then adequate tidal volumes can be delivered by pressure support; and PEEP is only indicated in few patients. Arterial O_2 saturation of 90% is adequate.

      Blood transfusion is indicated to improve oxygenation if haemoglobin level is < 7g/dl.

   C. *Metabolic support:*
      i. **Correction of metabolic acidosis:** Lactic acidosis is a consequence of low perfusion and hypoxia. It is corrected by bicarbonate administration if arterial PH is < 7.2. Electrolytes need constant monitoring and appropriate management.
      ii. **Coagulopathy or DIC:** Successful treatment of infection is essential for the reversal of both acidosis and DIC. For severe DIC with major bleeding, transfusion of fresh frozen plasma and platelets is indicated.
      iii. **Nutritional supplementation** is needed to reduce the impact of protein hypercatabolism. Nutrition is provided by enteral feeding (long-term management) or parenteral feeding (short-term management).
      iv. **Renal failure:** Many patients develop acute renal failure due to sepsis and require treatment with antibiotics, vasoactive substances and fluid therapy. Most of the patients improve and only a few of them may need dialytic support.

   D. *Other measures:*
   To reduce the mortality due to septic shock, two types of drugs i.e. anti-endotoxin agents (monoclonal antibodies to endotoxin, human neutrophil protein, a polymyxin B-dextran conjugate etc). and antimediators agents (anticytokines drugs, PAF antagonists, bradykinin antagonists and ibuprofen) are being investigated but still not been found successful. Use of high dose glucocorticoids have not improved survival. Recently recombinant activated protein C (aPC)—an anticoagulant agent has been cleaved by US

food and Drug Administration (FDA) to be used specifically in patients with septic shock who are > 18 years of age and who meet the APACHE II score ≥ 25 and have a low risk of haemorrhage related side effects. Dose of continuous infusion is 24 μg/kg/hr for 96 hours, clotting parameters should be monitored as haemorrhage is serious complication of this therapy.

E. **General measures** include good nursing care, prevention of nosocomial infection, good enteral nutrition, prevention of stress ulcer and GI bleed by H_2-blockers, care of skin and prevention of deep vein thrombosis. They contribute significantly to reduce the mortality.

Complications

1. *ARDS or shock lung.* ARDS develops in 20 to 25% cases of septic shock.
2. *Renal failure.* Oliguric and nonoliguric renal failure can develop.
3. *Coagulopathy or DIC.*
4. *Nutritional deficiencies.*

The treatment of these complications has already been discussed in the management.

Chapter 19

Dengue Fever

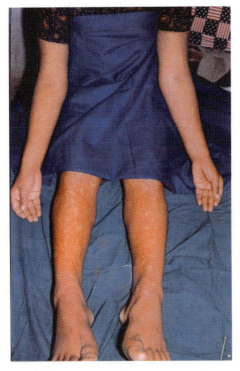

Fig. 19.1: Rash of classic dengue fever

DENGUE FEVER AND RELATED EMERGENCIES

Dengue Fever

It is a mosquito-borne virus infection characterised by febrile illness (classic dengue), bleeding manifestations (dengue haemorrhagic fever) and shock (dengue shock syndrome).

The disease is transmitted from human to human by bite of a female anopheles mosquito (*Aedes aegypti*) and is caused by one of the distinct 4 types of *flavi viruses (dengue virus 1 to 4)*. The disease occurs in endemic and epidemic forms. In India, many outbreaks have been reported, but recent one occurred in the capital (Delhi) in 1996.

The incubation period is 3 to 7 days. The viraemia begins 24 hours before the fever and subsides with the end of fever. The virus disseminates to the regional lymph nodes, then through the lymphatics throughout the body.

Clinical Characteristics

Three distinct entities of dengue fever have been described depending on the severity of infection and whether infection is primary or secondary.
1. Classical dengue fever. The clinical features of classical dengue are given in the Box 19.1.
2. Dengue haemorrhagic fever (DHF).
3. Dengue shock syndrome (DSS).

The secondary infection may be more severe due to circulating antibodies. Sequential infection by any 2 out of 4 sero types of dengue virus may lead to DHF and DSS in *hyperendemic* areas. Chronic infection by this virus is unknown. The features of classical dengue are described in the Box 19.1.

Dengue Fever

Treatment

The treatment of dengue fever is entirely symptomatic with analgesics for relief of pain and fever. Patient is advised rest during the stage of fever. Transfusion of blood or blood products is indicated in case of severe bleeding. The disease is self-limiting.

DENGUE HAEMORRHAGIC FEVER (DHF) AND DENGUE SHOCK SYNDROME (DSS)

Dengue haemorrhagic fever is characterised by all manifestations of classical dengue fever, thrombocytopenia, vascular instability and increased permeability resulting in leakage of intravascular fluid to interstitial space (hemoconcentration) and local haemorrhage (positive tourniquet test, spontaneous petechiae and/or purpura) or frank haemorrhage (epistaxis, gum bleeding, bleeding into GI tract i.e. malena and menometrorrhagia) have been described. The haemorrhage is inconstant and is thought to be a combined effect of vascular damage and thrombocytopenia.

As the plasma leakage increases, patient may become restless, irritable and develops hypotension and shock (cold extremities) called *dengue shock syndrome (DSS)*. In severe cases, frank shock is present with low pulse pressure (< 20 mmHg), cyanosis, hepatomegaly, pleural effusion and ascites. In some cases, severe ecchymosis and GI bleeding may be seen.

Diagnosis

The diagnosis is purely clinical and the full brown picture of dengue haemorrhagic fever is easy to recognise. The grading of DHF (WHO) is given in the Box 19.2. The laboratory findings that support the diagnosis include leucopenia, thrombocytopenia and raised serum aminotransferases. The diagnosis is helped by antibody detection (IgM-ELISA) or paired serology during recovery or by antigen detection (ELISA or RT-PCR) during acute phase. Virus can also be isolated from the blood by virus culture.

Management

Early recognition is necessary because of the need for virus-specific therapy and supportive measures. The treatment include:

1. *Judicious fluid therapy:* All patients do not require admission. Patients with mild circulatory

---

Box 19.1: Clinical features of classical dengue

Symptoms	Signs
• Sudden onset of fever, headache, retro-orbital pain, back pain with severe myalgia for which a common term '*break-bone fever*' is used. In children, there is associated cough, sore throat, nausea, vomiting and abdominal pain. • *Macular erythematous* rash (Fig. 19.1) which blanches on pressure may be seen on trunk within 24 hours of fever. There may be flushed facies with scleral injection (redness of eyes). The illness lasts for a week. At the time of defervescence—a maculopapular (see the figure 18.1 on front page) rash beginning on the trunk and spreading to the extremities and the face is characteristic. This fades over next few days. • Epistaxis, petechiae and purpura are often noted in uncomplicated dengue	• Pharyngeal congestion • Scleral congestion/injection • Suffused facies • Abdominal tenderness • Lymphadenopathy • A positive tourniquet test for capillary fragility (> 10 petechiae over 2.5 cm^2 area) • Cutaneous hyperaesthesia.

Infections

Box 19.2: WHO classification of Dengue and its related syndrome

Grade	Platelet nadir (per ml)	Plasma leakage	Circulatory collapse	Others
Classical dengue	Variable	Absent	Absent	• Tourniquet test variable
Dengue haemorrhage fever				
Grade I	< 1 lac	Present	Absent	• Tourniquet test positive
Grade II	< 1 lac	Present		• Tourniquet test positive and frank haemorrhage
Dengue shock syndrome				
Grade III	< 1 lac	Present	Pulse pressure < 20 mmHg	• Tourniquet test positive • Haemorrhage may be present
Grade IV	< 1 lac	Present	Blood pressure unrecordable	• Tourniquet test variable Haemorrhage may be present

collapse or hypotension require fluid replacement by mouth and close monitoring of the vital signs. Patients presenting with circulatory collapse (hypovolaemia, cold extremities, pallor, oliguria) and falling platelet count require hospitalisation for fluid replacement. Intravenous fluids (5% dextrose in half normal saline or Ringer's lactate) are given in the beginning. If no improvement occurs, or in severe cases, a plasma expander may be given as rapidly as possible to produce volume expansion. Fluids are to be continued till patient comes out of shock and vital parameters improve.

2. *Pressor agents:* Pressor agents along with fluid therapy may be used to resuscitate shock in severe cases. Blood pressure is to be maintained above 90 mmHg.
3. *Oxygen therapy* should be used to improve oxygenation.
4. *Blood transfusion* is given in the presence of massive bleeding with falling hematocrit.
5. *Coagulopathy or thrombocytopenia* may need cryoprecipitate and platelets transfusion.
6. *Corticosteroids* are of not much help.
7. *Antiviral therapy* has also not been found useful.

Prevention and Control

- Avoidance and eradication of mosquito vectors.
- During an epidemic, fumigation of insecticide by road vehicles or air crafts in the area affected.
- Removal of breeding sites/containers.
- Avoid the use of stored water and try to use piped water.
- No effective vaccine available.

Differential Diagnosis

Other conditions that produce haemorrhagic fever are:
1. Lassa fever.
2. Yellow fever.
3. Meningoccocaemia.
4. Kyasanur forest disease.
5. Rift-valley fever.
6. Rickettsioses.
7. Haemorrhagic fever with renal syndrome.

Chapter 20

Typhoid Fever and its Complications

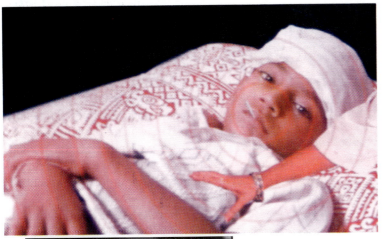

Fig. 20.1: A patient of uncomplicated typhoid fever being treated in the hospital

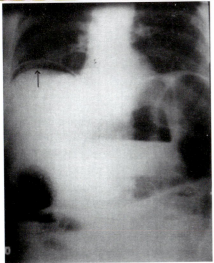

Fig. 20.2: Enteric perforation. Note the air under right dome of diaphragm

TYPHOID FEVER AND ITS COMPLICATIONS

Typhoid fever is an acute systemic illness caused by infection due to *S. typhi*. The disease is acquired by oro-faecal route through faecal contamination of food, water, drinks and other eatables. The reservoir of infection include; patients suffering or convalescing from typhoid or chronic carriers of typhoid (food handlers).

Typhoid fever is characterised by fever, malaise, abdominal pain, rash, splenomegaly and leucopenia (see Box 20.1). The untreated patients may develop complications during 2nd and 3rd week due to toxaemia and septicaemia. In some cases, it may be fatal.

Clinical Features

The incubation period is 10-14 days. The onset is usually insidious. The clinical manifestations are variable from mild illness to acute systemic illness which may last for 6-8 weeks if untreated. The symptoms and signs of typhoid fever (Fig. 20.1) are summarised in the Box 20.1.

> **Box 20.1: Clinical symptoms and signs of typhoid fever**
>
> 1. *During first week* (first 5-7 days)
>   - Remittent fever, headache, bodyache, malaise, constipation, leucopenia, relative bradycardia.
> 2. *Between first and second week*
>   - Rose spots, splenomegaly, bronchitis, abdominal pain, abdominal distension and diarrhoea. The fever reaches its maximum and persists. The patient looks ill and more toxic.
> 3. *Beyond second week:*
>   If everything is well and treatment is effective, patient recovers. In severe infection, the patient may develop stuporose state (typhoid encephalopathy). The temperature may remain slightly above normal in the convalescence period.
>   *Relapse* occurs in 5-10% cases after 7-14 days of defervescence. It is milder than the initial attack.

Complications

1. *Gastrointestinal* e.g. intestinal perforation (Fig. 20.2), or acute paralytic ileus, intestinal haemorrhage.
2. *Hepatobiliary* e.g. hepatitis, necrotising cholecystitis.
3. *Cardiovascular* e.g. myocarditis.
4. *Hematological* e.g. aplasia of bone marrow, pancytopenia, DIC, haemolytic anaemia.
5. *Renal* e.g. nephritis.
6. *Respiratory* e.g. bronchitis, pneumonia.
7. *Bone and joints* e.g. arthritis, osteomyelitis.
8. *Neurological* e.g. enteric encephalopathy, encephalitis, brain abscess, meningitis, peripheral neuropathy.

Diagnosis

The diagnosis is suggested by the clinical features; whereas the definite diagnosis still depends on the isolation of the organism from the blood or bone marrow culture, the overall yield of culture is disappointingly low about 90% in first week, falls to less than 50% in untreated patient during 3rd week. Yield can be approximately 100% when both blood and bone marrow culture are done in patients not receiving antibiotics. Stool culture may be positive in 75% cases during third week, while it is negative during first week. The culture of intestinal (duodenal) secretions aspirated through ryle's tube gives better results than stool culture.

DNA probe have been developed for identifying *S. typhi* from culture isolates and from blood. Recently a PCR based test using 2 pairs of oligo nucleotide from a fragment of *S. typhi* flagellum gene (HI-d) was found to be 93% sensitive and 100% specific on clinical trials, but still is not commercially available. Another test—PCR based on the nucleotides sequencing using Vi antigen (VaB region) has been developed. Serological diagnosis is made by widal test which is less reliable than culture. In the absence of immunisation, a higher titre of agglutinins on widal test (1:300) is suggestive but not diagnostic. A four-fold rise in antibody titre between paired sera samples is highly suggestive. Recently developed latex agglutination or coagulation tests for antibody to the Vi antigen appear to be much more specific and sensitive than classic widal test.

In addition there may be leucopenia or neutropenia is about 50% cases.

Treatment

With the emergence of chloramphenicol resistant strains, it no longer remains the drug of choice now-a-days. Fluoroquinolones and 3rd generation cephalosporins are antibiotic of choice due to development of multi-drug resistance.

1. 4-fluoroquinolones such as ciprofloxacin 500-750 mg bid or ofloxacin 400 mg twice a day or Gatifloxacin 400 mg once a day are sufficient to treat uncomplicated typhoid fever. Parenteral preparations (e.g. ciprofloxacin 200 mg I.V. bid) are used in typhoid with complications.

The third generation cephalosporins such as ceftriaxone and cefoperazone are equally effective in dosage of 1 g twice a day I.V. or 50 mg/kg/day for 7 to 10 days or at least 3 days after defervescence.

In pregnancy, the third generation cephalosporin is preferred drug over fluoroquinolone. Ampicillin 6-12 g/daily for adults or 100 mg/kg for children in divided doses is also useful. If sensitivity to chloramphenicol is present then it is given 2-4 g/day.

2. Antipyretics are used orally or I.V. for fever and pain. Hydrotherapy for high grade fever is indicated (Fig. 20.1).
3. Patient is advised to take oral liquids and semi-solid diet so as to avoid fluid loss/deficit due to fever during defervescence. I.V. fluids are to be given if there is state of dehydration.
4. Relapse and primary attack are similarly treated.
5. *High doses steroids:* In one Indonesian study, it has been reported that high doses of corticosteroids in typhoid fever with CNS manifestations and/or evidence of DIC if given along with antibiotic therapy, reduces the mortality rate. Dexamethasone 3 mg/kg I.V. as a bolus followed by 1 mg/kg I.V. every 6 hours for 24-48 hours should be considered in such a typhoid state.
6. *Treatment of carriers:* A person is said to be carrier if he/she excretes the organisms in the stool after one year following illness. Carrier state in the absence of gall stones is treated by oral ampicillin (100 mg/kg/day) *plus* probenecid 30 mg/kg/day for 6 weeks or cotriamoxazole 960 mg/day/for 4 weeks or ciprofloxacin 750 mg bid for 4 weeks to sterilise the gall bladder which is responsible for this state. Cholecystectomy may be necessary in some cases.

Management of Complications

Enteric Encephalopathy

It is a toxic complication, occurs commonly during second or third week of typhoid fever, is characterised by fever with an altered state of consciousness ranging from disorientation to coma and has a mortality rate exceeding 40%.

Treatment

It includes:
1. Care of semiconscious or unconscious state.
2. Intravenous fluids to treat dehydration and to maintain proper hydration and blood pressure so as to prevent other complications. Vitals are to be monitored.
3. Intravenous antibiotics specially third generation cephalosporin e.g. ceftriaxone 2 mg I.V. 12 hourly for 2-3 days then 1 g after every 12 hours over few days.
4. High dose corticosteroids: High dose corticosteroids have been recommended in this complication. Dose and duration of therapy has already been discussed.
5. If patient recovers, he/she has to be treated with one of the drug used to treat carrier state. This is given for 4 weeks to sterilise the gall bladder and to prevent relapse and to eradicate the organisms to prevent carrier state.

Intestinal Haemorrhage

It is characterised by bleeding per rectum in a patient of typhoid during 2nd and 3rd week, followed by development of anaemia. The patient is pale, dehydrated and has toxic look. There is tachypnoea and tachycardia. There may be hypotension or shock depending on the loss of blood.

Management

- Endoscopy, coeliac axis angiography, radioisotopic scanning to localise the site of bleeding.
- Supportive therapy by intravenous fluids and antibiotics.
- Blood or blood products transfusion.
- Surgical intestinal resection may be required occasionally.
- Monitoring of vital parameters.

Chapter 21

Rabies

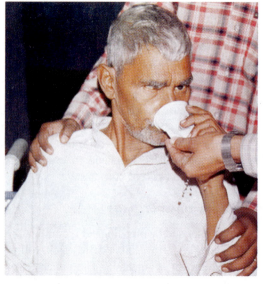

Fig. 21.1: A patient of rabies depicting hydrophobia. Note the severe phobic reaction following just holding of a glass of water by the observer while the patient is supported by his attendant. Patient ultimately died after 24 hours.

RABIES

It is an acute *viral* infection of the brain caused by RNA virus of rhabdoviridae family and affects all the mammals. It is transmitted by the infected secretions, commonly the saliva containing the virus through the bite of infected animal. In most areas of the world, the dog is the most important vector for rabies virus transmission to humans.

However other animals such as wolf, mongoose, vampire bat and cats may also be important vectors. Several cases of human-to-human transmission of rabies through corneal transplantation have been reported; otherwise human rabies (human bite) is exceedingly rare.

Clinical Features

They are given in the Box 21.1.

Diagnosis

The diagnosis of rabies is generally made on clinical grounds supported by investigations such as fluorescent antibody test to detect rabies antigen in corneal impressions or in salivary secretions and confirmation is done by classical *Negri bodies* at postmortem examination of brain.

Management

1. *Once the disease is established, therapy is symptomatic:*
   - The patient should be nursed in a quiet, isolated, darkened room with all facilities.
   - Nutritional, respiratory and cardiovascular support to be provided.
   - To reduce psychomotor excitation, morphine, diazepam and chlorpromazine should be used liberally in such patients.
   - Maintain water and salt balance because dehydration results due to aversion to drinking

Rabies

> **Box 21.1: Clinical features of rabies (hydrophobia)**
>
> **Prodromal symptoms**
> - Incubation period is 1-4 days
> - Fever, headache, malaise, myalgia, GI symptoms, paraesthesias and/or fasciculations around the site of inoculation of virus indicate multiplication of virus in dorsal root ganglia of sensory neve supplying the area
>
> **Encephalitic phase**
> - Agitation, excitation, enhanced motor activity
> - Confusion, hallucinations, bizarre thoughts
> - Fear of water (hydrophobia), muscles spasms, meningismus, opisthotonus
> - Seizures and focal paralysis
> - Hyperesthesia with excessive sensitivity to bright light, noise, touch and even gentle breeze is common
> - *Temperature is elevated*
> - Autonomic symptoms and signs e.g. dilated irregular pupils, lacrimation, salivation, postural hypotension and cardiac arrhythmias
> - Change in the voice (vocal cord paralysis)
> - Evidence of UMN paralysis e.g. exaggerated reflexes with plantar extensor is the rule
> - Dumb rabies or paralytic rabies presents with a symmetric ascending paralysis resembling Guillain-Barré syndrome
>
> **Brainstem dysfunctions**
> - Cranial nerve palsies
> - Hydrophobia (Fig.21.1)
> - Priaprism and spontaneous ejaculation
> - Unconsciousness or coma
> - Death

water and excessive perspiration. Intravenous fluids are to be administered liberally.
- Prednisolone and mannitol may be given in patients with raised intracranial pressure.

2. **Prevention of rabies:**
   A. *Post-exposure prophylaxis (see the algorithms in the Box 21.2):* Dramatic clinical features and fatal outcome in rabies makes the prevention of rabies essential. The steps of prophylaxis includes:
   - Local treatment of the wound.
   - Immunisation (active and passive).

   i. *Local treatment of the wound:* It consists of:
      - *Wound toilet with soap and water:* The wound is scrubbed with soap and flushed with water so as to remove the saliva from the wound.
      - *Chemical cleansing of the wound:* After removal of soap with water, chemical cleansing is done by any quaternary ammonium compound (1-4% benzalkonium chloride or 1% cetrimonium bromide) to inactivate the rabies virus.
      - Tetanus toxoid and antibiotics should be administered.
      - Wound must not be stitched.

   ii. *Passive immunisation with antirabies serum of either equine or human origin:* The antirabies serum provides passive immunity in the form of ready-made antibodies against rabies virus. Human rabies immunoglobulin (HRIG) is preferred because equine anti serum may cause serum sickness.
      Dose: Total dose of HRIG is 20 units/kg. and equine antiserum is 40 units/kg. Half the dose is infiltrated around the wound and remaining half is given by deep intramuscular injection into the gluteal region. The antirabies serum needs sensitivity test; while HRIG dose does not require any prior sensitivity testing.
      Warning: When a person is re-exposed to rabies virus after administration of antirabies vaccines, antirabies serum should not be injected.

   iii. *Active immunisation with antirabies vaccine:* In the developed world, human diploid cell vaccine (HDCV) is recommended which is

104 Infections

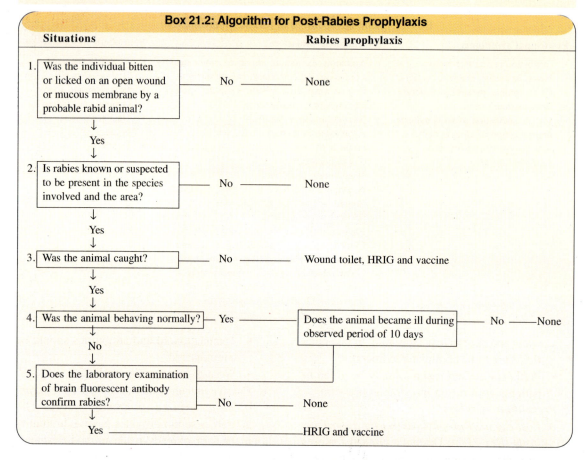

least antigenic and systemic (1-4%) and local reactions (15-20%) are uncommon.

In the developing world, several other rabies vaccines have seen licenced and used extensively. These include vaccines made in chick embryonic cells, vero-cells and duct embryonic cells. These preparations are safe but immunogenic and are effective for post-exposure prophylaxis. In India, HDCV is not available. Other tissue culture vaccines are; primary chick-embryo cell vaccine (PCECV) and purified vero-cells rabies vaccine (PVRV). The dose schedule of vaccine recommended by WHO is given in the Box 21.3.

Pre-exposure Prophylaxis

Some individuals who are at high risk of contact with rabies virus due to their profession such as

Box 21.3: Dose schedule of vaccine in post-exposure prophylaxis (WHO schedule)

- Five doses of the vaccine available are given intramuscularly, preferably in the deltoid region, the first dose is administered as soon as possible after exposure and should be accompanied by injection of HRIG. The five doses are to be given within 30 days on the following schedule; Days 0, 3, 7, 14 and 30. Day 0 indicates the day of vaccination started and the day of the bite.
  The 6th injection at 90th day has also been recommended by WHO in those persons who are either immunodeficient or are on steroid therapy and/or at the extremes of ages.
- Period of immunity conferred is 3-5 years.
- Adverse effects with tissue culture vaccines are minimal such as sore arm, headache, nausea, fever, localised oedema at the site of injection. Symptomatic treatment is advised to the patient.

veterinarians, laboratory research workers and animal handlers should receive pre-exposure prophylaxis with three doses of rabies vaccine on days 0, 7 and 21 or 30. Neutralising antibody titre is to be checked after vaccination. Depending on the level of risk, serological testing to be done at 2 to 6 years intervals. If titres of neutralising antibody falls below 1:5, booster doses should be given.

Post-exposure prophylaxis in individuals who have received pre-exposure prophylaxis consists of initial two injections on days 0 and 3. HRIG is not given.

Chapter 22

Tetanus

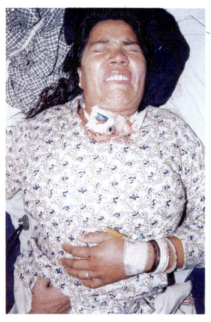

Fig. 22.1: Risus sardonicus in a patient with tetanus. A 40-year-old woman developed tetanus following injury. Note the grimacing or grinning appearance of the face due to facial muscle spasms.

TETANUS

It is a disorder of neuromuscular excitability caused by an exotoxin (e.g. tetanospasmin) elaborated by *Clostridium tetani*, characterised by rigidity and powerful muscle spasms. It manifests clinically in many forms i.e. *generalised, neonatal, cephalic* and *localised*.

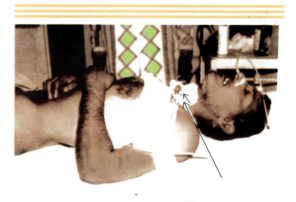

Fig. 22.2: A patient of tetanus being treated in the hospital. Note the tracheostomy tube indicated by arrows (↑)

Aetiopathogenesis

C. tetami—a causative organism of tetanus, is a motile, gram-positive spore forming obligatory anaerobic organism found in the soil and the environment. It is a normal commensal of animals and human GI tract and is excreted in the stool/excreta. The organism is heat-resistant but sensitive to penicillin and metronidazole. The spores can survive for many years in adverse circumstances.

The organism attacks the wound with low redox potential (low oxidation-reduction potential). The development of tetanus depends on the immune status of the individual. The tetanus occurs sporadically in non-immunised or partially immunised persons mostly through the contaminated wound having local anaerobic conditions. It is common in ruralites than urbanites, and during summer months. It is common in neonates and children in under developed countries where a comprehensive immunisation policy is not followed. It is common in extremes of ages.

The majority of cases occur after an acute injury with abrasion, laceration or punctured wound. The portal of entry is contaminated wounds containing the spores of C. tetani but sometimes entry cannot be identified as injury may be trivial or goes undetected. Following contamination, if local environment of the wound is anaerobic (low oxidation-reduction potential), the spores germinate and produce exotoxin.

Skin abrasions/ulceration, abscesses, gangrene are the wounds commonly predisposed to tetanus. The predisposing conditions include: burn, surgery, abortion, childbirth, drug abuse and tattooing presence of a foreign body in the wound.

The exotoxin (tetanospasmin) released from the wound, enters locally through the peripheral motor neurons to axons and travels to the nerve cell bodies in the brain stem and spinal cord. The length of the nerve determines the time of ascent and explains why the disease first manifests in the muscles supplied by short cranial nerves in cephalic tetanus.

The mode of action is to block the release of inhibitory neurotransmitter-GABA at myoneural junction or synapse. Therefore:

- *In tetanus*, central inhibition is abolished resulting in free play of alpha (α) and gamma (γ) neurones producing typical rigidity with its clinical manifestations.
- With lessened inhibition, the agonists and antagonists contract simultaneously resulting in spasms.
- The loss of central inhibition also affects the autonomic nervous system resulting in sympathetic overactivity and features of autonomic dysfunction.

In cephalic or local tetanus, the muscles supplied by involved local nerves are paralysed initially followed by rigidity of the affected muscle following central inhibition.

In tetanus neonatorum, the portal of entry is infected umbilical cord stump.

Clinical Features

The features of adult generalised tetanus are given in Box 22.1.

> **Box 22.1: Clinical features of general tetanus**
>
> 1. *Incubation period* is about 7 days (varies from 3-14 days).
> 2. *Hypertonia and rigidity of muscles:* Hypertonia of muscles of face (risus sardonicus—grinning expression of face Fig. 21.1), Jaw (lock jaw or trismus), neck, shoulder, chest pain and stiffness, abdomen (abdominal rigidity) and back (opisthotonus—arched back). These spasms occur spontaneously or are induced by noise, light and handling of the patient.
> 3. *Visceral manifestations:* Painful strong spasms of muscles of respiration may result in hypoventilation, apnoea and cyanosis. Oesophageal and urethral spasms result in dysphagia and urinary retention. The patient may be febrile due to strong muscular contractions. Deep tendon reflexes may be increased.
> 4. *Autonomic symptoms:* These include labile or sustained hypertension, tachycardia, arrhythmias, fever, sweating etc. and may require beta blockade if become severe.
> 5. *Nonimmunised or partially immunised status of an individual.*

Neonatal tetanus develops in children born to mothers who have been either not immunised or inadequately immunised during pregnancy. It follows infection of umbilical cord stump by unsterilised means. The onset is common during first 2 weeks of life. It occurs in generalised form, proves fatal if left untreated. Poor sucking, failure to thrive, grimacing and irritability followed by rigidity and spasms are its diagnostic features. Mortality is high.

Loal tetanus is characterised by rigidity and spasms restricted to the muscles around the wound, is thus a limited form of tetanus, hence, carries excellent prognosis.

Cephalic tetanus: It is an uncommon form and follows injury of face or head and neck region or the ear. The incubation period is short. The trismus (lock jaw) and dysfunction of one of the cranial nerve mostly the seventh nerve are its common manifestations. Generalised tetanus may or may not develop. The mortality is high due to early and severe involvement of brain-stem.

Investigations

There is no single test which can confirm tetanus including culture of the orgnism from the wound; however, recovery of the organisms from the wound in the symptomatic patients of tetanus is highly suggestive.

  i. *Other tests such as EMG* may show continuous motor units discharges and shortening or absence of silent interval (normally, these intervals, are seen).
  ii. *ECG:* It may be done frequently in patients with autonomic dysfunction.
  iii. *Muscle enzymes:* The CPK (creatinine phosphokinase), aldolases may be high during acute phase.
  iv. Serum anti-toxin levels ≥ 0.01 IU/ml is unlikely. This is protective antotoxin level.

Management

Aims

  i. To eliminate the source of toxin (care of the wound).
  ii. To neutralise unbound toxin.
  iii. To prevent muscle spasms.
  iv. To maintain patent airway by tracheostomy
  v. Ventilatory support if needed.

Treatment

1. *General measures:*
    a. *Good nursing* care is the single most important measure to reduce mortality significantly. The patient should be nursed in a dark, quiet, well ventilated isolated room.
    b. *Nutrition:* Initially or in case of diarrhoea, nutrition is given in the form of intravenous fluids. Calories expenditure is high in a patient with tetanus, hence more than 2500 Kcal and 70 g proteins are needed daily, may be given through nasogastric tube for long-term management.
    c. *Wound debridement:* Cleansing of the wound and its debridement is necessary to eliminate the anaerobic environment of the wound so as to eliminate the source of the toxin.
    d. *Care of the unconscious patient:* Meticulous care of the skin to prevent bed sores, proper urinary drainage, maintenance of vitals is necessary.
    e. *Patent airway or tracheostomy:* (Fig. 22.2): It is always required in the presence of laryngeal spasms or excessive secretions. Tracheostomy should be done electively and as early as possible. Frequent suction of the secretions is mandatory to prevent aspiration and to maintain patent airway.
2. *The role of antibiotic:* The penicillin is the drug of choice in doses of 10-12 millions units I.V. daily for 10 days or a single injection of benzathine penicillin 2.4×10^6 units provides bactericidal concentrations for a period of 2 weeks. Some physicians prefer metronidazole 500 mg 6 hourly or 1g 12 hourly due to its potent anaerobicidal action. Tetracyclines, clindamycin and erythromycin are alternative antibiotics.
3. *Antitoxin:* The antitoxin (ATS-anti-tetanus serum) is given as 10,000 IU intravenously after testing the sensitivity to neutralise the circulatory as well as unbound tetanus toxin in the wound.

Local infiltration of the wound is obsolete now-a-days.

Human tetanus immunoglobulin (TIG) should be given I.M. in doses of 3000-6000 IU in divided doses; however, 1500 IU is considered as optimal dose now-a-days. The intrathecal administered of TIG has no role.

4. *Control of muscle spasms:* Diazepam—a benzodiazepine derivative and GABA agonist is the drug of choice. Continuous I.V. infusion of 100-200 mg daily may be needed initially to control the painful spasms, then dose is reduced to maintenance dose. Lorazepam and midazolam are other alternatives. Barbiturates and phenothiazines are second-line agents.

The spasms that are unresponsive to medication or that threaten ventilation are best treated with mechanical ventilation and therapeutic muscular *paralysis by neuromuscular blockade e.g. curarisation.* Alternative agent is propofol but is expensive. Baclofen and dantroline are being investigated with the hope that their use will shorten the period of paralysis.

5. *Control of autonomic symptoms when and if they arise:* A hemodynamic monitoring is needed for autonomic dysfunction. Betablockers are used in case of sympathetic overactivity to control hypertension and prevent arrhythmias. Bradycardia or bradyarrhythmias may require pacemaker insertion. Hypotension responds to volume expansion and pressure agents.

6. *Vaccine:* Active immunisation before discharge of the patient from the hospital is considered necessary in view of the fact that patients of tetanus do not generate sufficient antitoxin in the blood after recovery.

7. *Other measures:*
   - *Maintain proper hydration* by adequate fluid replacement. Vitamins are to be supplemented.
   - *Care of bowel, bladder and skin* is of ulmost importance. Decubitus ulcer must be prevented by frequent change of posture, adequate urinary drainage by condom or catheter, proper disposal of excreta and frequent change of soiled clothes.
   - *Intercurrent infection* must be dealt appropriately by use of proper antibiotic after culture and sensitivity. Prophylactic antibiotic therapy has no role.
   - *Physiotherapy* is to be instituted to prevent contractures.

Prophylaxis

The prophylaxis in the injured person requires wound cleansing and a booster dose of tetanus toxoid. Previously unimmunised individuals or partially immunised individuals should receive vaccine similar to those recovering from tetanus i.e. 1500 IU of ATS or 250 IU of TIG intramuscularly.

Active immunisation schedule of tetanus consists of three doses during first year of life i.e. 3rd, 4th and 6-12th months. The booster dose is given at school-going age and then after 5-10 years intervals (Read the immunisation schedule from textbook).

Complications

1. *Pulmonary infection* occurs due to:
   - Aspiration of infected secretions.
   - Depressed cough and swallow reflex.
   - Impaired ventilation and mucociliary defense mechanisms following tracheostomy.
2. *Autonomic dysfunctions* such as hypertension, tachy and bradyarrhythmias and hypotension. They require monitoring and proper treatment.
3. *Vertebral fractures of the dorsal spine* during violent and severe spasms.
4. *Myositis ossificans* due to deposition of calcium in the ligaments around the joints (knee, elbow) can occasionally occur.
5. *Decubitus ulcer/pressure sores occur due to:*
   - Prolonged immobilisation
   - Skin contamination with urine and faeces.

Chapter 23

Myonecrosis (Gas Gangrene)

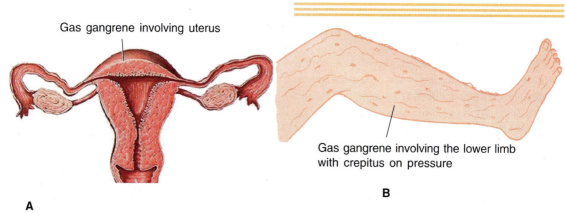

Figs 23.1A and B: Gas gangrene (myonecrosis). **A.** Uterus, **B.** Lower limb

MYONECROSIS (GAS GANGRENE)

Myonecrosis (gas gangrene) is produced from invasion of healthy muscle from adjacent traumatised muscle or soft tissue infected by anaerobes especially clostridial group of organism. About 80% cases are caused by *C. perfringes*; while remainders are due to *C. novyi*, *C septicum* and *C. histolyticum*. The finding of gas in the muscle, soft tissue or uterus is not pathognomonic of clostridial infection as other bacteria particularly anaerobes, mixed with aerobes can also produce gas.

Aetiopathogenesis

Gas gangrene is a serious complication seen in devitalised and devascularised muscle following trauma, surgery or amputation. The causative organisms are present in the soil and in the GI tract of animals and humans. The presence of necrotic tissue, foreign bodies or ischaemia in a wound reduce locally available oxygen (low oxidation-reduction potential) and permit the organism to grow and produce toxin.

The concerned toxins spread through tissue and expand them in aerobic area. The alpha toxins of *C. perfringens* results in the destruction of muscles fibres by disrupting the phospholipid in cell membranes. *Collagenases* and hyaluronidases destroy the partitions of connective tissue and enable the infection to spread, through muscles. In less virulent infection, local fascitis rather than myositis may result.

Clinical Features

The clinical features are summarised in Box 23.1.

Myonecrosis (Gas Gangrene)

> **Box 23.1: Clinical features of clostridial myonecrosis**
>
> - *Incubation period* is short i.e. less than 3 days, frequently less than 24 hours.
> - *Precipitating or incriminating factors* include; deep muscle trauma (lacerated wound), surgery or intramuscular injection which creates an anaerobic environment for growth of clostridia.
> - *The initial symptom* is pain of sudden onset, severe, localised to the infected area and then may spread. This is followed by local swelling, oedema and haemorrhagic exudation from the wound. There is associated elevation of temperature and marked tachycardia. There may be frothiness of the wound on compression at this stage. The symptoms progress rapidly i.e. swelling, oedema and toxaemia increase and a profuse serous discharge with sweetish smell appear. Gram-stain of the wound may reveal—Gram-positive rods with few inflammatory cells. At this stage, there is an evidence of suppuration, and gas in the soft tissues (subcutaneous crepitance) (Fig. 23.1) as well as overwhelming toxaemia.
> - *These patients preserve consciousness* in spite of hypotension, renal failure and body crepitance. They lapse into toxic delirium and coma in later phases. In untreated cases, skin become bronzed; bullae appear, become filled with dark red fluid and are accompanied by dark patches of cutaneous gangrene. Jaundice is rare, if present is associated with haemoglobinuria, haemoglobinaemia and septicaemia. DIC may be seen in severe infection.

Investigations

- There may be leucocytosis due to toxaemia.
- *Muscle enzymes*. There may be raised CK (creatinine phosphokinase).
- *Radiograph of the involved area* may show collection of gas with ill-defined soft tissue shadow.
- *USG and CT scan* may confirm badly damage muscle and presence of gas.
- *Isolation of the organism from scrapping from uterus, smears from the wound or cervical discharge. Blood culture* for isolation of the organism to be placed in anaerobic media.
- Frozen section biopsy of muscle confirms the diagnosis.

Diagnosis

The diagnosis of gas gangrene is primarily on the clinical findings with demonstration of gas in the muscles, soft tissue or uterus and isolation of the organism from the site involved (smears of wound exudates, uterine scrappings or cervical discharge) or from the blood cultures to be placed in selective media and incubated under anaerobic conditions. The diagnosis is confirmed by frozen section biopsy of the muscle.

Management

1. *Eradication of source of infection:*
   a. *Surgery:* It includes debridement of local soft tissue infection, debridement of all the involved muscles in abdominal myonecrosis or surgical removal of the source of infection such as amputation of a limb or hysterectomy for uterine myonecrosis.
   b. *Antibiotics:* Penicillin G (20 million units a day in adults) have been the drug of choice till now. Recently its role has become controversial because of increasing resistance to this drug. Clindamycin (600 mg every 6 hourly) and penicillin combination has been found to be superior than either of them alone. In case of penicillin allergy, other antibiotic should be used. Broad spectrum antibiotic with a aminoglycoside may be used for the aerobic gram-negative bacteria involved in mixed infections.
2. *Polyvalent gas gangrene antitoxin:* It is still recommended by some authorities but at present its role has become controversial because of questionable efficacy and risk of hypersensitivity to horse serum from which it is derived.
3. *Hyperbaric oxygen:* Its role has also become questionable because:
   i. Its efficacy is not proved but is believed to produce dramatic clinical improvement. Such therapy is usually associated with untoward effects of hyperbaric O_2.
   ii. Some authorities without hyperbaric chambers have reported acceptable mortality rates.
   iii. Expert surgical and medical management and control of complications are the most important factors in the treatment of gas gangrene.

Chapter 24

Cholera

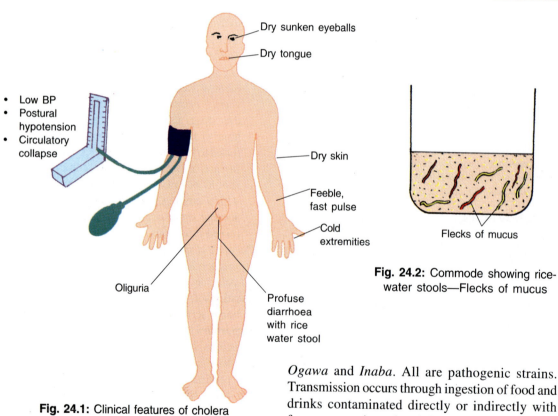

Fig. 24.1: Clinical features of cholera

Fig. 24.2: Commode showing rice-water stools—Flecks of mucus

CHOLERA

Cholera is an acute diarrhoeal illness caused by *vibrio cholerae* OI or *V. cholerae* U139. The two biotypes—classical and *El Tor* are major causes of cholera. Each biotype has two serotypes— *Ogawa* and *Inaba*. All are pathogenic strains. Transmission occurs through ingestion of food and drinks contaminated directly or indirectly with faeces or vomitus of an infected person (feco-oral route).

It is secretory acute watery diarrhoea produced by the action of exotoxins elaborated by V. cholera producing loss of fluids and electrolytes resulting in dehydration, acidosis, hyponatremia, hypokalaemia and renal failure as a complication.

Clinical Features (Fig. 24.1)

Cholera is a disease of children (most common during 1-5 years of age). The incubation period is few hours to 6 days.

The disease may be mild or remain asymptomatic but typical cholera presents with severe diarrhoea without pain or colic followed by vomiting. Following the evacuation of normal gut faecal contents, typical 'rice-water' material is passed consisting of clear fluid with flecks of mucus floating in the watery stool (Fig. 24.2). Classical cholera produces significant loss of fluids and electrolytes resulting in dehydration with muscle cramps. Later on, shock and oliguria (acute renal failure), develop but mental clarity is preserved. Improvement is rapid with proper treatment. Death occurs due to acute circulatory collapse in untreated patients. The clinical hallmarks of cholera are given in the Box 24.1.

Box 24.1: Clinical hallmarks of cholera
- Rapid onset of symptoms
- Profuse watery diarrhoea (liquid stools) typical rice-water stool
- Absence of fever
- Occasional vomiting
- Symptoms and signs of dehydration, hypovolaemic shock, acute renal failure, acidosis, hypokalaemia

Diagnosis

Diagnosis is easy during an epidemic and depends on clinical features. Confirmation is done by bacteriological culture of the stool for isolation, identification of agents—V. cholerae 01 and 0139 and antibiotic sensitivity. Stool specimens or rectal swabs must be taken for culture before antibiotic therapy.

It is better to collect the specimen and place it immediately in the transport medium viz *Cary-Blair, Venkataraman Ramkrishnan fluid (V.R. fluid)*. If transport medium is not available, then blotting paper strips soaked in liquid stool may be preserved in sealed plastic bags.

Management

Management of cholera is similar to acute watery diarrhoea from other causes (Read also acute diarrhoea as an emergency). The main aim of treatment is to maintain circulation by adequate replacement of fluids and electrolytes. It should be accomplished as early as possible to reduce the risk of hypovolaemic shock. The steps of treatment are:

1. Assessment of dehydration (e.g. restlessness, irritability, sunken eyeballs, dry tongue, excessive thirst, dry skin, weak pulse and low blood pressure).
2. Rehydration therapy: Rehydration is mainly oral by oral rehydration solution (ORS), but intravenous fluids therapy is necessary for severely dehydrated patients and for those with acidosis (pH < 7.2).

Replacement of fluids by ORS is highly effective and saves countless lives of dehydrated patients. The components of ORS are given in the Box 24.2. The fluid therapy and its type depend on the degree of dehydration:

1. **Mildly dehydrated patients** need ORS (75 ml/kg in 4 hours). Reassess after 4 hours and then further treatment depends on degree of dehydration. Hydration can be maintained by allowing liberal amount of fluids as much as he/she can take.
2. **Severely ill dehydrated patients** need I.V. Ringer's lactate and the diarrhoea treatment solution (NaCl 4.0 g, sodium acetate 6.5 g, KCl 1.0 g and glucose 9.0 g/L). If not available then normal saline (100 ml/kg I.V. in 3 hours and in 6 hours in infants), 30% of fluid rapidly within half an hour followed by ORS as soon as the patient can drink orally. Rehydration can be maintained after correction of dehydration by adequate amount of fluids in adults; 100 ml of fluid after each stool in < 2 years old; 200 ml after each loose stool in 2-9 years old.

- *Electrolytes to be monitored during treatment.*
- *Frequent assessment of dehydration to be done.*

114 Infections

Box 24.2: Oral rehydration solutions

Content	WHO/* UNICEF	Cereal based ORS*	UK/Europe ORS**
Sodium (mmol/L)	90	90	35-60
Potassium (mmol/L)	20	20	20
Chloride (mmol/L)	80	80	37
Bicarbonate (mmol/L)	—	—	90-200
Glucose (mmol/L)	111	—	90-200
Citrate (mmol/L)	10	10	10
Rice (g/L)	—	50-80	—

* Used in cholera
** ORS currently recommended in children UK/Europe

The maintenance of hydration by replacement of ongoing fluid losses to be continued until diarrhoea stops.

3. *Antibiotics:* Antibiotics are generally not essential for most of the cases of cholera but should be used in severely dehydrated patients. They reduce the loss of amount of fluids and duration of diarrhoea and shorten the period of V-cholera excretion. Tetracycline (250-500 mg 6 hourly for 3 days) or doxycycline (300 mg as a single dose) or ciprofloxacin 1g/day as single dose for 3 days are effective to eradicate the infection. Recently during an epidemic of cholera in Delhi (2000), the antimicrobial agents effective against both V. cholerae 01 and V. cholerae 0139 were nalidixic acid and furazolidine followed by cotrimoxazole.
4. *Feeding:* Feeding should be continued to the extent possible. Normal diet should be instituted as soon as vomiting stops. Breastfeeding in infants should be continued uninterruptedly even during rehydration with ORS.

Prevention

- Strict personal hygiene (wash your hands after defecation and before preparing and eating food. Use soap for washing hands).
- Drink water from a safe source or use boiled water or disinfected water.
- Store drinking water in clean, covered and narrow mouthed container.
- Avoid raw and uncooked food. Cook food thoroughly and eat it while it is hot.
- Keep the flies away from food.
- Old parenteral cholera vaccines are of limited use because of low efficacy and short duration of protection. New generation cholera vaccines (WC/rBS and CVD 103-HgR) provide convincing protection. The WC/rBS vaccine is given orally in 2 doses, 10-14 days apart, confers 80-90% protection for 6 months.
The level of protection is still about 50%, 3 years after immunisation in those who were > 5 years of age at the time of vaccination.
The vaccine is indicated in population believed to be at imminent risk (within a period of 6 months) of a cholera in an epidemic, but not to contain an epidemic once it has occurred. WC/rBS is currently licenced is some countries but is not available in India as yet.
- Mass chemoprophylaxis, immunisation with conventional parenteral vaccines and cordon sanitaire are useful measures during an epidemic but all are ineffective in preventing and controlling the epidemic.

Chapter 25

Bacterial Food Poisoning

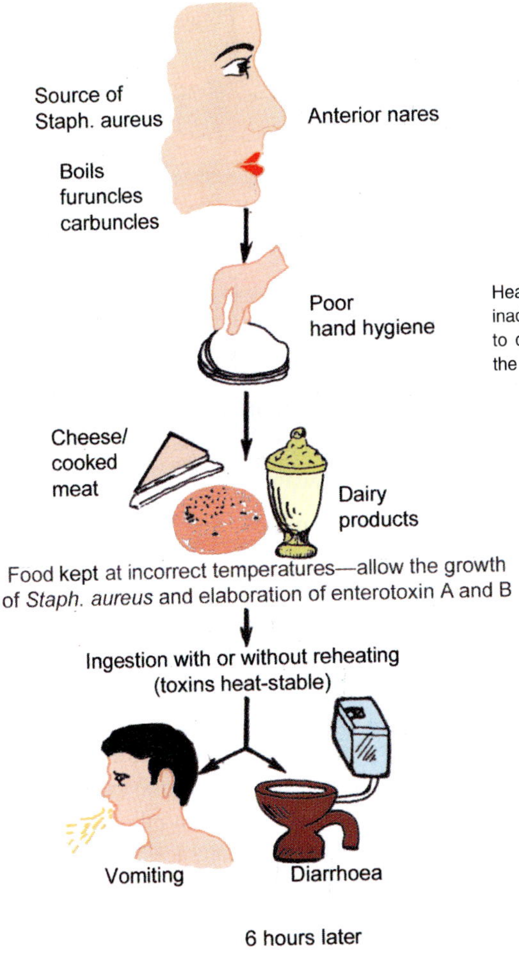

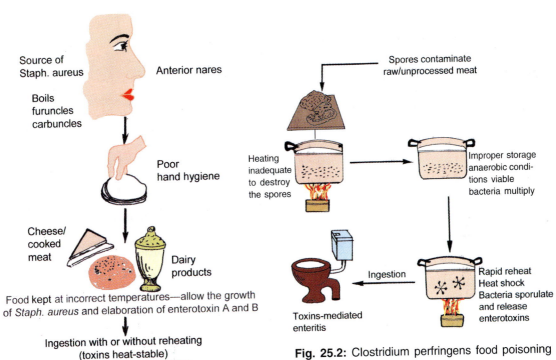

Fig. 25.1: Staphylococcal food poisoning

Fig. 25.2: Clostridium perfringens food poisoning

BACTERIAL FOOD POISONING

Bacterial food poisoning or enterocolitis is an acute short-lived infection of the intestine due to a wide variety of organisms. It is characterized by fever, malaise, cramping abdominal pain, bloody diarrhoea and vomiting. Occasionally cholera like picture may be present. The incubation period of this illness is

116 Infections

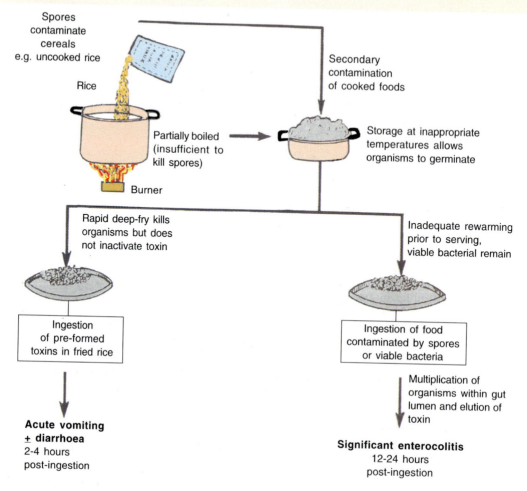

Fig. 25.3: Bacillus cereus bacterial food poisoning

variable. It is self-limiting illness that lasts for 2-3 days.

Aetiology and Clinical Features

They are given in the Box 25.1.

Staph. aureus is a common commensal in the anterior nares. Poor hygiene is the cause Transmission occurs via the food handlers who do not keep up hygiene to the food stuffs especially dairy products, cheese and cooked meat. Inappropriate storage of these eatables allows the growth of the organisms and production of one or more heat-stable exotoxins (Fig. 25.1).

Spores of C. perfringens are widespread in the gut of large animals and in soil. If contaminated meat products are incompletely cooked and stored in anaerobic conditions, spores germinate and viable organisms multiply. Sporulation is associated with production of enterotoxins. Botulism (food poisoning by *C. botulinum*) occurs due to ingestion of contaminated food stuffs, commonly the canned meat, fish and preserved vegetables (Fig. 25.2).

Bacillus cereus causes food poisoning by ingestion of pre-formed toxins in the contaminated food (Fig. 25.3). Fried rice or freshly prepared vanila sauces are frequent sources. The organisms grow and produce exotoxins during storge. The

Bacterial Food Poisoning

Box 25.1: Bacterial causes of acute diarrhoea (food poisoning)

Pathogen	Source	Clinical features	Investigations	Recovery
Staphylococcus aureus	Contaminated food or other eatables	Incubation period 2-6 hours. Diarrhoea, vomiting and dehydration are symptoms	Culture the organisms in vomitus or stool	Rapid within few hours
Bacillus cereus	Spores in food (often rice) resistant to boiling	Incubation period is 1-6 hours. Diarrhoea, vomiting and dehydration occur	Culture the organism in stool and food	Rapid
Clostridium perfringens	Spores in food survive boiling	Incubation period is 8-20 hours. Watery diarrhoea and abdominal cramps occur (toxin-induced enteritis) "Point source" outbreaks, in which a number of cases become symptomatic following ingestion, classically occurs following school or canteen lunches where meat stews are served	Culture the organisms in faeces and food	2-3 days
Clostridium botulinum	Canned or bottled food. Spores survive cooking and germinate in anaerobic conditions	Incubation period is long (24-36 hours). Brief diarrhoea and gut paralysis due to neuromuscular block by neurotoxin. There is bulbar or ocular nerves palsies (difficulty in swallowing, blurred or double vision, proptosis)	Demonstration of toxins in food and stool	10-14 days
Salmonella enteritidis (phage type 4), sometimes S. typhimurium	Bowel of animals Contaminated food and water	Incubation period is 12-24 hours. Fever vomiting and diarrhoea ($\pm$ blood) occur	Culture the organism in stool	Usually 2-5 days but may take 2 weeks
Campylobacter jejuni	Bowel of animals especially fowls; and cattle (Zoonotic infection). The most common source of infection is meat such as chicken or contaminated milk product	Incubation period is longest (1-3 days). Fever, pain abdomen and diarrhoea with or without blood occur. Campylobacter species have been linked to Guillain-Barré syndrome and reactive arthritis	Culture the organism in stool	3-5 days

Contd.

118 Infections

Contd.

Pathogen	Source	Clinical features	Investigations	Recovery
Vibrio cholera (enterotoxins)	Contaminated food and eatables	Incubation period is few hours to few days. Profuse, painless, watery diarrhoea (rice water stools), dehydration, hypotension or shock are its manifestations	Stool culture for organisms	Variable (may be fatal)
Chemical *(toxin produced by fishes)*				
• Shellfish toxin (Saxitoxin)	Ingestion of fish	Consumption produces gastrointestinal symptoms within 30 minutes followed by respiratory paralysis		
• Ciguatera fish poisoning (ciguatoxin)	Consumption of fish	Incubation period is 1-6 hours, G.I. symptoms are associated with paraesthesias of lips and extremities, distorted temperature sensation, myalgia, progressive flaccid paralysis	—	The gastrointestinal symptoms resolve rapidly but neuropathic features may persist for months
• Scomprotoxic fish poisoning (histamine and other chemicals)	Ingestion of fish-tuna bonito, skip jack and canned dark meat of sardines	Symptoms are immediate, occur within minutes, include flushing, burning, sweating urticaria, pruritis, colic nausea, vomiting and diarrhoea, bronchospasm and hypotension	—	Symptoms resolve with treatment with antihistamines and salbutamol; I.V. fluid replacement cures dehydration

Note: Toxins found in fishes or shellfish can produce food poisoning (by ingestion)

"Chinese restaurant syndrome" is caused by this organism, characterised by rapid onset of vomiting within hours of food ingestion followed by some diarrhoea.

Management

It is an emergency. Patient needs replacement of fluids and electrolytes to prevent the development of peripheral circulatory failure. The steps of management include:

1. **Fluid and electrolytes:** The patient should be given fluids to compensate the fluid loss in the stools and to correct dehydration which is commonly present in these cases. The pulse, BP, temperature and urinary output should be monitored. The electrolytes should be monitored and corrected accordingly.

2. **Antibiotics:** Specific treatment of bacterial diarrhoea includes oxytetracycline (500 mg after every 6 hours) for shigellae infection and ciprofloxacin 500 mg bid for E. coli, salmonella or other bacterial diarrhoea. Metronidazole 400-800 mg tid is effective against anaerobes.

Conventionally, it is better to start with ciprofloxacin *plus* metronidazole in such an acute situation so as to cover most of the causative organisms till a final report of stool culture is received. Parenteral antibiotic therapy is indicated if patient is not accepting orally. The treatment is continued for few days. Depending on the response, most of the patients show rapid recovery.

3. *Anticholinergic and antimotility* drugs have no role.

Chapter 26

Acute Dysentery

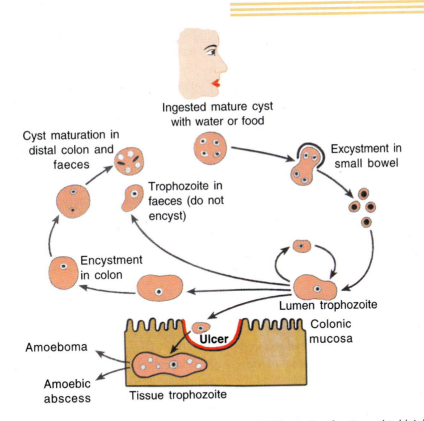

Fig. 26.1: Pathogenesis of amoebic dysentery with life cycle of entamoeba histolytica

ACUTE DYSENTERY

Acute dysentery is an acute inflammation of the large intestine characterised by diarrhoea with blood and mucus in the stool. Its causes are bacillary or amoebic infection. It has to be differentiated from bloody diarrhoea which may be due to infections and noninfectious causes (Read acute diarrhoea).

120 Infections

Box 26.1: Distinguishing features of two common types of dysentery

Amoebic dysentery (Fig. 26.1)	Bacillary dysentery
1. 4-8 motions (< 10 motions/day)	8-12 motions (> 10 motions/day)
2. Fairly large stools with streaks of dark blood and mucus seen on the surface	Small amount of stools mixed with fresh blood and mucus
3. Offensive (foul smelling) and acidic stools	Odourless, alkaline stools "red current Jelly"
4. Stools are semisolid or viscid, stick to the container or latrine sheet	Liquid or semisolid stools do not stick to the container
5. Tenesmus is not usual	Tenesmus is usual
6. A lot of mucus, scanty pus and RBCs present. Charcot layden crystals present. Trophozoites with ingested RBCs may be present	Microscopically, stool contain numerous pus cells, RBCs and macrophages with ingested RBCs. No charcot layden crystals. Few bacteria visible
7. Tenderness over the whole colon (diffuse)	Tenderness over the left colon and caecum
8. Fever, weakness but usually no signs of dehydration	Fever with dehydration and weakness common

Clinical Features

The clinical features between two types of dysentery are summarised in the Box 26.1.

Diagnosis

The diagnosis of acute dysentery is based on the clinical features and confirmation is done by stool examination and stool culture. Mixed infection (amoebic plus bacillary) is also common which will have features of both types of dysentery i.e. patient experiences acute bowel symptoms with more frequent stools, the passage of much blood and mucus. There may be fever with chills and rigors.

Management

The bacillary dysentery has to be differentiated from amoebic dysentery from therapeutic point of view (See Box 26.1). The stools are to be examined for trophozoites, pus cells, RBCs and culture be immediately sent. The steps of management include.

1. *Assessment of dehydration* should be done and oral rehydration therapy may be started if dysentery is mild or moderate. In severe cases, intravenous fluids and electrolytes should be given to correct fluid and electrolyte deficit. The pulse, BP, urine output, temperature and electrolytes be monitored.

2. *Antimicrobial therapy:* Ciprofloxacin 500 mg bid for 3 days is effective in bacillary dysentry, while amoebic dysentery needs metronidazole 800 mg 8 hourly for 5 days or tinidazole single dose of 2 g daily for 3 days. Diloxanide furoate 500 mg should be given orally 8 hourly for 10 days to eliminate the luminal cyst.

Parenteral antibiotics may be given if patient has associated vomiting or cannot take orally or has serious illness.

Before starting specific treatment and before the stool culture report, an empirical treatment with ciprofloxacin *plus* metronidazole or tinidazole is advised. The treatment is to be revised after report of stool culture.

Chapter 27

Cerebral Malaria

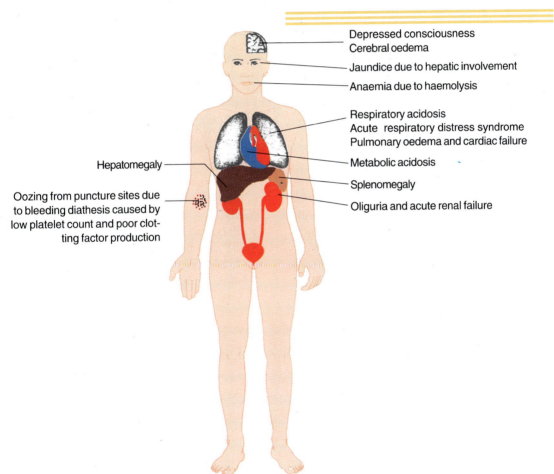

Fig. 27.1: Organ involvement in cerebral malaria

CEREBRAL MALARIA

Cerebral malaria is defined as an unarousable coma (for more than 6 hours after a generalised convulsion in adults) in the presence of a *P. falciparum* parasitaemia after correction of hypoglycaemia and exclusion of other encephalopathies.

It results from engorgement of cerebral capillaries and venules with parasitized and non-parasitized RBCs. As falciparum malaria attacks all stages of RBCs, hence, there is heavy parasitization, and red cells containing schizonts adhere to capillary (cytoadherence) in brain and other organs leading to vascular occlusion making them anoxic or hypoxic. Rupture of schizonts liberates toxic and antigenic substances which trigger cytokines production which may cause further damage. High levels of cytokine "tissue necrosis factor-TNF". upregulates the nitrous oxide synthetase activity. It is possible that large amounts of nitrous oxide produced locally due to sequestration of parasitized RBCs, diffuses across the wall of the affected cerebral vessels into the brain parenchyma where it interferes with the calcium influx mechanisms and synaptic transmission leading to coma.

> **Box 27.1: WHO criteria for severe falciparum malaria**
>
> - Cerebral malaria (unexplained unarousable coma)
> - Severe anaemia (Hb < 5 g/dl or haematocrit < 15%)
> - Renal failure (oliguria—urine output < 400 ml/day or < 12 ml/kg/day plus serum creatinine > 3 mg/dl or 265 μmol/L)
> - Pulmonary oedema (ARDS, hypoxaemia, respiratory failure)
> - Hypoglycaemia (whole blood glucose < 40 mg/dl or 2.2 mmol/L)
> - Circulatory collapse (systolic BP < 70 mmHg with cold clammy extremities)
> - Spontaneous bleeding and DIC (prolonged PT, PTT) and thrombocytopenia
> - Repeated generalised convulsions (> 3 in 24 hours)
> - Acidaemia (arterial pH < 7.25) or acidosis (plasma bicarbonate <15 mmol/L)
> - Haemoglobinura (not drug induced)
> - Jaundice (icterus or serum bilirubin > 3 mg/dl)
> - Hyperparasitaemia (> 5% in nonimmune patients or > 10,000/ml)

Clinical Features (Fig. 27.1)

Cerebral malaria is the most severe form of P. falciparum malaria with high levels of parasitaemia. The WHO criteria for severe malaria are given in the Box 27.1. About 1% patients with P. falciparum infection develop cerebral malaria or severe malaria.

Cerebral malaria is a diffuse encephalopathy in which focal neurological signs are unusual though reported in Indian series. Coma is a characteristic and ominous feature of falciparum malaria and carries high mortality rates (20% in adults and 15% in children). Therefore lesser degree of disturbance in consciousness barring coma should be taken seriously. The onset may be gradual or sudden following a convulsion. The following symptoms and signs occur in cerebral malaria:

1. *Symptoms:*
   - Fever, high grade, irregular.
   - Convulsions—generalised, common among children.
   - Disturbance in consciousness lapsing into coma.
   - Petechial haemorrhage in skin and mucous membrane occur rarely.
   - Haemetemesis presumably from stress ulcerations or acute gastric erosions can occur.
2. *Signs:*
   - Pulse rate is fast (tachycardia).
   - BP may be normal or low.
   - *Neurological manifestations* include signs of meningism (passive resistance to head flexion) but not of meningitis, divergent eyeballs and pout reflex are common. Other primitive reflexes are absent. Corneal reflexes are preserved except in deep coma. The pupils are normal and react to light. Motor system examination reveals variable muscle tone and deep tendon reflex are usually brisk and the plantar reflexes are usually extensor (UMN signs) but at times flexor. The superficial reflexes (abdominal and cremasteric) are absent. In advanced stages of the disease, there may be generalised hypertonia, opisthotonus and abnormal posturing in the form of decerebrate or decorticate rigidity.
   - *Associated other signs;* such as anaemia, jaundice, acidotic breathing, bleeding due to

DIC, tachypnoea and tachycardia (due to ARDS) and/or oliguria (due to acute renal failure).
- Hepatosplenomegaly.

Diagnosis

Diagnosis of cerebral malaria depends on the clinical manifestations (already discussed), the severity of falciparum infection to be decided by WHO criteria and confirmation of the diagnosis is done by demonstration of asexual forms (ring stage in case of falciparum) of the parasite in thick and thin film of peripheral blood. The parasite load or degree of parasitaemia is seen in thin film as percentage of infected red cells in PBF. Immuno chromatographic 'dipstick' tests for P. falciparum antigen are now available for detection of this infection. They should be used in parallel with blood film examination but are less sensitive than a carefully examined blood film. Other tests are done to detect complications. Hypoglycaemia is common.

Management

Severe malaria is a medical emergency and cerebral malaria is the common presentation and cause of death in adults. The management of severe malaria or cerebral malaria include:
1. Early appropriate antimalarial therapy.
2. Active treatment of complications or severe manifestations.
3. Correction of fluid, electrolyte and acid-base disturbances.
4. Avoidance of harmful ancillary treatments.
5. Supportive measures and care of unconscious patient.

1. *Appropriate antimalarial therapy:* Quinine is the drug of choice. Intravenous quinine is given as an infusion of 20 mg/kg over a period of 4 hours as a loading dose, followed by 10 mg/kg after every 8 hours till patient regains consciousness and starts accepting orally. Oral therapy (10 mg/kg after every 8 hours) to be given as soon as patient can take orally and be continued for total of 10 days including parenteral therapy. The loading dose should not be given if the patient has received quinine outside during the previous 24 hours. Tinnitus, nystagmus and ECG changes (prolonged QRS duration and QTc interval) should be looked for especially in the cardiac patients; and the dose of quinine reduced if these are present.

In some areas, the Chinese drugs derived from artemisinin (artemether, artesunate) have become first-line treatment for severe malaria as controlled trials have shown comparable efficacy of parenteral quinine and intramuscular artemether. In quinine-resistant cases, the artesunate or artemether is drug of choice. Artesunate should be given as a loading dose of 2.4 mg/kg I.V. or I.M. stat followed by 1.2 mg/kg (not exceeding 600 mg) at 12 and 24 hours interval and then daily. Artemether dose is 3.2 mg/kg (loading dose) I.M. stat then 1.6 mg/kg I.M. daily. Mefloquine should not be used for severe malaria as no parenteral formulation is available.

2. *Severe manifestations and complications of falciparum malaria* are to be actively treated as given in the Table 27.1.
3. *Maintenance of fluid, electrolyte and acid-base balance:* Intravenous fluids are given to replace fluid loss. If hypotension or shock present, saline should be given. 25% dextrose to be given in case hypoglycaemia develops. Blood transfusions to correct severe hemolytic anaemia and sodium bicarbonate for metabolic acidosis may be needed. Blood sugar, pH and electrolytes are to be monitored.
4. *Avoidance of ancillary treatments such as corticosteroids:* Decongestive therapy, low molecular dextran, heparin and adrenaline should be avoided as they have been proved of no value and even may be harmful.
5. *Care of unconscious patient:* Care of the skin, bowel and bladder should be taken. Frequent change of position, self-retaining catheter to measure urinary output and maintenance of pulse, BP and temperature chart should be undertaken.

Radical cure and chemoprophylaxis of malaria—Read antimalarial drugs.

124 Infections

Table 27.1: Management of complications/manifestations of falciparum infection

Lesion	Treatment
Coma (cerebral malaria)	• Maintain patent airway • Exclude other causes of coma (e.g. hypoglycaemia, bacterial meningitis) • Nursing on the side position • Care of skin, bowel, bladder • Monitor pulse and BP
Hypoglycaemia	• Measure blood glucose • Give 25-50% glucose injection stat followed by 10% glucose infusion
Hyperpyrexia	• Parenteral antipyretic • Cold sponging, fanning etc.
Convulsions	• Parenteral diazepam or phenobarbitone • Maintain patent airway
Severe anaemia and thrombocytopenia	• Transfuse fresh whole blood, packed cells, platelet concentrates
Acute pulmonary oedema	• Prop up position • Give O_2, diuretics • Stop I.V. fluids • Intubate and add PEEP/CPAP in life-threatening hypoxaemia • Haemofilteration
Acute renal failure	• Exclude pre-renal cause • Check fluid balance and urinary sodium • Give diuretics and dopamine if urine output falls • Peritoneal dialysis, haemofiltration or haemodialysis if available
Spontaneous bleeding and DIC	• Transfuse fresh whole blood/cryoprecipitate/fresh frozen plasma and platelets if available • Injection vitamin K
Metabolic acidosis	• Exclude or treat hypoglycaemia, hypovolaemia and gram-negative septicaemia • Give O_2
Shock	• Consider gram-negative septicaemia • Take blood cultures • Give parenteral antibiotics • Correct haemodynamic disturbances • Monitor pulse, BP, urine output
Aspiration pneumonia	• Take X-ray • Give parenteral antibiotics • Change posture • Physiotherapy • O_2 inhalation
Heavy parasitaemia e.g > 15% of circulating erythrocytes in a patient with malaria	Consider exchange transfusion

Part Four

Cardiology

Chapter 28

Acute ST-Elevation Myocardial Infarction (STEMI)

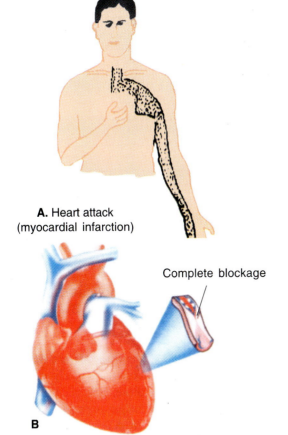

A. Heart attack (myocardial infarction)

B

Fig. 28.1: (A) A patient of acute MI showing character of pain by thrusting the fist into anterior chest at the site of pain and radiation of pain to left arm and forearm (B) Coronary angiogram showing coronary occlusion (diagram)—a common cause of acute MI

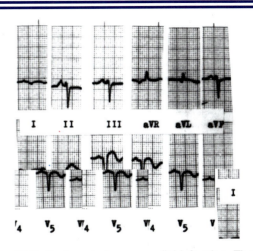

Fig. 28.2: Acute anterior myocardial infarction. The ECG showing ST elevation, QS pattern from V_1-V_6 and T wave intervion. There is left axis deviation (left anterior hemiblock)

ACUTE ST-ELEVATION MYOCARDIAL INFARCTION (STEMI)

Definition

Myocardial infarction is characterised by acute cardiac pain due to sudden and complete occlusion of a coronary artery due to thrombus. The thrombus is formed at the site of rupture of an atheromatous plaque in a coronary artery. The present hospital mortality of AMI is 6.5% which is significantly decreased from prethrombolytic era. Spontaneous thrombolysis can occur but takes time, and by this time, the damage has already

128 Cardiology

occurred, therefore, induced thrombolysis (revascularisation) is the mainstay of treatment now-a-days.

The myocardial infarction is more common in those having one or more risk factors enumerated in the Box 28.1.

Box 28.1: Risk factors for AMI

- Age (old age)
- Smoking
- Sex (males are more prone)
- Mental stress
- Family history
- Obesity
- Hypertension
- Hypercholestrolaemia
- Polyunsaturated fatty acid deficiency
- Diabetes mellitus
- Sedentary habits
- Hyperfibrinogenaemia and hyperhomocysteinaemia
- Low levels of antioxidant vitamins
- Low levels of protein C and S

Clinical Features

The myocardial infarction is characterised by typical anginal pain which is more severe and prolonged, radiates to left arm or to other sites and is associated with signs and symptoms of sympathetic overactivity (Fig. 28.1). About 25% of AMI may have atypical symptoms such as atypical chest pain, nausea, vomiting, dyspnoea, fatigue, exhaustion, etc. Myocardial infarction may also masquerade as the development or worsening of CHF, appearance of an arrhythmia (more common in anterior MI), an overwhelming sense of apprehension, profound exhaustion, acute indigestion, pericarditis, stroke or peripheral embolism. The symptoms and signs are given in the Box 28.2.

Diagnosis

It is very important to examine the patient of acute myocardial infarction before embarking on the treatment. The diagnosis of MI suspected clinically must be confirmed by ECG (Fig. 28.2), cardiac enzymes and/or radioisotope studies. For detection of complication, echocardiogram and X-ray chest may be carried out.

Management

It is divided under three heads:

Box 28.2: Myocardial infarction

A. **Symptoms**
   i. Prolonged and severe retrosternal chest pain radiating to left arm, throat, shoulder, epigastrium and back
   ii. Anxiety, fear, apprehension of impending death
   iii. Nausea, vomiting, sweating
   iv. Dyspnoea
   v. Giddiness or syncope or collapse

B. **Signs**
   i. *Signs of sympathetic overactivity* usually present, e.g. pallor, perspiration, tachycardia
   ii. *Signs of vagal stimulation* may be present as in inferior wall infarction, e.g. bradycardia
   iii. *Signs of myocardial dysfunction* and/or left heart failure may be evident if complicated:
       - Cold extremities, hypotension or shock
       - Oliguria
       - Low volume pulse, low pulse pressure
       - Quiet first heart sound
       - Diffuse apical thrust. Mid-systolic murmur of papillary muscles dysfunction may be present
       - Fine crepts at the bases
   iv. *Signs of tissue damage,* e.g. fever, leucocytosis and raised ESR
   v. *Signs of pericarditis,* e.g. pericardial rub may be present

1. Management of uncomplicated AMI:
   - Pre-hospital management.
   - In-hospital management.
2. Management of complications of AMI.
3. Secondary prevention of infarction.

I. Management of Uncomplicated AMI (See the Algorithm i.e. Fig. 28.3)

Pre-hospital management

Most out-of-hospital deaths from MI are due to development of arrhythmias (particularly ventricular fibrillation). Out of these, 50% occur in first one hour. Therefore, the major steps in management of suspected AMI in developed countries include:
   i. Recognition of the symptoms by the patient
   ii. Rapid deployment of an equipped emergency ambulance to provide advanced cardiac life support.

Acute ST-Elevation Myocardial Infarction (STEMI)

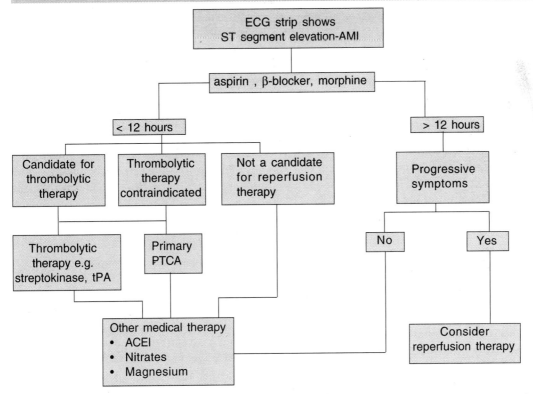

Fig. 28.3: Algorithm for management of ST segment elevation myocardial infarction (STEMI)

iii. Expeditious transportation of the patient to a hospital.

Pre-hospital Treatment Includes

a. Routine measures.
b. Aspirin.
c. Nitrates.
d. Thrombolysis.
   a. ***Routine immediate measures include:***
   - High-flow O_2.
   - I.V. access
     Nitroglycerine (0.3 mg) or isosorbide dinitrate (5 mg) sublingual to be given to relieve pain before morphine. The dose can be repeated at 5 minutes interval upto 3-4 doses. If no relief occurs after 15 minutes, patient should be hospitalised.
   - ECG monitoring and a 12-lead ECG.
   - Analgesia (opiates) and an antiemetic—

Adequate analgesia is essential not only to relieve severe distress, but also to lower adrenergic drive and thereby reduce pulmonary and systemic vascular resistance. Intravenous morphine 10 mg and an antiemetic (prochlorperazine 12.5 mg or cyclizine 50 mg) should be given stat through a cannula and to be titrated according to the response.

b. ***Aspirin:*** Oral administration of 75-300 mg of aspirin daily improves survival by 25% on its own, hence, is called '*poor man*'s streptokinase' and enhances the effect of thrombolytic therapy. The first tablet of 300 mg to be given in a soluble or chewable form and then daily dose should be continued indefinitely if there are no contraindications.

c. ***Nitrates.***

d. ***Acute reperfusion by thrombolysis:*** Earlier the thrombolysis, better the prognosis and the maximum benefit is achieved when it is given within first one to two hours. So, if possible, thrombolysis can be done out-of-hospital in a well-equipped ambulance by the trained staff.

In-hospital Management

Accidental and emergency department

1. *Routine measures include;* bed-rest, O_2 therapy, administration of analgesia and intravenous nitroglycerin if pain or ST segment elevation persists. Before morphine is administered, sublingual nitroglycerin (0.3 mg) or isosorbide dinitrate (5 mg) can be given. Upto 3-4 doses at an interval of 5 minutes can be given. Nitrates reduce myocardial O_2 demand (reduce preload) and increase myocardial O_2 uptake (by dilating the infarct-related artery or collateral vessels). If response occurs, nitroglycerin infusion (0.6-1.2 mg/hr) is given to relieve ongoing ischaemia diagnosed by persistent chest pain. Nitrates are avoided in hypotension and inferior or right ventricular infarction.

2. *Intravenous beta blockers*: They are useful in the control of the pain of AMI by reducing myocardial O_2 demand and hence ischaemia. Most important, there is evidence that I.V. beta blockers reduce in-hospital mortality. A commonly employed regimen is I.V. metoprolol 5 mg every 2 to 5 minutes or atenolol 5 mg given over 5 minutes for a total of 3 doses provided the patient has heart rate > 60/min and BP > 100 mmHg and P-R interval < 0.24 sec. Fifteen minutes after the last dose, an oral regimen consisting of 50 mg 6 hourly for 48 hours followed by 100 mg after every 12 hours may be started.

> *Avoid beta blockers if there is heart failure, heart block or severe bradycardia.*

Unlike betablockers, calcium channel blockers are of little help in AMI, rather they may be detrimental.

3. Aspirin (75-300 mg/day) and/or clopidogrel 75 mg/day.

4. Acute reperfusion (e.g. thrombolysis, primary percutaneous coronary intervention).

Thrombolysis: Coronary thrombolysis helps to restore coronary patency, preserves left ventricular function and improves survival. Mortality related benefit is maximum if window period is less than 6 hours. Beyond a period of 12 hours, there is no rationale for administration of thrombolytic therapy. Between 6-12 hours it has been realised that it may be beneficial in those selected patients who have on-going chest pain and persistent ST segment elevation of at least 1 mm in atleast two contiguous leads on ECG.

> *The benefit of thrombolysis is more in anterior myocardial infarction, non-diabetic patients and younger subjects (< 55 years of age).*

The thrombolytic agents i.e. tissue plasminogen activator (tPA), streptokinase and anisoylated plasminogen streptokinase activator complex (APSAC) have been approved by FDA for intravenous use in acute MI. These drugs act by promoting the conversion of plasminogen to plasmin which lyse the fibrin clot (fibrinolysis). The principal goal is prompt restoration of coronary arterial patency (TIMI-grade 3 flow).

"Streptokinase 1.5 million units in 100 ml of saline given as an I.V. infusion over a period of one hour, is a widely used regimen. It is cheap but antigenic and occasionally causes serious allergic reaction. The drug may cause hypotension, which can often be managed by stopping the infusion and restarting at a slower rate. Being antigenic, it induces antibodies which can render subsequent infusions of streptokinase ineffective, so it is advisable to use another non-antigenic agent if the patient requires further thrombolysis in future. The summary of thrombolytic therapy is given in Box 28.3.

Alteplase (human tissue plasminogen activator or tPA) is a genetically engineered drug, which is not antigenic but is more expensive than streptokinase. It seldom causes hypotension.

Acute ST-Elevation Myocardial Infarction (STEMI)

> **Box 28.3: Streptokinase therapy**
> - **Maximum benefit** is achieved when administered within few hours (< 6 hours) of infarction with ST segment elevation in more than 2 leads without Q waves.
> - **Thrombolysis** is not beneficial in patients with ST segment depression and even may be harmful.
> - **Parameters of success of thrombolysis** include:
>   — Relief of pain.
>   — Significant reduction (> 70%) or complete resolution of elevated ST segment.
>   — Transient arrhythmias e.g. idioventricular rhythm.
> - **The drawback and disadvantage of thrombolytic therapy** include stroke (1%), bleeding (7%) and re-infarction (5%).

Many ICU use tPA if streptokinase is contraindicated but there is evidence that it produces better survival rates than streptokinase.

The standard regimen given over 90 minutes includes bolus dose of 15 mg, followed by 0.75 mg/kg but not exceeding 50 mg over 30 minutes and then 0.5 mg/kg but not exceeding 35 mg over 60 minutes.

Tenecteplase (TNK) and *Reteplase* (rPA) are also as effective as alteplase.

The contraindication of thrombolytic therapy includes:
1. Active internal bleeding.
2. Previous subarachnoid or intracerebral bleed.
3. Uncontrolled hypertension.
4. Recent surgery (within 1 month).
5. Recent trauma.
6. Suspicion of active peptic ulcer.
7. Pregnancy.

5. *Heparin and thrombolysis*: Administration of heparin after thrombolysis with streptokinase and urokinase is controversial but it is now clear that there is no added advantage. However, heparin should perhaps be continued for 24-48 hours, when tPA is given as a thrombolytic agent.

> *Heparin is given to prevent reinfarction after successful thrombolysis and to reduce the risk of thromboembolic complications*

6. *Thrombolysis and new antiplatelet agents* such as inhibitors of platelet membrane IIb/IIIa glycoprotein fibrinogen receptor have potent antiplatelet activity and are being tested in acute ischaemic syndromes.

Primary percutaneous coronary intervention (PCI) or primary percutaneous transluminal coronary angioplasty (PTCA) without thrombolysis of the infarct-related coronary artery is a safe and effective alternative method of reperfusion therapy. The disadvantages of this therapy are that it needs sophisticated facilities, expertise, more time and more expense than thrombolysis. It is particularly suitable for patients who are high-risk cases of AMI (e.g. large infarct, cardiogenic shock) or in whom the hazards of thrombolysis are high or ineligible cases for thrombolysis.

Management in Coronary Care Units

These units are routinely equipped with a system of continuous ECG monitoring of each patient and haemodynamic monitoring of selected patients. Facilities of advanced life support, pacemaker and pacing catheters and flow-directed balloon tipped catheters are also available in addition to staff trained in the management of various aspects of AMI.

Patients should be admitted to a coronary care unit (CCU) early in their illness so that they can derive maximum benefit during the critical phase of infarction. The duration of stay in coronary care unit depends on the need for intensive monitoring. Patients in whom AMI have been ruled out should be shifted out of coronary care units after 8-12 hours of observation. Similarly patients with confirmed infarction who are considered to be at low risk (no prior infarction and no persistent chest pain or no complication and haemodynamically stable) may be safely shifted out of CCU within 24-36 hours.

Steps of Management in CCU

1. **Bed-rest** for first 12 hours is necessary in acute infarction. However, in the absence of complications, patient can resume an upright posture on bed within first 24 hours followed by sitting in a chair. Provided no complication occurs, patient can be made ambulatory in the room by the third day with increasing duration and frequency of movements. By day 4 to 5 after infarction, patient should be increasing their ambulation progressively to a goal of 600 feet at least 3 times a day.
2. **Diet:** Patient should receive either nothing or only clear fluids by mouth during first 6 to 12 hours. During first 4-5 days, a low caloric diet, low in sodium, high in K^+ and magnesium divided into multiple small frequent meals is advisable.
3. **Sedation:** Most patients require sedation in CCU in order to withstand the period of enforced inactivity with tranquillity. Diazepam (5 mg) or lorazepam (0.5 to 2 mg 3 to 4 times a day is effective. Appropriate sleeping medication may be given at night to ensure to dream free sleep. It should be given for few days.
4. **Bowels:** Constipation is a problem and occurs due to prolonged rest and use of opiates. Most patients are not comfortable using a bed pan, which frequently results in straining during defecation. A bedside commode, a fibre-rich diet, routine use of stool softener or a laxative are recommended.
5. **Other durgs (pharmacotherapy):** Several drugs are important in routine treatment of AMI. They need to be started early but may not be required on an emergency basis.
   i. *Betablockers:* They reduce both short and long-term mortality, hence, to be started as early as possible after AMI if there is no contraindication (such as heart failure, left ventricular dysfunction, heart block, orthostatic hypotension or a history of asthma).
   ii. *Angiotensin converting enzyme inhibitor (ACEI).* Now there is convincing evidence that ACEIs have additive advantages in reducing mortality in addition to those achieved with aspirin and beta blockers. Hence, recent recommendation is to start ACEI therapy in all patients of AMI within 24-48 hours, continue it during hospital phase and reassess after 4-6 weeks later to decide whether or not to continue for long-term benefits.
   iii. *Calcium channel blockers:* Current practice is not to use calcium channel blockers routinely after AMI as they have been shown to increase mortality rates.
   iv. *Nitrates:* They are beneficial in limiting the infarct size and may be used for this reason in addition to aspirin and thrombolysis. They have been shown to have added advantage over aspirin and thrombolysis. They are, otherwise, indicated in the presence of angina and heart failure (to decrease preload).
   v. *Glucose-Insulin-potassium, magnesium infusion:* Though some small studies have shown benefits, but it is difficult to justify the routine use unless a large trial show conclusive benefit. However, ISIS-IV trial has shown no benefit of such therapy.

II. Treatment of Complications of STEMI

They are given in the Table 28.1.

The common arrhythmias in acute MI are give in the box 28.4.

> **Box 28.4: Common arrhythmias in AMI**
>
> **Ventricular**
> - Ventricular premature complexes (VPCs)
> - Accelerated idioventricular rhythm
> - Ventricular tachycardia
> - Ventricular fibrillation
>
> **Atrial**
> - Atrial tachycardia
> - Sinus tachycardia
> - Atrial fibrillation
> - Sinus bradycardia especially in inferior wall infarction
> - Heart blocks

III. Secondary Prophylaxis (Secondary Prevention of Infarction)

- Control of risk factors and life-style modifications.

Acute ST-Elevation Myocardial Infarction (STEMI)

Table 28.1: Treatment of complications of STEMI

Complication	Corrective measures
I. Hypotension may result due to one or more causes	• Find out the cause and treat it accordingly. • Drugs like nitrates, betablockers and ACEI should either be stopped or their dose is reduced. • I.V. fluids and inotropic support if required. • If hypotension is due to rhythm disturbances, then correct arrhythmia. • Cardiogenic shock due to CHF is most serious cause of hypotension and also a marker of poor prognosis. Treat it urgently (Read cardiogenic shock as an emergency).
II. Arrhythmia and conduction disturbance i. VPCs	• Find out the cause and treat it accordingly. • VPCS may be asymptomatic but some forms of VPCs are markers of poor prognosis, hence, to be treated with either betablockers or amiodarone.
ii. VT	• Correction of aggravating factors such as ischaemia, electrolyte disturbance. • Antiarrhythmics like lidocaine, amiodarone. • DC shock. • VT occurring after 48 hours of AMI need long-term amiodarone or AICD implantation, while occurring within 48 hours does not require such a measure.
iii. VF	• Primary VF (occurring within 24 hours) does not alter long-term prognosis but requires immediate defibrillation. • Resistant VF may require bretylium or amiodarone. • Late VF is associated with an adverse long-term outcome and may recur, hence, use of AICD is recommended in such cases.
iv. Complete heart block (occurs in 5 to 15% cases)	• Complete heart block with idioventricular rhythm originating from infranodal or bundle of His (escape rhythm > 45/min) is common and may respond to atropine. If not responding to atropine, temporary pacing may be required. • When escape rhythm originates below the bundle of His (15-45/min), it requires an immediate pacing. • If complete heart block is persistent and irreversible, then a permanent pacemaker is indicated.

- Drug therapy such as betablockers and aspirin to be continued for life or for 5-7 years of infarction. Nitrates can be used for long-term if there is angina, left ventricular dysfunction, thrombus or recurrent sustained VT/SVT or AF.
- Revascularisation either by PTCA and adjuvant techniques like stenting, atherectomy, laser and rotablation is required in selected cases. Coronary artery bypass surgery may be required in few selected patients depending on the findings of stress-testing and angiography (e.g. left main coronary artery disease).

Chapter 29

Cardiogenic Shock

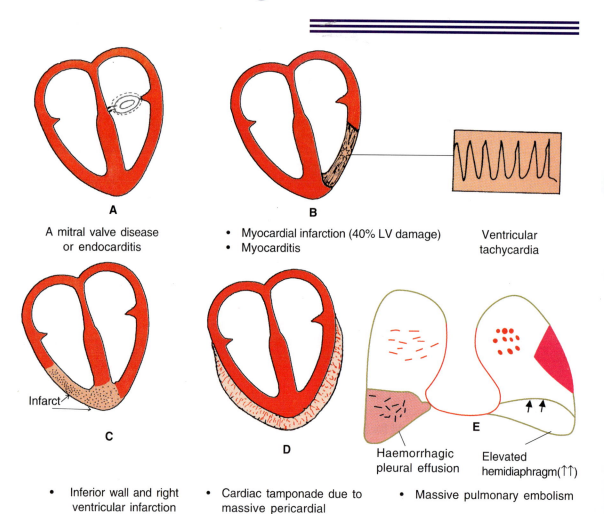

Fig. 29.1: Common conditions associated with cardiogenic shock

CARDIOGENIC SHOCK

Definition

Cardiogenic shock is a state of acute circulatory failure resulting from severe depression of cardiac performance leading to tissue hypoperfusion and dysfunction, which may become irreversible if not promptly corrected.

Haemodynamic Criteria of Cardiogenic Shock

1. Systolic BP < 90 Hg or > 60 mm fall below baseline level.
2. Cardiac index < 2.2 L/min/m^2.
3. Left ventricular filling pressure > 18 mmHg; and pulmonary oedema is usually present.

These haemodynamic parameters with clinical evidence of peripheral circulatory failure (e.g. altered mental state, cold clammy skin and oliguria with urine output < 20 ml/hr) constitute clinical syndrome of cardiogenic shock.

Causes (Fig. 29.1)

They are:
1. *Following myocardial infarction*
   i. Involvement of critical muscle mass (> 40%) and/or arrhythmias (80%).
   ii. *Mechanical complications of AMI*
      - Acute mitral regurgitation (6-7%).
      - Acquired ventricular septal defect (3-4%).
      - LV free wall rupture/tamponade.
      - Ventricular aneurysm
2. *Severe valvular lesions*
   - Severe aortic (stenosis/regurgitation) or mitral (stenosis/regurgitation) valve disease.
   - Left ventricular outflow tract obstruction obstructive cardiomyopathy.
3. *Extracardiac obstructive causes*
   - Pericardial effusion with tamponade (1-1.5% cases).
   - Massive pulmonary embolism.
   - Severe pulmonary hypertension (primary or Eisenmenger).
   - Severe restrictive cardiomyopathy.
4. *Inflammatory/infectious myocardial disease*
   - Severe myocarditis.
   - Acute endocarditis with myopathic or valvular involvement.
5. *Severe myocardial depression*
   - Septic shock.
   - Acidosis or alkalosis.
   - Hypoxia.
   - Drugs e.g. betablockers, calcium channel blockers, anaesthetics and anti-arrhythmics.
   - Post-cardiopulmonary bypass.
6. *End stage of myocardial disease*
   - Dilated cardiomyopathy
7. *Traumatic* e.g. pericardial, myocardial or valvular injuries.

Acute myocardial infarction with acute left ventricular failure is the most common cause of cardiogenic shock.

Clinical Features and their Pathogenesis

Irrespective of the cause of cardiogenic shock, it is characterised by severe myocardial (systolic and diastolic) dysfunction (Fig. 29.2). Systolic dysfunction results in fall in cardiac output, BP and thereby coronary perfusion pressure. Hypotension, oliguria, confusion or altered mental state, tachypnoea, tachycardia and cold, clammy extremities are the manifestations of low output state or acute circulatory failure.

Diastolic dysfunction causes a rise in left ventricular end-diastolic pressure, pulmonary congestion and oedema, leading to hypoxia which further worsens the myocardial ischaemia. Breathlessness, orthopnoea, PND, cyanosis, cough, haemoptysis, hypoxia, perspiration and inspiratory crackles at the bases of the lungs, and S3 and S4 gallops are features of acute pulmonary oedema. A chest X-ray may reveal signs of pulmonary oedema when clinical examination is normal. If necessary, a Swan-Ganz catheter can be used to measure the pulmonary artery wedge pressure which is > 18 mmHg.

> *Untreated shock leads to multiple organ dysfunction e.g. heart, brain, lungs, kidneys and liver.*

Diagnosis

It is based on the evidence of:
1. **Clinical features (Fig. 29.2):** The features of acute circulatory failure combined with features of the cause of cardiogenic shock such as:
   - *Acute MI* is diagnosed by cardiac pain, typical ECG changes and raised cardiac enzymes. Echocardiography will give estimate of extent of myocardial damage and is useful to detect mechanical complications such as acute MR and VSD
   - *Valvular heart lesions* are diagnosed by clinical features, echocardiography and cardiac catheterisation.
   - *Cardiac tamponade* presents with raised JVP, pulsus paradoxus and X-ray chest for pericardial effusion and echocardiography.
   - *Massive pulmonary embolism* with shock. Echocardiography may demonstrate a small vigorous left ventricle with dilated right ventricle. Sometimes a thrombus in right ventricular outflow tract may also be seen. Spiral CT confirms the diagnosis, which is now-a-day prefered over ventilation perfusion scan and pulmonary angiography.
   - *Myocarditis* is diagnosed by systemic illness supported by identification of the virus and endomyocardial biopsy can be used for confirmation.
   - *Aortic dissection* presents with classical tearing or stabbing pain with pulse deficit, acute AR and neurological manifestations. Echocardiography confirms the diagnosis.
2. **Haemodynamic parameters:** It includes BP < 80 mm, cardiac index < 1.8 L/min/m^2 and pulmonary capillary wedge pressure > 18 mmHg.
3. **Investigations:**
   - ECG and cardiac enzymes for myocardial infarction.
   - X-ray chest for signs of pulmonary oedema.
   - Arterial blood gas analysis may show hypoxaemia.
   - Echocardiogram will show depressed I.V. functions, and helps to find out the cause.

Management

1. The management of cardiogenic shock is difficult and complex and carries a mortality rate of 50-80% in spite of best resuscitative measures. The management is divided into:
   1. General principles of management of shock.
   2. Specific measures.

General Management

The major goals are:
  i. To recognise the condition as early as possible and to correct the initial insult so as to maintain adequate tissue perfusion and preservation of vital functions.
  ii. To find out and treat the underlying cause.

The steps of initial management include:
- Whenever possible, patient should be treated in ICU.
- ECG monitoring to assess heart rate and rhythm and for prompt diagnosis of arrhythmias.
- Monitoring of clinical parameters i.e. heart rate, rhythm, BP, cerebral function, skin temperature and urine output.
- Measure blood gases.
- Correct hypoxaemia.
- Consider intubation if $PaCO_2$ is > 6.5 kPa, respiratory rate > 25/min and impaired consciousness < 7 (glasgow coma scale).
- Correct acidaemia with I.V. bicarbonate if pH < 7.20 and $PaCO_2$ < 6 kPa.
- Measure CVP (off ventilator): If CVP < + 6 mmHg from mid-axillary line, give volume challenge (250 ml of normal saline or colloid). If CVP > + 6 mmHg or poor ventricular function, use 100 ml of fluid only as a challenge and consider the insertion of PA catheter to direct further treatment with

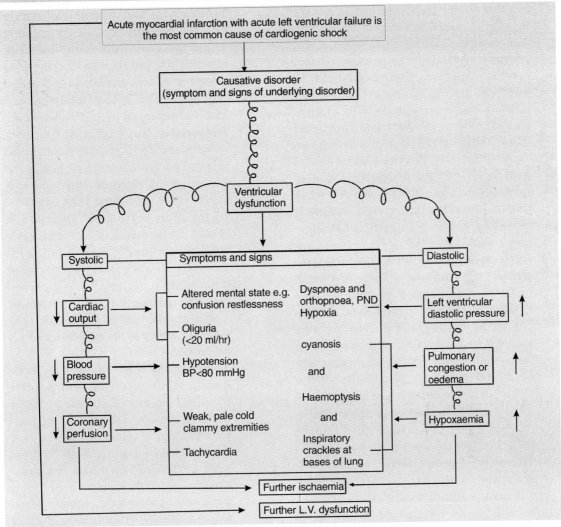

Fig. 29.2: The clinical features and their pathogenesis. The systolic dysfunction leads to fall in cardiac output, BP and coronary perfusion; while diastolic dysfunction causes pulmonary congestion and hypoxaemia

fluids and vasoactive drugs and to monitor the response to treatment.

Specific Measures

They are directed depending on the cause:

A. Cardiogenic shock due to AMI:

1. *Relief of pain and anxiety:* Pain should be relieved with judicious use of morphine or pethidine sulphate; but may be given cautiously as they may reduce BP.

2. *Oxygen inhalation:* O_2 inhalation should be delivered through nasal catheters at a rate of 5-10 L/min to relieve hypoxaemia and maintain O_2 saturation beyond 90%. Ventilatory support may be needed if there is apnoea or ventilatory failure leading to acute respiratory acidosis or there is failure to achieve adequate oxygenation with high flow system.

3. **Fluid therapy:** Hypovolaemia is not the important cause of hypotension and low cardiac output in patients with acute myocardial infarction (AMI) but may be a contributory factor in some cases. Hypovolaemia may be ruled out after assessing the pulmonary capillary wedge pressure (PCWP) which is normal or elevated in AMI with cardiogenic shock. The initial fluid therapy depending on the CVP has been described under general measure i.e. if CVP < + 6 mmHg, 250 ml of saline be given and if > + 6 mm 100 ml of fluid is given, the further fluid therapy is guided by monitoring of pulse, BP, urine output and CVP/PCWP.
4. **Early reperfusion with thrombolytic therapy:** If patient is seen within first 4 to 8 hours of the onset of infarction, early reperfusion either by thrombolytic therapy (TT) or by PTCA may reduce infarct size and improve LV function and thereby reduce the mortality rate in AMI (mortality was 58% in GUSTO trial). Thus, for hospitals without revascularisation facilities, a strategy of early TT and intra-aortic balloon pumping (IABP) followed by an early transfer for PTCA or CABG may be appropriate.
5. **Treatment of an arrhythmia:** Sustained VT in a patient with haemodynamic instability or VF, must be treated with DC shock and I.V. bolus lidocaine 1-2 mg/kg followed by an infusion at a rate of 1-2 mg/min.
6. **Vasoactive drugs:** A variety of intravenous vasoactive drugs may be used to augment arterial pressure and cardiac output in patients with cardiogenic shock. Inotropic drugs such as dopamine or dobutamine or combination improves haemodynamics (cardiac output and BP) in cardiogenic shock but does not improve hospital survival significantly.
   - **Dopamine:** At lower doses ($\leq$ 2 µg/kg/min), it has vasodilator effect and apparently has little effect on myocardial oxygen consumption. At low dose 2-5 µg/kg/min); it has both chronotropic (increase HR) and inotropic (increase contractility) effects as a consequence of beta-receptor stimulation. Intravenous dopamine is started at an infusion rate of 2-5 µg/kg/min and the dose is increased every 2 to 5 min to a maximum of 20-50 µg/kg/min.
   - **Dobutamine:** It is a synthetic sympathomimetic amine with positive inotropic and minimal positive chronotropic effects and less peripheral vasoconstrictive action. It should not be used alone when vasoconstrictor effect is required. Therefore, it should not be used alone in cardiogenic shock to raise the BP, but be given simultaneously with dopamine infusion. The dose is 2-10 µg/kg/min.
   - **Norephinephrine:** It is sympathomimetic amine, may be used to increase diastolic BP of 90 mmHg and to maintain coronary perfusion.
   - **Amrinone and milrinone** are phosphodiestrase inhibitors with both positive inotropic and vasodilator action. These drugs resemble dobutamine in their pharmacological action, but have a more potent vasodilator action. Both the drugs have longer half-live and can cause hypotension, so they are reserved for use when other agents have proven ineffective. Amrinone is given as a loading dose of 0.75 mg/kg/min over 2-3 minutes followed by an infusion of 5-10 µg/kg/min; if necessary dose can be increased further upto 15 µg/kg/min.

Other Mechanical Measures

Intra-aortic balloon pumping (IABP)

In cardiogenic shock, mechanical assistance with an intra-aortic balloon pumping capable of augmenting both diastolic pressure and cardiac output have been found useful in reducing the in-hospital mortality. This therapy is reserved for patients whose condition merits mechanical (surgical or

angioplastic) intervention. It is contraindicated in presence of aortic regurgitation or aortic dissection.
- **Percutaneous cardiopulmonary bypass support:** It is used where intra-aortic balloon pumping is ineffective, for example, in patients with unstable rhythm i.e. frequent VT/VF or those with severe LV dysfunction.
- **Hemopump** is a catheter mounted LV assist device which is capable of augmenting cardiac output and providing systemic perfusion without intrinsic LV function.
- **External ventricular assist device** such as pneumatically driven thoracic system can be used for intermediate terms (day or months) for support of either or both ventricles.

Treatment of complications of AMI:
1. *Intraventricular septum rupture:* Circulatory support by IABP and inotropic agents followed by surgical repair.
2. *Free wall rupture (pseudoaneurysm):* Pericardiocentesis to be done to relieve tamponade followed by coronary angiography and subsequent resection of necrotic and ruptured myocardium with primary reconstruction and CABG if required.
3. *Rupture of papillary muscle (acute MR):* Medical treatment (inotropic agent and IABP support) followed by surgical repair/mitral valve replacement usually accompanied by coronary revascularisation.

B. Management of cardiogenic shock due to other causes:
1. *Pericardial tamponade:* Only effective therapy is removal of pericardial fluid either by needle/catheter drainage or by surgery.
2. *Pulmonary embolism:* Read pulmonary embolism as an emergency). Massive pulmonary embolism with shock is treated with thrombolytic therapy i.e. streptokinase 2.5 lac I.V. over 30 min as a loading dose followed by 1 lac unit/hr for 24-48 hours. Other options are: suction embolectomy, mechanical fragmentation of the thrombus or surgical embolectomy with cardiopulmonary bypass.

Chapter 30

Shock (Acute Circulatory Failure)

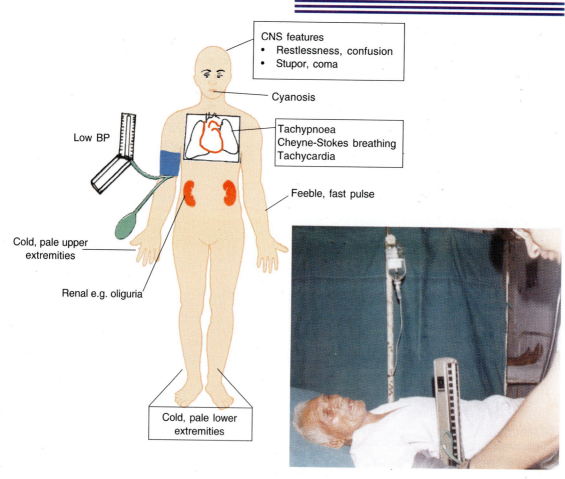

Fig. 30.1A: Clinical features of shock syndrome

Fig. 30.1B: A patient of peripheral circulatory failure due to gastroenteritis being treated in the hospital

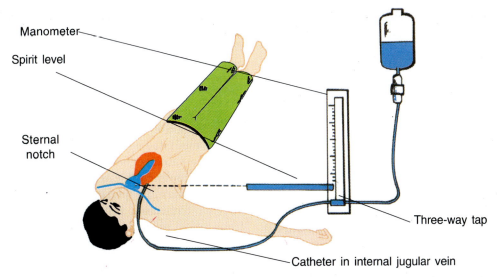

Fig. 30.2: Central venous pressure measurement using a manometer system. The reading must be referred to the level of the right atrium (indicated by the axillary fold or, provided the patient is supine, the sternal notch) using a spirit level

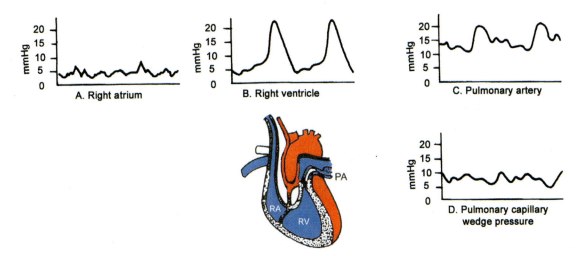

Fig. 30.3: Passage of a Swan-Ganz catheter through the chambers of the heart into the 'wedge' position (A) Once in the thorax, marked respiratory oscillations are seen. The catheter should be advaned further towards the lower superior vena cava/right atrium, where oscillations become more pronounced. The balloon should then be inflated and the catheter advanced (B) When the catheter is in the right ventricle, there is no dicrotic notch and the diastolic pressure is close to zero. The patient should be returned to the horizontal, or slightly head-up, position before advancing the catheter further (C) When the catheter reaches the pulmonary artery, a dicrotic notch appears and there is elevation of the diastolic pressure. The catheter should be advanced further with the balloon inflated (D) Reappearane of a venous waveform indicates that the catheter is 'wedged'. The catheter is deflated to obtain the pulmonary artery pressure. The balloon is inflated intermittently to obtain the pulmonary capillary wedge pressure

SHOCK OR ACUTE CIRCULATORY FAILURE

Definition

It is a clinical syndrome of low cardiac output characterised by hypotension, peripheral vasoconstriction, oliguria and impairment of consciousness. The basic underlying mechanism is low cardiac output followed by vasoconstriction and hypoperfusion of vital organs such as brain, lungs and kidneys.

Aetiology and Classification

Adequate organ perfusion, depends on arterial pressure which is determined by cardiac output and peripheral vascular resistance. Cardiac output is a product of stroke volume and heart rate. The stroke volume is dependent on *preload, afterload and myocardial contractility*. Hence, organ perfusion may be compromised by a decrease in cardiac output or its maldistribution.

Vascular resistance is proportional to length of vessel and viscosity of blood and inversely proportional to fourth power of the radius of the vessel, therefore, cross-sectional area of the vessel is major determinant of vessel resistance. Vascular resistance is regulated by arterial tone which depends on neural (sympathetic system), hormonal (adrenal) mechanisms and intrinsic or local factors (a variety of vasoconstrictor e.g. endothelin-II, angiotensin-II) and O_2 free radicals and vasodilators e.g. endothelial derived relaxation factor eicosanoids etc.

Microcirculatory failure is critical in pathogenesis of shock. Normal blood supply to an organ does not guarantee the fulfillment of adequate metabolic demands of all segments of that organ. Adhesion of leucocytes and platelets to the damaged or activated endothelium cause occlusion of microvasculature, activation of coagulation cascade and fibrin deposition (microthrombi) also contribute to vessel occlusion. Shunting of blood and decreased deformability of RBCs through vessel are also contributory factors for microcirculatory failure.

Microvascular flow depends on the balance between colloid osmotic pressure and capillary hydrostatic pressure, which, in turn, determines the balance between intravascular and extravascular fluid. Sympathetic stimulation decreases the capillary hydrostatic pressure by constricting the precapillary resistance vessels, results in movement of fluid from the extravascular compartment to intravascular compartment. As severe tissue hypoxia and acidosis supervene, then this sympathetically mediated responses are overcome by metabolic vasodilatation and this response along with vasoconstriction can cause extravasation of fluid into interstitial space resulting in reduction of effective circulatory volume. In addition, circulating toxins, adhesions of activated leucocytes can increase capillary permeability and further increase the tissue oedema. This process is increased by further loss of plasma proteins into the interstitium resulting in reduction of colloidal osmotic pressure, intravascular volume and tissue perfusion.

An aetiological classification of shock is given in the Box 30.1.

Box 30.1: Aetiologic classification of shock

1. **Hypovolaemic shock**
   (Low CVP; low PCWP, low cardiac output)
   - *Haemorrhage* (external or internal)
   - *Fluid loss* e.g. gastrointestinal (diarrhoea, vomiting); renal (diabetes mellitus, insipidus, and diuretics), and cutaneous (burn, perspiration)
   - Internal sequestration e.g. pancreatitis, acute intestinal obstruction, hemothorax, ascites, hemoperitoneum
2. **Cardiogenic shock:** (Read as a separate emergency) (raised CVP, raised PCWP low cardiac output)
3. **Obstructive shock (extracardiac obstruction)** (raised CVP, raised PCWP, low cardiac output)
   - Pulmonary embolism
   - Tension pneumothorax
   - Dissecting aneurysm of aorta
4. **Distributive shock (Low CVP, low PCWP, high cardiac output)**
   - Septic shock
   - Anaphylaxis (type I hypersensitivity reaction)
   - Neurogenic shock
   - Endocrinal shock (e.g. Addisonian crisis, thyrotoxic crisis, myxoedema)
   - Anaesthesia
   - Ganglion-blocking drugs

Shock (Acute Circulatory Failure)

The causes of acute circulatory failure are divided into two groups:
i. Those associated with low central venous pressure (CVP) such as hypovolaemic shock, anaphylaxis and septic shock.
ii. Those associated with raised central venous pressure such as cardiogenic shock, pulmonary embolism and cardiac tamponade.

Central venous pressure measurement (Fig. 30.2) before and during management of shock is mandatory.

Clinical Manifestations

Some symptoms and signs are similar for all types of shock, characterised by low cardiac output, hypotension (BP < 80 mmHg) and low tissue perfusion (Fig. 30.1). They are enumerated in the Box 30.2.

Box 30.2: Clinical manifestation of shock
1. **Cardiovascular**
   - Fast and feeble pulse
   - Systolic BP < 80 mmHg or a drop of > 50 mmHg from the baseline in hypertensive patients
   - Feeble heart sounds
2. **Respiratory**
   - Tachypnoea
   - Cheyne-Stokes breathing
   - Cyanosis
3. **CNS**
   - Listlessness, restlessness
   - Confusion, disorientation
   - Stupor and coma
4. **Renal**
   - Oliguria (urine output < 20 ml/hr)
5. **Skin**
   - Cold, pale extremities
   - Perspiration

Other manifestations are specific to the type of shock. They are given in the Table. 30.1

Diagnostic Evaluation

Shock is an emergency, needs full clinical assessment to understand the shock and target therapy

Table 30.1 Symptoms and signs of specific forms of shock

1. **Cardiogenic shock**
   (symptoms or signs of heart disease will be present)
   - Raised JVP
   - Pulsus alternans
   - Gallop rhythm
   - Basal crackles
   - Pulmonary oedema
2. **Hypovolaemic shock**
   (history of blood loss or fluid loss)
   - Dehydration
   - Haemoconcentration
   - Extreme pallor
   - Collapsed jugular veins
3. **Mechanical shock**
   - Elevated JVP
   - Pulsus paradoxus and muffled heart sound in cardiac tamponade
   - Kussmaul's sign (JVP rises in inspiration) in cardiac tamponade
   - Signs of pulmonary embolism (if present)
4. **Anaphylactic shock**
   i. Signs of profound vasodilatation
      - Warm extremities
      - Low BP
   ii. Erythema, urticaria, angioedema, pallor, cyanosis
   iii. Bronchospasm
   iv. Oedema of face, pharynx, larynx
   v. Pulmonary oedema
   vi. Hypovolaemia due to capillary leak
   vii. Nausea, vomiting, abdominal cramps, diarrhoea
5. **Septic shock**
   - Pyrexia, rigors or hypothermia
   - Nausea, vomiting
   - Warm extremities (vasodilatation)
   - Bounding pulse, hypotension
   - Other signs e.g. jaundice, coagulopathy or coma

to the cause. A practical approach is to make a clinical diagnosis based on the clinical features and a rapid diagnostic evaluation by specific diagnostic procedures directed towards determining the cause as well as severity of shock. The investigations for initial evaluation include:
1. A complete hemogram and blood culture.
2. X-ray chest.

Box 30.3: Haemodynamic changes in shock

Diagnosis	CVP	PCWP	CO
Cardiogenic shock	↑↑	↑↑	↓↓
Cardiac temponade (pericardial effusion)	↑	↑	↓ or ↓↓
Pulmonary embolism	N or ↑	N or ↑	↓↓
Hypovolaemic shock	↓↓	↓↓	↓↓
Septic shock	↓ or N	↓ or N	↑ or N rarely ↓
Anaphylactic shock	↓ or N	↓ or N	↑ or N

↑↑ or ↓↓ designates moderate to severe increase or decrease
↑ or ↓ designates mild to moderate increase or decrease

- CVP is central venous pressure N. means normal
- PCWP is pulmonary capillary wedge pressure
- CO is cardiac output

3. ECG.
4. Measurement of arterial blood gas.
5. Serum electrolytes (Na^+, K^+, Ca^{++}, Mg^{++}).
6. Haemodynamic parameters such as central venous pressure (CVP—Fig. 30.2), pulmonary capillary wedge pressure (PCWP—Fig. 30.3) and cardiac out (CO). They are given in the Box 30.3 in relation to specific shock.

Management

Goals of treatment

1. To maintain adequate arterial BP above 90 mmHg to ensure adequate tissue perfusion.
2. Reduction of elevated serum lactate levels.
3. Specific therapy directed against the cause.

1. Initial Resuscitation

Delay in making the diagnosis and initiating treatment as well as inadequate resuscitation may lead to multiorgan failure, hence, must be avoided. The initial resuscitation include:
- Intravenous access and to start fluid administration unless the patient is in pulmonary oedema
- Maintain patent airway e.g. endotracheal tube may be inserted as it will prevent aspiration of the gastric contents.

Blood volume is a critical factor in shock hence 'fluid first' strategy to be adopted for all patients irrespective of aetiology.

2. Monitoring

Once initial resuscitation has been started, efforts should be made to find out the underlying cause and to recognise the pattern of shock by haemodynamic studies (already discussed). Based on the CVP, cardiac output and pulmonary capillary wedge pressure measurements, the nature of shock can be defined. The other investigations needed to be done in case of a shock have been already discussed. Parameters to be monitored in shock are given in the Box 30.4.

Box 30.4: Parameters to be monitored in shock

Clinical	Biochemical
• Pulse, BP, temperature, respiration	• Haemoglobin
• Urine output (self-dewelling catheter to be put)	• Oxygen saturation
• Level of consciousness	• CVP and PCWP, cardiac index
	• Platelets, PTI, PTTK
	• Blood urea, creatinine
	• Blood lactate

3. Fluid Therapy

Optimizing preload by infusion of fluid is the fundamental treatment of acute hypovolaemia and to increase cardiac output. The challenge is to restore adequate ventricular filling pressure to optimal levels promptly and adequately without inducing pulmonary oedema and compromising oxygenation. Volume replacement is mandatory in hypovolaemic shock but is also essential in anaphylactic and septic shock. In cardiogenic shock, the CVP and PCWP may be high and volume expansion need utmost care in these patients (Read cardiogenic shock).

In hypovolaemic shock (low CVP, low PCWP and low CO) the most important step is to replace fluids lost from the circulation quickly (in minutes or hours) to reduce tissue damage and to prevent acute renal failure. Fluid is administered through a wide-bore intravenous cannula to allow large amount to be given quickly and the effect is continuously monitored.

Care must be taken to prevent fluid overload with a risk of pulmonary oedema.

Choice of fluid

Crystalloids either normal saline or Ringer's lactate are used for initial resuscitation for most forms of hypovolaemic shock. Patient may need several litres of crystalloid to replace fluid deficit. Colloids such as albumin or starch solution has been advocated after initial treatment with crystalloids for fluid repletion and to maintain colloid osmotic pressure. However, they are expensive and numerous studies have not revealed convincing results.

The goal of fluid therapy is to restore systolic BP above 90 mmHg in a previously normotensive person and CVP to be kept around 12-15 mmHg but should not exceed 18 mmHg.

Initially, it matters a little whether isotonic saline, blood or plasma are given, but when large amount of fluid is to be used then the nature of fluid lost should determine the nature of its replacement.

When large transfusions are needed rapidly, it is important to warm the fluid to body temperature before use.

In haemorrhagic shock, the blood or packed RBCs are transfused to maintain haemoglobin concentration of 10 g/dL.

4. Vasopressor Agents

Vasoactive drugs dobutamine, dopamine, noradrenaline though widely employed in treatment of shock but are not much helpful. Dopamine or dobutamine are the inotropes of choice in most critically ill patients. Most patients respond to an infusion of dopamine 2.5-10 µg/kg/min. The combination of dopamine and noradrenaline is currently popular for the management of patients who are in shock with a low systemic resistance. Dobutamine is substituted to achieve an optimal cardiac output, once arterial pressure is restored while noradrenaline is used to restore an adequate BP by reducing vasodilatation. However, this combination can only be used safely when guided by full haemodynamic monitoring. Large doses of steroids (hydrocortisone 400 mg 4-6 hourly) have been used to restore the response to endogenous catecholamines and to retain salt along with water due to their salt-retaining properties.

5. Treatment of Precipitating Factors and Underlying Illness

Following immediate improvement of perfusion in patients with shock, efforts should be made to findout the cause and to treat it such as gastrointestinal haemorrhage, gastroenteritis, diabetic ketoacidosis or septicaemia. *Metabolic acidosis* is corrected by administration of sodabicarb to restore normal pH and serum electrolytes. Gram-negative septicaemia to be treated with appropriate antibiotic after culture and sensitivity (Read septic shock). Tissue hypoxia is to be corrected by administration of 100% O_2 through nasal catheters. In case of cardiac tamponade, pericardiocentesis should be done to remove pericardial fluid.

6. Care of Other Systems

To prevent acute tubular necrosis and acute renal failure, renal perfusion pressure must be maintained by adequate hydration. Acidosis and electrolyte disturbance must be corrected.

To prevent the development of progressive hypoxia and subsequent development of ARDS, oxygen therapy should be given to maintain oxygen saturation more than 90% Mechanical ventilation may be required as respiratory support.

Coagulopathy (disseminated intravascular coagulation) should be looked for and BT, CT, PTTK should be done.

Chapter 31

Heart Failure

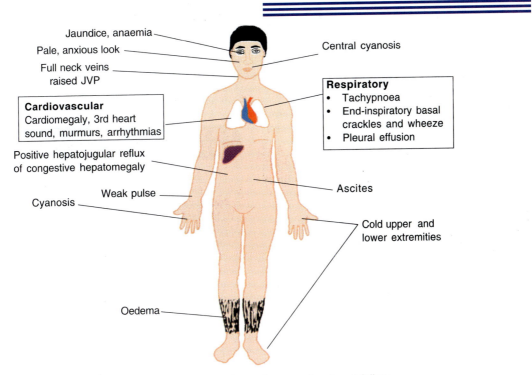

Fig. 31.1: Physical signs of congestive heart failure

HEART FAILURE

Definition

Heart failure is designated term to describe a state when heart is not able to maintain its cardiac output (pump action) to meet the demands of the body despite normal venous return, or can do so only at the expense of raised filling pressures. It may be mild or severe. In mildest form, cardiac output is adequate at rest but becomes insufficient during stress or exercise.

Pathophysiology

Cardiac output depends on (i) *preload* (ii) *afterload* and (iii) *myocardial contractility*. The heart failure results due to interactions of these three basic mechanisms depending on the *Starling law of forces* which states that "overstretching of the heart leads to deterioration of its functions".

Heart failure is frequently, but not always caused by a defect in the myocardial contractions leading to a fall in cardiac output. This activates counter regulatory neurohormonal mechanisms such as:
  i. Activation of renin-angiotensin-aldosterone system.
  ii. Sympathetic nervous system.

At first, both these systems try to compensate normal cardiac function by altering the preload, afterload, and augmenting myocardial contractility. Later on, these mechanisms become counterproductive and often reduce cardiac output by increasing peripheral vascular resistance which further stimulates renin-angiotensin-aldosterone system. Thus a vicious circle is set up on left heart failure.

Retention of salt and water due to secondary hyperaldosteronism leads to development of peripheral oedema. These mechanisms also operate in combination with elevated left atrial pressure to produce pulmonary oedema (Read pulmonary oedema).

Causes

For management of congestive heart failure, it is important to identify the underlying cause of the heart disease and also the precipitating factors of heart failure. The causes are tabulated (Table 31.1).

Precipitating Factors

A patient with compensated heart failure (impaired cardiac function without an overt heart failure) becomes decompensated with development of frank signs and symptoms of heart failure under the effect of acute illness such as an infection or development of an arrhythmia which jeopardies the ventricular function. Patients with chronic heart failure follow a remitting and relapsing course, with period of stability and episodes of decompensation leading to worsening of symptoms and repeated hospitalisation. The precipitating factors are summarised in the Box 31.1.

Table 31.1: Causes of heart failure
1. *Ventricular pressure overload:*
   i. *Left ventricular pressure overload*
      - Systemic hypertension
      - Aortic stenosis
   ii. *Right ventricular pressure overload*
      - Pulmonary hypertension (cor pulmonale)
      - Pulmonary stenosis
2. *Disturbance in ventricular filling*
   - Mitral stenosis (left ventricular inflow obstruction)
   - Tricuspid stenosis (right ventricular inflow obstruction)
   - Endomyocardial fibrosis (stiff ventricles)
3. *Ventricular volume overload*
   - Mitral regurgitation, mitral valve prolapse
   - Aortic regurgitation
   - ASD and VSD (Eisenmenger's syndrome and complex)
   - High output states
4. *Depressed myocardial contractility*
   - Myocarditis
   - Cardiomyopathy
   - Myocardial ischaemia/infarction

Box 31.1: Precipitating factors that aggravate CHF in patients with pre-existing heart disease
- Infection
- Myocardial ischaemia or infarction
- Thyrotoxicosis
- Rheumatic and other forms of carditis
- Pulmonary embolism
- Inappropriate reduction or discontinuation of therapy for CHF
- Anaemia
- Arrhythmias (e.g. atrial fibrillation)
- Pregnancy
- Infective endocarditis
- High sodium intake, blood transfusion, fluid overload, emotional stress etc.

Clinical Features

Congestive cardiac failure is a clinical syndrome of right heart failure associated with left heart failure leading to low cardiac output. The congestion of various viscera is a characteristic feature, hence, the name.

Symptoms

1. **Dyspnoea and orthopnea:** Dyspnoea is the earliest symptom of CHF, occurs as a result of increased effort in breathing, first observed during strenuous exercise, then with progression of heart failure, it appears first with less exertion

and then at rest. This is due to reduced compliance of the lung and increased cost of breathing Orthopnoea (dyspnoea in recumbent position) occurs later than exertional dyspnoea. Patients with orthopnoea may elevate their heads on several pillows at night to get relief. Frequently, they feel short of breath at night when their head slips off their pillow and disturb their sleep. The breathlessness is usually relieved by sitting upright since this position reduces venous return and pulmonary venous congestion. In advanced heart failure, patient with orthopnea cannot lie down at all and may spend the whole night in sitting position. On the other hand, long standing left heart failure may lead to right heart failure which relieves the pulmonary congestion and breathlessness.

2. *Paroxysmal nocturnal dyspnoea (PND):* Attacks of breathlessness and coughing occur at night, usually awaken the patient from sleep and is not relieved by sitting position.
3. *Cough with expectoration and wheezing:* This is due to left heart failure with pulmonary congestion and oedema. The cough and wheezing accompany the dyspnoea in CHF.
4. *Cheyne-Stoke respiration:* It is periodic breathing in which periods of apnoea alternate with periods of hyperventilation. It is a sign of CHF, can also be seen in raised intracranial tension, respiratory failure and uraemia.
5. *Fatigue, weakness, poor effort tolerance:* These are nonspecific but common symptoms of heart failure, are related to low cardiac output with hypoperfusion of skeletal muscles.
6. *Oliguria and nocturia:* It is a sign of CHF, occurs due to hypoperfusion of kidneys leading to acute renal failure.
7. *Cerebral symptoms:* Disturbed consciousness, confusion, impairment of memory, headache, insomnia, difficulty in concentration are due to low cerebral perfusion.

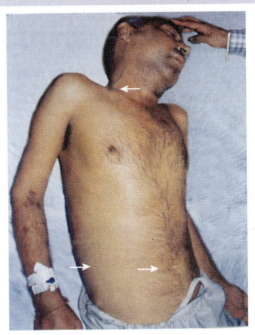

Fig. 31.2: Congestive cardiac failure in a 40-year-old male (1) An arrow at the level of neck shows distended veins and raised JVP (2) An arrow at abdomen indicates ascites

Physical Signs (Fig. 31.1)

The general physical examination reveals, pallor, anxious look, cyanosis, anaemia and pitting oedema over legs, sacrum, abdominal wall. Jaundice may be present. Neck veins are full and JVP is raised (Fig. 31.2). Cardiovascular system examination shows cardiomegaly, 3rd heart sound, murmurs, arrhythmia. Respiratory system examination reveals tachypnoea, end-inspiratory basal crackles and wheeze. Pleural effusion is seen in severe cases. Abdominal examination may reveal congestive hepatomegaly and ascites.

Diagnosis

The diagnosis of CHF may be established by observing some combinations of the clinical manifestations of heart failure together with findings characteristic of underlying heart disease and precipitating illness/factor. The *Framingham criteria* for diagnosis of CHF are given in the Box 31.2.

> **Box 31.2: Framingham criteria for diagnosis of CHF**
>
> | Major | Minor |
> |---|---|
> | • Paroxysmal nocturnal dyspnoea | • Peripheral oedema |
> | • Distended neck veins | • Nocturnal cough |
> | • Rales | • Exertional dyspnoea |
> | • Cardiomegaly | • Congestive hepatomegaly |
> | • Acute pulmonary oedema | • Pleural effusion |
> | • S3 gallop | • Reduced vital capacity by one third |
> | • Increased venous pressure (> 16 cm H_2O) | • Tachycardia (HR > 120/min) |
> | • Positive hepatojugular reflux | • Weight loss |
>
> Δ **For diagnosis:** At least one major and two minor criteria are required

Investigations

These are done to establish the nature and severity of the disease and to detect complications.

1. **Electrocardiogram:** It will reveal ventricular hypertrophy, arrhythmias and myocardial ischaemia/infarction.
2. **Chest X-ray** will show enlargement of heart, peripheral lung congestion, presence of *Kerley's lines*, pulmonary oedema, hydrothorax, pulmonary hypertension, double atrial shadow in mitral valve disease and calcification of valves.
3. **Two-dimensional echocardiography** is useful to detect unsuspected valvular lesion, assessing the dimensions, left atrial myxoma and a thrombus or aneurysm.
4. **Blood urea, creatinine and electrolytes** for renal failure and electrolyte disturbance.

Management

Aims of treatment

- Removal of precipitating factor(s).
- Correction of underlying cause.
- Control of congestive state.

To control congestive heart failure, following measures are taken:
1. Reduction of afterload on the heart.
2. Improvement of myocardial contractility.
3. Control of salt and water retention.

Hospitalisation of all severe cases is essential to control the heart failure as early as possible.

1. **Reduction of cardiac workload:** The heart size can be decreased by reducing physical activity or by enforcing rest at home or in the hospital for 1-2 weeks in patients with overt heart failure. Anxiety relieved by anxiolytics and reassurance. Meals should be small. In many cases, bed rest and sedatives often result in effective diuresis.
2. **To improve myocardial contractility:**
   A. **Digitalis:** It is a cardiac glycoside, acts by increasing the force of contraction (positive inotropic action), delays conduction through AV node, slows the heart rate (negative chronotropic effect) and increases the excitability of heart, hence, is a proarrhythmic agent also.

   It is useful in CHF to improve ventricular emptying i.e. it improves cardiac output, ejection fraction, reduces end-diastolic pressure, thus improves symptoms resulting from pulmonary vascular congestion. It is most beneficial in patients in whom myocardial contractility is impaired secondary to chronic ischemic heart disease, hypertensive heart disease or when valvular or congenital heart disease imposes an excessive volume overload. It is less useful in CHF due to high output states (thyrotoxicosis, beri beri, cor pulmonale) or CHF due to stenotic valvular lesions or myocarditis. However digoxin is used to slow ventricular rate in atrial fibrillation or to convert atrial fibrillation to atrial flutter due to any cause.

   Digitalis dosage: Rapid digitalisation is now-a-days not preferred but 0.5 mg digoxin I.V. may be given stat in an emergency situation followed by 0.25 mg orally after 4-6 hours not exceeding total dose of 1 mg/24 hours. When there is no urgency, 0.25 mg orally/

day may be given to control CHF-called *slow digitalisation*.

Toxic effects: These occur due to large dose administration. Hypokalaemia, hypothyroidism, renal and hepatic failure potentiate digitalis effects as well as toxic effects. They are given in the Box 31.3.

Box 31.3: Digitalis (Digoxin) toxic effects

A. Cardiac
- Arrhythmias e.g. ventricular ectopics, ventricular bigeminy, non paroxysmal atrial tachycardia with block
- Bradycardia
- AV blocks (e.g. first degree) second degree and complete AV block

B. Extracardiac
- Gastrointestinal e.g. nausea, vomiting, anorexia
- Gynaecomastia
- Yellow vision
- Cachexia
- Neuralgia
- Fatigue, headache, confusion, hallucinations

The clinical digoxin toxicity occurs when its serum level is > 2.0 ng/ml.

Treatment of digitalis toxicity if develops, include its discontinuation along with diuretic and administration of potassium to treat hypokalaemia; and phenytoin, lidocaine and aminodarone for digitalis induced arrhythmias. A specific antidote for digitalis toxicity is digoxin-specific antibody (*Fab fragments*).

B. *Amrinone:* It is a noncatecholamine, non-cardiac glucoside that exerts positive inotropic effect similar to digitalis and is a vasodilator. It reverses major hemodynamic abnormalities associated with heart failure by stimulating the cardiac contractility and dilating the vascular bed. It is indicated in selected patients not responding to digoxin, because it may worsen myocardial ischaemia or ventricular ectopy.

3. Control of fluid and salt retention
A. *Salt restriction:* Considerable improvement in symptoms and signs occurs by restricting the dietary intake of salt by 50% of normal intake i.e. simply by excluding salt-rich foods and *no use of salt at the table in any form*. In moderate to severe heart failure, dietary intake of salt should be less than 1.0 g.

B. *Diuretics:* They are usually the first line of treatment. Diuretics increase urine volume and sodium excretion leading to reduction of preload and improvement in symptoms and signs of pulmonary and systemic venous congestion. Of the commonly used agents, fursemide, torsemide and bumetanide act as loop diuretics, hence, are potent to be used during an emergency. Whereas thiazides, metolazone and potassium-sparing agents act in the distal tubule.

Dose: For mild to moderate heart failure, oral fursemide 20-80 mg or torsemide 10-20 daily in single or divided doses is sufficient. For severe or advanced congestive heart failure fursemide 40-100 mg or Torsemide 10 mg I.V. may be given initially and then to be repeated 8 hourly depending on the response. Large single daily doses are to be avoided because of risk of acute reduction in blood volume. The ethacrynic acid is given as 50/100 mg i.v. two or three times a day. Potassium is to be monitored during fursemide therapy. For long-term management, a combination of a loop diuretic and potassium-sparing diuretic is useful.

4. Reduction of afterload by vasodilators: The vasodilators reduce afterload, left ventricular end-diastolic pressure and volume, and raise stroke volume and cardiac output by reducing aortic pressure. Vasodilators are contraindicated in CHF with hypotension.

Angiotensin-converting enzyme (ACE) inhibitors are potent vasodilators (dilatation of both venous and arterial bed), act by antagonising the action of stimulated renin-angiotensin system in CHF, therefore, all patients with heart failure due to LV systolic dysfunction should receive an ACE inhibitor.

Dose: Treatment with ACE should be initiated at very low doses followed by gradual increments in dose. The starting dose i.e. captopril 6.25 mg, enalapril 2.5 mg, lisnopril 2.5 mg should be given twice or thrice a day for 3-5 days and then dose may be increased if needed. Renal function and potassium should be assessed during the therapy.

The side-effects of ACE include hypotension, worsening renal function and hyperkalaemia, intractable cough and angioedema. Less common side-effects are rash, mouth ulcers, taste disturbance and blood dyscrasias.

Contraindication: Intrinsic renal disease, bilateral renal artery stenosis and systemic hypotension are their contraindications. In case of cough and angioedema due to ACE, another class of drug-*angiotensin receptor blocker* (losartan, irbesartan candesartan) may be used whose effects are similar to ACE).

5. ***Other drugs:***
   A. *Beta-adrenergic receptors blocker:* So far beta blockers were considered to be contraindicated because of blunting of sympathetic response in CHF, but recent clinical trials have shown beneficial effects. Out of several beta blockers, only carvedilol bisoprolol and nebivolol have been approved by FDA for management of class II or III chronic heart failure. Treatment with betablockers should be initiated in very low doses followed by gradual increments in dose if lower doses have been well-tolerated. For example, therapy should be started at a dose of 3.125 mg of carvedilol twice daily, followed by doubling the dose after 2 to 4 weeks. Patients should be monitored closely for evidence of hypotension, bradycardia, fluid retention or worsening heart failure.
   B. *Antiarrhythmic and device therapy:* Because patients with heart failure have frequent and complex ventricular arrhythmias, and being at high risk of sudden death, may require antiarrhythmics therapy for their suppression, but recent recommendation is to use them only in life-threatening ventricular arrhythmia refractory to treatment in hemodynamically stable patients. The results of use of a device-implantable cardioverter defibrillator (ICD) are promising in clinical trials, in cardiac arrest survivors and high risk postinfarction patients, but at present there is little evidence that ICD placement prevents sudden death or prolongs life in patients with chronic heart failure who have asymptomatic arrhythmias.
   C. *Pacemaker:* Although pharmacotherapy is the primary therapy for patients with heart failure, the use of pacemakers to improve cardiac haemodynamics is under investigation. Despite promising initial results, controlled studies have not verified the benefits of dual-chamber pacing in a non-selected population of severely symptomatic congestive heart failure.

The overview of treatment of heart failure is given in the Figure 31.3

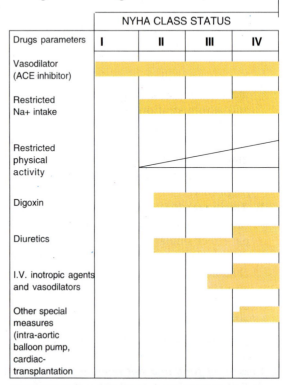

Fig. 31.3: Overview of treatment of CHF according to NYHA functional class (I to IV)

Chapter 32

Left Ventricular Failure (Pulmonary Oedema)

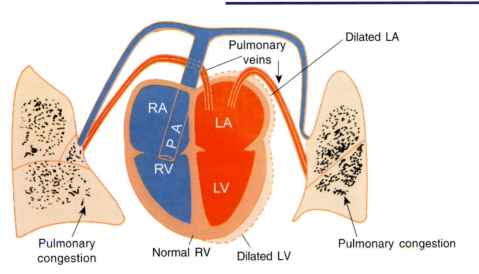

Fig. 32.1: Pathophysiology of left ventricular failure leading to acute pulmonary oedema
(i.e. rise in left ventricular end-diastolic pressure, left atrial and PCWP)
LA = Left atrium, RA = Right atrium, LV = Left ventricle, RV = Right ventricle, PA = Pulmonary artery
PCWP = Pulmonary capillary wedge pressure

LEFT VENTRICULAR FAILURE (ACUTE CARDIOGENIC PULMONARY OEDEMA)

Definitions

Left ventricular failure (LVF) is defined as failure to maintain an effective left ventricular output for a given pulmonary venous or left atrial pressure or can do so at the cost of an elevated left atrial filling pressure. Acute pulmonary oedema is a haemodynamic consequence of LVF.

Acute Pulmonary Oedema

It refers to collection of fluid into alveoli, its wall and alveolar sacs due to transudation as a result of elevated pulmonary capillary venous pressure (> 25 mmHg) consequent to elevated left atrial pressure. This is called backward failure. Acute pulmonary oedema can be cardiogenic or noncardiogenic. Cardiogenic pulmonary oedema will be discussed here. The elevated hydrostatic pressure within capillaries more than oncotic pressure leads to transudation from capillaries into lungs (Fig. 32.1).

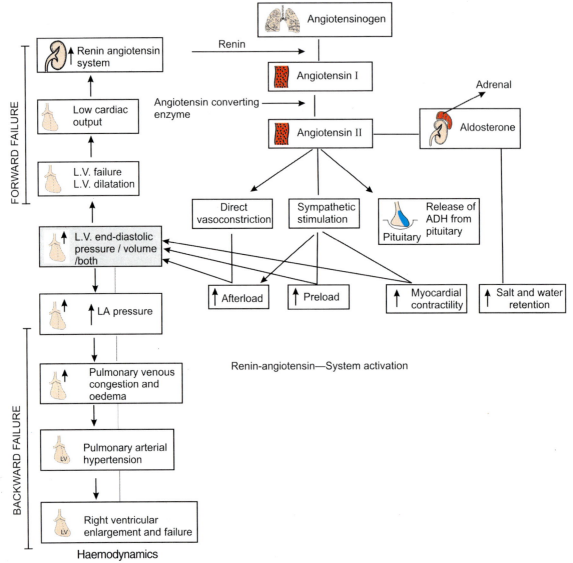

Fig. 32.2: Pathogenic mechanism and haemodynamics of left ventricular failure. LA = Left atrium, LV = Left ventricle ↑ Increase or stimulation

Pathophysiology

Left ventricular output depends on *preload, afterload* and *myocardial contractility*. Left ventricular failure occurs due to interactions of these complex mechanisms. Low cardiac output due to LVF leads to complex neuroendocrine changes in which there is stimulation of renin-angiotensin-aldosterone system as well as stimulation of sympathetic system. At first, these try to optimise the left ventricular function-called *compensatory mechanism*; but when these mechanisms also fail, then LVF sets in. The activation of renin-angiotensin-aldosterone system increases *afterload* due to vasoconstriction and salt and water retention. Stimulation of sympathetic system increases both preload and afterload (peripheral vasoconstriction). This also increases myocardial contractility. By these complex mechanism LVF is produced (Fig.32.2).

Left Ventricular Failure (Pulmonary Oedema)

By backward failure mechanism, due to rise in left ventricular end-diastolic pressure/volume due to increased afterload, there is rise in left atrial pressure and subsequently rise in pulmonary venous and capillary pressure (> 25 mmHg). This raised pulmonary venous pressure is more than plasma oncotic pressure in the capillaries leading to transudation and development of acute pulmonary oedema (Fig.32.1). In long standing cases or in chronic heart failure, hypoxia produced by edematous lungs is potent vasoconstrictor of pulmonary vessels leading to pulmonary arterial hypertension and ultimately oedema is relieved slowly. Development of pulmonary arterial hypertension is protective mechanism for acute pulmonary oedema.

Causes

They are given in the Table 32.1. The precipitating factors are listed in the Box 32.1.

Clinical Features

The clinical features result from low cardiac output, pulmonary venous congestion and rise in left ventricular end-diastolic volume/pressure. They are given in the Table 32.2.

Box 32.1: Precipitating factors of LVF
- Infection
- Anaemia
- Acute coronary ischaemia
- Pregnancy
- Rapid I.V. infusions
- Tachyarrhythmias
- Undue physical exertion
- Increase in blood volume

Table 32.1: Causes of left ventricular failure
1. **Left ventricular outflow obstruction (pressure overload)**
   - Systemic hypertension
   - Aortic valvular stenosis (congenital or acquired)
   - Hypertrophic cardiomyopathy
2. **Left ventricular inflow obstruction**
   - Mitral stenosis
   - Left atrial myxoma
   - Endomyocardial fibrosis (left ventricle)
3. **Left ventricular volume overload**
   - Mitral regurgitation or mitral valve prolpase.
   - Aortic regurgitation (rheumatic and non-rheumatic).
   - Ventricular septal defect.
   - Patent ductus arteriosus.
   - High output states (anaemia, thyrotoxicosis, beri-beri, AV fistula, Paget's disease).
   - Papillary muscle dysfunction.
4. **Reduced left ventricular contractility**
   - Dilated cardiomyopathy (LV predominant)
   - Anterior wall MI
   - Myocarditis and left ventricle endocarditis

Investigations

1. *Full blood count*, blood urea, creatinine, electrolytes etc.
2. *Arterial blood gas analysis* may show low PaO_2 with normal or low $PaCO_2$ and low blood pH (metabolic acidosis).
3. *The ECG* may show LVH, arrhythmias, evidence of ischaemia or myocardial infarction, LBBB or ventricular strain pattern depending on the cause of LVF.
4. *Chest X-ray*: It will show pulmonary oedema (haziness extending from the hilum to periphery Fig. 32.3) and cardiomegaly. Kerley's B lines may be seen due to alveolar oedema. Hydrothorax or left-sided pleural effusion may be evident.
5. *Echocardiogram:* It is most useful investigation and is mandatory in all patients with acute cardiogenic pulmonary oedema. It gives valuable information regarding;
   i. Unsuspected yet correctable valvular lesion(s).
   ii. Unsuspected cardiac aneurysm.
   iii. Hypertrophic or dilated cardiomyopathy.
   iv. Systolic or diastolic LV dysfunction.
6. *Pulmonary capillary wedge pressure:* It is elevated, may be above 25 mmHg. The pulmonary capillary wedge pressure indirectly reflects left atrial pressure.

Differential Diagnosis

It has to be differentiated from bronchial asthma. Acute pulmonary oedema is also called cardiac

Table 32.2: Symptoms and signs of LVF with their pathogenic mechanisms

Underlying mechanism	Symptoms and signs
1. Rise in left ventricular end-diastolic volume or pressure and subsequent rise in left atrial pressure	• Tachycardia • Murmurs depending on the cause • Gallop rhythm • Low BP • Heaving apex beat • Low volume pulse or pulsus alternans
2. Pulmonary venous hypertension, pulmonary congestion/oedema	• Dyspnoea, orthopnoea, PND, tachypnoea • Cough, haemoptysis (pinkish, frothy sputum) • Basal pulmonary crackles and rales • Central cyanosis • Hydrothorax/pleural effusion • Cheyne-Stokes respiration
3. Low cardiac output leading to hypo-perfusion and hypoxia of various organs	• Oliguria and nocturia • Cerebral symptoms e.g. confusion, difficulty in concentration, anxiety, insomnia etc. • Fatigue and weakness • Peripheral cyanosis • Pale, cold extremities

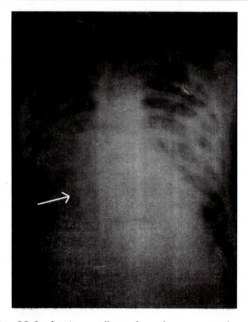

Fig. 32.3: Acute cardiogenic pulmonary oedema. Chest X-ray (PA view) shows enlarged heart shadow. There is bilateral diffuse haze extending from hila to periphery. An arrow indicates outline of right border of the heart

asthma. The difference between bronchial asthma and cardiac asthma are given in Box 32.2.

Management

Cardiogenic pulmonary oedema is life-threatening emergency, may be precipitated by arrhythmias and infection, need immediate attention and urgent treatment.

Aims of Treatment

1. To reduce venous return (preload) to the heart by upright posture, narcotics.
2. To lower pulmonary capillary pressure and decrease transudation e.g. O_2, positive pressure ventilation, diuretics.
3. To improve myocardial contractility by digitalis if systolic LV dysfunction is the cause.
4. To reduce afterload by vasodilators e.g. I.V. nitroprusside, ACE inhibitors.
5. To find out the precipitating cause such as an arrhythmia or infection and treat them appropriately.

Left Ventricular Failure (Pulmonary Oedema)

Box 32.2: Differentiation between cardiac and bronchial asthma	
Cardiac dyspnoea (asthma)	**Bronchial asthma (dyspnoea)**
1. History	
• Clinical evidence of heart disease	• Clinical evidence of respiratory disease
2. Symptoms	
• Acute onset	• Gradual onset or there can be an acute exacerbation of chronic asthma
• Non-seasonal, no evidence of atopy	• Atopic or nonatopic and seasonal
• Associated symptoms are e.g. chest pain, orthopnoea palpitation, sweating	• Associated symptoms include e.g. cough, wheeze, haemoptysis, stridor
• Attacks of PND are common, relieved by sitting or recumbent position	• Attacks of PND are less common, relieved by cough and expectoration
• Wheeze is less frequent	• Wheezing is marked and even audible
• Dyspnoea is out of proportion than cough	• Cough is out of proportion than dyspnoea
Signs	
• Tachypnoea, tachycardia, cyanosis (central, peripheral)	• They are less marked
• Trachea central, normal in length	• Trachea is central but palpable part is decreased
• No retraction of supraclavicular fossae or intercostal spaces	• Retraction of supraclavicular fossae and/or intercostal spaces is marked
• Percussion note is dull at the bases	• Hyper-resonant note may be present
• Crackles at the bases	• Both crackles and rales throughout the lungs
• Apex beat is normal or displaced	• Apex beat may not be visible or normal
• Breath sounds are normal	• Normal breath sounds with prolonged expiration
• 3rd heart sound (gallop rhythm) may be present	• No 3rd heart sound
Investigations	
• Chest X-ray shows cardiomegaly with acute pulmonary oedema	• Heart size normal, or may be tubular. There is increased translucency of lungs with low flat diaphragm
• ECG may show LVH, LBBB, MI, arrhythmias or conduction defect	• Sinus arrhythmia
• Echocardiogram shows depressed ejection fraction, enlarged LV	• Normal ejection fraction
• Arterial blood gases; low PaO_2 and $PaCO_2$	• PaO_2 low but $PaCO_2$ is normal

Steps of Management

i. ***Upright or prop up posture of the patient on the bed*** with legs dangling along the side of the bed, if possible. This reduces venous return.

ii. ***Morphine*** is given I.V. in dosage of 5-10 mg with an antiemetic (metoclopramide 10 mg I.V.) and repeated frequently as desired. This drug, in addition to reducing anxiety, also reduces adrenergic drive to arteriolar and venous bed, leads to arteriolar and venous dilatation (capacitance vessels) thereby reduces venous return. Naloxone should be available in case respiratory depression occurs.

iii. ***Oxygenation:*** There is arterial hypoxaemia due to lowered oxygen diffusion as a result of alveolar oedema, hence, 100% O_2 should be given through the mask preferably under positive pressure (it will stop transudation of fluid into alveoli by reducing venous return and thereby lowering pulmonary capillary pressure). Positive pressure ventilation has been found beneficial in refractory cases of pulmonary oedema.

iv. ***Diuretics:*** The high potency loop diuretics such as fursemide (40-100 mg I.V.) or bumetanide (1 mg) or torsemide 10 mg I.V. may be given to reduce the circulating blood volume and clear fluid overload by profuse diuresis. Fursemide, when given I.V. also exerts vasodilator action, thereby reduces venous return.

v. ***Vasodilators:*** Intravenous sodium nitroprusside 20-30 µg/min may be given to reduce afterload in patients whose systolic BP is above 100 mmHg.

vi. ***Digitalis:*** It is given to improve left ventricular myocardial contractility, hence, is useful in patients of LVF failure due to systolic dysfunction. If the patient has not taken digoxin within the last 5-6 days then 0.5 mg I.V. may be given stat followed by 0.25 mg (half the initial dose) after 6 to 8 hours, if necessary, to a maximum of 1 mg/24 hours. This therapy is also beneficial if pulmonary oedema has been precipitated by one of supraventricular tachyarrhythmia such as supraventricular tachycardia or atrial fibrillation with rapid ventricular rate.

vii. ***Nitrates:*** Now-a-days, sublingual nitrate (0.4 mg × 3 every 5 min) is considered as first line therapy for acute cardiogenic pulmonary oedema, I.V. nitroglycerine can be given if patient is not in hypotension. I.V. nitroprusside can be used if patient has hypertension with pulmonary oedema.

viii. ***Bronchodilatation:*** Sometimes aminophylline (theophylline ethylenediamine), 240 to 480 mg given I.V. is effective in relieving bronchospasm, and in addition may lower pulmonary venous pressure. It has also a mild diuretic and positive inotropic effect (augment myocardial contractility).

ix. If above measures fail, ***rotating tourniquets*** may be applied, but its efficacy is doubtful.

x. After instituting the above measures, attempt should be made ***to find out the precipitating factor*** such as an arrhythmia or infection which should be treated by appropriate antiarrhythmic and antibiotic therapy respectively.

xi. ***For future management***, the diagnosis of underlying disease must be established and if possible to be removed such as mitral valvotomy for MS, or surgical treatment for atrial myxoma, aneurysms or papillary muscle dysfunction.

After discharge from the hospital, patient should be advised salt restriction, avoid exertion; and the dose of diuretic, digitalis and an ACE inhibitor should be properly adjusted to prevent further episode.

Chapter 33

Management of Tachyarrhythmias

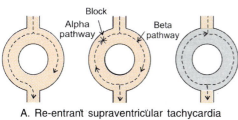

A. Re-entrant supraventricular tachycardia

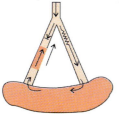

B. Re-entrant Ventricular tachycardia

Fig. 33.1: Mechanisms of re-entry (circus movement) (A) Re-entrant supraventricular arrhythmia. (1) shows the impulses passing down both limbs of the potential tachycardia circuit. (2) shows that impulse is blocked in alpha pathway but proceeds slowly down the beta pathway and returns along the alpha pathway. The diagram (3) shows the impulse travels so slowly along the beta pathway that when it returns along the alpha pathway to its starting point, it is able to travel down the beta pathway producing a circus movement tachycardia. (B) Re-entrant ventricular tachycardia (anatomical re-entry). The Purkinje fibres splits into two pathways. An impulse travelling through lower common pathway (a), gets blocked in antegrade conduction at site (b) (arrow followed by bar), but travels down slowly at (c) (serpentine arrow) to excite the ventricle. The impulse now re-enters the Purkinje system of myocardium, excites it and then re-enters at site (d) as a result of which ventricular extrasystole results. Continued re-entry in this manner produces ventricular tachycardia.

AV node
- Adenosine
- β-blockers (II)
- Digoxin
- Verapamil (IV)
- Diltiazem (IV)

SA node
- β-blocker (II)
- Atropine
- Verapamil (IV)
- Diltiazem (IV)

Bypass tract
- Disopyramide (Ia)
- Procainamide (Ia)
- Quinidine (Ia)
- Flecainide (Ic)
- Amiodarone (III)

Atrium
- Disopyramide (Ia)
- Quinidine (Ia)
- Procainamide (Ia)
- Flecainide (Ic)
- Propafenone (Ic)
- Amiodarone (III)
- Digitalis

Ventricles
- Disopyramide (Ia)
- Quinidine (Ia)
- Procainamide (Ia)
- Lidocaine (Ib)
- Mexiletine (Ib)
- Flecainide (Ic)
- Propafenone (Ic)
- β-blocker (II)
- Sotalol (II and III),Bretylium (III)
- Amiodarone (III)

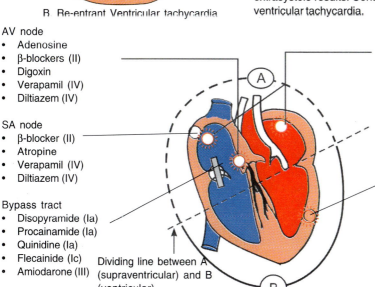

Dividing line between A (supraventricular) and B (ventricular)

Fig. 33.2: Tachyarrhythmias: Division into A (supraventricular) and B (ventricular) indicates their origin. The drugs acting at different sites are depicted with their classification (given in the bracket)

TACHYARRHYTHMIAS

Definitions

Tachyarrhythmias result from disorders of impulse propagation and disorders of impulse formation. Tachyarrhythmias due to disorders of impulse propagation (re-entry) are generally considered to be most common (Fig. 33.1). Disorders of impulse formation can be subdivided into tachyarrhythmias caused by enhanced automaticity and those caused by triggered activity. Sinus tachycardia, escape rhythms, accelerated AV nodal rhythms and ectopic tachycardias are its examples. The classification of antiarrhythmics is given in the Table 33.1. The sites of action of antiarrhythmics are depicted in Figure 33.2.

Table 33.1: Vaughan William's classification of antiarrhythmics

Class I: They block fast Na+ channels
A. Prolong action potential duration
- Quinidine, procainamide, disopyramide

B. Shorten duration of action potential
- Lidocaine, phenytoin, tocainide mexiletine,

C. No effect on action potential, slow the conduction
- Flecainide, encainide, propafenon

Class II-Beta blockers
- Propranolol metoprolol, atenolol, timolol, sotalol

Class III. They block K+ channel
- Amiodarone, sotalol, bretylium

Class IV: Ca++ channel blockers
- Verapamil, diltiazem

TACHYCARDIAS

Definition

Tachycardias refer to arrhythmias in which three or more complexes occur in a row at a rate exceeding 100 beats/min. They occur more often in diseased rather than normal hearts. Those tachycardias that are initiated by an APC or a VPC are considered to be due to an re-entry mechanism except digitalis induced arrhythmias which are due to triggered activity.

In a hemodynamically stable patient, an attempt should be made to find out the mechanism and origin of tachycardia by examining the patient clinically and by recording a 12 lead surface ECG. This is important for appropriate therapeutic decision.

The ECG will give informations regarding:
1. The presence or absence of P wave, frequency, morphology and regularity of P waves as well as QRS complexes.
2. Relationship of P waves to QRS complexes.
3. A comparison of QRS morphology can be made during sinus rhythm and during an episode of tachycardia. It is useful to summon the ECG before tachycardia i.e. recorded during sinus rhythm.
4. If necessary, an oesophageal lead may be used to define supraventricular tachycardia by the recording the atrial activity (P waves).
5. The response to carotid sinus massage or other vagomimetic maneuvers such as Valsalva maneuver, immersion of face in cold water and administration of 5-10 mg endrophonium.

Clinical Observations

1. Examination of jugular venous pulse is important because 'a' wave will be absent in atrial fibrillation.
2. Arterial pulse will reveal regularly irregular pulse in ventricular ectopy and irregularly irregular pulse in atrial fibrillation. The pulse deficit is < 10 beats min in frequent VPCs but is > 10/min in atrial fibrillation.
3. Cannon 'a' wave suggest AV dissociation, complete AV block and nodal rhythm.
4. Variable intensity of first heart sound during an arrythmia suggest AV dissociation, or heart block or atrial fibrillation.

PAROXYSMAL SUPRAVENTRICULAR TACHYCARDIA (PSVT)

Supraventricular tachycardias (atrial or nodal in origin) occurring in paroxysms (paroxysmal) are due to re-entry (circus movement); while non-paroxysmal supraventricular tachycardia is digitalis induced.

Re-entry or circus movement is only possible when:
i. There is functional difference in conduction and refractoriness in the AV node.
ii. *Unidirectional block.* In the presence of two pathways, one shows antegrade unidirectional block, which later on becomes responsive to retrograde conduction.
iii. *The presence of re-entry circuit (circular conduction pathway).* A re-entry circuit is formed by two pathways that are connected at the upper as well as lower ends, providing an uninterrupted circuit for impulse conduction.

The re-entry circuit may involve the AV node called *micro re-entry* circuit responsible for AVNRT (Fig. 33.1A) or may be around AV node connecting an atrium and a ventricles by an accessory pathway (*Kent bundle*) which is a *macro re-entry* circuit responsible for atrio-ventricular re-entrant tachycardia (AVRT). In re-entrant tachycardia, the supraventricular impulse enters through one pathway, and while in the way to ventricle, gets conducted retrogradely back to atria resulting in the activation of atria again. This sets up a vicious circle perpetuating the tachycardia. The various types of supraventricular tachycardias are given in Box 33.1.

AV Nodal Re-entrant Tachycardia

> **Box 33.1: Supraventricular tachycardias**
> 1. **AV nodal re-entry** (Atrioventricular nodal reentrant tachycarida-AVNRT). This is commonest form of PVST.
> 2. **Atrioventricular re-entry:** (atrioventricular re-entrant tachycardia-AVRT). This is less common. It may be;
>   - *Orthodromic AVRT:* In this type, impulses are conducted to the ventricles via AV node, and the retrogradely back to atria through an accessory pathway. This is a narrow QRS complex tachycardia.
>   - *Antidramic AVRT:* In this type, impulses are conducted abnormally through an accessory pathway, and then rogadely via AV node. This produces wide QRS tachycardia simulating VT.
> 3. **SA nodal or atrial re entrant tachycardias.**
> 4. **Non-paroxysmal supraventricular tachycardia.** It is commonly due to digitalis.

It is the most common form of PSVT characterised by regular narrow QRS complexes at a rate of 120 to 250/min. It occurs commonly in females. Age is no bar. It is invariably initiated by an APC with prolonged P-R interval (marked AV nodal conduction delay-prolonged AH interval) which may be visible on ECG followed by narrow QRS complexes with embedded P waves or distortions of QRS at the terminal parts by P waves.

The pathogenesis is explained by dual pathway hypothesis, AV node has two pathways: (i) a beta (fast) pathway and (ii) slow alpha pathway. During sinus rhythm, only conduction over the fast pathway manifests resulting in a normal P-R interval. An atrial premature complex (APC) with critical coupling interval is blocked in beta pathway but is conducted slowly through alpha pathway. This beat while passing through alpha pathway may find beta pathway recovered, gets conducted through it retrogradely into atria resulting in setting up of a vicious circle resulting in sustained tachycardia.

Clinical Features

It may produce palpitation, syncope and heart failure depending on the rate and duration of an arrhythmia. The signs and symptoms of underlying heart disease are present. Hypotension may occur due to loss of atrial boost to ventricular filling due to rapid rate. There may be visible cannon 'a' wave due to simultaneous atrial and ventricular contractions.

Treatment

1. Vagal maneuvers (e.g. carotid sinus massage, Valsalva maneuver, immersion of face in cold water) can be performed to block the conduction in the AV node. They may terminate tachycardia.
2. If vagal maneuvers are unsuccessful, the intravenous injection of a drug that prolongs the refractory period of AV node (adenosine, verapamil, diltiazem, propranolol or metoprolol) and digitalis may be administered. The dose of adenosine is 6 to 12 mg I.V., verapamil 2.5-10 mg I.V., diltiazem 0.25/kg I.V. Out of these, adeno-

sine is preferred because of its extremely short half-life and less side-effects.

3. When these drugs fail to terminate the tachycardia or when tachycardia is recurrent but patient is still hemodynamically stable, atrial or ventricular pacing via a temporary pacemaker may be used to terminate tachycardia called *overdrive suppression*.
4. If the patient is symptomatic and has compromised state (e.g. hypotensive or in acute distress), synchronised cardioversion may be performed.
5. For chronic recurrent AVNRT, radio-frequency ablation of micro re-entry circuit may be indicated. The chronic drug therapy include use of class 1A, class 1C and class III (amiodarone) antiarrhythmic drugs.

For AVRT

- Vagal maneuvers as discussed above.
- Antiarrhythmic drugs that block conduction in the accessory pathway (e.g. procainamide, amiodarone, ajmaline) should be used.
- Synchronised DC shock in haemodynamically unstable patient (e.g. hypotension, acute distress).
- Surgical interruption or ablation of accessory pathway.

Note: Vagal maneuvers and drugs such as adenosine, beta blockers, calcium channel blockers, digoxin used in treatment of AVNRT may be effective in orthodromic AVRT but not in antidromic AVRT. The algorithm of narrow QRS complex tachycardia is given in (Fig. 33.3).

NON RE-ENTRANT ATRIAL TACHYCARDIA

Nonparoxysmal atrial tachycardia is commonly digitalis-induced or may be associated with severe pulmonary or cardiac disease, with hypokalaemia or with administration of theophylline or adrenergic drugs. Multifocal atrial tachycardia (MAT) is not digitalis induced, occurs commonly following theophylline administration.

The atrial tachycardia is characterised by atrial rate of 150-200/min and the P wave contour is different from that of sinus P wave. In MAT, three different types of P wave from three different atrial foci will be seen. As atrial rate increases, the degree of AV block increases and Wenckebach second degree AV block may ensue i.e. atrial tachycardia with block (a manifestation of digitalis toxicity).

The ECG shows isoelectric line between the P waves which are abnormal is shape and differ from sinus P waves. The ventricular complexes are narrow and there is normal intraventricular conduction.

Treatment

1. Digoxin withdrawl is sufficient to terminate it if it is the cause of the arrhythmia.
2. Automatic atrial tachycardia not caused by digitalis is difficult to terminate. Radio-frequency ablation should be attempted since control of this form of tachycardia with drugs such as digitalis, beta blockers, calcium channel blockers is usually unsuccessful.

ATRIAL FIBRILLATION

It is characterised by rapid atrial rate > 350 beats/min, uncoordinated atrial contractions and irregular rapid ventricular response. It is a common supraventricular arrhythmia which may occur in paroxysms (paroxysmal atrial fibrillation) and persistent forms (chronic atrial fibrillation). Atrial re-entry is the common underlying mechanism.

In atrial fibrillation, the AV node is bombarded by numerous excitatory stimuli from the atria (atrial re-entry) but all supraventricular (atrial) impulses do not reach the ventricles due to refractoriness of AV node which produces physiological block to these impulses and protects the ventricles from going to chaos. On the other hand, if AV node is bypassed such as in accessory pathway conduction (WPW syndrome), then the atrial fibrillation will be dangerous because there will be 1:1 conduction without any AV nodal interference.

Management of Tachyarrhythmias

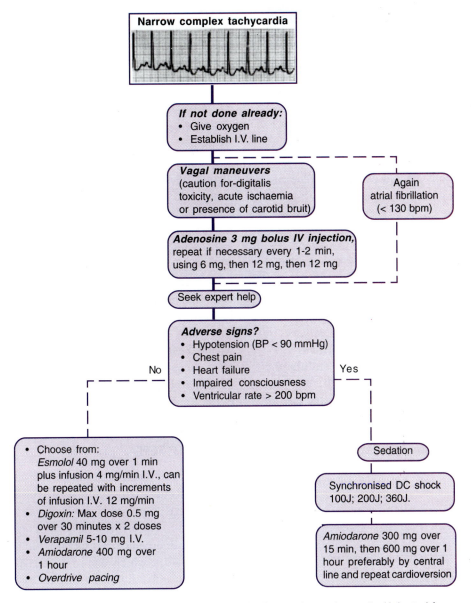

Fig. 33.3: Algorithm for treatment of narrow QRS complex tachycardia (Adapted from European Resuscitation Council endorsed by British Resuscitation Council)

Causes

They are given in the Box 33.2:

Clinical Features

Atrial fibrillation may produce palpitation, syncope due to rapid ventricular rate and the pause following cessation of AF. Loss of contribution of atrial contractions may lead to fatigue. AF may lead to hypotension, pulmonary congestion due to precipitation of angina pectoris in susceptible individuals. It may manifest as systemic embolisation producing

164 Cardiology

> **Box 33.2: Causes of Atrial fibrillation**
>
> - Rheumatic heart disease (MS, MR etc.)
> - Mitral valve prolapse
> - Hypertensive heart disease
> - Cardiomyopathy, alcohol induced (holiday heart syndrome)
> - Thyrotoxicosis
> - Congential heart disease (ASD, Ebstein's anomaly)
> - Constrictive pericarditis
> - Cor pulmonale
> - Left atrial myxoma
> - Idiopathic (lone atrial fibrillation)

hemiplegia, monoplegia, peripheral gangrene and infarction of various organs in patients with underlying rheumatic or ischaemic heart disease.

Patients with AF exhibit loss of 'a' wave in the jugular venous pulse and variable pulse deficit. The arterial pulse is irregularly irregular. The first heart sound varies in intensity. In addition, there may be signs of underlying heart disease.

Diagnosis

It is made on ECG which shows fibrillatory (f) waves instead of normal P waves, undulating baseline, atrial rate > 400 bpm and ventricular rate > 100/min. The R-R intervals are variable due to irregular ventricular response. The morphology of QRS is narrow unless there is phasic aberrant ventricular conduction called *Ashman's phenomenon*. On echocardiography, the left atrium is frequently enlarged and may even contain a thrombus.

Treatment

1. Find out the precipitating factor or cause and treat it accordingly.
2. If the patient's clinical status is severely compromised, cardioversion is the treatment of choice.
3. In the absence of cardiovascular compromise, drug therapy is indicated to slow the ventricular rate. Digoxin, beta blockers (propanolol, metoprolol) and calcium channel blockers (verapamil, diltiazem) may be used for this purpose.
4. Conversion to sinus rhythm may then be attempted by using class IA (quinidine, procainamide, disopyramide) or flecainide (class 1C) drugs.
5. If medical therapy fails to convert AF within 24 hours, electrical cardioversion is useful.
6. In situations where AF has been present for 48-72 hours or more or when there is evidence of systemic embolisation, anticoagulants may be used.
7. In patients of AF with enlarged (giant) left atrium, it is difficult or even impossible to convert AF into normal sinus rhythm, in such patients, drug therapy may be used to control the rapid ventricular response.
8. In occasional patient, it may not be possible to slow the ventricular rate by drugs what to talk of conversion of AF to sinus rhythm. Such a case may require creation of complete heart block by radiofrequency ablation of the AV node followed by implantation of permanent pacemaker.
9. Once sinus rhythm is restored by any means described above, quinidine or related drugs (1A) or flecainide (1C) or amiodarone (class III) may be used to prevent recurrence.

ATRIAL FLUTTER

It is a supraventricular arrhythmia characterised by rapid atrial rate (250-350/min) due to intra-atrial re-entry (circus movement), involves commonly the right atrium. The arrhythmia occurs commonly in patients with organic heart disease. Flutter may be paroxysmal in which there is a precipitating factor such as pericarditis, acute respiratory failure, or it may be persistent. Atrial flutter if lasts for more than a week, it will usually convert into atrial fibrillation.

Causes

The causes of atrial flutter are more or less same as that of atrial fibrillation with the exception that pericardial disease, severe pulmonary disease commonly lead to atrial flutter than atrial fibrillation.

Diagnosis

It is diagnosed on ECG which shows rapid atrial rate of > 300 bpm with ventricular rate either half or one third (2:1, 3:1 block) which is regular. The P waves produce saw-tooth appearance of the baseline between R-R intervals.

Treatment

When the diagnosis of atrial flutter is made, then there are three therapeutic modalities to treat it:
1. Drug therapy.
2. DC cardioversion.
3. Overdrive pacing.

    Out of these options, DC cardioversion or pacing is the preferred treatment because drugs are less effective than these techniques. The initial effective treatment in acute setting is low-energy DC shock (25-50J) under mild sedation. Higher energy 100 J shock is virtually always successful and never harmful, hence, may be considered as initial shock.

    The *indications* of drug therapy in this condition are:
    i. To slow the ventricular rate either by a beta blocker or a calcium channel blocker.
    ii. To enhance the efficacy of overdrive pacing in restoring normal sinus rhythm. In this regard, quinidine or procainamide or sotalol is used.
    iii. To prevent the recurrence after DC shock.

VENTRICULAR TACHYCARDIA (VT)

Definition

It is a wide QRS tachycardia at a rate of > 100 bpm. The sudden onset of a wide QRS tachycardia usually rings an alarm bell if the patient is symptomatic. If left untreated, VT may degenerate into fatal ventricular flutter. VT may be sustained (persists for > 30 sec) or nonsustained (does not persist beyond 30 second). The sustained VT requires termination because of haemodynamic consequences.

Causes

VT generally accompanies some form of structural heart disease. The causes are:
1. Acute myocardial infarction or ischaemia.
2. Cardiomyopathy (ischaemic or idiopathic).
3. Electrolyte disturbance (e.g. hypokalaemia, hypomagnesemia).
4. Drugs (e.g. digitalis and other proarrhythmics)
5. Myocarditis.
6. Reperfusion.
7. Ventricular aneurysm.
8. Pacemaker mediated (e.g. DDD pacemaker).
9. Mechanically induced by a pacing catheter or flow directed pulmonary artery catheter.
10. Idiopathic.
11. Miscellaneous such as right ventricular dysplasia, Bergada syndrome, sarcoidosis.

Diagnosis

Sustained VT occurs in association with a cardiac disease; while nonsustained VT can occur in the absence of heart disease. Sustained VT is almost always symptomatic; while nonsustained VT (3 VPCs in a row or VT lasting for < 30 sec) does not produce symptoms. Sustained monomorphic VT is commonly encountered in patients with chronic or old myocardial infarction. A fixed anatomical lesion producing ischaemia is responsible for recurrent sustained monomorphic VT.

The symptomatic patients of sustained VT present with palpitations, dizziness, syncope or even a cardiac arrest. The presence of cannon waves, changing intensity of first heart sound with rapid ventricular rate suggest AV dissociation and favour the diagnosis of VT. A history of previous infarction and first episode of tachycardia after infarction is highly suggestive of VT: while long history of tachycardia with frequent attacks, absence of organic heart disease and presence of preexcitation suggest PSVT with aberrant conduction.

The ECG helps in the diagnosis. Wide QRS complexes (>0.14 sec), at a regular rate of > 100 bpm with presence of AV dissociation (independent P wave not related to wide QRS complexes), concordant pattern, superior QRS axis, capture beats and fusion complexes favour the diagnosis of VT. It must be stressed here that in spite of all these criteria, the ECG diagnosis of VT is not only difficult but may be impossible to differentiate it from PSVT with aberrant conduction (another common cause of wide QRS tachycardia) because there is no single electrocardiographic sign which confirms the diagnosis. The causes of wide QRS tachycardia are given in Box 33.3.

Box 33.3: Common causes of wide QRS tachycardia

- Ventricular tachycardia
- Supraventricular tachycardia with aberrant intraventricular conduction (common)
- Supraventricular tachycardia with pre-existing bundle branch block (less common)
- Atrioventricular tachycardia (antidromic WPW conduction)

Management

See the algorithm for wide QRS tachycardia (Fig. 33.4).

Treatment of VT depends on the clinical setting and the ability of the patient to tolerate it. Proceed as follows:

1. First of all establish intravenous line and give oxygen.
2. Check the pulse: If there is no pulse in presence of VT on ECG (pulseless VT), treat it as for ventricular fibrillation (see the algorithm of cardiac arrest Chaper 38).
3. If there is pulse, evaluate vital signs and clinical symptoms. Look for adverse signs:
   - If patient is not tolerating the tachycardia and adverse signs (BP < 90 mm, ischaemic chest pain, heart failure, unconsciousness, ventricular rate > 150 bpm) are present, attempt to convert rhythm with a single precordial thump (thump-version) if onset of VT is witnessed on monitor and then proceed immediately with defibrillation. After that begin therapy with xylocaine or bretylium.
   - If patient is tolerating the tachycardia and no adverse signs present, then proceed with drug therapy. Intravenous lidocaine (50-100 mg) is given as bolus over 2 minutes with second injection of one half of the dose given after half an hour (total dose not exceeding 200 mg). The infusion has to be maintained at 1-4 mg/minute.

The efficacy of other agents such as procainamide, and amiodarone is higher than lidocaine. Procainamide can be given as I.V. bolus in the dose of 10-15 mg/kg at a rate of 50 mg/min, following which a maintenance infusion dose of 2-6 mg/min is necessary. During procainamide therapy monitoring of BP (for hypotension), QRS duration (prolongs QRS) and QTc interval (prolongs the QTc interval) is necessary.

Intravenous amiodarone has also been found successful for management of VT but the time taken for the response is longer. The usual intravenous dose is 15 mg/min for 10 minutes followed by 1 mg/min for 6 hours and then 0.5 mg/min for next one hour for next few days. *Bretylium* is also approved for use in patients with life-threatening VT.

If unresponsive to drug therapy, sedate the patient and perform cardioversion (100 J: 200 J: 360J).

Treatment of chronic recurrent VT includes therapy with oral antiarrhythmic drugs. Long-term treatment options for recurrent VT include the use of implantable cardioverter defibrillator (ICD), catheter ablation and surgery after specialised electrophysical studies and endocardial mapping.

VENTRICULAR FIBRILLATION (VF)

It is a catatrophic arrhythmia characterised by a rapid, irregular, disorganised ventricular rhythm resulting in lack of cardiac output, absent pulses and unrecordable BP. In the absence of ECG monitoring, VF cannot be distinguished from ventri-

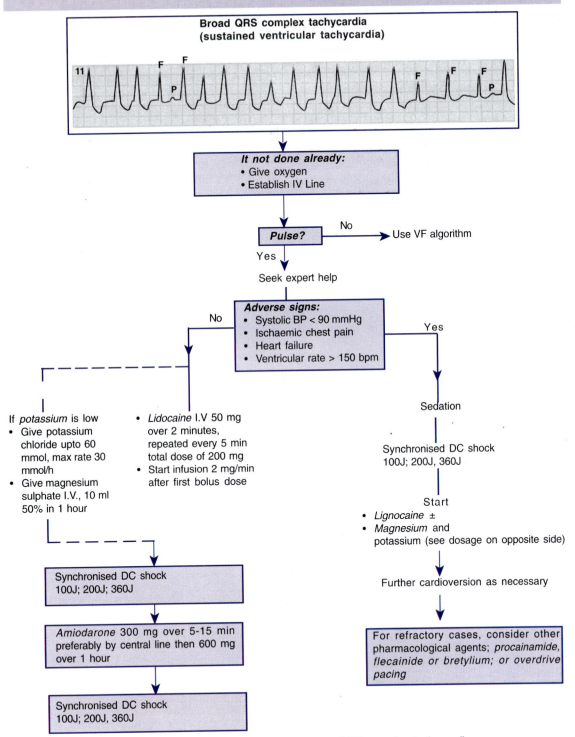

Fig. 33.4: Algorithm for treatment of broad QRS complex tachycardia

cular asystole because both rhythm disturbances result in clinical cardiac arrest.

Causes

They are given in the Box 33.4:

Management

On ECG ventricular fibrillation has no identifiable waveform or pattern with undulating wavy. baseline. Clinically it is indistinguishable from cardiac arrest, hence, management is like cardiac arrest (see The Algorithm of Cardiac Arrest—Ch-38).

Box 33.4: Causes of ventricular fibrillation

- Myocardial ischaemia/infarction
- Electrolyte disturbance (e.g. hypokalaemia, hypomagnesaemia)
- Electric shock
- Atrial fibrillation with rapid ventricular rate may degenerate to VF
- Congenital prolonged QT syndrome
- Severe hypothermia
- Cardiomyopathy
- Drugs (digitalis, proarrhythmics
- Failure to proper synchronisation of cardioversion
- As a terminal cardiac event in dying heart

Chapter 34

Management of Bradyarrhythmias and Stokes-Adam Attacks

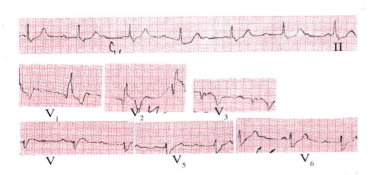

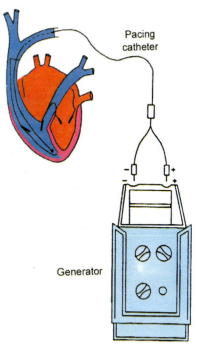

Fig. 34.1: Complete AV block in myocardial infarction. The upper strip (lead II) shows complete heart block (P-P and R-R intervals constant and P wave has no relation to QRS which is wider than normal). The precordial leads (V_1-V_6) show ST elevation anterior myocardial infarction (wide abnormal Q waves in leads V_1-V_2 with QS complexes in V_3. There is reduction of R wave from V_4-V_6. The T is wide and inverted from V_1-V_3 with ST segment elevation). There is evidence of complete AV block in precordial leads. The site of block is below the bundle of His because there is RBBB pattern in V_1-V_2 (wide qR pattern in V_1 and wide slurred S wave in V_4-V_6.)

Fig. 34.2 Temporary pacing (diagram). A pacing catheter is connected to a temporary generator. A bridging cable or pacemark extension cord (not shown) can be used between the generator and the catheter

MANAGEMENT OF BRADYARRHYTHMIAS

Definitions

These are disorders of impulse formation or of impulse conduction manifesting with slow ventricular rate (< 60/min). These occur due to disorders of SA node and AV node.

1. *Sinus node dysfunction (sick sinus syndrome)*
   - First degree sinoatrial block.
   - Second degree sinoatrial block.
   - Third degree sinoatrial block.
   - Bradycardia-tachycardia syndrome.
2. *AV conduction disturbances*
   - First degree AV block.
   - Second degree AV block.
   - Third degree AV block (Fig. 34.1).
   - AV dissociation.

SINUS NODE DYSFUNCTION

1. *Sinus node dysfunction:* The sinus node is a natural dominant pacemaker. Its intrinsic rate of discharge is highest than other potential cardiac pacemakers (e.g. atrium, AV node, ventricle), hence, suppresses the activity of all these pacemakers, hence called *king of his own empire*. It is influenced by autonomic nervous system; alterations in autonomic nervous system is responsible for the normal acceleration of heart during exercise and the slowing that occurs during rest and sleep. Sympathetic stimulation increases its discharge rate; while parasympathetic stimulation slows the discharge rate. *Sinus bradycardia* refers to heart rate of less than 60 bpm which can be physiological (e.g. athletes) or pathological. In case the SA node defaults, the lower subsidiary pacemaker, i.e. AV node or ventricle may take up the control of cardiac rhythm. The SA node lies in the right atrium and has dual blood supply. The causes of structural sinus nodal disease are given in Box 34.1.

> **Box 34.1: Causes of structural nodal disease**
> - Acute MI (inferior wall infarction)
> - Cardiomyopathies
> - Metastatic disease involving the heart (right atrium)
> - Primary muscular dystrophies
> - Amyloid heart disesae
> - Tuberculosis involving the heart
> - Degenerative fibrotic disease of atria

Clinical Manifestations

The clinical manifestations of sinus node dysfunction are due to marked sinus bradycardia (HR < 50/min), sinus pauses due to intermittent sinus arrest or sinoatrial exit block. In either case, the ECG manifestation is prolonged period (> 3 sec) of atrial asystole. The symptoms include weakness, fatigue, paroxysmal dizziness or syncope, confusion and congestive heart failure.

In some patients, there may be abnormality in AV node conduction (dual nodal disease) hence, there is failure of the AV node to take up the control of rhythm in case of sinus node defaults resulting in periods of ventricular asystole and syncope.

Occasionally, SA node dysfunction is manifested by an inadequate increase in heart rate in response to stress such as exercise or fever (inadequate normal response).

Sick sinus syndrome is a hallmark of sinus node dysfunction, refers to include a combination of symptoms (dizziness, confusion, fatigue, syncope and CHF) and manifested by marked sinus bradycardia, SA blocks, or sinus arrest on ECG or Holter's monitoring.

The ECG manifestations of sick sinus syndrome:

1. Sinus bradycardia with or without sinus arrhythmia.
2. Sinus pauses due to intermittent sinus arrest or SA blocks.
3. SA block, and AV blocks.

Management of Bradyarrhythmias and Stokes-Adam Attacks

4. Failure of emergence of escape rhythm after prolonged bradycardia.
5. Presence of nodal rhythm automatically indicates failure of sinus rhythm.
6. Bradycardia-Tachycardia syndrome.

Diagnosis

The diagnosis of sick sinus syndrome is suspected on clinical grounds and correlated with ECG manifestations of sinus node dysfunction. SA node dysfunctions manifest three types of SA blocks (first, second and third degree) out of which the second degree SA block is seen intermittently or constantly on the ECG as a pause created by cessation of atrial activity (the whole P-QRS-T complex is dropped). The *tachycardia-bradycardia syndrome* is also a manifestation of sick sinus syndrome characterised by alternating periods of tachyarrhythmias and bradyarrhythmias. The atrial tachyarrhythmias e.g. atrial tachycardia, flutter, fibrillation occurring during tachycardia phase of this syndrome suppresses the automaticity of SA node resulting in its failure to recover leading to bradyarrhythmia (e.g. bradycardia).

The most important step in diagnosis of sick sinus syndrome is to correlate symptoms with ECG manifestations of sinus node dysfunction. While ambulatory ECG (Holter) monitoring remains a mainstay in evaluation of sinus node dysfunction, most of the episodes of syncope are paroxysmal and unpredictable. Single and multiple 24-hour monitoring may fail to record a symptomatic period, therefore, provocative tests (carotid sinus pressure, exercise test and pharmacological tests) are frequently helpful. *Carotid sinus pressure* for 5 seconds producing a sinus pause > 3 second on ECG indicates sinus node dysfunction. Similarly injection of *atropine* 1-2 mg I.V. will not accelerate the heart beyond 90/min in case of sinus node dysfunction but will do so in vagotonaemia (normal response). Similarly isoprenaline 1-2 mg I.V. may be employed to test structural nodal disease.

Electrophysiological studies (sinus node recovery time and sinoatrial conduction time) help in establishing the diagnosis. The normal values are given below. These parameters are recorded following pacing.

1. Sinus node recovery time (corrected for spontaneous heart rate) normally is < 550 ms; prolongation indicates sinus node dysnfunction in a symptomatic patient.
2. Sinoatrial conduction time: It is one half of the difference between the pause following termination of brief period of pacing and the sinus cycle length.

Management

- Treat the underlying cause.
- Administer atropine (if necessary).
- Insertion of permanent pacemaker is the mainstay of treatment for symptomatic patients. Patients with intermittent paroxysms of bradycardia or sinus arrest are usually adequately treated by demand ventricular pacemaker. Patients with symptomatic chronic sinus bradycardia or frequent prolonged episodes of sinus node dysfunction do better with dual chamber pacemakers that preserve the normal AV activation sequence (AV synchrony). For the management of bradycardia as an emergency, see the Fig. 34.3 (Algorithm for management of bradycardia and conduction block).

AV Conduction Disturbances

The impulses from the SA node travel through atria to AV node where there is slight physiological delay before they are conducted to the ventricles. Abnormalities of conduction of sinus impulses to the ventricles occur due to block at the level of AV node (heart blocks) which can ultimately lead to syncope or cardiac arrest.

EVALUATION OF CONDUCTION ABNORMALITIES

The physician must assess:
  i. The site of conduction disturbance.
  ii. The risk or possibility of progression to complete heart block.

iii. The probability that an emergence of escape rhythm arising distal to site of block will be haemodynamically stable. This is the most important since the rate and stability of the subsidiary pacemaker will determine what symptoms result from heart block. This is because a pacemaker arising from bundle of His or above will discharge at a rate of 45-60 bpm and will be stable and asymptomatic. On the other hand, pacemaker distal to bundle of His will generate impulses at a slower rate (15-45 bpm), produces wide QRS complexes, and symptoms of syncope, dizziness, and will be unstable. There will be chances of developing ventricular asystole.

The morphology of QRS determines the site of block in AV node.

Causes of Heart Blocks

1. Vagotonaemia.
2. Acute rheumatic carditis.
3. Myocarditis (diphtheric, chagas' disease).
4. Coronary artery disease (e.g. inferior wall infarction, right ventricular infarction).
5. Drugs (e.g. digitalis, beta blockers, calcium channel blockers).
6. Aortic valve disease (e.g. syphilitic aortitis).
7. Infiltrative heart disease (e.g. amyloidosis, myxoedema).
8. Idiopathic fibrosis of conduction system (*Lenegre's disease*).
9. Idiopathic calcification and sclerosis of fibrous ring of aortic and mitral valve called *Lev's disease*.

Classification of Heart Block

1. *First degree AV block* is characterised by prolongation of P-R interval beyond 0.20 sec at normal heart rate and 0.22 at heart rate of 60/min. It does not cause any symptoms and is detected on the ECG. It does not require specific treatment except the underlying cause or when bundle of His ECG shows block in the infranodal region.

2. *Second degree AV block:* (intermittent AV block). In this block, some of the atrial impulses (P waves) are conducted while others are blocked. It is of two types i.e. *mobitz type I* (Wenckebach) and *mobitz type II* (fixed).

In *mobitz type I*, there is progressive lengthening of P-R intervals with each successive beat till one atrial impulse (P wave) is blocked. In this type, first P-R interval is always shorter than the last P-R interval prior to blocked P wave. The pause that follows the blocked P wave is less than twice of the normal sinus intervals. This type of block is always localised to AV node and is followed by normal QRS complex. It occurs transiently in inferior wall infarction or with drugs toxicity, particularly digitalis, beta blockers etc. This type of block can occur normally in athletes or normal individuals with high vagal tone. It usually does not progress to complete heart block, except in setting of acute inferior wall infarction. Even when it does, it is well tolerated because the escape pacemaker lies in the proximal part of bundle of His and provides a narrow QRS stable rhythm. As a result, Mobitz type I block rarely requires aggressive therapy. Therapeutic decision depends on the ventricular rate and symptoms of the patient. If ventricular rate is adequate and the patient is asymptomatic, observation is sufficient.

In *Mobitz type II second degree AV block*, conduction fails suddenly and unexpectedly without a delay in preceding P-R intervals. It is always due to the disease of His-Purkinje system and most often associated with wide QRS. It has a high incidence of progression to complete heart block, leading to unstable wide QRS (idioventricular) rhythm. Therefore, pacemaker implantation is necessary in this condition. The causes of AV blocks have already been discussed in the beginning.

In *high grade AV block* (Fig. 34.2) there are periods of three or more consecutively blocked P waves (e.g. > 3:1 AV block) but intermittent conduction can be demonstrated. Block is usually in the His-Purkinje system, but simultaneous block in AV node is also present. The escape rhythm arises from the focus below the His-Purkinje system which produces wide QRS (idioventricular) slow rhythm. It is unstable and usually the patient is symptomatic and a cardiac pacemaker implantation is mandatory.

3. ***Third degree (complete) AV block*** is said to be present when no atrial impulse (e.g. P wave) is propagated to the ventricles, therefore, there are two independent pacemakers in complete heart block i.e. one in the atria and other in the ventricle. The duration of QRS decides the site of pacemaker in the ventricle. If QRS duration is normal, and heart rate is 40-55 beats/min, the pacemaker is situated in the AV node above the bundle of His. Congenital complete AV block is usually localised to AV node. If pacemaker lies below the His bundle (block is within His bundle), the escape rhythm is wide (one of bundle branch block pattern) and is usually less responsive, occurs at a slow rate (15-45 beats/min) and requires immediate pacemaker implantation.

AV dissociation exists whenever there are two pacemakers in the heart i.e. one in the atrium (SA node) and other in the ventricle. Complete AV dissociation exists in complete heart block as described above. Incomplete AV dissociation manifests as AV dissociation with interference where two pacemakers interfere with each other's progression resulting in frequent fusion complexes on ECG. The AV dissociation occurs under two conditions:

1. Nodal rhythm in a patient with severe bradycardia where the rate of nodal rhythm and sinus rhythm are more or less equal with the result P waves occur just before, in, or following QRS complex-called iso-rhythmic AV dissociation. Treatment is removal of the cause usually a drug (digitalis, betablockers etc.), acceleration of sinus rhythm by vagolytic agents or insertion of a pacemaker if escape rhythm is slow and patient is symptomatic.
2. AV dissociation with interference occurs when the lower subsidiary pacemaker (nodal or ventricular) accelerates its rate and competes with the normal sinus rhythm and usually its rate is higher than sinus rate. Interference dissociation is usually seen during VT, accelerated nodal or ventricular rhythm seen with digital intoxication, myocardial ischaemia and/or infarction. Treatment of AV dissociation is removal of the offending drug or correction of metabolic abnormalities or ischaemia.

BRADYCARDIA AND CONDUCTION BLOCKS

The bradycardia (HR < 60/min) or conduction blocks with impending asystole or with an appreciable risk of asystole is important to be recognized from treatment point of view. The following are the situations where the risk of developing asystole is high and there is need to recognize them before starting the treatment:

1. History of previous episode of asystole.
2. A pause equal or greater than 3 seconds regardless of the cause.
3. Presence of AV block with idioventricular rhythm (Fig. 34.1 on front page).
4. Dual nodal disease with an idioventricular escape rhythm.
5. Trifascicular and bifascicular block in AMI.

First of all, assess the patient for developing risk of asystole.

1. ***When there is risk for asystole:*** If there is definite risk of developing asystole, I.V. line should be established and atropine administered as indicated in the algorithm (Fig. 34.4) In the meantime, arrangements should be made for transvenous pacing. In many cases, expert help will be required for this purpose. If situation demands an early pacing and if necessary equipment is available, then external pacing (Fig. 34.2 on front page) should be done. Isoprenaline (initial dose 1 µg/min is used by dissolving 2.5 mg in 500 ml of carrier solution and 0.2 ml/min delivered by an infusion pump) is an alternative mode of treatment. Isoprenaline also increases the O_2 demand and may even cause serious hypokalaemia, therefore, its use must balance the benefits versus risks.

174 Cardiology

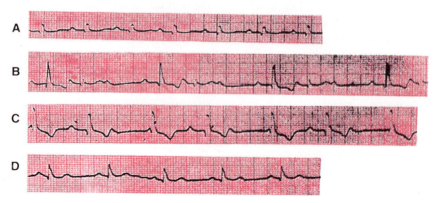

Fig. 34.3: Transient high grade AV block degenerating into complete AV block followed by restoration of normal sinus rhythm with treatment. (A) First degree AV block (P-R interval = 0.24 sec) (B) Second degree 3:1 AV block (high grade) (C) Complete AV block (D) Restoration of normal sinus rhythm

2. *When there is no risk of asystole:* If there is no risk of asystole, proceed on the other side of algorithm and look for the presence or absence of adverse signs.
   a. *When adverse signs are absent*, the patient should be just monitored and observed.
   b. *When one or more adverse signs present*, then atropine should be given I.V. as initial dose of 0.5 mg, increased at an interval of few minutes if required, but not exceeding a total dose of 3 mg. If a satisfactory response to atropine is achieved, then observe the patient; if no response, then proceed for transvenous pacing. If there is likelihood of an appreciable delay in instituting pacing, then interim measures as discussed in the algorithm may be adopted.
   When the successful effect of atropine is short-lived or higher doses are required, transvenous pacing will usually be indicated for long-lasting stabilization.

STOKES-ADAM SYNDROME

It is defined as transient loss of consciousness due to hypoxia of the brain as a result of sudden fall in cardiac output.

Causes

The underlying pathogenic mechanism is sudden fall in cardiac output which may be due to:
1. *Marked bradycardia (HR < 30 min) due to:*
   - Sinoatrial dysfunction e.g. sinus pauses, sinoatrial block, high grade or complete AV block (Fig. 34.3).
2. *Depressed ventricular contractions e.g.* ventricular tachycardia, ventricular fibrillation or asystole.

The causes are summarized in Box 34.2.

Box 34.2: Cause of Stokes-Adam attacks
- Acute myocardial infarction (inferior wall)
- Acute myocarditis
- Complete heart block due to any cause
- Sinus node dysfunction (structural disease)
- Syphilitic aortitis
- Aortic stenosis
- Drugs e.g. beta-blockers

Clinical Features

The typical attacks of Stokes-Adam syndrome are characterised by frequent faintings without any warning symptoms; and in majority of the cases, high grade or complete AV block is detected. In patients with these attacks, the block may be

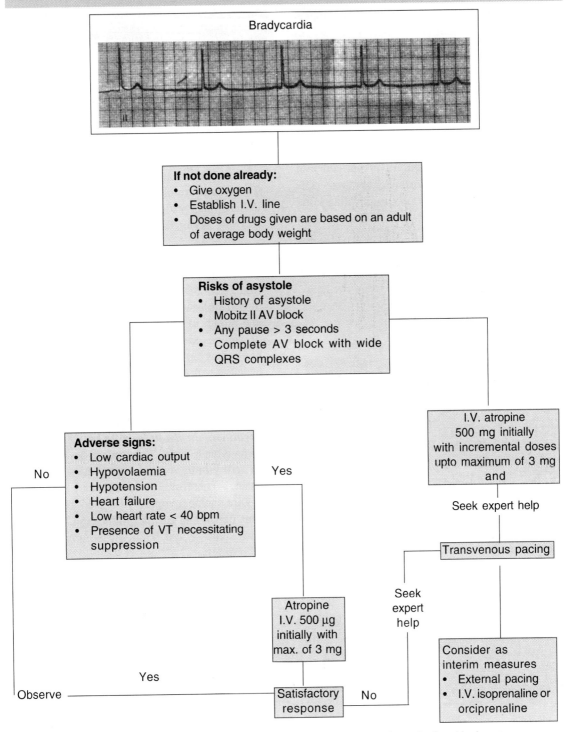

Fig. 34.4: Algorithm for management of bradycardia and conduction blocks

persistent or temporary with a subsidiary pacemaker below the block which either fails to function or functions at slow rate producing bradycardia. If the attacks occur during standing, the patient may fall and hurt himself/herself. Should the attack persists more than 8 to 10 seconds, the patient turns pale, falls unconscious and may exhibit few clonic jerks. If an attack persists with longer period (2-3 minutes) asystole results leading to irregular breathing, cyanosis, fixed pupils, incontinence of urine and bilateral plantar extensor response. The giant T waves in leads V_2-V_4 is virtually diagnostic of recent syncopal attack (Box 34.3). The recovery from such attacks is also prompt and complete without permanent impairment of mental functions. After recovery, patient does not recall presyncopal symptoms.

Diagnosis

In between *Stokes-Adam attacks*, the patient appears normal or may be slightly confused, does not remember what happened before the attack. A careful history, clinical and electrocardiographic evidence of basic heart disease with conduction defect or an arrhythmia help in the diagnosis. If routine ECG fails to reveal an arrhythmia or conduction defect, a 24-hour Holter monitoring may be useful to find out the underlying cause.

Syncopal attacks have to be differentiated from epileptic fits and transient ischemic attacks.

1. *Epileptic fits* are abrupt in onset, longer in duration, are preceded by an aura or cry, and followed by post-ictal phenomenon (e.g. confusion, mental cloudiness, headache etc.).
2. *Transient ischaemic attacks:* They are recurrent, longer in duration (persist for hours but < 24 hr) and are characterised by neurological deficit which is identical during each attack and recovers within 24 hours.

> **Box 34.3: Pathognomic sign of Stokes-Adam attacks on ECG**
>
> Large, broad, bizarre and inverted T waves-called giant 'T' in leads V_2-V_4 is visually pathognomic sign of recent syncopal attack; if present. This is associated with prolonged QTc interval

Management

1. *Treatment of an attack:* This is just similar to treatment of cardiac arrest e.g. precordial thump, followed by external cardiac massage and mouth to mouth breathing (See algorithm of cardiac asystole). Most of the attacks are so brief; may not be witnessed by the physician because it may disappear before a physician arrives. In such a situation, the future plan to prevent such an attack is warranted, therefore, find out the underlying cause and treat it.
2. *Treatment in-between attacks:* Most of the patients have either a complete heart block or an arrthythmia as underlying cause for such attacks. Therefore, complete heart block may require pacing; temporary (Fig. 34.2) or permanent depending on the underlying cause. An arrhythmia should be identified and managed accordingly.

Chapter 35

Acute Coronary Syndrome

Presenting symptom	→	Ischaemic chest pain			
Provisional diagnosis	→	Acute coronary syndrome (ACS)			
ECG	→	Persistent ST elevation	Non persistent ST elevation	Normal	
Cardiac markers (CPK + MB, troponin)	→	Positive	Positive	Negative	Negative
Final diagnosis	→	ST elevation MI (STEMI)	Non-ST elevation MI (NSTEMI)	Unstable angina	Not ACS

Fig. 35.1: Spectrum of acute coronary events

ACUTE CORONARY SYNDROME

Definition

Clinically coronary artery disease manifests as stable angina pectoris, unstable angina pectoris or acute coronary syndrome and acute myocardial infarction (catastrophic presentation). Unstable angina pectoris is an intermediate coronary syndrome between angina pectoris on one side and acute MI on the other side of spectrum of ischaemic heart disease. Acute coronary syndrome (Fig. 35.1) includes unstable angina, acute MI without ST elevation–NSTEMI and ST segment elevation MI (STEMI).

Etiopathogenesis

Almost all cases of acute coronary syndrome occur as a result of plaque rupture or hemorrhage, leading

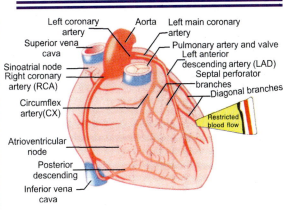

A. Acute coronary syndrome (ACS)

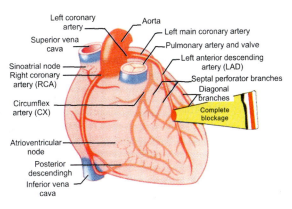

B. Acute myocardial infarction

Figs 35.2A and B: Pathogenesis of acute coronary artery disease
NB: Stable angina pectoris is not shown

to thrombus formation and incomplete occlusion of a major vessel (See Figs 35.2A and B). The thrombus often forms over a tear or fissuring on the surface of a cholesterol plaque. A severe narrowing of a coronary artery i.e. stenosis > 70% of the diameter is generally required to produce angina.

Clinical Presentation

Symptomatically, the following three patient's groups may be said to have unstable angina (acute coronary syndrome):
1. Patient with recent onset of angina (< 2 months). The angina is severe and/or frequent (> 3 episodes/day).
2. Patients with accelerating angina i.e. those patients of chronic stable angina who develop pain which is more severe, frequent and prolonged or precipitated by less exertion as compared to previous level.
3. Angina at rest or after recent myocardial infarction is also often taken as unstable angina.

Symptoms and Signs

Patients of unstable angina may have symptoms of atypical angina with no relation to exertion or mental stress, or may have anginal equivalents (jaw, neck, arm or upper abdominal discomfort). Occasionally, patients with acute coronary syndrome may present with unexplained breathlessness on exertion, unexplained nausea, vomiting, sweating, fatigue and exhaustion. There is usually no physical sign but patients with rest pain frequently develop third or fourth heart sound during the episodes, and in some instances exhibit transient left ventricular failure (murmur of mitral incompetence).

Patients with unstable angina should be explored for the precipitating cause such as uncontrolled hypertension, anaemia, occult thyrotoxicosis, and presence of atherosclerosis (carotid, aortic or peripheral artery disease).

Investigations

1. *The electrocardiogram (ECG):* The ECG taken during an episode of pain is highly valuable. Its diagnostic accuracy further improves if a prior ECG is available for comparison.

Transient ST segment depression and T wave inversion occurring during an episode of pain that resolves when the patient becomes asymptomatic is highly suggestive of acute coronary syndrome. Therefore, patients presenting with ST segment depression belong either to unstable angina or non-ST elevation myocardial infarction (see Fig. 35.2 on front page), the distinction between the two rests on the detection of biochemical serum cardiac markers. Deep, symmetric T wave inversion strongly suggests acute ischaemia and indicates critical narrowing of a coronary vessel especially acute anterior descending coronary artery in 85% cases. Nonspecific ST-T changes are frequent and less helpful. Preexisting Q waves of prior MI suggest post-myocardial angina.

> A completely normal ECG in a patient with chest pain does not exclude the possibility of acute coronary syndrome. One to six percent of such patients are found to have non-ST elevation MI and 4% have unstable angina.

2. *Biochemical serum cardiac markers:*
   - Troponins (T and I).
   - CPK-MB.
   - Serum myoglobin.
   i. *Troponins:* Immunoassays are used to detect cardiac specific troponins T and I. Both troponins (T and I) have equal sensitivity and specificity in detection of muscle damage. Normally troponins are not present in the blood of healthy persons, detectable troponin indicates muscle damage whether CPK-MB is *elevated or not.*
   Troponins are not helpful in very early detection of myocardial necrosis (< 6 hours) after the onset of symptoms, hence, if an early troponin test is negative, another sample should be taken after 8-12 hours after the onset of symptoms for confirmation. The another disadvantage of troponin is their persistence for long time (10-14

days), hence, if a patient who had recent infarction 7-10 days before and again presents with chest pain, a slightly elevated troponin level is unable to differentiate whether MI is old or new. An additional disadvantage of troponins is nonspecific elevation in conditions other than MI such as pulmonary embolism, sepsis, CHF etc.

ii. *Serum CPK-MB:* It is less sensitive and less specific than troponins for detection of minor myocardial damage (micro-infarct). It is elevated in non-ST segment elevation myocardial infarct in which 25% cases develop acute Q-wave MI (See Fig. 35.2). If CPK-MB is elevated, it suggests a significant myocardial damage.

iii. *Serum myoglobin:* Serum myoglobin may be helpful in this situation. Even though it is nonspecific, a negative myoglobin test indicates that raised troponins is not due to acute event.

> Note: CPK-MB and myoglobin are useful for detection of an early infarction (< 6 hours) whereas troponins are useful for late diagnosis of MI.

Management

The patients with rest pain or severe angina developing after MI should be admitted for observation, further diagnosis and treatment. Concomitant conditions that may accelerate ischaemia such as uncontrolled tachycardia, hypertension, diabetes, thyrotoxicosis, heart failure, cardiomegaly, arrhythmias and any acute febrile illness should be looked for and treated.

Patients with definite or possible acute coronary syndrome are observed with cardiac and hemodynamic monitoring. An ECG, CPK-MB and troponin tests are repeated after 8-12 hours of the onset of symptoms. If the follow up ECG and biochemical markers are also normal, the patient may be discharged.

Acute MI should be ruled out by serial ECGs and measurements of serum cardiac enzymes. A stress ECG may be performed before and after discharge to assess the prognosis. If stress test is negative, then patient is managed as outpatient; if the patient is unable to exercise or has persistent ST-T changes, should undergo dobutamine stress echocardiography.

Steps

1. *Continuous ECG monitoring* should be carried out and the patient should receive reassurance and sedation. Sudden ventricular fibrillation is the major cause of death in early period.
2. *Bed rest* should be enforced while ischaemia is ongoing, but patient can sit in a chair and use commode when symptom free.
3. *Oxygen therapy:* Oxygen therapy is given to improve arterial oxygen saturation.
4. *Intravenous nitroglycerine:* Patients whose symptoms are not relieved with three doses of 0.4 mg sublingual nitrate and I.V. beta blockers, may get benefit from I.V. nitroglycerine (NGT). Intravenous NTG (10 µg/min as a starting dose; increase the dose to titrate the response) is recommended in each and every symptomatic patient of acute coronary syndrome to relieve ischaemia and pain. It can be given in the presence of low BP. Side-effects include headache, fall in BP and tolerance. To avoid tolerance, intermittent infusion may be used once the patient is free of pain or oral nitrate may be started.
5. *Morphine:* Intravenous morphine sulphate, (2.5 to 10 mg) is recommended for patients whose pain is not relieved by sublingual NTG and anti-ischaemia therapy. It is repeated after 3-5 minutes if needed.
6. *Anti-thrombotic therapy:* Intravenous heparin should be given for 3 to 5 days to maintain partial thromboplastin time at 2 to 2.5 times than control, together with or followed by oral aspirin at a dose of 325 mg/day.
7. *Intravenous betablockers:* Beta-blockers reduce myocardial contractility and decrease the oxygen demand of myocardium, hence, are useful in high risk patients and in patients

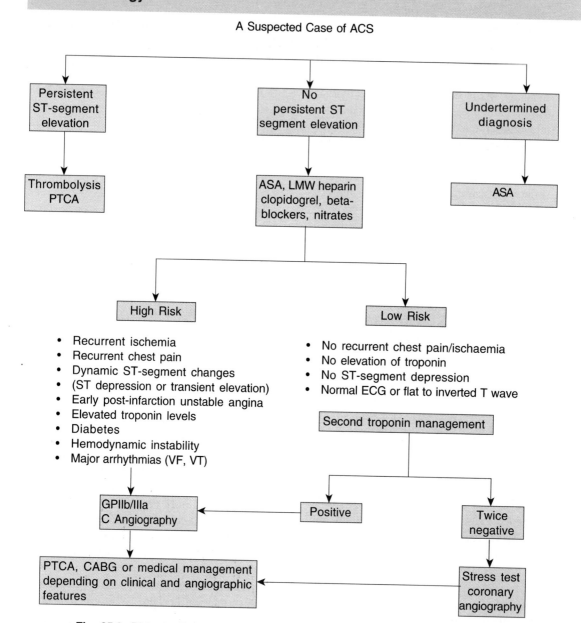

Fig. 35.3: Risk stratification and management protocol for acute coronary syndrome. PTCA Percutaneous transcoronary angioplasty. CABG. Coronary artery by pass graft

with rest pain. If there is no contraindication (e.g. heart block, asthma, CHF etc.), then I.V. metoprolol or atenolol may be used in rapid increasing doses and the patient must be observed carefully to avoid bradycardia, heart failure and hypotension. After initial I.V. dose, it is possible to change to an oral beta blocker. The target resting heart rate during beta, blockers therapy is between 50-60 bpm.

8. *Calcium channel blocker:* Calcium antagonists are reserved as a second or a third choice after the initiation of nitrates and/or

beta blockers. Definite evidence to their benefit is symptom relief, hence, are used in combination with nitrates or beta blockers to relieve pain. These drugs may control hypertension in patients with acute coronary syndrome. I.V. verapamil or diltiazem is preferred if calcium antagonist is to be used. Side effects include fall in BP, precipitation of heart failure and heart blocks. A combination of a beta blocker and calcium antagonist may act in synergy to depress LV contractility.

9. *Potassium channel openers* (e.g. nicorandil): In one study, nicorandil has been claimed to significantly reduce the number of episodes of transient myocardial ischaemia and arrhythmias.

   The majority of the patients (about 80%) improve with such treatment over a period of 48 hours.

10. *Urgent revascularisation:* If angina and/or ECG evidence of ischaemia do not diminish within 24-48 hours of the comprehensive therapy discussed above, then the patient should undergo cardiac catheterisation and coronary angiography if there is no contraindication for revascularisation procedures. If anatomy of coronary artery is suitable, PTCA (percutaneous transluminal coronary angioplasty) can be performed. If angioplasty can not be done, coronary artery bypass surgery should be considered to relieve symptoms and myocardial ischaemia, and as a means of preventing myocardial damage.

European society of cardiology Guidelines for management of ACS according to risk stratification are depicted in Figure 35.3.

Hospital Discharge and Follow-up

If patient's symptoms and signs are controlled on medical therapy, a diagnostic stress ECG should be obtained at the time of hospital discharge. If there is evidence of severe myocardial ischaemia and/or a high risk of coronary events, cardiac catheterisation should be done followed by revascularisation if needed. Many patients in whom unstable state is controlled with medical therapy, are left with severe chronic stable angina and ultimately require mechanical revascularisation (angioplasty with stenting).

Chapter 36

Cardiac Tamponade

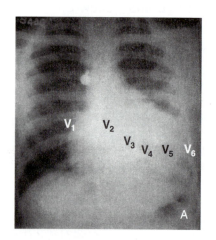

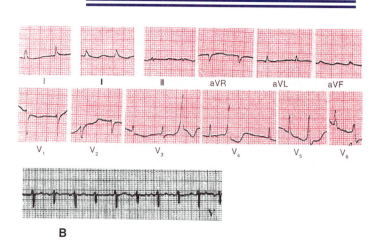

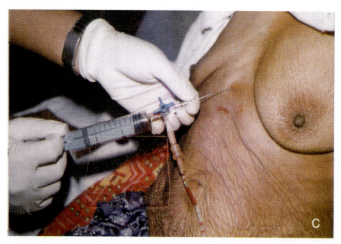

Figs 36.1A to C: Cardiac tamponade due to acute massive pericardial effusion. (A) The X-ray chest showing pericardial effusion with labelling of ECG leads (B) The 12 lead ECG shows: (i) Low voltage of QRS complexes in standard leads I, II, III, aVR, aVL and aVF (ii) There is ST segment depression in leads I, II, aVL, aVF, V_1-V_6 with low flat T wave (iii) VPCs are seen in lead V_3-V_6 (shown). The lead V_1 recorded from some other patient shows electrical alternans—a characteristic feature of pericardial effusion with cardiac tamponade. In electrical alternans, one short QRS complex alternates with a large QRS complex (C) Procedure of pericardiocentesis

CARDIAC TAMPONADE (Figs. 36.1A to C)

It is defined as clinical syndrome occurring due to compression of heart from outside by rapid, large accumulation of fluid in the pericardial sac leading to obstruction to the inflow of blood to the ventricles. It is a life-threatening emergency where cure can be achieved by pericardiocentesis (removal of pericardial fluid).

Causes

Acute pericardial tamponade occurs either due to trauma with penetrating or blunt abdominal or thoracic injury or due to iatrogenic causes such as following cardiac surgery, cardiac catheterization, pacing etc.

Most cases are subacute or chronic. Tuberculosis is the most common cause followed by viral pericardial effusion. The causes of cardiac tamponade are given in the Box 36.1.

Clinical Features

The clinical manifestations result due to acute elevation of intracardiac pressure, restricted ventricular filling and reduction of cardiac output. The amount of fluid required to produce cardiac tamponade may be as small as 200 ml if it collects rapidly or may be 2000 ml if it collects slowly to allow the pericardium to stretch and adapt to the increasing volume of fluid.

The manifestations of tamponade range from asymptomatic or mild disease to shock like state (acute onset). Tamponade may also develop more slowly, and the clinical manifestations resemble those of heart failure (e.g. dyspnoea, orthopnoea, congestive hepatomegaly, raised JVP). Tamponade, sometimes, may be so sudden that symptoms may not be experienced or reflect only vague symptoms. A high degree of suspicion of cardiac tamponade is required since, in many instances when there is no apparent cause of pericardial disease; and tamponade should even be considered in any patient with hypotension, low volume pulse, raised JVP with prominent X descent. A widened area of dullness on percussion on anterior aspect of chest wall, a paradoxical pulse, clear lung fields, diminished cardiac pulsations over precordium, nonvisible apex beat, should raise the suspicion of cardiac tamponade and patient should be subjected to investigations for confirmation of the diagnosis. The clinical features are summarized in the Fig. 36.2 and Box. 36.2.

Diagnosis

Cardiac tamponade should be suspected in a patient who appears to be in shock but has high

---

Box 36.1: Causes of cardiac tamponade

Acute cardiac tamponade	Subacute or chronic cardiac tamponade
1. *Trauma* • Penetrating or blunt thoracic injury • Iatrogenic e.g. pacing, catheterisation, pericardial tapping, post-resuscitation 2. *Cardiac rupture* • Acute MI-free wall rupture • Aortic aneurysm rupturing into pericardium	1. *Infections* • Tuberculosis • Bacterial (pneumococal, streptococcal, staphylococcal) • Viral, fungal, parasitic • AIDS-associated 2. *Malignancy*-secondaries 3. *Uraemic* pericarditis 4. *Systemic* disorders e.g. SLE, myxoedema, Dressler's syndrome (Post-MI or postcardiotomy), amyloidosis 5. *Radiation* 6. *Idiopathic* 7. *Drugs* e.g. anticoagulants, procainamide, isoniazide hydralazine, daunorubicin etc.

184 Cardiology

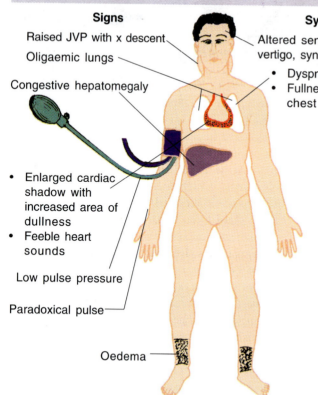

Fig. 36.2: Clinical manifestations of cardiac tamponade (diagrammatic illustration)

Box 36.2: Clinical features of cardiac tamponade

1. **Symptoms:**
   - Progressive dyspnoea, tachypnoea
   - Fullness, tightness of chest
   - Cerebral symptoms e.g. altered sensorium, confusion, dizziness, vertigo, syncope.
   - Pain chest if pericarditis present
2. **Signs:**
   - Tachycardia, low blood pressure with low pulse pressure
   - Elevated JVP with x descent
   - Kussmaul' sign (paradoxical rise in JVP during inspiration) is less common
   - Pulsus paradoxus,
   - Increased area of dullness over anterior chest on percussion
   - Feeble heart sounds
   - Congestive hepatomegaly
   - Dry lung fields on auscultation
   - Pericardial knock can sometimes be present

jugular venous pressure and distended neck veins. This is especially true in setting of trauma. The physical signs of low cardiac output with silent heart, enlarged area of dullness further strengthen the diagnosis which is confirmed by demonstrating the fluid in the pericardial sac on echocardiography. The investigations that help in the diagnosis are:

1. ***Chest X-ray*** may show enlarged globular heart (money-bag appearance) with oligaemic lungs (Fig. 36.1A).
2. ***Fluoroscopy*** may show diminished cardiac pulsations with enlarged cardiac shadow.
3. ***The electrocardiogram*** (Fig. 36.1B) may show low voltage graph, sinus tachycardia and electrical alternans (QRS alternans).
4. ***The echocardiogram:*** shows:
   i. Significant anterior and posterior echo-free space.
   ii. Right ventricular and right atrial diastolic collapse due to high pericardial pressure.
   iii. Enlarged inferior vena cava with absence of respiratory variations.
   iv. *Doppler study*: The characteristic and diagnostic feature on Doppler study is the exaggerated respiratory variations in inflow velocity. Venous flow is prominently systolic with exaggerated respiratory variations in inferior vena cava (IVC) and hepatic vein flow (diminished forward flow during expiration).
5. ***CVP monitoring*** helps in the diagnosis, differential diagnosis and serves as a guide to fluid therapy. CVP is raised in pericardial effusion with shock, hence, differentiates it from hypovolemic shock where CVP is low.

Table 36.1: Features that distinguish cardiac tamponade from other similar clinical disorders

Features	Tamponade	Constrictive	Restrictive	CHF
A. Clinical				
• Pulsus paradoxus	Common	Absent	Rare	Absent
• Prominent X descent on JVP	Present	Usually present	Present	Absent
• Prominent Y descent on JVP	Absent	Usually present	Rare	Present
• V and Y collapse on JVP	Absent	Absent	Absent	Present
Kussmaul's sign	Absent	Present	Absent	Present
Third heart sound	Absent	Absent	Rare	Present
Pericardial knock	Absent	Present often	Absent	Absent
B. ECG				
• Low voltage graph	May be present	May be present	May be present	May be present
• Electrical alternans	May be present	Absent	Absent	Absent
C. Echocardiography				
• Thickened pericardium	Absent	Present	Absent	Absent
• Pericardial calcification	Absent	Often present	Absent	Absent
• Pericardial effusion	Present	Absent	Absent	May be present in small amount
• RV size	Usually small	Usually normal	Usually normal	Enlarged
• Myocardial thickness	Normal	Normal	Usually increased	Normal or decreased
• Right atrial collapse and RVDC	Present	Absent	Absent	Absent
• Increased mitral flow velocity	Absent	Present	Absent	May be present
• Exaggerated respiratory variations in inflow velocity	Present	Present	Absent	Absent
D. CT/MRI				
Thickened or calcific pericardium	Absent	Present	Absent	Absent
E. Chest X-ray				
Cardiac shadow	Enlarged	Normal or enlarged	Normal	Enlarged
Cardiac pulsations on fluoroscopy	Absent	Diminished	Diminished	Normal or diminished
F. Cardiac catheterisation				
Square root's sign in ventricular pressure pulses	Absent	Present	May be present	Absent

6. *Other investigations* are done to find out the cause such as biochemical, microbiological and cytological examination of pericardial fluid.

Differential Diagnosis

The conditions that simulate the cardiac tamponade have to be differentiated from therapeutic point of view. The differential diagnosis of cardiac tamponade is tabulated (Table 36.1).

Management

It includes:
1. *Treatment of shock:* If patient is in shock state, treat it like cardiogenic shock (Read cardiogenic shock). After assessment, maintain basic life support measures i.e. airway, breathing and circulation. Fluid therapy is given to maintain preload under CVP monitoring. Inotropic agent may be used if fluid therapy alone is insufficient

to restore the shock. Metabolic acidosis may be corrected.

2. ***Pericardiocentesis (removal of pericardial fluid):*** It is the mainstay of management because it provides rapid relief and restores the circulation and diastolic filling of the ventricles. Unless situation is immediately life-threatening, tapping should be done by an experienced personnel under echo or fluoroscopic guidance with ECG monitoring.

   Procedure: Left subxiphoid approach with patient propped upto 45° is preferred (Fig. 36.1C on front page). Rarely apical or parasternal approach may be required in loculated effusions. The procedure is as follows:

   1. The patient is made to lie in propped up position with back rest.
   2. The patient is premedicated with atropine and diazepam.
   3. The skin over the precordium and upper part of the abdomen is shaved.
   4. Under aseptic precautions and local anaesthesia, a large bore long needle or I.V. cannula connected to a syringe is inserted and then connected to a 3-way stopcock for rapid aspiration. The fluid is continuously aspirated. Fluid is removed as much as possible till patient feels relief in dyspnoea and BP is restored above 90 mmHg.
   5. If at any stage during procedure, frank blood is seen entering the syringe, the tip of the needle should be repositioned.
   6. Always look at the ECG monitor for any VPC as this may indicate the presence of the needle in the myocardium.
   7. If the fluid drawn is purulent, then it should be drained by an indwelling catheter connected to an underwater seal.
   8. After removal of the fluid, patient is made to lie comfortably on the bed and observed for pulse, BP for few hours. The I.V. line is maintained during this period.

3. ***Surgical pericardiotomy or pericardiectomy:*** It is indicated for recurrent, frequent, disabling pericardial effusion.

Chapter 37

Acute Chest Pain

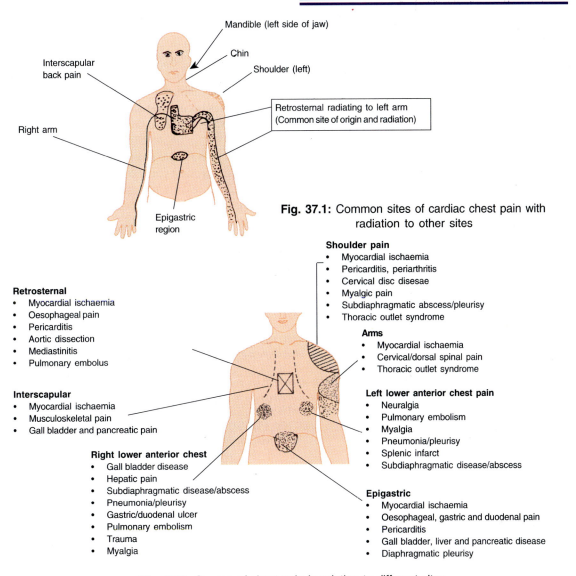

Fig. 37.1: Common sites of cardiac chest pain with radiation to other sites

Retrosternal
- Myocardial ischaemia
- Oesophageal pain
- Pericarditis
- Aortic dissection
- Mediastinitis
- Pulmonary embolus

Interscapular
- Myocardial ischaemia
- Musculoskeletal pain
- Gall bladder and pancreatic pain

Right lower anterior chest
- Gall bladder disease
- Hepatic pain
- Subdiaphragmatic disease/abscess
- Pneumonia/pleurisy
- Gastric/duodenal ulcer
- Pulmonary embolism
- Trauma
- Myalgia

Shoulder pain
- Myocardial ischaemia
- Pericarditis, periarthritis
- Cervical disc disesae
- Myalgic pain
- Subdiaphragmatic abscess/pleurisy
- Thoracic outlet syndrome

Arms
- Myocardial ischaemia
- Cervical/dorsal spinal pain
- Thoracic outlet syndrome

Left lower anterior chest pain
- Neuralgia
- Pulmonary embolism
- Myalgia
- Pneumonia/pleurisy
- Splenic infarct
- Subdiaphragmatic disease/abscess

Epigastric
- Myocardial ischaemia
- Oesophageal, gastric and duodenal pain
- Pericarditis
- Gall bladder, liver and pancreatic disease
- Diaphragmatic pleurisy

Fig. 37.2: Causes of chest pain in relation to different sites

Cardiology

ACUTE CHEST PAIN

Definitions

Acute chest pain (central or peripheral) is a common emergency encountered in clinical practice. Chest pain is a common presentation of cardiac disease, but can also be a manifestation of anxiety, or of disease of respiratory system, musculoskeletal system or gastrointestinal system. Correct assessment and management is essential because failure to recognise a life-threatening situation such as myocardial infarction may result in unnecessary delay in instituting the treatment resulting in adverse outcome. On the other hand, erroneous diagnosis may result in psychological tension and economic consequences.

Chest pain results due to a variety of causes, has a little correlation with seriousness of the disease, hence, to be taken seriously unless proved otherwise.

Causes

A variety of causes that can lead to chest pain are divided mainly into two major categories i.e. central and peripheral (see Box 37.1).

Differential Diagnosis of Acute Chest Pain

A detailed history and physical examination would help in distinguishing cardiac pain from that of non-cardiac chest pain (Figs. 37.1 and 37.2). Recording the ECG is essential in each and every case of acute chest pain or discomfort. It is important to differentiate between central and peripheral chest pain as it will help in assessing the cause of origin of pain as already listed in the Box 37.1.

The characteristics of cardiac and noncardiac chest pain are tabulated (Table 37.1).

Once it has become established that it is cardiac chest pain then its cause has to be established as follows:

1. *Anginal pain (stable vs unstable):* Stable angina is defined as chest pain brought on exertion and relieved by rest and/or sublingual nitrate. The provoking factors include; anaemia, thyrotoxicosis, exposure to cold, heavy meals, stress and sexual activity.

Box 37.1: Common causes of chest pain

Central	Peripheral
a. **Psychological** e.g. anxiety or cardiac neurosis	a. **Lungs pleura**
b. **Cardiac**	• Pneumonia (consolidation)
• Myocardial ischaemia (angina)	• Pneumothorax
• Myocardial infarction	• Malignancy
• Myocarditis	• Pleurisy
• Pericarditis	b. **Musculoskeletal**
• Mitral valve prolapse syndrome	• Osteoarthritis
• Aortic dissection	• Costochondritis (Tietz's syndrome)
• Aortic aneurysm	• Injury (muscle/rib)
c. **Gastroesophageal**	• Epidemic myalgia (Bornholm disease)
• Oesophagitis	c. **Neurological**
• Diffuse oesophageal spasms	• Prolapse intervertebral disc
• Peptic ulcer disease	• Neurolagia e.g. herpes zoster
• Hiatus hernia	• Thoracic outlet syndrome
• Mallory-Weiss syndrome	
d. **Massive pulmonary embolism**	
e. **Mediastinal**	
• Tracheitis	
• Malignancy	

Note: The musculoskeletal disorder have such a wide clinical presentation that they may produce central, and/or peripheral or both types of chest pain.

Table 37.1: Some important conditions producing acute chest pain

Conditions/disorders	Associated symptoms/signs
1. Ischaemic chest pain	Centrally located, retrosternal or across the chest, radiating to left arm, shoulder, neck, jaw or even right arm. Patient describes such a pain either as discomfort or tightness, pressure, squeezing or like a band rather than actual constriction pain. Clenching of fist in front of chest (Levine's sign) is highly suggestive of cardiac pain
2. *Inflammatory/musculoskeletal* • Myalgia • Costocondritis (Teitz's syndrome)	There is tenderness of chest on applying pressure. Pain increases on movements and is constant. Tenderness and swelling of costochondral junctions present in Teitz' syndrome
3. *Neurological* • Herpetic neuralgia	There are either vesicles or scabs present along the distribution of intercostal nerves. Pain increases with chest movements
4. *Gastrointestinal* • Hiatus hernia • Reflux esophagitis • *Diffuse oesophageal spasms*	Pain is retrosternal, occurs during lying down, relieved on sitting or by antacids and H_2 blockers. Pain is in the form of heart burn, occurs after heavy meals on lying down. It causes retrosternal pain, intermittent in character, relieved by prokinetics drugs. Sometimes, it is difficult to distinguish it from angina at rest
5. *Cardiovascular* • Acute aortic dissection • Pericarditis	Acute severe 'tearing' pain across the chest, asymmetric pulses, bradycardia are its features. Pain varies in intensity, does not increase with respiration. Audible pericardial rub may be present
6. *Respiratory* • Pleurisy (pleurodynia) • Pneumothorax	Pain increases with breathing and a pleural rub is present Sudden onset of pain with breathlessness. Hyperresonant percussion note. Chest X-ray is diagnostic
7. *Psychological* • Cardiac neurosis	Tachycardia, pain not related to exertion but related to anxious moments. They can pinpoint the site of pain

Unstable angina is *crescendo angina* or rapidly worsening angina with changing pattern of pain during the past 6 weeks (occurs on minimal exertion or at rest and pain is prolonged) without an evidence of myocardial infarction on ECG or cardiac enzyme elevation (CPK-MB).

2. **Prinzmetal's angina or variant angina**, occurs at rest without any provoking factor and is due to coronary vasospasm. The characteristic features of this type of angina is marked ST segment elevation > 4 mm with increase in the height the R wave in same leads during attack of pain and return of ST segment to normal with relief of pain.

3. **Myocardial ischaemia:** Prolonged chest pain lasting for 10-20 minutes may be present due to myocardial ischaemia and these patients even have no abnormalities on ECG and cardiac

enzymes are normal. Others may have ST-T changes with elevation of cardiac markers like Troponin-T or Troponin I.

Exceptions: Atypical anginal symptoms such as fatigue, exhaustion, fainting sensation or dyspnoea may occur. These are called anginal equivalents. Older patients and patients with distress may not have chest pain but may have anginal equivalents as described above.

4. **Myocardial infarction:** It is characterised by central retrosternal pain which is prolonged and severe and is associated with nausea, vomiting, sweating and dyspnoea. Initial ECG and levels of cardiac enzymes may be normal but subsequent ECGs show serial changes of infarction (i.e. ST segment elevation, q wave and T wave inversion in more than 2 leads) and elevation of cardiac markers i.e. troponin T and I and raised cardiac enzymes (CPK-MB).

5. **Pain due to dissecting aneurysm of aorta:** A centrally located excruciating tearing pain lasting for hours and radiating to the back into thoracic region is a characteristic feature. Examination may show acute aortic regurgitation (early diastolic murmur in the aortic area) and evidence of hypertension (the condition is common in hypertensive). X-ray chest may show mediastinal enlargement. ECG may be normal.

6. **Pain of pericarditis:** Acute pericardial pain is not related to effort, is constant and continuous, not aggravated by deep breathing. The pain is 'sharp' located in the precordial region and may radiate to the left or right shoulder. To relieve pain, patient may sit leaning forward (Muslims' prayer sign). The pericardial rub is often present but its absence does not rule out pericarditis.

7. **Pain of pulmonary embolism:** Only large embolism produce pain similar to myocardial infarction. The triad; *pain*, *hemoptysis* and *pleuritic pain* in a patient with deep vein thrombosis suggests acute pulmonary embolisms. The pain is mostly peripheral but may be central, gets aggravated by respiration and coughing.

8. **Noncardiac chest pain:** The causes and characteristics are discussed in the Table 37.1 and elaborated in the Figure 37.2.

Management

The patients of acute chest pain should be managed appropriately depending on the cause.

Chapter 38

Cardiac Arrest and Sudden Cardiac Death

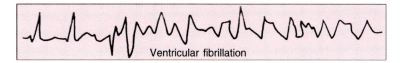

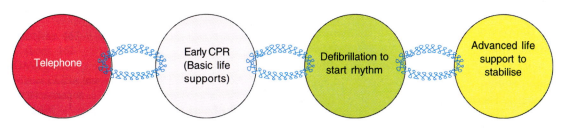

Fig. 38.1: A chain of measures for survival in cardiac arrest. CPR = Cardiopulmonary resuscitation

CARDIAC ARREST AND SUDDEN CARDIAC DEATH (SCD)

Cardiac Arrest

It is defined as sudden and complete loss of cardiac pump function leading to no pulse, no respiration and sudden loss of consciousness. Death is virtually inevitable if prompt intervention is not done.

Sudden Cardiac Death (SCD)

It is defined as the unexpected natural death due to cardiac causes within a short period of time (usually within one hour) from the start of symptoms in an individual who may have pre-existing heart disease but in whom the *time* and *mode* of death are unexpected.

Death means irreversible loss of all biological functions.

Sudden and unexpected cardiac death is usually due to development of a catastrophic arrhythmia and accounts for 25-30% of cardiovascular deaths. Arrhythmias may complicate many types of heart diseases and may, sometimes, occur in the absence of a heart disease. Ventricular fibrillation (VF), followed by bradyarrhythmias or asystole, and sustained ventricular tachycardia (VT) are responsible for SCD. Other less common mechanisms include acute mechanical catastrophes such as electromechanical dissociation, cardiac rupture, cardiac temponade and acute disruption of a major blood vessel (e.g. aortic dissection).

Risk Factors

1. **Advanced age:** The incidence of sudden cardiac death increases with age in both the sexes and in all races; though it is more common in males. The first peak incidence of sudden cardiac death occurs within 6 months after birth and is due to sudden *infant death syndrome*; and again between 45-75 years as a result of coronary artery disease (CAD).
2. **Altered coronary anatomy** such as atheroma, plaque rupture or both are the common underlying mechanisms of SCD due to coronary causes.
3. **Other risk factors are:**
   - Hypertension
   - LVH
   - Conduction defects
   - Hyperlipidaemia
   - Smoking
   - Glucose intolerance
   - Decreased vital capacity.

   In *Fragmingham study*, the incidence of SCD in smokers was two and half times more than in non-smokers.
4. **Depressed left ventricular function:** It is an independent risk factor for SCD in heart patients. There is an increased risk of sudden cardiac death in patients with cardiac disease having ejection fraction < 30%.
5. **Reversible risk factors:** Certain factors such as transient myocardial ischaemia and reperfusion, electrolyte disturbances (hypokalaemia, hypomagnesemia), drugs (diuretics, digitalis), alteration in pH or blood gas may provoke SCD if not taken care of immediately.

Causes

Structural coronary or myocardial abnormality provides a plateform for other risk factors to operate. The causes are enumerated in Table 38.1. Structural coronary artery disease is the single most common cause of SCD (90%). The myocardial causes (cardiomyopathies) account for another 10-15% cases; the remaining are due to other causes given in Table 38.1.

Table 38.1: Common causes of sudden cardiac death

1. *Coronary artery diseases (80%)*
   - Myocardial ischaemia
   - Acute MI
   - Previous MI with myocardial scarring
   - Anomalous coronary artery anatomy
2. *Myocardial diseases*
   - Ventricular hypertrophy e.g. LVH, RVH, CHF
   - Hypertrophic cardiomyopathy e.g. obstructive and nonobstructive
   - Dilated cardiomyopathy
   - Inflammatory or infiltrative diseases e.g. myocarditis, arrhythmogenic right ventricular dysplasia.
3. *Valvular heart diseases*
   - Aortic stenosis/regurgitation
   - Mitral valve prolapse
   - Endocarditis
4. *Congenital heart diseases*
   - Stenotic lesions (aortic or pulmonary)
   - Eisenmenger's syndrome
   - *Postoperative* repair of Fallot's tetralogy
5. *Nonstructural heart disease (e.g. electrophysiological abnormalities):*
   - Prolonged QT syndrome (congenital or acquired)
   - Brugada syndrome. It is characterised by a defect in sodium channels function and an abnormal ECG (RBBB and ST elevation in V_1 and V_2 without prolongation of QT interval)
   - Wolff-Parkinson-White syndrome (Kent bundle conduction)
   - Adverse drug reactions leading to *torsade de pointes*
   - Electrolyte disturbances (severe hypokalaemia)
   - Acid-base disturbance e.g. severe acidosis.
6. *Miscellaneous*
   - Massive pulmonary embolism, air embolism
   - Aortic dissection
   - *Cafe* coronary

Aetiology of Cardiac Arrest

Cardiac arrest may be due to:
- Ventricular fibrillation.
- Pulseless ventricular tachycardia.
- Asystole.
- Electromechanical dissociation.

Ventricular fibrillation (VF) and pulseless ventricular tachycardia: This is most common and most easily treatable cause of sudden death. It is characterised by uncoordinated rapid, bizarre ventricular contractions which are ineffective to produce a pulse. The ECG shows rapid irregular ventricular rhythm with no identifiable complexes. (Fig.38.1 on front page) Ventricular tachycardia may also cause loss of cardiac output (pulseless VT) and may further degenerate into VF.

Ventricular asystole: It is characterised by no electrical activity of the ventricles producing more or less straight line on ECG. It is usually due to failure of the conducting tissue or massive ventricular damage complicating MI. A sudden blow to the chest (precordial thump) or cardiac massage can sometimes restore the cardiac activity. An artificial pacemaker may be needed to prevent further attacks (see the algorithm).

Electromechanical dissociation: There is dissociation between electrical activity (it is normal or near normal) and mechanical events (no effective cardiac output). It is mostly due to extraneous causes such as hypovolaemia, tension pneumothorax, cardiac rupture or massive pulmonary embolism. It carries poor prognosis.

Clinical Characteristics of Cardiac Arrest

1. *Prodromal symptoms and signs:* These complaints are nonspecific, presaged by days, weeks or months and are indicative of any major cardiac event. These include increasing angina, dyspnoea, palpitation, easy fatiguability etc.
2. *Onset of terminal events:* Any change in cardiovascular status one hour before cardiac arrest constitutes onset of terminal events. The more rapid is the onset of terminal events, the more is the probability of cardiac arrest. Continuous ECG recordings fortuitously obtained at the onset of a cardiac arrest commonly demonstrate changes in cardiac electrical activity (ECG changes of dying heart) within the minutes or hours before the event. Most cardiac arrest occurring by the mechanisms of VF begin with a run of sustained or nonsustained VT degenerating rapidly into VF and asystole.
3. *Disturbed consciousness:* Arrhythmic cardiac arrest is characterised by a high likelihood of the patients being awake and active prior to arrest and VF is the mechanism of cardiac arrest; while on the other hand cardiac arrest due to circulatory failure is characterised by patients who are inactive or comatosed, have long duration of terminal illness and cardiac arrest is asystolic.

> *Compete loss of consciousness with no pulse and BP are sine qua non of cardiac arrest.*

4. *Forewarning symptoms and signs* may occur in setting of acute MI; such as prolonged angina or pain of AMI, acute onset of dyspnoea, orthopnoea, sudden onset of palpitation, sustained tachycardia or light headedness. In MI, cardiac arrest may be *primary* (no haemodynamic instability) or *secondary* (presence of haemodynamic instability) and has clinical significance because majority or all patients survive with primary cardiac arrest while majority (70%) die in secondary cardiac arrest immediately or during the hospitalization.
5. *Progression to biological death* is a function of the mechanism of cardiac arrest. The length of the delay before interventions. VF or asystole without CPR within first 4-6 minutes have a poor outcome.

Management

The treatment of a patient with cardiac arrest is divided into 5 stages:
1. Initial response.
2. Basic life support.
3. Advanced life support.
4. Post-resuscitation management/care.
5. Long-term management.

Initial Response

The first step is to establish from the person who has witnessed the sudden collapse of the patient whether it is due to cardiac arrest. Ask the patient, ***Hello! Are you O.K.*** and immediately shout for help. Observe for respiratory movement, pulse and skin colour, sweating etc. The absence of pulse and respiration are primary diagnostic criteria and can be confirmed accurately by a trained lay person.

Thumpversion (a sudden discharge of a blow to the precordium) and clearing the airway are the steps of initial management before CPR can be carried out.

Basic Life Support (Fig. 38.1)

See the algorithm. It means maintenance of:
A. Airway.
B. Breathing.
C. Circulation hence, called ABC of cardiopulmonary resuscitation.

Advanced Life Support Measures

Advance life support aims at:
1. To restore normal cardiac rhythm by defibrillation when the cause of cardiac arrest is tachyarrhythmias.
2. To restore cardiac output by correcting other reversible causes of cardiac arrest (*4 Hs and 4 Ts*) given in the Box 38.1:

Box 38.1: Potentially reversible causes of cardiac arrest	
4Hs	**4Ts**
• Hypovolaemia	• Tension pneumothorax
• Hypoxia	• Temponade
• Hypo or hyperkalaemia	• Toxic disturbance or therapeutic disturbances
• Hypothermia	
	• Thromboembolism

3. To provide additional support to basic life saving measures by administering intravenous drugs and by inserting an endotracheal tube to administer positive pressure ventilation.

Measures/Actions

If cardiac arrest is witnessed, a thumpversion (precordial thump) may sometime convert VF/ VT to normal sinus rhythm. It is of no use if the cardiac arrest has lasted longer than few seconds.

The priority of advanced life support (ALS) is to assess basic cardiac rhythm by attaching a defibrillator/monitor. Defibrillation is indicated if VF or pulseless VT is observed on monitor. Defibrillation is started first with 200 Joules, if normal sinus rhythm is not restored within few seconds, then next shock of 200 Joules is given; if unsuccessful, this is followed by a third shock of 360 Joules. If all the three shocks remain unsuccessful, then 1 mg of adrenaline intravenously *plus* CPR is given for full one minute to prepare the patient for next cycle of three shocks each at 360 Joules (Fig. 38.2).

If cardiac arrest is due to asystole, which can occasionally be confused with VF of low amplitude or fine VF, in such a situation, it should be treated like VF and should be defibrillated. Definite asystole is treated without defibrillation like electromechanical dissociation.

If electromechanical dissociation is the cause of cardiac arrest, then it is treated without defibrillation by only maintaining the CPR and treating or correcting the reversible causes of cardiac arrest (4 Hs and 4Ts) which have already been discussed (Box 38.1).

Postcardiac Arrest Care

After successful resuscitation of cardiac arrest, the patient is admitted and observed in intensive care unit for continuous monitoring for a minimum period of 48-72 hours. Treat the underlying cause if found out.

Long-term Management

Patients who survive a cardiac arrest caused by AMI need no specific treatment other than routinely given to those recovering from an infarct. Those with reversible causes such as exercised induced ischaemia or aortic stenosis should have the underlying cause treated if possible. Survivors in

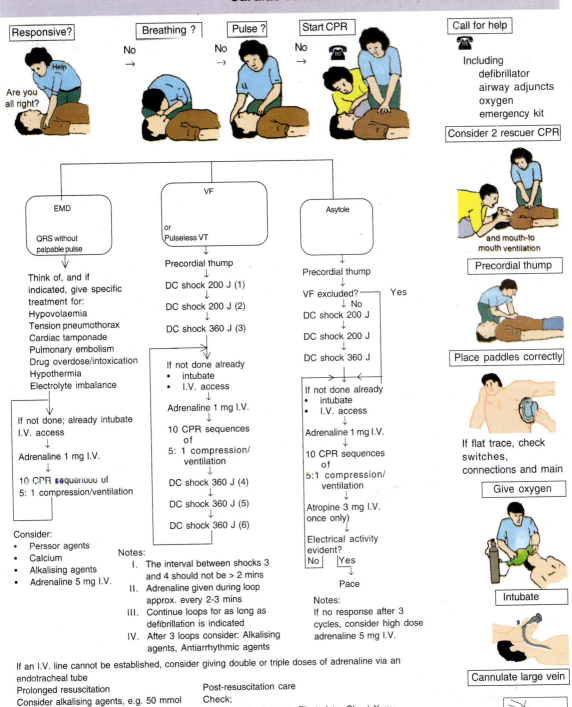

Fig. 38.2: Advanced cardiac life support (Recommended by the European Resuscitation Council and Resuscitation Council of UK)

whom no reversible cause can be found out and treated are at higher risk of developing another episode, such patients are treated either by antiarrhythmic therapy or implantation of implantable cardioverter defibrillator (ICD). Superiority of ICD over antiarrhythmic drug therapy (predominantly amiodarone) has been shown in AVID trial and in other studies (CIDS and CASH).

ICD is the initial treatment of choice for long-term management in patients revived from VF in whom no reversible cause could be found out.

Chapter 39
Hypertensive Emergencies/Urgencies

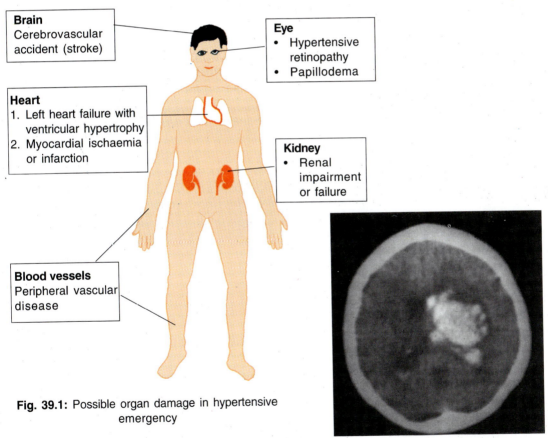

Fig. 39.1: Possible organ damage in hypertensive emergency

Fig. 39.2: CT scan showing intracranial bleed

HYPERTENSIVE CRISES

Terms used Related to Hypertension

Hypertension: The 7th JNC (Joint National Committee) report on prevention, detection, evaluation and treatment of hypertension has defined normal and abnormal values of BP (see Box 39.1) superseding the recommendation of VI JNC report (< 130/85 mmHg was taken as normal).

Cardiology

Box 39.1: JNC VII classification of hypertension

Category	Systolic (mmHg)	Diastolic (mmHg)
Normal	< 120	< 80
Prehypertension (previous term high normal replaced)	120-139	80-89
Hypertension Stage 1st	140-159	90-99
Stage 2nd	≥ 160	≥ 100

The VIIth JNC report describes < 120/80 mmHg as normal BP in patients aged 18 years or above; beyond 120/80 mmHg, this patient is either prehypertensive or hypertensive.

HYPERTENSIVE EMERGENCIES/URGENCIES

Hypertensive emergency: According to JNC VI report, a hypertensive emergency was defined as a severely elevated BP with signs or symptoms of acute target organ damage (Fig. 39.1), requiring parenteral drug treatment, close observation in ICU and immediate reduction is blood pressure.

Hypertensive urgency: It is a state of severely elevated blood pressure which is not associated with severe symptoms or progressive organ dysfunction wherein BP can be reduced within hours, often with oral drug therapy given in an outpatient setting.

> JNC VI stressed acute target organ damage irrespective of blood pressure reading as hypertensive emergency rather than urgency.

With this report, previously used term, (i) accelerated hypertension (diastolic BP > 130 mmHg with Grade 3 fundus changes e.g. exudates and hemorrhage-Keith-Wegner retinopathy) and malignant hypertension with diastolic BP > 130 mm associated with papilloedema (Grade IV Keith-Wegner retinopathy) have been replaced by stage 2 VIIth (Stage 2 and 3 of VI JNC report combines) of JNC report. The fundoscopic differentiation. between accelerated and malignant hypertension has no relevance with respect to clinical picture and prognosis, hence, may be taken hypertensive emergency or urgency. JNC VII report has not changed these definitions.

Most authors treat hypertensive emergency as hypertensive crisis.

Common Hypertensive Emergencies and Urgencies

Hypertensive encephalopathy is defined as sudden, marked rise in blood pressure associated with encephalopathic features i.e. headache, vomiting, visual disturbances, transient paralysis, convulsions, stupor and coma. These manifestations have been attributed to spasm of cerebral vessels and to cerebral oedema. (Read the management at the end). The other examples of hypertensive emergency and urgency are given in the Table 39.1.

Table 39.1: Hypertensive emergencies and urgencies

Emergencies	Urgencies
• Hypertensive encephalopathy or malignant hypertension	• Hypertension associated with coronary artery disease
• Acute aortic dissection	• Accelerated hypertension
• Phaeochromocytoma crisis	• Severe hypertension in patients with kidney transplantation
• MAO inhibitors with tyramine interaction	• Postoperative hypertension
• Intracranial haemorrhage	• Uncontrolled hypertension in patients requiring surgery
• Pre-eclampsia	

The pathophysiological basis of hypertensive crisis is loss of autoregulation on the vascular beds (cerebral, cardiac, renal) with the result they are not able to constrict appropriately to maintain perfusion. This leads to ischaemia and tissue damage. This forms the basis that BP should be lowered as early as possible (within minutes or hours) with parenteral drugs during hypertensive emergency so as to restore autoregulation. The blood pressure should not be drastically reduced to normal because it can give rise to serious consequences, hence, should be kept near normal rather than normal.

Other factors that predispose to crisis are:
1. Elevated plasma renin, angiotensin and natriuretic peptides levels.
2. Discontinuation or inadequate dose adjustment in hypertensive patients without monitoring BP levels.
3. Sometimes ingestion of substances i.e. tyramine containing foods may cause crisis in patients receiving MAO inhibitors.
4. Renovascular hypertension, phaeochromocytoma and primary hyperaldosteronism may frequently present as hypertensive emergency.

Clinical Evaluation

It includes:
1. Careful history with respect to duration, severity of preexisting hypertension and symptoms of any target organ damage should be asked.
2. Record the type of drug therapy received and compliance of treatment.
3. Examination of BP in both lying and standing positions, in both the arms. Significant difference between two arms suggests aortic dissection.
4. Examine cardiovascular, renal and nervous system for any organ damage.
5. Fundus examination for retinopathy.
6. Blood biochemistry i.e. urea, creatinine, sodium, K^+.
7. Chest X-ray for cardiomegaly.
8. ECG for LVH, prior MI.
9. Urine examination for proteinuria
10. CT scan/MRI for neurological damage.

COMMON HYPERTENSIVE EMERGENCIES

Cerebrovascular Emergencies

It includes:
1. Hypertensive encephalopathy diagnosed on clinical picture, fundus examination.
2. Intracranial bleed (Fig. 39.2 on front page) or subarachnoid haemorrhage is diagnosed by altered mental state, signs of meningeal irritation, symptoms and signs of raised intracranial tension; and confirmed on lumbar puncture, CT scan and MRI.
3. Transient ischaemic stroke/stroke-in-evolution.

Treatment

The risks and benefits of acute lowering of BP during an acute stroke or cerebrovascular disease is still unclear, but control of BP at intermediate level (160/100 mmHg) is appropriate until the condition has stabilized or improved (JNC report VII). Sudden drastic lowering of BP in hypertensive emergency is counterproductive, may increase ischaemia of watershed areas of brain. The drug therapy used is discussed at the end for all emergencies. However a short-acting intravenous drug is preferred which can be stopped at ease.

Renal Emergencies

Most patients who present as hypertensive emergencies have already dearranged renal functions, i.e. reduction in GFR, rise in serum creatinine, microalbuminuria or overt albuminuria.

The therapeutic goals are to slow deterioration of renal functions and prevent cerebrovascular disease (CVD). Hypertension appears in majority of patients and should receive aggressive BP management often with combination of drugs (3 or more) to reach target BP value of < 130/80 mmHg.

Cardiovascular Emergencies

It includes:
1. Acute myocardial ischaemia/infarction in hypertensive patient is diagnosed on ECG and echocardiography.
2. Left heart failure or pulmonary oedema due to HT is diagnosed on clinical examination, chest X-ray and echocardiogram.

Table 39.2: Parenteral drugs used in hypertensive emergencies

Drug	Dosage and route	Onset of action	Duration of action	Side-effects
Nitroprusside (Veno-arteriolar dilator)	I.V. infusion 0.25-8 µg/kg/min	Immediate	2-3 minutes	Nausea, vomiting, sweating muscle twitchings, thiocyanate toxicity with high doses for prolonged period
Diazoxide (arteriolar dilator)	50-150 mg I.V. as bolus every 5-10 minutes or 15-30 mg/min I.V. infusions	2-4 minutes	6-12 min	Nausea, hypotension, flushing, tachycardia, chest pain and hyperglycaemia
Hydralazine	10-20 mg/I.V. or IM 0.5-1 mg/min I.V infusion	10-20 minutes	3-8 hours	Tachycardia, flushing, headache, vomiting, aggravation of angina
Nitroglycerine (predominant venous than arteriolar dilator)	5-100 µg/min I.V. infusion	2-5 min	2.5 minutes	Headache, methemoglobinaemia, nitrate tolerance requiring an increase in dose
Enalaprilat (ACE inhibitor)	0.625-1.25 mg every 6 hourly	10-15 min	Within 6 hours	Hypotension, angioedema, renal failure (if bilateral renal artery stenosis)
Nicardipine (Ca++ channel blockers)	2-8 mg/hour I.V.	5-10 min	30-60 minutes	Tachycardia, headache, flushing, rhinitis
Esmolol (betablocker)	200-500 µg/kg/min for 4 minutes then 50-300 µg/kg/min	1-2 min	10-20 minutes	Hypotension, bronchospasm, nausea, bradycardia, AV blocks
Labetolol (alpha and beta adrenergic blocker)	20-80 µg/I.V. bolus every 10 min; 2 mg/min I.V. infusion	5-10 minutes	3-6 hours	Nausea, vomiting, burning in throat, dizziness, bronchospasm postural hypotension
Trimethaphan (ganglion blocker)	0.5-5 mg/min I.V. infusion	1-5 minutes	10 minutes	Postural hypotension, bowel paresis, blurring of vision and tachycardia

3. Aortic dissection is suspected clinically and echocardiogram is helpful in diagnosis.

The goal of therapy is to reduce BP < 140/90 mmHg. The choice of drugs are vasodilators i.e. ACE inhibitors and/or angiotensin receptor blockers (ARBs), beta blockers and diuretics.

In aortic dissection, a BP of < 120 mmHg should be achieved quickly within minutes using beta blockers and a vasodilators to decrease aortic stress. Surgical management thereafter is mandatory.

DIABETES AND HYPERTENSION

Pregnancy Related States

1. *Gestational hypertension* is defined as transient hypertension occurring after 20 weeks of gestation without any other symptoms of pre-eclampsia. Such women need close observation.
2. *Pregnancy induced hypertension (PIH)* means a previously normotensive woman develops hypertension after 20 weeks of pregnancy. *Pregnancy induced hypertension* is the earliest

sign of pre-eclampsia syndrome. Increasing blood pressure as compared to the BP during first half of pregnancy is more important than any exact figure. BP after delivery returns to normal.

3. **Pre-eclampsia/Eclampsia**: Pre-eclampsia is diagnosed clinically by the development of hypertension, proteinuria, oedema which may be associated with convulsions (eclampsia) or hemolysis, hepatic dysfunction i.e. elevated liver enzymes and thrombocytopenia (HELLP syndrome) even in the absence of significant hypertension.

Blood pressure declines during pregnancy and therefore, emergencies occur at much lower level of BP in pregnancy. As the risk of eclampsia is real, BP control has to be much stricter in pregnant patients. Therefore, women with hypertension who become pregnant should be followed carefully because of increased risk to mother and foetus. Methyldopa, β-blockers and vasodilators are preferred drugs; while ACEs and ARBs should be avoided. The target blood pressure to be achieved is < 140 /90 mmHg by drug therapy.

Drug Therapy for Hypertensive Emergencies

Drugs used for hypertensive emergencies are generally given parenterally in an ICU where the progress can be easily monitored. The drugs (see the Table 39.2) used are those which have rapid onset and offset of action and their effects can easily be reversed.

Choice of An Antihypertensive Drug During An Emergency

Each drug has its own advantages and disadvantages, hence, choice of an antihypertensive drug during an hypertensive emergency depends not only on its action but its suitability during that situation. The various drugs suited to various hypertensive emergency are given in the Box 39.2.

Treatment Targets

In the hypertension optimal treatment (HOT) trial, the optimal BP for reduction of major cardiovascular events was found to be 130/83 mmHg, or even lower in patients with diabetes. Now-a-day a consensus opinion is to achieve the target BP of < 130/80 mm in all patients of hypertension without diabetes and < 130/75 mm in patients with diabetes.

Follow-up

Patients taking antihypertensive drugs require follow-up at an interval of 3 months to monitor BP, minimise side-effects, implement life style modifications.

Drugs Therapy in Hypertensive Urgencies (see Box 39.3)

As already discussed, the hypertensive urgencies require oral administration of drugs to control hypertension as there is no target organ damage. The drugs are:

1. *Oral or sublingual nifedipine:* This was the most common and most popular drug for immediate control of hypertension and is available in gelatinous capsule. It fell into controversy for some period due to its adverse effects (e.g. sudden fall in BP following sublingual use leading to hypoperfusion of organs), but recently the use of this drug in obstetrics have given an indication that it provides a good BP control with acceptable rates of adverse effects. It is given as 5 mg sublingual to be repeated after 10-15 minutes according to the response.

2. *Oral clonidine:* It is given as oral loading dose of 0.2 mg followed by 0.1 mg every hour thereafter till BP falls to a target level. It can be given on outpatient basis.

3. *Oral captopril:* It can be used in hypertensive urgencies in the dose of 12.5 to 25 mg.

MALIGNANT HYPERTENSION

It is characterised by marked rise in BP (≥ 200/140 mmHg) associated with grade IV fundal changes (haemorrhage, exudate and papilledema

Box 39.2: Preferred parenteral drugs during hypertensive emergencies

Emergency	Recommended drug	To avoid
Hypertensive encephalopathy	• Labetolol • Nicardipine, Nimodipine • Nitroprusside • Trimethophan	• Diazoxide • Methyldopa
Stroke	• Labetolol • Trimethophan • Nitroprusside • Esmolol	• Methyldopa • Diazoxide • Hydralazine
Heart failure	• Enalaprilat • Nitroglycerine • Nitroprusside • Loop diuretics (Fursemide)	• Labetolol • Beta blockers (e.g. esmolol)
Coronary artery disease	• Nitroglycerine • Nitroprusside • Labetolol • Nicardipine	• Hydralazine • Diazoxide
Phaeochemocytoma	• Phenotolamine • Labetolol	All others
Postoperative	• Labetolol • Nitroglycerine • Nicardipine	Trimethophan
Eclampsia	• Hydralazine • Labetolol	• Nitroprusside • Trimethophan • Diuretics
Aortic dissection	• Nitroprusside • Trimethophan • Esmolol	• Hydralazine • Diazoxide

Box 39.3: Oral drugs for hypertensive urgencies

Drug	Dose and route	Duration of action	Side-effects
Nifedipine	5-10 mg sublingual or bitten and swallowed	Action starts within 5-15 min: remains for 3-6 hours	• Hypotension • Tachycardia
Clonidine	0.1-0.2 mg every hour	Action starts within 45-60 min: and remains for 6-8 hours	• Dry mouth • Sedation
Captopril	6.25-20 mg	Action starts within 15-30 min and lasts for 4-6 hours	• Acute renal failure • Angioneurotic oedema
Labetolol	100-300 mg	Action within 30-60 min: lasts for 6-12 hours	• Bronchospams, nausea, vomiting, tingling of scalp burning in throat, dizziness, postural hypotension
Prazosin	1-2 mg	Onset of action 15-60 min; remains for 6 hours	• Flushing • Hypotension

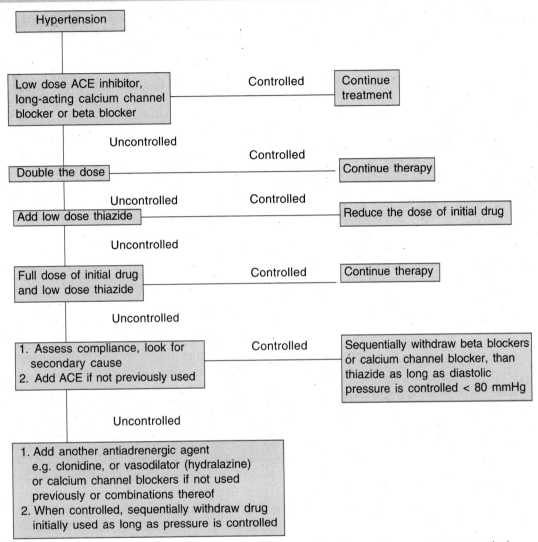

Fig. 39.3: Schematic approach to hypertension (fresh case who does not have volume expansion)

of optic fundi) and features of hypertensive encephalopathy. Cardiac decompensation and rapidly declining renal function are other critical features of malignant hypertension. The characteristic lesion of malignant hypertension is fibrinoid necrosis of walls of small arteries and arterioles.

The clinical manifestations have been attributed to spasms of cerebral vessels and to cerebral oedema (The clinical features of hypertensive encephalopathy have been discussed).

Perhaps less than 1% of hypertensive patients develop malignant phase, which can occur in the course of both essential and secondary hypertension. Rarely, it is the first recognised manifestation of hypertension. With the advent of effective antihypertensive therapy, now 50% patients survive more than 5 years after development of malignant hypertension.

Treatment

Aims

1. **To reduce the diastolic BP around 95 mmHg:** It is unwise to reduce the BP too rapidly because there may occur further deterioration of cardiac, cerebral and renal functions.
2. **Treatment of associated organ dysfunction:** i.e. LHF, encephalopathy or renal impairment.

Steps

1. Hospitalise the patient and put the patient on railing bed if there are convulsions.
2. Maintain I.V. line; give O_2.
3. Drug therapy.
1. **Antihypertensive drug therapy** The drugs to be used are chosen on the basis of onset of action and availability as I.V. preparation. The first line drug of choice is *nitroprusside* I.V. infusion (0.3-1.0 mg/kg/min) but requires constant supervision preferably in an intensive care unit. *Nitroglycerine* I.V. infusion (5-100 µg/min) is used in treatment of hypertension following coronary bypass surgery, myocardial infarction, left ventricular failure, or unable angina pectoris. *Diazoxide* is an alternative immediate acting drug, can be used as 50-150 mg I.V. rapidly as bolus, can be repeated after every 5-10 min (max dose 600 mg). This drug should not be used in patients in whom aortic dissection or myocardial infarction is being suspected.

   Other drugs that have slight delayed action than the drugs mentioned above, can be used such as I.V. Enalaprilat (ACE inhibitor), I.M. labetolol (2 mg/min to maximum of 200 mg) or hydralazine (5-10 mg aliquot repeated at half an hour interval; dose titrated according to response). In some patients, especially in severe hypertension, sublingual nifedipine 10 mg has been used previously to produce a graded reduction in BP and was best option for treatment of patients outside the hospital. It is still widely used drug in third world countries.
2. **Intravenous fursemide or torsemide:** to induce sodium diuresis and thus reduce the BP and to speed recovery from encephalopathy.
3. **Digoxin:** It is used to treat LHF, if present.
4. **Sedation:** Intravenous diazepam is given for effective sedation.
5. In the mean time, investigate the patient and find out the cause such as phaeochromocytoma, if suspected. This can be treated by appropriate measures if proved.
6. In patients who fail to respond to above mentioned measures, there is still hope to improve with peritoneal or hemodialysis as removal of extracellular fluid has resulted in better blood pressure control and impairment of renal functions.
7. Once patient comes out of emergency situation, oral conventional antihypertensive drugs may be instituted.

A schematic approach to hypertension (fresh case who does not have volume overload) is represented in Figure 39.3 (see previous page).

Part Five

Neurology

Chapter 40

Acute Confusional State (Delirium)

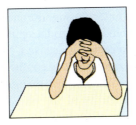 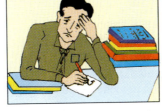

Thought reduced   **Concentration impaired**

Fig. 40.1A: Acute confusional state

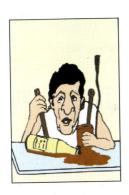 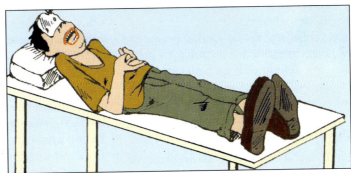

Fig. 40.1B: Delirium due to substance abuse

ACUTE CONFUSIONAL STATE (DELIRIUM)

Confusional state and coma are the most common disorders of consciousness encountered in clinical practice. It has been estimated that 5% of all emergency admissions of large municipal hospitals are due to diseases that cause disorders of consciousness.

Although the interpretation of consciousness is a psychological but distinction between the level of consciousness or wakefulness, and content of consciousness or awareness, have neurological significance. Wakefulness or alertness is maintained by reticular activating system (RAS) and its broad connections to the cerebral hemispheres, therefore, the reduced wakefulness results from the depression of neuronal activity of RAS or cerebral hemispheres. On the other hand, awareness and thinking are dependent on integrated and organized thoughts, subjective experiences, emotions and mental processes. There are certain anatomically defined areas in the brain for this purpose. The inability to maintain a coherent sequence of thoughts accompanied by inattention and disorientation is called *confusion* which is a disorder of content of consciousness.

Definition

Confusional state or confusion is a state of reduced mental clarity, coherence, comprehension and thinking compounded by inattention and disorientation (Fig. 40.1A and B). As this state worsens, there is deterioration in memory, perception, comprehension, decision making, language, praxia and visuospatial functions.

Encephalopathy means confusion with an element of drowsiness. The drowsiness caused by systemic changes or by brain lesions is typically accompanied by confusion.

While psychiatrists use the term *delirium* and *confusion* interchangeably but neurologists prefer to use the term delirium for an agitated, hyper-sympathotonic, hallucinatory state, most often due to alcohol, or substance abuse.

Pathophysiology

Acute confusional state of metabolic origin occurs due to interruption of energy substrate delivery. The substrate for neuronal functions is oxygen and glucose. The cerebral blood flow carries these substrate to neurons. Therefore reduced substrate supply such as O_2 (hypoxia), glucose (hypoglycaemia) or reduced blood supply (ischaemia) or alteration of neurophysiological responses of neurons by drugs or alcohol intoxication, toxic endogenous metabolites, anaesthetics or epilepsy produce acute confusional state and coma by widespread neuronal dysfunction in the cortex (cerebral hemispheres and RAS) and reduces all aspects of mentation.

Confusion and coma due to hyponatraemia, hyperosmolality, hypercapnia and encephalopathies of hepatic and renal failure result from metabolic derangements of neurons and astrocytes, but the nature of reversible toxic effects of these conditions is not understood, could be due to change in ion fluxes across the neuronal membranes and neurotransmitters abnormalities. **In hepatic coma**, raised brain NH_4 level interferes with cerebral energy metabolism and Na^+, K^+, ATP-ase pump, results in abnormalities of neurotransmitters including possible 'false' neurotransmitters. Ammonia and other toxic metabolites may bind to benzodiazepine-gamma-aminobutyric acid receptors to cause CNS depression.

In **renal failure**, confusional state is not related to urea itself, but results due to an increased permeability of the blood-brain barrier to toxic substances such as organic acids and an increase in brain Ca^{++} or CSF phosphate content.

Hypercapnia produces disturbance in consciousness due to rise in $PaCO_2$ in the blood resulting in CSF acidosis. The pathophysiology of other metabolic encephalopathies such as hypercalcaemia, hypothyroidism Vit B_{12} deficiency and hypothermia are incompletely understood but are related to derangements of CNS biochemistry and membrane functioning.

Abnormalities of **osmolality** caused by several medical disorders such as diabetic coma, non-ketotic hyperosmolar state and hyponatraemia are involved in pathogenesis of confusional state, seizures and coma. In **hyponatraemia**, brain water content correlates well with level of consciousness. Sodium levels below 120 mmol/L cause convulsions and coma. Serum osmolality above 350 moSm/kg is associated with hyperosmolar coma.

Certain drugs (CNS depressants), anaesthetics, and some endogenous toxins produce confusion and/or coma by suppression of RAS and the cerebral cortex.

Postictal confusion or coma following seizures is probably due to exhaustion of energy metabolites or be secondary to locally toxic metabolites produced during the seizures, and recovery occurs when neuronal metabolic balance is restored.

Causes

They are given in Box 40.1.

> **Box 40.1: Causes of actue confusional state**
>
> 1. *CNS disorders*
>   A. *Vascular*
>   - Transient ischaemic episode
>   - Cerebral, subarachnoid, subdural, haemorrhage
>   - Hypertensive encephalopathy
>   B. *Infections*
>   - Meningitis, encephalitis
>   - Typhoid, malarial encephalopathy
>   C. *Nutritional/ Vitamin deficiency*
>   - Thiamine (Wernicke-Korsakoff syndrome)
>   - Vit. B_{12}
>   D. *Head injury/trauma*
>   E. *Epilepsy (postictal)*
>   F. *Degenerative*
>   - Multiple sclerosis
>   - Alzheimer's disease
> 2. *Metabolic*
>   - Hepatic failure
>   - Renal failure
>   - Post-operative state
>   - Hypoxia
>   - Fluid and electrolyte disturbance
> 3. *Endocrinal*
>   - Hypo or hyperthyroidism
>   - Hypopituitarism
>   - Adrenal crisis (Addison's disease)
> 4. *Cardiopulmonary*
>   - Myocardial infarction
>   - Cardiac arrhythmias
>   - Congestive heart failure
>   - Respiratory failure
>   - Shock
> 5. *Systemic illness*
>   - Substance intoxication or withdrawal (see Fig. 40.1 on front page)
>   - Systemic infection
>   - Heat injury (hypo or hyperthermia)
>   - Hypoglycaemia

Clinical Features

Acute confusional state is a nonspecific neuropsychiatric clinical syndrome of varied aetiology. Disorientation with hypoactive presentation is called *confusion*; while hyperactive disoriented patients are called *delirious*. There is an acute onset and fluctuating course. Its characterstic features are:

1. **Impaired consciousness or clouding of consciousness:** Usually, there is decreased awareness of surrounding, decreased ability to respond to external stimuli, disturbance in sleep-wake cycle (insomnia at night with day-time drowsiness).
2. **Disturbance in memory:** There is impairment of registration, and retention of new memories and recall. Disorientation of time, place and person is the earliest or presenting manifestation, may be associated with inattention and distractibility.
3. **Disturbance in perception:** Normal perceptions are distorted i.e. objects may appear larger (macropsia) or smaller (micropsia) than normal. Illusions and hallucinations are common.
4. **Thought disorder:** Difficulty in thinking and slowness of thought is present. Fleeting delusions are common.
5. **Psychomotor disturbance:** Psychomotor activity is reduced. Speech is slow, slurred and incoherent. Motor symptoms include tremors and myoclonus. Motor and verbal preservation, agraphia and impaired comprehension are seen.
6. **Emotional changes:** There may be anxiety, irritability and depression. In severe cases, emotional responses become apathetic.
7. **Autonomic disturbance:** Pallor, sweating, tachycardia, dilated pupils, raised temperature, piloerection and G.I. disturbance may occur.

Diagnosis and Differential Diagnosis

The diagnosis of acute confusional state involves:
1. To find out the cause of confusion/ delirium by detailed history and physical examination (see the Tables 40.1 and 40.2).

Table 40.1: Substance induced or withdrawl confusion/delirium

1. **Substance abuse**
   Alcohol, cannabis, hypnotics, opiates, sedatives hallucinogens, cocaine, inhalants

2. **Toxins**
   - Anticholinesterases
   - Organophosphorus
   - Insecticides
   - Carbon-monooxide
   - Volatile substances
   - Organic solvents

3. **Therapeutic agents**
   Anaesthetics, analgesics (opiates, salicylates) theophylline, anticonvulsants (barbiturates, valproate), anticholinergics, antidepressants (lithium), antispasmodic (atropine), antihypertensives (beta blockers, clonidine), digitalis, antiarrhythmics (disopyramide, lidocaine, mexiletine) anti-inflammatory (NSAIDs), antibiotics, antimalarial (chloroquine, mefloquine), antitubercular (isoniazid, rifampicin), antipsychotics (phenothiazines), sedatives, hypnotics, muscle relaxant (scopolamine) corticosteroids, sympathomimetics

Table 40.2: Clinical clues to the aetiology of confusional state/delirium

Finding	Clinical clues to
Smell of breath	Diabetic ketoacidosis, uraemia, alcohol, aluminium phosphide poisoning
Fever	Septicaemia, thyroid crisis, vasculitis
Autonomic hyperactivity	Anxiety, thyrotoxic crisis, hypoglycaemia
Bradycardia	Hypothyroidism, Stokes-Adam attacks, OP poisoning
Tachycardia	Hyperthyroidism, shock, CHF, infections
Hypotension	Shock, Addison's disease, AMI, drug intoxication, internal haemorrhage etc.
Hypertension	Encepholopathy, intracranial mass, cerebral haemorrhage etc.
Tachypnoea	Diabetes, metabolic acidosis, pneumonia, infections
Shallow breathing	Alcohol, acidosis
Dilated pupils	Anxiety, autonomic hyperreactivity
Papilloedema	Hypertensive encephalopathy brain-tumour, subarachnoid haemorrhage
Neck rigidity	Meningitis, subarachnoid haemorrhage, meningism
Tongue/Cheek bite	Seizures, postictal delirium
Cardiomegaly	CHF, hypertensive heart disease
Arrhythmia	Myocardial infarction, CHF
Pulmonary rales and crackles	Pulmonary oedema, CHF, pneumonia
Hepatomegaly	CHF, hepatic failure
Asymmetric deep tendon reflexes	CVA, subdural haematoma, mass lesion
Plantar extensors	Raised intracranial pressure, hypoglycaemia
Primitive reflexes present	Dementia, frontal lobe lesions

2. Exclusion of other psychiatric disorders associated with confusion, delirium such as acute functional psychosis, dementia and affective (mood) disorders (Table 40.3).

In general, metabolic encepholopathies and intoxication with sedative drugs tend to produce quiet confusion where as clinical conditions accompanying fever, withdrawl states and CNS stimulant drug intoxication produce delirium.

Investigations

1. *Laboratory investigations:* They are done in all cases with delirium:
   - Complete blood counts.
   - Routine blood biochemistry.
   - Blood sugar.
   - Serum electrolytes (e.g. K^+, Na^+, Ca^{++}, Mg^{++}) and phosphate.

Acute Confusional State (Delirium)

Table 40.3: Differential diagnosis of acute confusional states

Feature	Acute confusional state	Delirium	Dementia	Acute functional psychosis
Onset	Acute	Acute	Insidious	Sudden
Course	Fluctuating	Fluctuating	Stable	Stable
Consciousness	Clouded	Clouded	Clear	Clear
Attention	Globally impaired	Globally impaired	Globally impaired	Variably affected
Cognition	Globally affected	Globally affected	Globally affected	Selectively affected
Hallucinations	Usually visual and tactile	Usually visual and tactile	Often absent	Mainly auditory
Delusions	Fleeting, poorly systematized	Fleeting	Often absent	Sustained and systematized
Orientation to time, space and person	Usually impaired	Mostly impaired	Often impaired	May be impaired
Psychomotor activity	Reduced or impaired	Increased	Often normal	Varies from retardation to hyperactivity
Speech	Slow, slurred incoherent	Incoherent, confabulations	Difficulty in finding the words	Normal, slow or rapid
Involuntary movements	Often asterixis, flapping tremors	Tremors, delirium tremens	Absent	Absent
Physical illness	Often present	May be present	Absent	Absent
Drug toxicity	May be present	May be present	Often Absent	Absent

- ECG and X-ray chest.
- Arterial blood gases analysis.

2. **Additional tests indicated on suspicion of specific conditions:**
   - Urine culture and sensitivity.
   - Blood levels of drugs and their estimations in urine.
   - Serum folate, Vit. B_{12} levels, ammonia.
   - HIV testing.
   - Urinary porphyrins.
   - Blood culture.
   - EEG.
   - Imaging e.g. CT scan, MRI etc.

Diffuse slowing of EEG has a good correlation with diagnosis of delirium but absence of EEG abnormalities does not rule out the diagnosis. Fast activity is seen in benzodiazepine and alcohol withdrawal delirium.

Management

1. **Supportive treatment**
   i. Identification of the cause and its immediate correction e.g. 25-50% glucose I.V. for hypoglycaemia, O_2 therapy for hypoxia, 100 mg of Vit. B_1 for thiamine deficiency, physostigmine 1 to 2 mg parenterally for anticholinergic overdosage. The fever must be reduced with fans, ice-packs and antipyretics.
   ii. I.V. fluids and electrolytes to correct dehydration and electrolyte disturbance. Dehydration is the common cause of delirium is elderly patients.
   iii. The patient should be placed near the nurse's station for close observation and monitoring. The patient's safety must be ensured by use of side-rails. The patients who use glasses and hearing aids, the same must be provided to reduce visual and auditory misperceptions. The level of noise in the patient environment should be minimum. A close family member should be advised to stay with the delirious patient. This strategy, if followed, can have calming effect on the patient and help in her/ his

re-orientation. The patient should not be allowed to sleep in the day by engaging him/her in day-time activities.

2. **Specific treatment**: A number of strategies are available for the specific (drug) treatment but each has to be individualised in the light of clinical circumstances of the case. All the current therapy should be reviewed and wherever possible stopped and replaced with drugs which have least psychoactive action.

Antipsychotics: Antipsychotics are the drug of choice for treatment of delirium. Neuroleptics are superior to benzodiazepines in patients with both hyperactive and hypoactive clinical profiles. Haloperidol is commonly employed drug because of its short half-life and lower anticholinergic side-effects. It has the advantage of being available as oral, intramuscular and intravenous preparations.

Abrupt discontinuation may result in rebound delirium. Droperidol is similar to haloperidol but is more sedating, hence, is preferred in agitated patients. The usual starting dose of haloperidol is 2 to 10 mg depending on the level of agitation. Dose may be repeated every 2-4 hours as needed. For elderly patients, dose is 0.5 to 1 mg.

Benzodiazepines: Usually benzodiazepines are useful for the treatment of deliriums caused by withdrawal from alcohol or CNS depressants, although they may cause further clouding of the sensorium. They can be used as beneficial adjunctive treatment in patients who cannot tolerate antipsychotics. Further benzodiazepines have anxiolytic, sedative and hypnotic effects which must be kept in mind while using these drugs.

Lorazepam has a rapid onset of action, intermediate half-life and is suitable for patients with impaired liver functions. The standard dose of lorazepam for delirium tremens is 2 mg every 2 hours. Additional doses are administered for agitation, tremors, and changes in vital signs. For severe agitation, lorazepam 2 mg I.M. may be given every hour until a calming effect is produced. Diazepam may also be used instead of lorazepam. After control of symptoms, the drug should be withdrawn slowly.

In patients unable to tolerate full doses of haloperidol, a combination of I.V. lorazepam and haloperidol in the same syringe may be considered. This combination is also useful when prominent symptoms are anxiety or agitation.

Electroconvulsive Therapy (ECT)

It is a standard treatment for delirium in Scandinavia. One to four ECT treatments are rapidly effective in the control of delirium regardless of the cause.

Prevention

i. Appropriate treatment of medical and surgical condition known to be associated with delirium.

ii. Alcohol or other substance dependence need appropriate treatment, i.e. de-addiction therapy. and

iii. In the instance of known delirious reactions to medications, great caution must be exercised not to prescribe the offending drug.

Chapter 41

The Unconsciousness or Coma

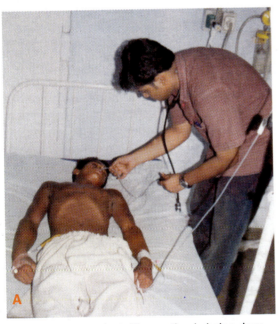
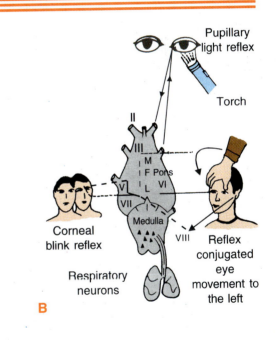

Unconscious patient. The suction is being done by the resident doctor

Fig. 41.1: (A) Unconscious patient (B) Brainstem reflexes in coma examination (read the text)

THE UNCONSCIOUSNESS OR COMA
(Fig. 41.1)

Definition

Coma is defined as persistent loss of consciousness in which the subject lies with eyes closed and shows no understandable response to external stimulus or inner need. The coma may vary in degree; and in its deepest stage no reaction of any kind is obtainable i.e. corneal, pupillary, pharyngeal. The tendon and plantar reflexes are absent. With lesser degree of coma, pupillary reflexes, reflex ocular movements and other brainstem reflexes are preserved and there may or may not be rigidity of the limbs and extensor plantar response.

The term 'semicoma' refers to that state when an individual responds to the painful stimuli by groaning, opening the eyes or with irregular respiration.

Coma Like Syndromes

Coma is characterized by complete unarousability. Several other syndromes render the patients apparently unresponsive or insensate, are considered separately because of their special significance.

1. *Vegetative state:* This is state of coma in which the eyelids have, after a time, opened giving the appearance of wakefulness. There is an absolute absence of response to commands and an inability to communicate. This is also called *'awake coma'*. There may be yawning, grunting and random movements of limbs and head. There are accompanying signs of extensive bilateral cortical damage i.e. Babinski signs, decerebrate or decorticate limb posturing and absent response to visual stimuli. Autonomic nervous system functions are preserved. The vegetative state results from global damage to the cerebral cortex most often following cardiac arrest or head injury.
2. *Akinetic mutism:* It refers to the state of partial or full awakefullness in which patient lies immobile with eyes open and is unable to talk. It results from hydrocephalus, mass in the region of third ventricle, bilateral frontal lobe lesions.
3. *Locked-in-state:* It is a state of pseudocoma in which patient appears to be unconscious, immobile and unresponsive but can open and move the eyes on command. Often these patients communicate with movements of eyes, a form of 'sign language'. These individuals are thus locked in, or **imprisoned within** their own bodies. It results **from infarction or hae**morrhage of ventral pons **due to basilar artery** occlusion.
4. *Coma vigil:* It indicates a state of impaired consciousness with muttering. The unconsciousness is not such as to amount coma. It is observed in infectious fevers such as typhoid, dengue or pneumonia.
5. *Catatonia:* It is hypomobile syndrome associated with major psychosis. In its typical form, the patients appear awake with eyes open but make no voluntary or responsive movements, although they blink spontaneously and may not appear distressed. The characteristic feature is that the limbs maintain their posture when lifted or moved by the examiner.
6. *Hysterical pseudocoma:* It indicates voluntary attempt to appear comatosed. Patient resists to examination. Eyelid elevation is actively resisted. Blinking occurs to visual threat when the lids are held open. The eyes moves concomittantly with head rotation. All these signs belie brain damage.

Pathophysiology of Coma

A normal level of consciousness depends on the activation of the cerebral hemispheres by neurone located in brainstem reticular activating system (RAS). Both these components and the connections between them must be preserved for maintenance of normal consciousness. The principal causes of coma are therefore:

i. Widespread damage to both hemispheres (i.e. disease, ischaemia, trauma).
ii. Depression of cerebral functions by drugs, toxins, hypoxia or metabolic derangements.
iii. Brainstem lesions involving RAS.

Causes

They are given in the Box 41.1.

Clinical Evaluation of A Patient with Coma

Proper management of a case of coma depends on the recognition of the cause of coma, an interpretation of certain clinical signs such as brainstem reflexes, proper use of diagnostic tests. It is a common practice that acute respiratory and cardiovascular problems should be attended to on priority basis than neurological examination. Therefore, vital signs must be maintained such as clear airway, pulse, BP before subjecting the patient to further

The Unconsciousness or Coma

> **Box 41.1: Common causes of coma**
>
> **A. Brainstem lesions**
> - Infarction
> - Haemorrhage
> - Infections e.g. encephalitis, brain abscess, meningitis
> - Tumour
> - Trauma
> - Cerebellar infarction or haemorrhage
>
> **B. Lesions of cerebral hemisphere with oedema and brainstem compression**
> - Infarction
> - Haemorrhage
> - Encephalitis, meningitis
> - Tumour
> - Trauma (subdural, extradural)
> - Hydrocephalus
> - Hypertensive encephalopathy
> - Status epilepticus
> - Cerebral malaria
>
> **C. Metabolic abnormalities**
> - Diabetes mellitus
> - Hepatic failure
> - Renal failure
> - Cardiac failure
> - Respiratory failure
> - Hyponatraemia (severe)
> - Hypokalaemia
> - Hyper and hypo-calcaemia
> - Hypoxia
> - Hypothyroidism
> - Hypopituitarism
> - Adrenal crisis
> - Vitamin deficiencies (e.g. B_1, nicotinic acid, B_{12})
>
> **D. Drugs and physical agents**
> - Anaesthetic agents
> - Drug overdose and alcohol ingestion Hyper and hypothermia
>
> **E. Psychogenic e.g.** hysteria

evaluation; otherwise appropriate resuscitative measures should be adopted immediately.

The clinical evaluation consists of:

1. **History:** In many cases, the cause of coma is immediately evident (e.g. trauma, cardiac arrest or known drug ingestion); while in others informations have to be gathered from friends, relatives and witnesses accompanying the patient regarding the:
   i. Mode of onset of coma.
   ii. Details of preceding neurological symptoms (confusion, weakness, headache, seizures, dizziness, diplopia etc.).
   iii. Use of medications, illicit drugs or alcohol
   iv. History of liver, kidney, lung, heart disease or other medical illness such as diabetes, hypothyroidism, Addison's disease.
2. **Physical examination:** The temperature, pulse, respiratory rate and pattern, and BP should be noted. The smell from the breath may be noted.

The clinical clues to the cause of coma are same as already discussed in the earlier chapter on acute confusional state (Table 40.2). High body temperature 42°C or above associated with dry skin indicate heat stroke or anticholinergic drug intoxication. Hypothermia is observed in alcoholic, barbiturate, sedative or phenothiazine intoxication. Hypothermia itself causes coma if temperature falls below 31°C.

3. **Neurological examination:** Systemic assessment of the unconsciousness patient is an important part of neurological examination. An application of Glasgow coma scale not only provides a grading of coma by numerical scale but allows serial comparisons to be made for prognostic information particularly in traumatic coma (see Box 41.2). This scale should be

> **Box 41.2: Glasgow coma scale**
>
> | Scale | Score |
> |---|---|
> | **Eye opening (E)** | |
> | • Spontaneous | 4 |
> | • To loud voice | 3 |
> | • To pain | 2 |
> | • Nil | 1 |
> | **Best Motor Response (M)** | |
> | • Obeys | 6 |
> | • Localises | 5 |
> | • Withdraws (flexion) | 4 |
> | • Abnormal flexion | 3 |
> | • Extensor response | 2 |
> | • Nil | 1 |
> | **Verbal response (V)** | |
> | • Oriented | 5 |
> | • Confused, disoriented | 4 |
> | • Inappropriate words | 3 |
> | • Incomprehensible sounds | 2 |
> | • Nil | 1 |
> | **Coma score (E+M+V)** | |
> | • Minimum | 3 |
> | • Maximum | 15 |
>
> **Note:** Patients with head trauma scoring 3 or 4 have an 85% chance of death or vegetative state; while scores above 11 indicate only 5-10% chance of death or vegetative state and 85% chance of moderate disability or good recovery. Intermediate scores have intermediate prognosis.

applied in each and every patient under observation and should be charted out from time to time for comparison.

4. ***Abnormal posturing:*** The patient posture should be observed first without examiner intervention.
   - Decorticate rigidity or posturing describes stereotyped arm and leg movements either occurring spontaneously or induced by sensory stimulation. It is characterised by flexion of elbows and wrists and arm supination against the rigid body; suggests bilateral cerebral damage above the midbrain.
   - Decerebrate rigidity or posturing describes extension and adduction of elbows and wrists with pronation; suggest corticospinal damage in the midbrain or caudal to diencephalon.
   - Arms extension with flaccid legs have been associated with low pontine lesions.
   - Total flaccidity of all the four limbs and hypotonia indicate the involvement of ponto-medullary junction.
   - Multifocal myoclonus is almost always an indication of a metabolic disorder.

   Note: Acute lesions of any type frequently cause limb extension regardless of location, and almost all extensor posturing become flexion as the time passes, so posturing alone cannot be utilized to pinpoint the anatomical site of the lesion.

5. ***Pattern of respiration:*** Respiration patterns though received much attention in the coma diagnosis, but are of little help in localisation of the lesion:
   - Slow, shallow, regular breathing suggest metabolic or drug effect.
   - Rapid, deep (kussmaul) breathing suggests metabolic acidosis, but can occur in ponto-mesencephalic lesions.
   - Cheyne-Stokes breathing in classic cyclic form ending with a brief apnoea suggests bihemispherical damage or metabolic coma.
   - Agonal gasps (gasping respiration) is a terminal respiratory pattern, suggests bilateral lower brainstem damage.

6. ***Pupillary size and reaction:*** The size, equality and inequality of pupils and their reaction to light provide valuable information regarding the site of lesion in an unconscious patient.
   - With cortical lesion, the pupils are small but react to light.
   - Symmetrically reactive round pupils usually exclude the midbrain lesion.
   - With early midbrain lesion, the pupils become mid-dilated and non-reactive to light. As the damage to the midbrain increases, the pupils become dilated and fixed. The cilio-spinal reflex is also lost at this stage. The use of mydriatic eye drops by a previous examiner, self administration by patient or direct ocular trauma may cause misleading pupillary enlargement.
   - Very small (pinpoint) pupils with reaction to light characterize narcotic or barbiturate poisoning but also occurs in bilateral pontine lesions (haemorrhage). The response to naloxone and the presence of reflex eye movements distinguishes the two.
   - Unilateral 3rd nerve palsy causes unilateral pupillary enlargement which could be due to ipsilateral lesion (mass lesion of midbrain) or due to contralateral compression of 3rd nerve in midbrain against the opposite tentorial margin (contracoup effect).
   - Unilateral small pupil of a *Horner's syndrome* is detected by failure of the pupil to enlarge in the dark, is seen in cerebral haemorrhage that affects the thalamus. (sympathetic system).

7. ***Eye movements:*** These are cornerstones of physical diagnosis in coma because they allow a large portion of the brainstem to be analysed (Fig. 41.1B).
   - The eyes are first observed by elevating the lids and noting the resting position and spontaneous movements of the globes. Horizontal divergence of the eyes at rest is nor-

The Unconsciousness or Coma

mally observed in coma. An adducted eye at rest indicates lateral rectus palsy due to 6th nerve in the pons; and when bilateral, it is often a sign of raised intracranial tension. An abducted eye with pupillary dilatation indicates 3rd nerve palsy in the midbrain.

- *Skew deviation* i.e. vertical separation of the eyes (ocular axes) results from pointine or cerebellar lesions.
- *Oculocephalic reflex (Doll's eye movement):* Normally sudden passive turning of the head to one side produces conjugate deviation of the eyes to the opposite side. Absence of this reflex in a comatosed patient implies dysfunction of pons where the 6th nerve nucleus or lateral gaze centre is located. However this reflex does not pinpoint the cause of coma, can occur both in structural and toxic metabolic causes of coma. Spontaneous conjugate horizontal deviation in a comatosed patient indicates pontine damage on the same side or frontal lobe damage on opposite side.
- *Oculovestibular reflex:* It tests the integrity of pathway from the labyrinth in the ear to the midbrain via medial longitudinal fasciculus (this connects the 6th nerve and 8th nerve to contralateral 3rd nerve). This reflex is tested by cold water irrigation into a ear. Normally there is deviation of eyes towards irrigated side. The absence of this reflex carries same significance as oculocephalic reflex.
- *Ocular bobbing* describes a brisk downward and slow movements of the eyes, indicates bilateral pontine damage.
- *Ocular dipping* describes a slower downward and faster upward movements of the eyes, denotes anoxic damage to the cerebral cortex.

8. **Motor responses:** Presence of local signs or unilateral paralysis indicates focal structural damage to the brain. The only evidence of paralysis may be abnormal flaccidity on the affected area. Alteration of deep tendon jerks and plantar extensor response on the paralysed size indicate contralateral corticospinal involvement; but in deep coma, plantar reflexes lose their significance because they may become extensor on both the sides.

Investigations

1. **Laboratory investigations** done are same as discussed in acute confusional state.
2. **Specialised investigations:**
   i. *CT scan and MRI:* The CT scan and MRI give valuable informations regarding radiologically detectable lesions e.g. haemorrhage, tumours, hydrocephalus etc. These investigations are not useful in toxic or metabolic causes of coma, but are done to exclude the radiological evident lesion.
   The CT scan and MRI is also useful to detect mass effect of the lesion by midline shift of the pineal body (a calcified lesion).
   ii. *The EEG:* It gives valuable informations:
   - Diffuse slowing of EEG indicates diffuse encephalopathy.
   - Predominent high-voltage slowing (delta waves) in the frontal regions is typical of metabolic coma (hepatic coma).
   - Alpha coma (8 to 12 Hz activity) indicates high pontine or diffuse cortical damage.
   iii. *CSF examination* is done in those cases where CT scan has ruled out mass lesion(s) or raised intracranial tension. It is valuable in the diagnosis of meningitis, encephalitis, subarachnoid haemorrhage (xanthochromic CSF) etc.

Management

I. Immediate treatment

Hospitalise each and every case of coma. Immediate treatment is to maintain patent airway, I.V. access and to stabilise vital signs i.e. pulse, BP before proceeding to clinical evaluation. An emergency sample of blood for biochemistry, sugar, electrolytes may be taken. Tracheostomy or endotracheal intubation and frequent suction be done to keep the airway patent (Fig. 41.1A on front page).

II. General supportive measures

A. Care of the patient

i. *Position of unconscious patient:* An unconscious patient should be nursed on one side rather than in supine position to minimise the risk of aspiration.

ii. *To prevent bed sores*: The position of the patient on bed must be changed frequently so as to minimise pressure at pressure points to prevent bed sores. The position should be changed every 1-2 hourly. A water or air mattress should be used if the course of illness is prolonged.

iii. *Gental movements on the bed:* The clothes of the patient should be loosened and rings to be removed. The limbs should be kept in optimal position. The limbs should be moved passively through full range frequently so as to avoid contractures and deep vein thrombosis.

iv. *Oral hygiene:* Proper oral hygiene to be maintained by mouth washes and suction.

v. The patient should be kept in *railing bed* so as to prevent falling.

vi. *Eye care:* e.g. tapping of lids, prevention of corneal damage.

vii. *Chest physiotherapy* should be carried out as soon as patient improves.

B. Feeding or nutrition:
Nasogastric feeding (liquid diet of 3000 kcal) should be given if there is no contraindication. The fluid balance should be maintained. Oral fluids through Ryle's tube should be administered to maintain the adequate renal perfusion. I.V. fluids to be given if patient does not accept much fluid orally. Serum electrolytes to be monitored and corrected wherever necessary. To avoid aspiration:
- Aspirate the gastric contents before each feed so as to ensure that the tube is in the stomach.
- The patient should be nursed in the sitting or propped up position.
- Each feed should be small (200 ml) to avoid distension of the stomach.

C. Maintenance of vital signs/parameters

i. *Respiration:* Adequate respiration must be ensured by patent airway. Denture should be removed and oral airway (mouth gag) inserted to prevent the falling of tongue backwards. Frequent suctions to be done to remove the secretions. If patient does not have cough reflex and is likely to stay in a coma for a long period, the endotracheal intubation or even tracheostomy may be done for proper removal of secretions. Intermittent O_2 therapy by nasal catheter may be given. In case of severe hypoxia, assisted ventilation may be required.

ii. *Circulation:* The circulation should be maintained by proper fluid balance and intake and output chart. A positive balance of 600-1000 ml should be kept as insensible loss over and above the daily output.

Drastic changes or fluctuations in the BP are to be avoided. If hypertension is present, it should be treated appropriately. Hypotension should be resuscitated by fluids and inotropic agents.

iii. *Care of bowel and bladder:* Urinary incontinence should be managed by condom drainage in men and indwelling catheter in women. Fecal impaction should be avoided and bowels to be kept open by frequent isotonic enemas or laxatives. Digital removal of fecal impaction may be needed sometimes.

III. Specific measures

Specific therapy should be directed against the cause of coma such as dextrose is given for hypoglycaemia, naloxone is administered for narcotic overdose. Thiamine is administered for Wernicke's encephalopathy in malnourished patient. The cause of coma should be appropriately dealt with. It is not possible to discuss the management of individual condition.

In cases with progressive cerebral compression due to raised intracranial pressure, decompressive therapy should be instituted. Seizures may be controlled with phenytoin. If these measures fail, surgical decompression may be required.

Chapter 42

Acute Headache

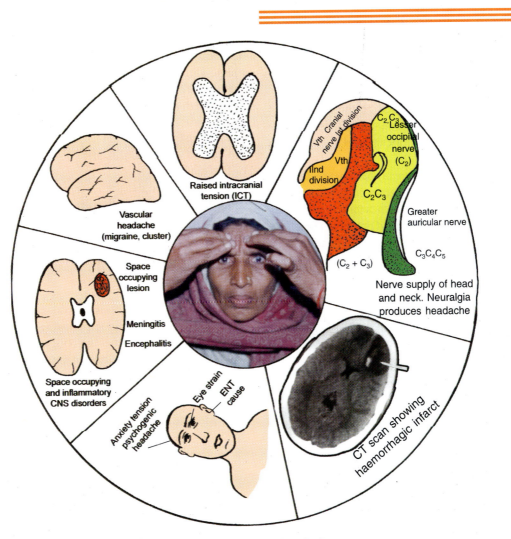

Fig. 42.1: Common headaches

ACUTE HEADACHE

Definition

Headache means ache or pain over the head. It is chronic and usually a benign symptom. Occasionally it can be a manifestation of a serious illness such as brain tumour, intracranial haemorrhage, meningitis etc. Even in emergency setting, only 5% patients presenting with acute headache have been found to have serious underlying neurological disorder; while most of them present with acute exacerbation of an underlying primary disorder like migraine. Nonetheless, it is imperative that in a patient presenting with headache these serious conditions be recognised and treated appropriately.

Causes (Fig. 42.1)

A useful classification based on the aetiology of headache, adapted from recommendations of the International Headache Society (IHS) is given in the Table 42.1.

Groups 1 to 4 cover the primary headaches and from groups 5 to 13 cover the secondary headaches. The IHS classification is much detailed and appears to be difficult to use in clinical practice. Therefore, a simple practical approach to headache is reproduced in the Table 42.2 and Fig. 42.1.

Mechanisms of Production of Headache

The following are the pain sensitive structures inside or outside the head, the stretching of which leads to pain or headache.
1. Skin, subcutaneous tissue, muscles, arteries and periosteum of the bone.
2. Intracranial dural venous sinuses or veins.
3. Tissues of eye, ears and nasal sinuses.
4. Duramater at the base of brain and the arteries within dura and pia-arachnoid mater.

   Headache commonly occurs due to:
   i. Distortions, inflammation, distension and dilatation of intracranial or extracranial vessels.
   ii. Traction or displacement of large intracranial veins and/or dural sinuses.
   iii. Compression, traction and inflammation of cranial and spinal nerves.
   iv. Muscle spasms (voluntary or involuntary) or trauma to cranial or cervical muscles.
   v. Meningeal irritation and raised intracranial tension. Headache due to mass lesions occurs only if they distort, displace or put traction on the blood vessels, dural structures or cranial nerves, hence, it may occur early before the raised intracranial tension develops, and produce typical bitemporal or bifrontal headache.

Clinical Evaluation of a Patient with Headache

Headache is a prominent symptom associated with a large variety of disorders, hence, to find out its cause is not only difficult but impossible some time. To establish the diagnosis, one has to go through a long list of causes of headache (Table 42.1 and 42.2) on history. The main issues to be addressed in a patient with headache are:
1. The diagnosis.
2. To look for the dangerous signals that suggest a serious underlying disorder.
3. Investigational plan.
4. Line of management and the follow up recommendations to prevent recurrence.

History

A careful detailed history is the most important tool in the headache diagnosis. Moreover, headache is complaint, where symptoms outweigh the signs and abnormal investigations are obligatory not the rule. Ascertain the followings on the history:
1. *Onset, duration and progress*
   i. Acute onset of severe headache commonly suggests subarachnoid haemorrhage and meningitis.
   ii. Progressively worsening headache suggests raised intracranial pressure or uncontrolled systemic disease. Focal or lateralizing signs make the diagnosis easier.
   iii. A chronic recurrent headache or chronic non-progressive daily headache represents a primary headache such as migraine, cluster headache or tension-type headache.

Table 42.1: Classification of headache (modified version of IHS, 1988)

Primary headaches
1. *Migraine*
   - Migraine without aura
   - Migraine with aura
   - Ophthalmoplegic migraine
   - Basilar migraine
   - Retinal migraine
   - Childhood migraine syndromes
   - Complications of migraine e.g. status migrainosus, migraine associated with stroke
2. *Tension-type headache*
   - Episodic tension-type headache
   - Chronic tension-type headache
3. *Cluster headache and chronic paroxysmal hemicrania*
   - Cluster headache (episodic, chronic)
   - Chronic paroxysmal hemicrania
4. *Miscellaneous headache not associated with structural lesion*
   - Idiopathic stabbing headache
   - External compression headache
   - Cold stimulus headache
   - Benign cough headache
   - Benign exertional headache
   - Headache associated with sexual activity (coital cephalgia)

Secondary headaches

5. *Post traumatic headaches*
6. *Headache associated with vascular disorders*
   - Acute ischaemic cerebrovascular disorders
   - Intracranial haematoma
   - Subarachnoid haemorrhage
   - Unruptured vascular malformations
   - Arteritis e.g. giant cell arteritis
   - Venous thrombosis
   - Arterial hypertension
7. *Headache associated with nonvascular intracranial disorder*
   - High CSF pressure syndromes e.g. benign intracranial hypertension, hydrocephalus
   - Low CSF pressure syndrome e.g. postspinal headache, CSF fistula
   - Intracranial infections e.g. meningitis, brain abscess
   - Sarcoidosis and other non-inflammatory diseases
   - Intracranial neoplasm
8. *Headache associated with substances or their withdrawl*
   - Acute use or exposure
     —Nitrate, nitrite-induced
     —Monosodium glutamate induced
     —CO-induced
     —Alcohol/induced
   - Chronic use or exposure
     —Ergotamine-induced
     —Analgesic abuse headache
9. *Headaches associated with noncephalic infection*
   - Viral infection
   - Bacterial infection
   - Other infection
10. *Headache associated with metabolic disorders*
    - Hypercapnia
    - Mixed hypoxia and hypercapnia
    - Hypoglycaemia
    - Dialysis
11. *Headache or facial pain associated with facial or cranial structures*
    - Disorders of cranial bone, eye, ear, nose, sinuses, teeth, mouth etc.
12. *Cranial neuralgias*
    - Persistent pain of cranial nerve origin
    - Trigeminal neuralgia
    - Glossopharyngeal neuralgia
    - Occipital neuralgia
    - Central causes of headache and facial pain
13. *Headache not classifiable*

> **Table 42.2: A practical classification of headache**
>
> 1. **Acute primary headaches**
>   - Migraine
>   - Tension-type
>   - Benign exertional headache
>   - Cluster headache
>   - Benign orgasmic headache
> 2. **Secondary headaches**
>   A. *Intracranial causes*
>   - *Vascular disorders* e.g. embolic thrombotic; arterial or venous, haemorrhagic, acute dissection
>   - *Infections* e.g. meningitis, encephalitis, sinusitis, brain abscess
>   - *Inflammation* e.g. vasculitis, arteritis
>   - *Tumours* e.g. primary, metastatic
>   - *Non vascular disorders* e.g. benign intracranial hypertension, postspinal headache, post-traumatic headache
>
>   B. *Extracranial causes*
>   - Eye, ear, sinuses, teeth, neck, temporomandibular joint involvement
>
>   C. *Systemic illnesses and acute intoxications*
> 3. **Neuralgias** e.g. trigeminal, glossopharyngeal and occipital

The frequency and duration of headache also help to differentiate the episodic headaches from chronic progressive headaches. Many attacks of headache of short duration in the day would favour the diagnosis of cluster headache or chronic paroxysmal hemicrania (a variant of cluster headache).

2. *Site and quality of pain*
   i. Unilateral pulsating/throbbing headaches are usually vascular such as migraine and cluster headache (occur at the same location unilaterally).
   ii. Bilateral diffuse dull headache is usually of tension-type headaches.
   iii. With secondary headaches of organic cause, the nature, location and severity of headache vary according to cause and mechanism of production.

3. *Associated symptoms*
   i. Associated features such as nausea, vomiting, hypersensitivity to light and noise along with headache suggest migraine but one should also consider the underlying organic cause in the absence of such associated symptoms.
   ii. Fever, arthralgia and malaise suggest a systemic illness or meningitis.
   iii. Transient visual symptoms (auras) is characteristic of migraine but can occur in transient ischaemic attacks, vascular anomalies or focal epilepsy secondary to space occupying lesions.
   iv. Behaviour following an acute attack of headache distinguishes migraine (patient tries to sleep undisturbed in a dark room) from cluster headache in which a patient is up and moving about.
   v. Headache may be related to menstruation, more common in morning (hypertensive) and worst on bending (sinusitis related), may occur towards the evening (eye strain headache) or follow a period of inactivity (cervical pain).

4. *Provoking and relieving factors*: Primary headaches such as migraine can be triggered by

iv. The headache that develops over weeks or months (slowly evolving recurrent headache) may have a benign cause such as migraine or tension type headache or it could even be due to a serious underlying cause (unruptured aneurysm).

v. Some headaches may show nocturnal frequency and awaken the patient at night or may occur at the same time of the day (cluster headache) or at specific occasion such as during menstruation or may increase towards the evening such as tension-type (psychogenic) headache.

The age of the patient is also a prime importance as migraine generally begins at a younger age, tension headache is more common in middle age and headache originating in older persons are usually due to organic causes.

various stimuli including food items (see Box 42.1). Headache due to intracranial pathology or raised intracranial tension worsens during coughing, straining or adopting the head in low posture.

> **Box 42.1: Provoking factors for migraine**
>
> 1. *Food item* — Cheese, dairy products, fruits, chocolates, ice-cream etc.
> 2. *Food additives* — Caffeine (coffee), nitrates
> 3. *Alcohol* — Beer, red wine
> 4. *Hormonal changes* — Menstruation, pregnancy, ovulation, oral contraceptive
> 5. *Visual triggers* — Bright lights, glare
> 6. *Auditory triggers* — Noise and music
> 7. *Olfactory triggers* — Perfumes, odours
> 8. *Sleep, hunger, exertion, head and neck trauma, stress and anxiety, cough*

Note: The clinical interview of an acute headache patient should be quick and systematic including onset, location of pain, the character, severity, duration of pain, precipitating and relieving factors. Past history of similar episodes, history of trauma, exertional aspect of headache, physical tests done earlier, any treatment taken earlier and relief obtained therefrom should be noted.

Physical examination
A thorough physical and neurological examination includes:
1. The physical examination should evaluate vital signs (pulse, BP), the cardiac status, the extracranial structures (to palpate over the head and neck for detection of tender trigger-point, to auscultate over the skull, carotid vessels for bruit, to palpate the temporal artery for pulsation) and cervical spine for pain and limitation of movements. Examine the nose and sinuses, the teeth and temporo-mandibular joint, the ear and throat.
2. *The neurological examination*:
   - Mental status and level of consciousness.
   - Cranial nerve examination including optic fundi.
   - Motor system examination e.g. power, tone, reflexes etc.
   - Look for neck stiffness and other signs of meningitis.

Investigations

Certain features in the history or examination should raise the suspicion of ominous disease warranting investigations. These danger signals are listed in Box 42.2.

> **Box 42.2: Danger signals warranting testing**
>
> 1. First severe headache ever
> 2. Subacute worsening or progressive over days and weeks
> 3. Disturbs sleep or presents immediately after awaking
> 4. Abnormal neurological examination
> 5. Fever, nausea, vomiting or other systemic signs
> 6. Headache precipitated by Valsalva maneuver (cough, sneeze, bending, straining, position change, exercise and sexual activity)
> 7. New-onset headache in adult life (>40 years) or a significant change in a long-standing headache problem.

The investigations to be done are:
1. Complete blood count, ESR and blood biochemistry.
2. *CSF examination:* CSF examination is indicated in acute onset of headache with fever or when there are associated cranial nerve involvement. The lumbar puncture should be done after a CT scan has ruled out the possibility of raised intracranial tension.
3. *Neuroimaging:* The choice of MRI or CT scan will depend on the clinical suspicion. CT scan is indicated in patients of headache with abnormal neurological examination (e.g. neck stiffness, focal deficits, diminished consciousness, signs of raised intracranial pressure) or progressive worsening headache, acute first severe headache etc. An MR scan has advantage over CT scan in a patient with headache of organic cause. It helps in identification of the lesions in the brainstem and pituitary region better than

CT scan. It also helps in ruling out or confirming the nature of the lesions i.e. demyelinating, ischaemic or inflammatory disease.
4. *EEG:* It is not of great value in the investigation of headache.
5. Temporomandibular joint and dental evaluation for malocclusion of teeth. X-rays or MRI of TM joint is useful for displacement.

Management

1. *Symptomatic relief of pain:* It involves the use of standard drugs that reverse or abort the headache and the accompanying symptoms. Treatment is dictated by the specific diagnosis for patients with serious secondary causes of headache. Acute migraine, tension-type headache and cluster headache need to be treated with both standard and specific drugs.

   Patients need symptomatic relief when the headache is severe or incapacitating or there is an acute exacerbation of an underlying primary headache or an acute infective neurological disorder or some more sinister underlying disorder.
   - *Analgesics and simple analgesic combinations* are more useful for mild to moderate headache such as migraine, tension-type or cluster headache. Opiate analgesics are used for more severe headache or when other measures fail. They should be avoided in benign recurrent headache due to their addicting properties. Aspirin, acetoaminophen and opiates are some of the drugs used. Aspirin should be avoided in children (potential to produce Reye's syndrome).
   - Non-steroidal anti-inflammatory drugs (NSAIDs) such as naproxen, indomethacin, diclofenac, meclofenamate, ketorolac are useful drugs to treat mild to moderate headache. Some of them are available in parenteral preparation e.g. diclofenac, ketorolac can be used in acute situation.
   - *Use of corticosteroids:* Corticosteroids (4-6 mg dexamethasone I.M. or I.V.) are recommended in acute headache due to raised intracranial pressure, but is also useful to abort the pain of cluster headache and migraine.
   - *Anticonvulsants* e.g. carbamazepine, phenytoin, or gabapentine may be needed to control trigeminal neuralgia in addition to analgesics.
   - *Ergot derivatives and triptans:* The ergot derivatives (ergotamine and parenteral dihydroergotamine) are useful in symptomatic relief of moderate to severe migraine, cluster headache and intractable chronic daily headache. Dihydroergotamine (DHE) can be given I.M. or I.V. alone or in combination with promethazine and dexamethasone (1 mg DHE plus 50 mg promethazine and 4 mg dexamethasone I.M.) to abort most migraine headaches. All ergotamine preparations produce nausea, vomiting, muscle cramps, paraesthesias and precipitate angina.
   Triptans (sumatriptan, zolmitriptan, naratriptan, rizatriptan) are useful in the treatment of migraine and cluster headache. Sumatriptan (25-50 mg orally or 6 mg subcutaneously) gives fastest relief in acute attack of migraine.
   - *Neuroleptics* (e.g. metoclopramide and domeperidone) are useful to control the associated nausea and vomiting associated with migraine and cluster headache.

2. *Specific management:* Certain conditions need specific management in addition to pain relief.
   - Subarachnoid haemorrhage needs angiographic confirmation and surgical intervention.
   - Meningitis needs confirmation by CSF and aggressive antibiotic therapy.
   - Raised intracranial tension needs diagnostic evaluation by CT scan or MRI. For control, I.V. mannitol or steroids may be helpful.
   - For suspected temporal arteritis, corticosteroids are beneficial.
   - Use of oxygen by a mask at 8 to 10 L for 10-15 min for acute cluster headache.

3. *Long-term management and follow-up:* One must plan to prescribe non-habituating therapy.

Chapter 43

Acute Syncope

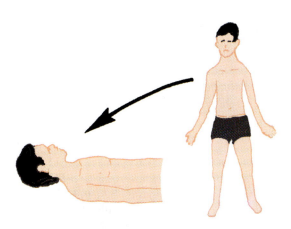

Fig. 43.1: A fall during syncope

ACUTE SYNCOPE

Definition

It is defined as sudden transient loss of consciousness with loss of postural tone (collapse or fall—Fig. 43.1) due to acute reduction in cerebral blood flow, followed by spontaneous recovery. There is no or minimal injury, no incontinence and no regular tonic—clonic movements. Exceptionally, there can be few clonic jerks.

Presyncope or near syncope is defined as premonitory symptoms such as feeling of weakness, nausea, visual blurring, light headedness, tinnitis, sweating, pallor and heaviness of lower limbs that occur before syncope. These symptoms increase in severity until consciousness is lost or ischaemia to the brain is corrected often by assuming the recumbent posture.

Causes

Syncope results from transient ischaemia of the brain usually in upright position, brought about by reduction in cardiac output or hypotension due to any cause. Depending on the pathophysiologic mechanisms, syncope may be vasodepressor (vasovagal, neurocardiogenic), postural (orthostatic), cardiac, carotid sinus, and may be due to neuralgia, cough and stretch. The causes of syncope are given in the table 43.1.

Clinical Features

It includes:
1. Symptoms and signs of syncope *per se.*
2. Symptoms and signs of the underlying disease/cause.
1. **Symptoms and signs of syncope:** A syncopal attack begins when the patient is usually in an upright position (sitting or standing) except in Stokes-Adam attack (this can occur in any position). The patient is warned of impending faint by premonitory symptoms:
    - There may be a sense of giddiness or vertigo (swaying of the floor or surrounding objects).
    - Confusion, yawning and blurring of vision.
- Perspiration or ashen-gray colour of the skin.
- Nausea, headache, light headedness may occur.

Table 43.1: Causes of syncope

1. **Decreased cerebral perfusion**
   A. *Inadequate vasoconstrictive mechanisms*
      - Vasovagal (vasodepressor)
      - Postural hypotension
      - Carotid sinus
      - Antihypertensive drugs e.g. hydralazine, alpha methyldopa etc.
      - Autonomic neuropathy
   B. *Hypovolaemia*
      - Fluid or blood loss
      - Addison's disease
   C. *Reduction in venous return*
      - Cough syncope
      - Micturition
      - Mediastinal compression
      - Defecation (straining at stool evacuation)
      - Valsalva maneuver
   D. *Reduced cardiac output*
      - Left ventricular outflow obstruction e.g. aortic stenosis, hypertrophic cardiomyopathy.
      - Right ventricular or pulmonary outflow obstruction e.g. pulmonary stenosis, pulmonary hypertension, pulmonary embolism
      - Myocardial disease e.g. myocardial infarction with pump failure
      - Pericardial disease e.g. cardiac tamponade
   E. *Arrhythmias*
      - Various grades of AV blocks
      - Sinoatrial blocks (sinus bradycardia), sinus arrests
      - Ventricular asystole
      - Supraventricular and ventricular tachy arrhythmias (tachycardia, fibrillation).
2. **Other causes**
   A. *Altered state of blood to the brain*
      - Hypoxia
      - Anaemia
      - Hyperventilation, anxiety state
      - Prolonged bed rest
      - Hypoglycaemia
   B. *Cerebral vascular disturbance*
      - Cerebrovascular disturbance (TIAs)
      - Vertebro-basilar insufficiency
      - Hypertensive encephalopathy

In some patients, syncope occurs without warning symptoms. The onset varies from 10-30 seconds, rarely longer.

The depth and duration of unconsciousness varies i.e. partly awareness to profound coma. The patient remains in the state for few seconds to minutes. Usually during the attack, patient lies motionless but sometimes a few clonic jerks may be noticed in the beginning of unconsciousness. There is no incontinence. Pulse is feeble and BP is low to undetectable and breathing is imperceptible. Following recovery in recumbent position, the volume of pulse improves, colour of skin begins to return, breathing becomes quicker and deeper and consciousness is regained. There is recovery with no residual symptoms.

2. **Symptoms and signs of underlying disease/condition** such as cardiac disorders with low cardiac output, arrhythmias or infarction with pump failure. There may be an evidence of hypovolaemia or dehydration. Certain syncopes are related to specific circumstances e.g. cough, menstruation, posture, etc. There may be history of cerebrovascular disease i.e. TIAs.

Diagnosis

The common causes of syncope have already been listed in Table 43.1. Diagnosis may be difficult but analysis of patient symptoms by careful analysis of history is useful. For example, a history of vertigo is suggestive of labyrinthine or central vestibular disorder.

History

Whenever possible, an accurate description of the attack (already discussed) should be obtained from the patient, relative or attendant and a witness. Particular attention should be paid to the predisposing factors or triggers such as medication, exercise, alcohol, the period of unconsciousness and the recovery phase.

In vasodepressor (vasovagal) syncope, there may be history of prolonged standing, fatigue, venepuncture, minor surgery etc., while certain situations e.g. cough, micturition, menstruation are related to an attack of syncope. In cardiac syncope, there may be history of structural heart disease or the presence of an arrhythmia at the time of an attack.

Acute Syncope

The period of recovery is important. Patients with cardiac syncope recover fast without residual symptoms; the patients with vasovagal syncope often feel nauseated and unwell for several minutes and patients with neurogenic syncope usually take more than 5 minutes to recover.

The typical features of three common types of syncope are summarised in the Table 43.2.

The syncope has to be differentiated from an epileptic attack (Table 43.3).

Table 43.2: Salient features of common syncope

Feature	Cardiac syncope	Vasovagal syncope	Neurogenic syncope
1. Premonitory symptoms	• Light headedness • Palpitation • Chest discomfort • Breathlessness • Convulsions may occur	• Nausea • Perspiration • Pallor • Light headedness	• Headache • Confusion • Hyperexcitability • Visual or olfactory hallucinations • Aura
2. Period of unconsciousness	Extreme, death like pallor	Pallor, Ashen-grey skin	• Prolonged (> 1 minutes) unconsciousness • Motor-seizure activity • Urinary incontinence • Tongue-biting
3. Recovery	Rapid recovery	• Slow recovery with nausea and light headedness	• Prolonged confusion • Headache • Focal neurologic signs

Table 43.3: The distinguishing features between syncope and epilepsy

Feature	Syncope	Epilepsy
• Precipitating factors	Emotional, painful or stressful event	Unusual
• Position	Upright (usual)	Any position
• Diurnal pattern	Daytime	Day and night
• Onset	Subacute or gradual	Abrupt
• Aura	Absent	Present
• Motor symptom and signs	Motionless, flaccid, may have short clonic spasms or jerks	Often tonic or tonic-clonic, clonic movement
• Colour of skin	Pale or ashen-gray	Pale or flushed
• Cyanosis	Absent	May be present
• Breathing	Slow, shallow foaming	stertorous
• Incontinence of urine and stool	Rare	Common
• Biting of tongue	Rare	Common
• Injury	Rare	Common
• Post-ictal	Rare	Confusion, headache, drowsiness, sleep
• Period of unconsciousness	Brief (few seconds)	Short (few minutes)

Physical Examination

1. *Observations* of pulse rate, BP, and symptoms in the recumbent and standing position for postural or orthostatic hypotension.
2. *Valsalva maneuver* to induce cough syncope, if suspected.
3. *Carotid sinus massage* for vasodepressor syncope. It is done under BP and ECG control commonly in supine position, and if response is negative in sitting and standing position. Generally massage is done for 5 seconds on one side, bilateral massage must never be done. Reproduction of the symptoms indicate carotid sinus hypersensitivity. If there is 50 mmHg or more fall in systolic BP associated with bradycardia, vasodepressor response is diagnosed.
4. *Head tilt testing* is useful provocative technique for diagnosis of vasodepressor (neurocardiogenic) syncope. Upright lift to a maximum of 60° to 70° usually precipitates symptomatic hypotension or syncope within 30 to 60 seconds in patients with this syndrome. In normal

subjects, passive tilting to 60° causes fall in systolic and increase in diastolic BP and heart rate. Sublingual nitroglycerine administered during head-tilt test may unmask vasovagal-induced syncope.

A positive result on upward head tilt is indicated by bradycardia, hypotension or both.

Investigations

1. **Resting ECG:** Resting ECG may be helpful in diagnosis of arrhythmias or coronary artery disease. However, a normal ECG does not rule out these as a cause of syncope. ECG done during carotid sinus massage indicates positive response (vasodepressor syncope) if a sinus pause of 3 seconds or more is produced.
2. **Holter monitoring:** Ambulatory ECG (Holter ECG) is mainly useful to correlate the symptoms with arrhythmias recorded on Holter ECG which could not be recorded on resting or serial ECGs. Continuous loop event recorders can be used for long-term monitoring for weeks to months; these are activated by the patient at the time of symptoms, freezing in its memory for analysis. In particularly difficult cases, tiny implantable ECG recorders may be used.
3. **Signal-averaged ECG:** It is helpful in detecting the late potentials for predicting inducible sustained VT.
4. **Electrophysiological studies:** In cases with recurrent syncope of unknown aetiology where Holter monitoring is noncontributory and there is underlying heart disease particularly ischaemia or prior MI, the detailed electrophysiological studies like sinus node recovery time (for sick sinus syndrome), His bundle electrocardiography for conduction delays and inducible VT by prolonged stimulation may be helpful.

Electrophysiological clues to syncope
- SNRT (sinus node recovery time) > 3 seconds or more
- Pacing induced infranodal block
- HV interval > 100 msec on His-bundle ECG
- Paroxysmal SVT with symptoms

5. **Autonomic function tests** in patients with diabetes and familial dysautonomia.
6. **EEG and CT scan** not helpful except in differentiating syncope from epilepsy.
7. **Psychiatric evaluation for anxiety disorders** may reveal hyperventilation and syncope.

A simple guide to investigation and diagnosis of recurrent syncope is given in the Figure 43.2.

Treatment

It depends on the aetiology. Wherever possible, the precipitating or triggering factors should be avoided.

1. **General supportive emergency measures:** During an attack of syncope, the patient should be placed in a position which allows maximal blood flow to the brain i.e. with head lowered between the knees, if sitting; or, preferably in the supine position. Clothings of the patient should be loosened. Head is turned to one side so that tongue does not fall back into the throat. Peripheral irritation such as sprinkling of cold water over face or application of cold moist towel may be helpful. If temperature is subnormal, the body should be covered with warm blanket. Aspiration of vomitus may be prevented by turning the patient to one side and nothing is allowed orally until the patient regains consciousness. Patients should not be allowed to rise immediately after regaining consciousness but should be observed for few minutes in supine position so that physical weakness has passed off.
2. **Treatment of the specific cause:**
   A. *Cardiac syncope*: In elderly patients, a sudden faint without obvious cause, should arouse the suspicion of complete heart block or a tachyarrhythmia, even though all findings are negative when the patient is examined. The treatment of cardiac syncope includes treatment of underlying structural disorder and appropriate management of arrhythmias (brady or tachyarrhythmias) and conduction defects.

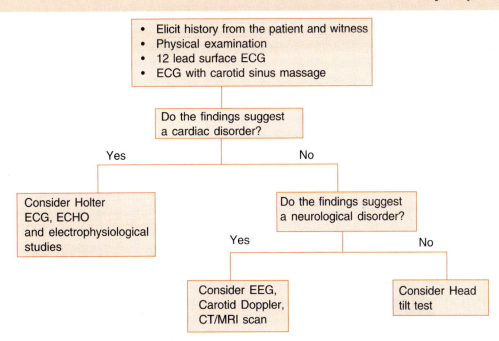

Fig. 43.2: A valuable guide to investigations, diagnosis and differential diagnosis of syncope

B. *Carotid sinus syncope:* It is better prevented than treated. Patient is advised to avoid measures that cause pressure on the carotid sinus such as tight cervical collar. Patient is advised to turn the whole body rather turn the head alone when looking to one side. Atropine or the ephedrine group of drugs should be used if there is profound bradycardia or hypotension during attacks. Dual-chamber pacing relieves the symptoms due to bradycardia unresponsive to other measures.

C. *Vasovagal syncope:* This is mediated by the Bezold-Jerisch reflex and is usually triggered by a reduced venous return due to prolonged standing, excessive heat or a large meal. Some variants of vasovagal syncope occur in the presence of identifiable and remediable triggers (e.g. cough syncope, micturition syncope etc.) are collectively called *situational syncope*.

Treatment is unnecessary is mild cases. In severe cases, beta-blockers or disopyramide (a vagolytic agent) may be helpful. Cardiac pacing alone is rarely indicated or effective in the prevention of this type of syncope. A dual-chamber pacing may be used in case profound bradycardia is the cause of intractable symptoms. Finally, patients with salt depletion syndrome (urinary excretion of less than 170 mmol/24 hours) may respond to salt loading. Paroxetine (a selective serotonine reuptake inhibitor) has been found effective in reducing the recurrence rate of refractory vasovagal syncope.

D. *Postural syncope:* Whenever possible, the underlying cause should be found out and treated such as control of diabetes. Dehydration should be avoided. Simple measures such as keeping the head-end of the bed elevated; gradual arising from the recumbent position, avoidance of prolonged standing flexing the calf muscles during standing to improve venous return, wearing a snug elastic abdominal binder and elastic stockings and volume expansion by liberal salt intake or 9α-fluorohydrocortisone (oral dose 0.1-0.2 mg/day) may be helpful.

Chapter 44

Acute Vertigo

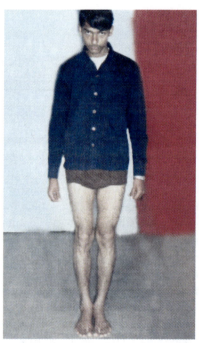 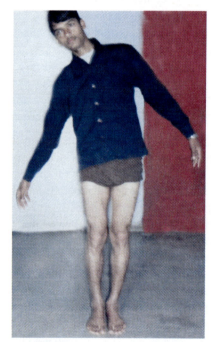

Fig. 44.1: Acute vertigo

ACUTE VERTIGO

Definition

Vertigo is an illusory or hallucinatory sense of self or environmental movement, most commonly due to a disturbance in the vestibular system (Fig. 44.1).

It is important to differentiate *true vertigo* from more common symptom of '*dizziness*' which is most often not due to vestibular causes.

Dizziness is common and often vexing symptom that patients use to describe a variety of sensations such as light-headedness, faintness, spinning, giddiness etc. Some patients use this term too loosely and inappropriately to describe symptoms such as confusion, blurring of vision, headache, tingling or walking on cotton and gait disturbances. Operationally, dizziness is classified into four categories: (i) faintness, (ii) vertigo, (iii) miscellaneous head sensations, and (iv) gait disturbances.

Acute Vertigo

Table 44.1: Common causes of vertigo

1. Peripheral (labrynthine and vestibular causes)
A. *Hereditary*
B. *Acquired*
  i. Physiological
   - Motion sickness
   - Height vertigo
   - Space sickness
  ii. Pathological
   - Infections e.g. labyrinthitis, vestibular neuronitis, meningitis
   - Benign paroxysmal positional vertigo
   - Meniere's disease/syndrome
   - Post-traumatic
   - Drugs induced e.g. ototoxic (aminoglycosides), nerve involvement (diuretics)
   - Cerebropontine angle tumours e.g. acoustic neuroma, meningioma, cysts (epidermal or arachnoid)
   - Vascular compression of vestibular nerves
   - Toxic e.g. ethyl alcohol

2. Central (brainstem and cerebellum causes)
- Brainstem ischaemia/infarction, embolism, haemorrhage
- Transient ischaemic attacks
- Multiple sclerosis
- Vertebro-basilar insufficiency
- Acute cerebellitis
- Posterior fossa tumour
- Migraine (basilar artery)
- Epilepsy (temporal lobe focus)

Causes

Vertigo is a symptom complex of any type of vestibular lesion whether situated in the vestibular receptors (semicircular canals, the utricle and saccule) or in the pathways (vestibular nerves) or projections to the cerebral cortex via thalamus-called 'central vertigo'.

The causes of both central and peripheral vertigo are given the Table 44.1.

Applied Anatomy and Physiology of Vertigo

The spatial orientation and maintenance of posture and equilibrium depends on three sensory systems:
1. *Vestibular system:* There are two basic vestibular system reflexes subserving this function: (i) vestibulo-ocular reflexes that stabilise the position of the eyes with respect to space so that images on the retina remain stationary (ii) vestibulospinal reflexes that stabilise the head and body position for motor control and maintaining upright posture.
2. *Visual system* (retina to occipital cortex) that conveys the informations from the eyes to the cortex.
3. *The somatosensory system* that conveys peripheral informations from the skin, joint muscle receptors.

Vertigo may represent either physiological stimulation or pathological dysfunction in any of the three systems.

Nystagmus is useful indicator of vestibular dysfunction in patients with vertigo. Inhibition of the canals (caloric test) results in nystagmus to the side of the lesion, while excitation of canals results in nystagmus away from the canals (lesion).

Clinical Evaluation of a Patient with Vertigo

The most important diagnostic tool is careful history focussed on the meaning of 'dizziness' to the patient and true vertigo. As already discussed, dizziness is used in broad sense, hence when the meaning of dizziness is uncertain; provocative tests may be helpful such as:

1. *Checking of orthostatic hypotension.* Duplication of symptoms during orthostatic hypotension indicate cerebral ischaemia.
2. *Valsalva maneuvers* exacerbate vertigo in patients with cardiovascular disease.
3. Sudden turns when walking or spinning the patients while standing reproduce true vertigo.
4. The simplest provocative test for vestibular dysfunction is *rapid rotation and abrupt cessation of movement in a swivel chair.* This always induces vertigo that the patient can compare with the symptomatic dizziness.
5. *Hyperventilation* is the cause of dizziness in many anxious patients. *Forced hyperventilation* for 1 minute is indicated for patients with enigmatic dizziness and normal neurological examination.

Once, it has been established that it is true vertigo rather than dizziness, then find out whether vertigo is central in origin or due to peripheral causes. Rapid unilateral injury to either peripheral or central vestibular structures produces the acute vestibular syndrome consisting of severe vertigo, nausea and vomiting, spontaneous nystagmus and postural instability.

The time course and duration of vertigo also help in the diagnosis:
1. Recurrent episodes of brief positional vertigo (lasting less than a minute) indicate benign positional vertigo, or post-traumatic vertigo. It can be psychogenic.
2. Recurrent spontaneous vertigo lasting for minutes or hours indicates Meniere's disease, vertebrobasilar insufficiency, migraine or autoimmune ear disease.
3. Spontaneous prolonged attacks of vertigo lasting for a day or longer suggest labyrinthitis, multiple sclerosis or infarction in the vertebrobasilar artery territory.

The differences between peripheral and central vertigo are given in Box 44.1.

A central vascular cause can be suspected on history in elderly patients with positive history of hypertension, smoking, IHD and past history of CVA. Patients with central cause cannot stand or walk and direction of fall is variable. Central nystagmus is multi-directional (nystagmus that changes direction with direction of gaze i.e. gaze evoked) in the brainstem and cerebellar disorders. Vertical nystagmus (upbeat-or downbeat nystagmus) is almost pathognomonic of brainstem or midline cerebellar disorders. Most common central disorders producing nystagmus and imbalance are vascular (brainstem ischaemia/infarction or basilar artery insufficiency or inferior cerebellar infarction).

A peripheral cause is suspected when there is a history of ear discharge or pain, unilateral deafness or tinnitus. Peripheral nystagmus due to labyrinthine disorders results in unidirectional nystagmus with slow phase (component) moving towards the affected ear and fast phase (component) opposite to the lesion. Vertigo is severe with direction of spin towards fast phase, while tendency to fall is toward slow phase. The nystagmus is spontaneous and unidirectional with a torsional component. It continues in the same direction when the direction of gaze changes. It increases in intensity as the eyes are deviated towards the normal ear. Visual fixation inhibits nystagmus and vertigo—a bed side diagnostic test.

Bed Side Test used for Evaluation of Vertigo

1. *Visual fixation:* The effect of visual fixation is tested at the bed side with an ophthalmoscope focussed on the optic disc of one eye while the patient covers and uncovers the other (fixating) eye. The intensity of the nystagmus and velocity of its slow phase are increased by covering the fixating eye in peripheral vestibular lesions.
2. *Caloric test:* Caloric stimulation test is applied to each ear separately. The test is performed by making the patient in recumbent position and head flexed at 30°. Cold water stimulation normally induces horizontal nystagmus with slow phase towards the cold water stimulation and fast phase to the opposite side. Warm water

Acute Vertigo

Box 44.1: Differentiation between central and peripheral vertigo

Feature	Peripheral vertigo	Central vertigo
Postural instability (imbalance)	Mild	Severe
Direction of nystagmus to lesion	Unidirectional, fast phase opposite	Bidirectional or unidirectional
Purely horizontal nystagmus without torsional component	Uncommon	Common
Vertical nystagmus	Never present	May be present
Visual fixation and vertigo	Attenuates or inhibits nystagmus	No change
Direction of spin	Towards fast component	Variable
Direction of fall	Towards slow component	Variable
Nausea and vomiting	Severe	Mild to moderate
Tinnitus and/or hearing loss	Common	Rare
Duration of symptoms but recurrent	Finite (minutes, days, weeks)	May be chronic
Neurological dysfunction	Rare	Common

stimulation has opposite effect. A reduced response indicates vestibular disorder on the same side.

3. **Auditory testing:** It gives informations regarding the hearing loss or tinnitus or other auditory symptoms that accompany vertigo in peripheral nerve lesions. CNS disorders rarely accompany auditory symptoms.

Specific Common Vertigo

Benign paroxysmal positional vertigo (BPPV): Positional vertigo is precipitated by a recumbent head position either to the left or to the right. BPPV is the most common positional vertigo. Benign positional vertigo is common in middle aged females and the episodes are precipitated by turning over in bed, getting in or out of bed, bending over and straightening up, extension of neck to look upwards, to reach an object placed overhead shelf. The duration of vertigo lasts for more than one minute. The common causes of BPPV include idiopathic, post-traumatic and viral neurolabrinthitis.

Diagnostic Clue to BPPV

The most important positive sign in paroxysmal positional nystagmus is elicited by Dix and Hallipike method. A rapid change of position from sitting to a sudden head hanging to left or right positions (30-45° on one side) induces nystagmus within 2 seconds. This nystagmus has fast component away from the undermost ear and disappears within few seconds.

The recognition of positional nystagmus by above described method is important from therapeutic point of view, because specific exercise programmes can cure it dramatically.

The vertigo and accompanying nystagmus have a distinct pattern of latency, fatiguability and habituation that differs from the less common central positional vertigo (Table 44.2).

Management

Aims

1. To abolish vertigo.
2. To enhance vestibular compensation to allow brain to find a new sensory equilibrium despite a vestibular lesion.

Treatment of acute vertigo consists of bed rest and vestibular suppressant drugs such as antihistaminics (meclizine—12.5 to 50 mg every 4-6 hrs; dimenhydrinate—25-50 mg every 4-6 hours, promethazine 25 mg 6 hourly), central-

234 Neurology

Table 44.2: Distinguishing features between benign paroxysmal positional vertigo and central positional vertigo

Feature	Benign paroxysmal positional vertigo (BPPV)	Central positional vertigo
Frequency	Common	Less common
Latency*	3-40 sec.	None, immediate vertigo and nystagmus
Fatiguability**	Yes	No
Habituation +	Yes	No
Intensity of vertigo	Severe	Mild
Reproducibility ++	Variable	Good

* Time between achieving head position and onset of symptoms
** Disappearance of symptoms with maintenance of offending position
+ Lessening of symtpoms with repeated trials
++ Reproduction of symptoms during each examination

acting anti-cholinergics (scopolamine, homatropine), histaminergic drugs (betahistadine—an antivertigo drug causing vasodilation of microcirculation of internal ear), or a trunquilliser with GABA-ergic effects (diazepam) or calcium channel antagonists (flunarizine, cinnarizine). If the vertigo persists beyond few days, most authorities advise ambulation, despite short-term discomfort to the patient.

Vestibular rehabilitation: Vestibular exercises should begin as early as possible as the acute phase ends; and vestibular suppressants should be avoided because dizziness is required for compensation. The exercise programme should be systematized to facilitate compensation. While nystagmus is present, fixation should be exercised in the direction with greatest dizziness. When nystagmus decreases then eye-head coordination exercises should be done.

Box 44.2: Treatment of recurrent spontaneous vertigo

Disease	Treatment
Meniere's disease	• Low salt diet
	• Diuretics
Migraine	• Anti-migraine treatment
Autoimmune inner ear disease	• Steroids and immunosuppressants
Vertebrobasilar insufficiency	• Antiplatelets
TIAs	• Anticoagulants
Syphilitic labrynthitis	• Antibiotics
	• Steroids

The treatment of recurrent spontaneous vertigo depending on the cause is summarised in Box 44.2. Prophylactic measures to prevent vertigo are variably effective. *Antihistamines* are commonly utilised.

Chapter 45

Acute Ischaemic Stroke

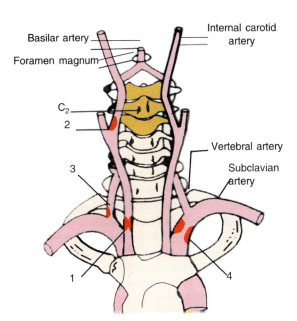

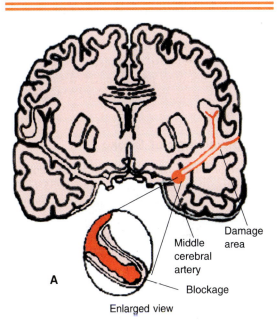

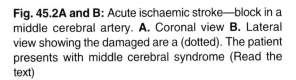

Fig. 45.1: The principal sites of atheroma in extra-cerebral vessels (1) common carotid artery (2) internal carotid artery; (3) vertebral artery; (4) subclavian artery

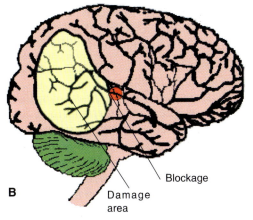

Fig. 45.2A and B: Acute ischaemic stroke—block in a middle cerebral artery. **A.** Coronal view **B.** Lateral view showing the damaged are a (dotted). The patient presents with middle cerebral syndrome (Read the text)

ACUTE ISCHAEMIC STROKE OR CEREBROVASCULAR ACCIDENT (CVA)

Definitions

Stroke is defined as sudden onset of focal neurological symptoms and signs resulting from diseases of the cerebral vasculature, lasting for more than 24 hours or leading to death with no apparent cause other than vascular accidents. The term *transient ischaemic attack (TIA)* implies complete recovery of such a deficit within 24 hours. It is the largest single cause of morbidity and disability in developing countries after cancer and heart diseases.

After an acute attack, 20-30% of patients die within first few days. Amongst the survivors, about 25% become permanently disabled or handicapped. Recurrent attacks of CVA are not uncommon.

Pathophysiology of Stroke

The normal functions of the brain are dependent on a relatively constant blood supply of 55 to 70 ml/100 g of brain/min. Ischaemic stroke results due to occlusion of a cerebral artery or less often due to reduction in perfusion due to severely stenosed artery (atherosclerosis). When the cerebral blood flow is critically reduced below 20 ml/100 g/min., the resulting cerebral ischemia with hypoxia results in loss of neuronal electrical excitation due to failure of Na^+, K^+ and ATP mechanism leading to cytotoxic oedema. This stage is reversible.

Further fall of cerebral blood flow to below 10 ml/100g/min causes failure of cellular aerobic metabolism and lactic acidosis and ultimately death. This stage is irreversible.

Truely speaking, in any infarction, there is central core where the cerebral blood flow is drastically reduced (<10 ml/100 mg/min) which cannot be salvaged. A large area surrounds this area where cerebral blood flow is sufficiently reduced (between 10-50 ml/100 g/min) and the clinical symptoms are as a result of this reduction. The area is salvageable, if adequate timely intervention is done to improve the perfusion. This area is called "*ischaemic pneumbra*" which can be rescued.

The variable effects of reduction of cerebral blood flow is given in the Table 45.1. The area with blood flow of about 20 ml/100 g/min. is salvageable, hence, efforts should be directed to improve circulation in this area to provide neuroprotection.

Therapeutic time window (window period): This is a period between reversible stage (ischaemic pneumbra) to irreversible stage of cellular death (homeostatic failure). This period is important from therapeutic point of view because intervention at this stage can protect the brain from damage (neuroprotection is possible). This window period is one to three hours which means that all intervention should be done within 3 hours and the earlier it is done the better are the results. However it is not possible to reach the hospital within this period soon after the stroke, some studies include patients upto 6 hours of stroke. It is estimated that about 50% pneumbra may still survive upto 72 hours.

Brain Ischaemia and Free Radicals Mediated Toxicity

Cellular ischaemia leads to cascade of free radicals mediated changes which are deleterious to the tissues. Ischaemic depolarisation results in membrane failure and in an uncontrolled release of excitatory neurotransmitters which are neurotoxic.

Table 45.1: Progressive reduction in cerebral blood flow and their variable effects

Cerebral blood flow	Effects
1. > 55 ml/100 g/min	Normal
2. ≤ 20 ml/100 g/min	Cytotoxic oedema, failure of Na^+, K^+, ATPase mechanism. The stage is reversible.
3. 10-20 ml/100g/min	Ischaemic pneumbra (read text) This can be rescued with timely intervention.
4. ≤ 10 ml/100g/min	Cellular failure or cellular dealth. This stage is irrevesible

A lot of substances such as prostaglandins, thromboxanes and leukotrienes are also released which are toxic to cell membrane causing lysis and generation of free radicals. The free radicals lead to neurotoxicity.

An inflammatory response to ischaemic neuronal damage leads to elaboration of interleukins, leucocyte adhesion, production of arachidonic acid and toxic free radicals formation.

Reperfusion either achieved by endogenous thrombolysis, thrombus migration or therapeutic intervention may aggravate ischaemic damage by production of toxic free radicals from reperfused tissue.

Causes

Three types of major strokes are now recognised. These are:
1. **Ischaemic stroke:** It is characterised by cerebral infarction resulting from atherothrombosis or embolism to cerebral vessel. The transient ischaemic attack (TIA) implies cerebral ischaemia with subsequent complete recovery within 24 hours. This results from platelet-fibrin microemboli (embolic hypothesis).
2. **Haemorrhagic stroke:** It results from bleeding within central nervous system, occurs due to ruptured aneurysm in the young and hypertensive intracerebral bleed in the elderly.
3. **Stroke due to undetermined origin:** *Lacunar or small vessel strokes* are deep, small, cerebral infarcts located deep in the basal ganglion or cerebral white matter resulting from lipohylinosis of small penetrating vessels leading to its obliteration.

The causes of various types of stroke are given in the Table 45.2.

Ischaemic Stroke (Fig. 45.1)

Ischaemic stroke results from thrombotic or embolic occlusion of a cerebral vessel or may result due to prolonged systemic hypotension with underperfusion of cerebral vessels (ischaemic-anoxic-encephalopathy). In the latter group, the areas of the

Table 45.2: Aetiological classification of stroke

1. *Ischaemic strokes*
   A. *Thrombotic stroke*
      - Atherosclerosis
      - Lacunar infarcts (small-vessel infarct)
      - Vasculitis (collagen vascular disease, temporal arteritis, PAN, rheumatic, tubercular, Takayasu's disease)
      - Dissecting aneurysm of brachiocephalic vessels
      - Haematological diseases (polycythaemia, thrombocytosis, sickle cell disesae, DIC, procoagulant states like protein C and S deficiency, dysproteinaemia)
      - Angiographic complication
      - Infarction of undetermined cause (AIDS related syndrome)
   B. *Transient ischaemia*
      - Transient ischaemic attacks (TIAs)
      - Cardiac diseases with arrhythmias
   C. *Embolic stroke*
      - Cardiac source (coronary artery disease, arrhythmias, rheumatic heart disease, cardiomyopathies, endocarditis)
      - Atherothrombotic arterial source
      - Unknown source
   D. *Vasospasm*
      - Cerebral vasospasm following subarachnoid haemorrhage
      - Reversible vasospasm (idiopathic, migraine eclampsia, trauma)
   E. *Venous thrombosis (thrombophlebitis)*
      - Drugs and oral contraceptive
      - Dehydration and infection
      - Postpartum state
      - Postoperative state
      - Systemic cancer
2. *Haemorrhagic stroke*
   - Hypertensive cerebral haemorrhage
   - Ruptured aneurysm (saccular, mycotic)
   - Ruptured angioma (arterial, venous, mixed)
   - Trauma
   - Blood dyscrasias (leukaemia, purpura, hyperviscosity syndrome)
   - Complications of anticoagulant or thrombolytic therapy
   - Haemorrhage in brain tumour
   - Miscellaneous (bleeding in haemorrhagic infarct, arteritis)
3. *Stroke of undetermine origin*
   - Multi-infarct dementia in lacunar syndromes
   - Moyamoya disease
   - Aortic arch syndrome (noninflammatory)
   - Fibromuscular dysplasia

brain with marginal blood supply are commonly affected.

Depending on the time course and reversibility of neurological signs, ischaemic stroke is divided into:
1. *Transient episode of ischaemia (transient ischaemic attacks—TIA).* This is reversible within 24 hours.
2. *Reversible ischaemic neurologic deficit:* This is an infrequently employed term, denotes an ischaemic event in which the neurological deficit usually recovers over a period of 24 to 72 hours but may take even one week to resolve.
3. *Completed stroke (thrombo-embolic stroke):* It evolves with a maximum neurological deficit at the onset (within few hours). Often, the patient awakens with a completed deficit. A completed stroke may be thrombotic or embolic, is sometimes heralded by one or more TIAs in the preceding days, weeks or months. The mechanism of ischaemic stroke resolves around the pathophysiology mechanisms responsible for TIAs.

Thrombotic strokes (completed stroke) are generally due to underlying atherosclerosis (Fig. 45.2); while embolic stroke results as a result of embolism from the proximal atherosclerotic vessel (ruptured plaques, clot) or the heart (cardiovascular cause).

Clinical Features

Symptoms and signs of TIAs: These are brief episodes of stroke symptoms or focal neurological deficit of vascular origin, lasting for less than 24 hours without any residual sign. The episodes may be isolated and infrequent, or may occur many times a day and tend to be consistent in their symptomatology in affected individuals suggesting that recurrent ischaemia consistently involves the same side of the brain. Recovery is the rule in TIA.

The embolism of platelet—fibrin clot formed over atheromatous plaques within a great vessel is the most common (90%) cause of TIAs.

Attacks are more common in older persons. The clinical features depend on the vascular system involved (see Box 45.1). TIAs cause sudden loss of function in one region of the brain, symptoms reach their peak within seconds and last for minutes or hours but not beyond 24 hours (by definition). Consciousness is usually preserved.

Physical signs: As signs may recover completely within a short period, hence, the clinical examination may be normal. Therefore, the description of the event that led to an attack may be diagnostic. In addition, there may be clinical evidence of a source of embolus such as:
1. Carotid atheroma may lead to arterial bruit.
2. Arrhythmia (atrial fibrillation) may produce irregularly irregular pulse.
3. Evidence of valvular heart disease, myocardial infarction (fresh or old) or endocarditis.
4. Difference of blood pressure between two arms suggesting dissecting aneurysm or subclavian stenosis.

In addition, there may be clinical evidence of associated disease such as:
- Atherosclerosis of carotid artery leading to weak pulsation.

Box 45.1: Features of transient ischaemic attacks	
Carotid system	**Vertebrobasilar system**
• Amaurosis fugax (sudden transient loss of vision in one eye due to embolisation of retinal artery)	• Diplopia, vertigo, vomiting, dysarthria
• Aphasia	
• Hemiparesis	• Hemianaesthesia and analgesia
• Hemianaesthesia and analgesia	• Hemianopic visual loss
• Hemianopic visual loss	• Transient global amnesia (loss of memory)
	• Quadriparesis
	• Disturbed consciousness (rare)

- Hypertension, diabetes, arteritis, polycythaemia.
- Postural hypotension, low cardiac output.

Thrombotic Stroke

Thrombosis with arteriosclerosis accounts for most of the cases of thrombotic stroke. Atherosclerosis affects extracranial and intracranial arteries at a specific locations (at branchings or divisions and curve of large vessels Fig. 45.1). The thrombus forms in the vessels where plaque narrows the lumen most. The platelet fibrin-endothelial clot is formed due to (i) fragmentation of endothelial lining by underlying atherosclerosis and the divided surface acts a nidus for thrombus formation, or (ii) there is dissection of plaque by blood column forming an ulcer crater that acts a nidus, or (iii) an hemorrhage within a plaque critically narrows a vessel and leads to superadded thrombosis.

Thrombosis of a major cerebral vessel typically produces a large stroke; whereas occlusion of a small penetrating artery results in a small infarction called (*lacunar stroke*). The clinical pictures varies in these two types:

1. ***Thrombotic stroke due to a large vessel involvement:*** The clinical picture varies depending on the size and site of infarction. In about 60% cases, prodromal warning symptoms may precede in the form of TIA. In some cases, the stroke evolves slowly in a stepwise fashion i.e. *stroke-in-evolution*, the symptoms may appear in each limb in succession or simultaneously. The stuttering or intermittent manifestation is characteristic of thrombotic infarction. Not infrequently, the stroke may manifest as a sudden completed stroke (a catastrophic event). The major neurovascular syndromes resulting from major arterial occlusion are given in the Table 45.3.
2. ***Lacunar stroke (occlusion of small perforating end arteries):*** Lacunar stroke results either from thrombotic occlusion of deep penetrating branches of carotid or vertebrobasilar system. Any of the perforating or penetrating branch can get blocked at its origin or by marked lipohyalinosis of intima in patients with hypertension. The infarcts produced in such a way are small ranging from 3 to 4 mm to 1 or 2 cm, often cavitate leaving small holes traversed by fine fibrous strands—'*lacunae*' hence, the name lacunar infarcts. Such infarcts are primarily located in basal ganglia or pons.

The symptoms and signs of lacunar infarct varies with size and site. Small infarct < 1 cm^3 are usually asymptomatic. Larger infarcts produce the following clinical syndromes:

1. *Pure motor hemiplegia* due to lacuna in internal capsule or pons on the side opposite to hemiplegia.
2. *Pure sensory stroke* (hemianaesthesia) results due to lacuna in posterior limb of internal capsule or thalamus of opposite side.
3. *Ataxic-hemiparesis stroke* results due to lacuna in opposite pons or internal capsule.
4. *Sudden dysarthria* and *clumsy hand syndrome*.
5. Pseudobulbar palsy due to brainstem infarct.

Embolic Infarct (Stroke)

On account of sudden impaction of an embolus, compensatory mechanisms do not get sufficient time to come into action to protect the brain from ischaemia, hence, the neurological deficit is instantaneous and maximum at the onset. Frequently, these embolic plugs break away thereby restoring the normal circulation, hence, recovery is almost complete in these patients of strokes.

The clinical feature is similar to thrombotic infarct (stroke) but differs in some aspects (see Box 45.2).

Hemorrhagic Stroke

This is discussed separately as intracerebral bleed.

Table 45.3: Clinical features of major vascular syndromes due to thrombotic occlusion of large vessels

1. **Internal carotid artery**
   - May be asymptomatic
   - Symptomatic cases have warning symptoms such as brief episodes of confusion, speech disturbance (aphasia, dysarthria) and paraesthesias (sensory symptoms) with or without contralateral hemiplegia.
   - Transient monocular blindness on the same side with contralateral hemiplegia or hemianaesthesia is pathognomonic of carotid occlusion
   - Bilateral lesion produces quadriplegia with coma, a picture indistinguishable from basilar artery syndrome
   - In fact, the clinial symptoms and sign of acute carotid occlusion resemble acute middle cerebral artery syndrome (Read middle cerebral syndrome)
   - Feeble carotid, poor pulsations of retinal vessels with or without optic atrophy, dilated pupil on the side of lesion and a cervical bruit are diagnostic clues to carotid artery occlusion

2. **Anterior cerebral syndrome:**
   - Sensori-motor weakness of opposite lower limb (monoplegia) with or without weakness of upper limb (incomplete hemiplegia)
   - Mental features
   - Urinary incontinence
   - Gait disturbances
   - Appearance of primitive reflexes (sucking, grasp)
   Occlusion of unimpaired (single) artery
   - Cortical type of paraplegia
   - Urinary incontinence
   - Akinetic mutism

3. **Middle cerebral syndrome** (Fig. 45.2)
   - Contralateral hemiplegia
   - Contralateral hemianaesthesia
   - Homonomous hemianopia may or may not be present on opposite side
   - Aphasia if dominant hemisphere is involved
   A. *Occlusion of upper division:*
      - Contralateral hemiplegia
      - Contralateral hemianaesthesia
      - Expressive aphasia (Broca's aphasia)
   B. *Occlusion of lower division*
      - All above features with
      - Wernicke's aphasia
   C. *Occlusion of perforating (es)*
      - Lacunar (pure sensory or pure motor syndrome)

4. **Posterior cerebral artery syndrome**
   - Contralateral homonomous hemianopia
   - Visual disturbances e.g. distorted vision, visual agnosia, dyslexia
   - Central vision is spared even in bilateral disease The pupillary reflexes are preserved
   - Contralateral hemiplegia
   - Thalamic syndromes
   - Memory loss (amnesia)

5. **Verbetrobasilsar (brainstem infarction syndromes)**
   - Hemiparesis or quadriparesis (pyramidal tracts involved)
   - Sensory loss due to involvement of medial leminscus and spinothalamic tracts
   - Diplopia (3rd nerve involvement)
   - Facial numbness (5th nerve involvement)
   - Nystagmus, vertigo (vestibular connections involvement)
   - Dysphagia, dysarthria (9th and 10th cranial nerves involvement)
   - Ataxia, dysarthria and hiccups (brainstem and cerebellar connections)
   - Horner's syndrome (sympathetic fibres involvement)
   - Altered consciousness or coma (reticular formation involvement)

Investigations

The preliminary investigations done to find out the cause in a patient with stroke are given in Box 45.3.

Further investigations done in patients with stroke are:

1. **Cerebrospinal fluid (CSF) examination:** It is done for inflammatory disease of the brain or for haemorrhagic infarct. It is useful in 80% cases of haemorrhagic strokes and in 90% of subarachnoid haemorrhage, where CSF contains blood. A three vials test should be done to rule out traumatic tap. Red cells and leucocyte counts/mm^3 of CSF in three vial citrated blood will differentiate traumatic tap. The availability of CT scan and MRI have obviated the need of invasive lumbar puncture except in subarachnoid haemorrhage or inflammatory cerebral lesions.

2. **CT scan:** This is now widely available and is indicated in usually all patients with stroke or TIA. CT scan will demonstrate the site of the

Box 45.2: Differentiation between thrombotic and embolic strokes

Feature	Thrombotic stroke	Embolic stroke
Prodromal symptoms	Often present	Absent
Onset of stroke	Slow onset, stuttering or intermittent progression or may be sudden	Acute catastrophic
Neurological deficit	Slowly evolves • Step-ladder fashion called stroke-in-evolution • Symptoms and signs may appear intermittently	• Deficit is maximum at the onset
Consciousness	Confusion, disorientation may be present. Coma may supervene	Consciousness is usually preserved
Convulsion	Common, occur during the course or at the onset	Uncommon
Cause	Underlying atherosclerosis of a large vessel with or without thrombosis	Cardiac source or artery to artery embolisation
Recovery	Incomplete recovery may occur with residual symptoms and signs	Recovery is complete. Residual symptoms and signs are rare

Box 45.3: Preliminary tests in stroke

- Urinalysis and blood glucose for diabetes mellitus
- Haemoglobin, platelets for polycythaemia
- WBC count for any evidence of infection
- ESR and C-reactive protein for inflammation
- Serological tests for neurosyphilis
- X-ray chest for neoplasm, tuberculosis etc.
- ECG for an evidence of myocardial infarct, ventricular aneurysm and arrhythmias
- Antinuclear factor (ANF), double stranded DNA, cardiolipin antibodies for stroke in young patients.
- Blood culture for endocarditis in patients with underlying heart disease

lesion and will also differentiate between haemorrhage and an infarction. It will detect an unexpected space occupying lesion i.e. tumour, abscess, hematoma, parasitic cyst. It can also detect surrounding oedema and less consistently haemorrhagic infarction. It cannot differentiate early (within 6 hours) ischaemic tissue from normal tissue, nor can it detect cases of early infarction (less than 24 hours). Detection rate increases over the succeeding few days and 90% of all infarcts are detected at one week.

CT scan with angiography (contrast CT scan) will differentiate enhancing from non-enhancing lesions.

3. ***Carotid doppler study:*** This ultrasound study is of value in screening for carotid artery disease (TIA, reversible ischaemic neurological deficit). In skilled hands, it is highly useful in demonstrating internal carotid artery occlusion.

4. ***Cerebral angiography or digital substraction angiography:*** These are most useful than doppler study to define the cerebral microvasculature with areas of stenosis and ulcerated atheromatous lesion. It may demonstrate aneurysm(s) or an angiomatous malformation. Angiography should not be done in a ruptured intracerebral aneurysm.

5. ***Magnetic resonance Imaging (MRI).*** It is supplement to CT scan. MRI can often visualise anoxic lesions missed on CT scan. It usually becomes abnormal within few hours of cerebral infarction, hence, useful in early diagnosis because the peri-infarction parenchyma which appears normal on CT scan often shows abnormality (ischaemic demyelination) on MRI. MR angiography (MRA) in hyperacute (within 6 hours) ischaemic strokes defines the extent and severity of cerebral lesions which are usually missed on CT (Fig. 45.3). Thus MRI and MRA help a great deal in taking decision about thrombolytic therapy.

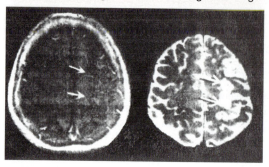

A. T1-weighted image   B. T2-Weighted image

Fig. 45.3: MRI findings in acute cerebral stroke. Acute onset of right hemiparesis. (A) The postcontrast T_1-weighted image (left) demonstrates contrast enhancement within the vascular bed (white arrows) distal to a high-grade stenosis or occlusion. (B) 24h later, abnormal prolongation of T2-weighted signal is seen in the cortex supplied by the middle cerebral occlusion (right image, white arrows). This is due to enhancement of vessels distal to occlusion due to percolation of contrast (gadolinium) into these vessels

Management of Stroke

Goals of Therapy

To avoid the development of cerebral infarction; if already present, then to retard its progression or recurrence. It is divided into three phases:
Phase I: To save life and to speed up recovery.
Phase II: Physical, occupational and social rehabilitation for a gainful employment.
Phase III: To prevent recurrence of stroke.

Phase I — General Measures and Intensive Care

In a patient with stroke, maintenance of vitals (pulse, BP, temp, respiration), patency of airway, fluid and electrolyte balance and prevention of complications such as lung aspiration, seizures, thrombophlebitis and bed sores are essential. The treatment in early stage in intensive stroke care unit is beneficial:

i. *Ventilation:* Cerebral hypoxia predisposes to cerebral oedema, raised intracranial pressure and brain herniation. Patent airway must be maintained to prevent accidental aspiration and for continued suction of tracheobronchial secretions to prevent hypoxia.

ii. O_2 *administration* (4-6 litres/min) through a nasal catheter or venturi mask is advocated. Ventilatory support in a comatosed patient is necessary if signs of hypoxia secondary to hypoventilation are present, or there is rising $PaCO_2$. Long-term ventilatory support warrants tracheostomy.

iii. *Blood pressure:* In acute stage of cerebral ischaemia/infarct, blood pressure should not be lowered unless moderate to severe hypertension (diastolic BP > 90 mmHg) persists despite the decongestive therapy and diuretics.
On the other hand, in hypertensive CVA with encephalopathy, or malignant hypertension, sublingual use of calcium channel blockers (nifedipine 10 mg) or parenteral beta blockers and diuretics may be employed to reduce the blood pressure keeping in mind that diastolic BP does not fall below 100 mmHg. Hypotensive episode may be treated by vasopressors (dopamine), by I.V. fluids and corticosteroids.

iv. *Cardiac arrhythmias:* In acute CVA, the pulse can be irregular. Frequent ventricular premature beats may be treated by diphenylhydantoin sodium (100 mg three times a day). Bradyarrhythmias may point to raised intracranial pressure or cerebral oedema which will disappear with parenteral fursemide or 100 ml bolus dose of mannitol.

v. *Fluid and electrolyte balance:* Ischaemic tissue with break in blood brain barrier retains fluid, predisposes to cerebral oedema. Judicious restriction of fluids intake (oral or parenteral) during first 2-3 days or even a negative balance is beneficial. On the other hand, excessive diuresis should not be attempted which may produce cerebral hyponatraemia.

vi. *Reduction of cerebral oedema and increased intracranial pressure:* In first week of massive cerebral infarction, I.V. mannitol is used to reduce the vasogenic cerebral oedema. High doses of corticosteroids can reduce cerebral oedema but their role in treatment of ischaemic strokes is doubtful. A controlled trial of I.V. glycerol infusion in acute stroke has demonstrated reduced mortality in treated patients probably due to reduction in cerebral oedema.

vii. *Measures to improve cerebral blood flow:* Hyperviscosity reduces cerebral blood, if present, should be treated with low molecular dextran, or 5% albumin infusion to bring down the hematocrit to 30-33%. Such treatment if employed, should be monitored in patients with cardiovascular disease and in those at risk of developing cerebral oedema.

A. **Specific therapy**: It is directed against the cause and to prevent recurrence and complications.

i. *Antiplatelet agents:* Antiplatelet agents (aspirin, dipyridamole, ticlopidine, clopidogrel) are used to inhibit platelets aggregation and useful in cerebral thrombotic infarction, embolism and transitory ischaemic episodes. Aspirin is widely employed drug for primary and secondary prevention of strokes. Higher doses of aspirin (300 mg/day) have been found more useful than low dose (100 mg/day).

Ticlopidine (a thienopyridine derivative) inhibits platelet aggregation, reduces plasma fibrinogen and increases red cell deformability. It is found more effective than aspirin. Subjects with diabetes mellitus, those on anti hypertensives and those with high creatinine levels benefit more with ticlopidine than aspirin. However, the drug is expensive and relatively toxic (transient neuropenia, diarrhoea). Now-a-days a combination of clopidogrel plus aspirin is preferred over either alone.

ii. *Anticoagulants:* Parenteral heparin and long-term oral anticoagulants have extensively been tried in acute ischaemic stroke to prevent extension of thrombosis but its value in completed or established stroke is doubtful, and its use is often fraught with dangers. Its use has been recommended in recurrent TIAs, thrombosis-in-evolution, in cerebral embolisation due to atrial fibrillation or a cardiogenic cause or carotid artery thrombosis.

Danger: A diagnosis of ischaemic infarct must be confirmed on the CT scan and CSF examination before start of anticoagulation therapy, otherwise, haemorrhagic complications will pose a danger

During heparinisation, thromboplastin time (aPTT) is kept twice the control. Heparin (3000-5000 units) is given after every six to eight hours or an I.V. bolus dose of 100 units/kg body weight followed by continuous infusion of 1000 units/hour for 24 hours is recommended under supervision in acute care unit. Oral anticoagulant-coumadine sodium (2-5 mg/day) is generally given keeping the PTI around 50%. Oral therapy can be continued upto 6 months or longer. A bleeding ulcer, malignant hypertension, hepatic failure and poor compliance constitute its contraindication.

iii. *Neuroprotective or cytoprotective agents:* Voltage dependent calcium channel blockers i.e. nimodipine has cytoprotective action in ischaemic stroke. To obtain best results, therapy should be started within 6-8 hours of ischaemic stroke with oral nimodipine 120 mg/day. Blood pressure should be monitored during the therapy.

Antioxidants to prevent free radicals mediated neuronal damage have been advocated.

iv. *Treatment of complications:* Infections (chest, urinary etc), dehydration, hyponatraemia, hypoxaemia, seizures, hyperglycaemia, deep vein thrombosis may occur and they should be treated appropriately. Avoid pressure sores by frequent turning and good nursing care. Use lexative for constipation.

Surgical treatment: Thrombo-endarterectomy with or without reconstructive surgery has been recommended within few hours or days after acute episode in select number of cases. Best results are

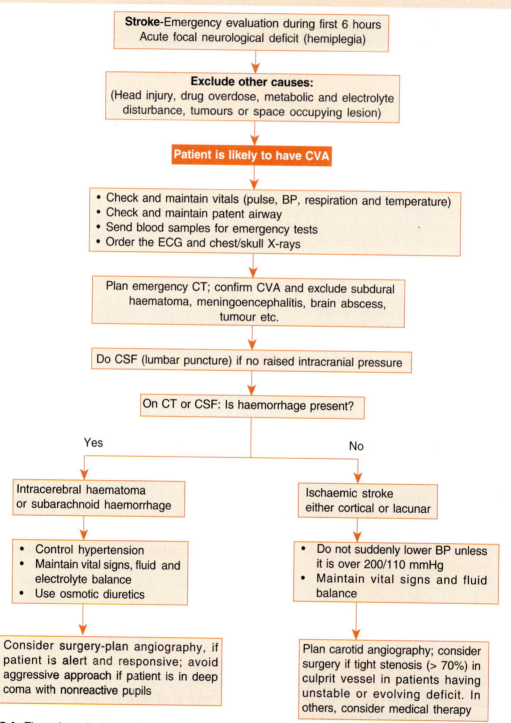

Fig. 45.4: Flow chart depicting diagnostic evaluation and emergency management plan of an acute stroke (hemiplegic syndrome). Modified from US national association recommendations for the emergency evaluation and treatment of stroke

obtained when endarterectomy is combined with best medical care. During the immediate postoperative period, higher doses of aspirin and control of all risk factors are mandatory. Carotid enarterectomy is useful for TIAs caused by carotid stenosis.

Extracranial to intracranial bypass surgery is necessary to create alternate blood channels in symptomatic patients with distal occlusion of either internal carotid or middle cerebral artery.

Recently, percutaneous angioplasty with stent has been tried in carotid artery stenosis with good results. In carotid circulation, angioplasty may find a place in treating accessible stenotic lesions and in postoperative stenosis.

An emergency management based on US national association recommendation is depicted in Fig. 45.4

Phase II—Rehabilitation Phase

Finally, the role of physiotherapy, occupational therapy, good nursing care and other modes of rehabilitation are useful in first few months following stroke. Exercise, re-education, the provision of walking-aids where appropriate, toe-raising springs or calipers and other appliances, adaptation to home and surroundings, speech therapy in aphasia, attention to diet and vitamins intake and care of bowel and bladder are invaluable. Treatment in specialised unit and well organised outpatient physiotherapy and occupation therapy in aphasic patients hastens the return of speech and this may be accomplished by patient's relative or by a therapist. Special attention should be paid to shoulder pain and immobility in the hemiplegic patients. The risk of deep vein thrombosis in the legs and consequent pulmonary embolisation should be recognised. With appropriate and intensive treatment many patients with stroke, can resume useful life and employment despite residual disability. Many problems such as driving of motor vehicles, operation of the machinery etc. can be resolved depending on the patient improvement and ability.

Depression is common after acute stroke and will often respond to antidepressant medication.

Aims of Physiotherapy

- To relieve spasticity and to prevent contractures.
- To teach patients to use walking-aids.
- To bring the patient in mainstream of life and to suggest useful means of employment and to teach them to lead independent life.
- To keep self-esteem and to prevent psychological upset.

Following recovery from stroke, various aids and modifications may be necessary at home, for example, stair rails, portable levatories, bath rails, sliding boards, wheel chairs tripods, modification of doorways and sleep arrangements, stairs lift and kitchen modifications.

Phase III—To Prevent Recurrence of Stroke

Chances of recurrence of stroke are high in survivors during first few weeks (80%) and then decreases to 10% during first year. Therefore modification of risk-factors is mandatory because it has shown significant reduction in morbidity and mortality. The risk modifications strategies include:

- Effective control of hypertension.
- Use of tobacco in any form (smoking, chewing) should be prohibited.
- Prophylactic antiplatelet (aspirin) therapy.
- Dietary modifications for hyperlipidaemia and diabetes.
- Carotid endarterectomy.
- Regular physical exercises and to maintain ideal body weight.
- All other treatable and/or modifiable risk-factors should be looked into and corrected wherever possible such as protein C and S deficiencies, anticardiolipin antibodies, lupus anticoagulants and homocysteinaemia.
- Prophylactic anticoagulant to prevent stroke in patients with cardio-embolic stroke in elderly having atrial fibrillation has been suggested.

Chapter 46

Subarachnoid Haemorrhage

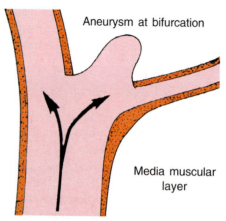

Fig. 46.1: Pathogenesis of formation of saccular aneurysm in intracranial arterial system under haemodynamic stress and its subsequent rupture produce SAH

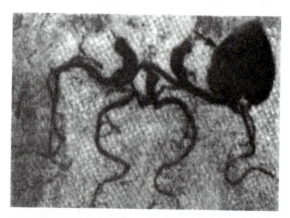

Fig. 46.2: MR angiogram showing a large (giant) aneurysm at the middle cerebral artery bifurcation (indicated by an arrow)

SUBARACHNOID HAEMORRHAGE

Definition

Subarachnoid haemorrhage (SAH) is defined as bleeding into subarachnoid space irrespective of its cause. The condition has high mortality due to various levels of neurological involvement. It can be traumatic in origin or spontaneous caused by rupture of a saccular aneurysm which is upto 5% in the normal population.

Causes

It may be traumatic following head trauma (cortical contusions and laceration) or spontaneous due to rupture of an aneurysm or arteriovenous malformation. The causes are given in the Table 46.1.

Precipitating Factors for SAH

1. Sudden rise in BP causes rupture of an aneurysm by haemodynamic stress (Fig. 46.1).
2. Physical exercise.
3. Emotional stress and strain.

Pathogenesis of Saccular Aneurysm

1. *Congenital (berry) aneurysm:*
   - Defect in the muscular and elastic layers at cerebral arterial bifurcations and branching (Fig. 46.2).

Subarachnoid Haemorrhage

Table 46.1: Causes of subarachnoid haemorrhage (SAH)

Spontaneous	Traumatic SAH
• Ruptured cerebral aneurysm (congenital or saccular and mycotic) • Arteriovenous malformation(s) • Leakage of intracerebral bleed into subarachnoid space • Haemorrhagic cerebral infarction • Rupture of atherosclerotic vessel • Bleeding disorder • Clotting disorder • Vasculitis	• Skull fracture (cerebral contusion and laceration) • Penetrating foreign body • Bleeding from traumatic AV fistula • Traumatic aneurysms (false aneurysm)

- Defect in the internal elastic lamina with a genetic influence as in polycystic kidneys, Ehler-Danlos syndrome, Marfan's syndrome and Rendu-Osler-Weber syndrome.

2. *Acquired:*
   - *Traumatic aneurysms:* They form as false aneurysms of meningeal vessels as a complication of major head injury. True aneurysms in the internal carotid or anterior or middle cerebral artery can occur from penetrating brain injury or bony fractures when intima herniates through the musculo-elastic layers. These are rare.
   - *Mycotic aneurysms:* Are secondary to infective microemboli in the vasanervosa of an artery which in turn predisposes to septic degeneration of its muscular and elastic coats.
   - *Arteriosclerotic aneurysms:* These aneurysms arise from weakness of arterial wall due to extensive arteriosclerotic degeneration in the large arterial trunks (basilar, internal carotid and middle cerebral). These aneurysms vary in appearance such as 'fusiform', globular or diffuse. They seldom rupture. They cause neurological deficit by compressing the nearby structures. They predispose to thrombus formation within its sac.
   - *Dissecting aneurysms:* Primary dissections between elastica, media, or adventitia of internal carotid, middle cerebral or vertebrobasilar arterial walls have now been documented in the absence of injury or atherosclerosis. They present like stroke syndrome without SAH. Such dissections can be treated by "trapping" of its proximal vessel some time by a by pass procedure.
   - Giant aneurysms (> 25 mm in diameter) may be congenital or atherosclerotic, represent 5% of all aneurysms. They produce symptoms due to mass effect like space-occupying lesion.

The most common mechanism of aneurysms formation is thus a combination of several causes as discussed, starting with a congenital defect in the media at the bifurcation of cerebral vessels (Fig. 46.2). These weak spots are present at branchings of these vessels. Hemodynamic stress in the form of local turbulence of blood at this site causes hyperplasia and splitting of internal elastic lamina. This combination of a congenital defect with acquired loss of elastic membrane under the effect of blood pressure may predispose to outpouching of the fragmented elastica leading to saccular aneurysm formation which produces clinical features due to its rupture at the weakest spot.

Clinical Features

They are divided into:
1. Symptoms and signs during acute phase.
2. Symptoms and signs in later phase (delayed neurological deficit).

1. *Symptoms and signs in acute phase of SAH:* Most aneurysms rupture without a warning and the most frequent presentation is sudden unexplained headache if rupture is small; while aneurysmal rupture with major subarachnoid

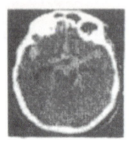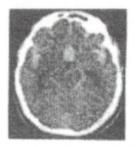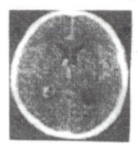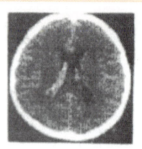

Fig. 46.3: Subarachnoid haemorrhage (a, b, c, d). CT axial images without gadolinium hyperdensity in the subarachnoid spaces due to extravasated blood. A more pronounced collection of blood is seen in the anterior part of the frontal interhemispheric cistern indicating the source of haemorrhage which was a ruptured anterior communicating artery aneurysm. Intraventricular blood is seen in the third and lateral ventricles.

haemorrhage (Fig. 46.3) produces rise in intracranial pressure leading to severe, headache, vomiting and sudden loss of consciousness (patient may collapse suddenly on the floor). The headache at the time of rupture or immediately after that is so severe that patient describes it as "the worst headache of my life" and is unforgettable. Fundus examination may show subhyaloid haemorrhage. The symptoms of SAH in order of frequency are given in Box 46.1.

Box 46.1: Symptoms of SAH in order of frequency	
Symptoms	*Percentage*
Headache	> 50%
Sudden loss of consciousness	20-22% (approx)
Convulsions	5% (approx)
Funny feeling in head	4% (approx)
Pain in back and limbs	2% (approx)
Paralysis or paresis	2% (approx)
Confusion	1% (approx)
No information	4% (approx)

Physical signs depend on the site of an aneurysm, amount of bleed and rapidity with which subarachnoid haemorrhage develops. Sudden death from massive bleed is not uncommon. Majority of the patients develop initial coma, wake up from coma, and continue to remain confused, disoriented and may have transient amnesia for few days. During this period intermittent lethargy and headaches are common.

Although sudden headache without focal neurological symptom is the hallmark of rupture of an aneurysm but focal neurological deficit may occur in addition to formation of hematoma that may produce mass effect. In posterior communicating aneurysmal bleed, 3rd nerve palsy is common and dilatation of pupil on side of lesion is the earliest sign. In SAH of internal carotid or middle cerebral aneurysmal bleed, hemiplegia with or without aphasia and slow mentation (abulia) has been described. Temporary paraplegia, urinary incontinence and akinetic mutism indicate aneurysmal rupture of anterior communicating artery. In aneurysmal bleed of vertibro-basilar system produce lower cranial nerve palsies with pyramidal signs. The clinical findings in SAH are given in Box 46.2.

Box 46.2: Common clinical findings in SAH

- Neck stiffness or rigidity (meningismus)
- Pyrexia
- Transient hypertension
- Bradycardia (HR < 60 min)
- Pre-retinal (subhyaloid) haemorrhage
- Confusion, restlessnes, memory loss
- Symptoms and signs of raised intracranial pressure i.e. headache, vomiting, papilloedema, pupillary change, 6th nerve palsy, bilateral plantar extensor response
- Irregular respiration (Cheyne-Stoke breathing)
- ECG shows nonspecific ST-T changes. There may be deep, symmetric T wave inversion, QTc prolongation, the cause of which is unknown

Subarachnoid Haemorrhage

2. *Symptoms and signs in later phase (delayed neurological deficit):* These are primarily due to:
   i. *Re-rupture:* The risk of re-rupture in untreated aneurysm is maximum within first 2-3 days; but few cases may have re-rupture within 4 weeks. Early surgery eliminates this risk.
   ii. *Hydrocephalus:* Acute hydrocephalus due to intraventricular bleeding may cause stupor and coma. Subacute hydrocephalus (developing over few days) produces progressive drowsiness and lethargy with incontinence. Chronic hydrocephalus (developing over few weeks or months following bleed) presents with gait difficulty, incontinence, slow mentation and lack of interest in surroundings.
   iii. *Vasospasm:* Vasospasm usually occurs following SAH. It causes symptomatic ischaemia or infarction, presents with symptoms referable to arterial territories involved as follows:
      a. Spasm of middle cerebral artery causes contralateral hemiplegia and aphasia (if dominant hemisphere is involved).
      b. Proximal anterior cerebral artery vasospasm causes abulia (slow mentation) and incontinence.
      c. Vasospasm of posterior cerebral artery produces characteristic hemianopia.
      d. Basilar or vertebral artery vasospasm produces variable focal brain-stem signs.

Investigations

1. *CSF examination:* A uniform blood stained or sanguinous CSF under raised pressure is diagnostic, to be done if CT scan does not show bleed or signs of raised intracranial pressure. Microscopically, it may show RBCs (crenated) and pleocytosis. On standing, CSF supernatant is xanthochromic.
2. *Cerebral angiography:* Cerebral angiography or digital substraction angiography is not only diagnostic but defines the site of bleed and outlines the aneurysm if seen.
3. *CT scan:* CT scan is diagnostic. Contrast CT demonstrates the aneurysm. Over 75% cases of SAH are detected on non-contrast CT within 48 hours of rupture.
4. *MRI* is better than CT scan in imaging the aneurysm.
5. *Transcranial doppler:* It is useful for proximal, middle, anterior and vertebro-basilar system flow detection and response to management of vasospasm.
6. *ECG:* The ECG frequently shows tall T waves, or deep symmetric inversion of T waves, widening of QRS and prolongation of QTc.

Complications of SAH (See Box 46.3)

Management

Aims of Treatment
1. Stabilisation of patient.
2. Prevention of recurrence of bleeding.
3. To control cerebral vasospasm.
4. Treatment of symptomatic hydrocephalus.

1. Stabilisation of Patient

Patient is stabilised by:
- Complete bed rest in a quiet room for 3-4 weeks if surgical treatment is not done.
- All sorts of physical strains (coughing, sneezing, straining at stool) or manipulations must be avoided.
- Mild sedation may be prescribed to prevent acute elevation of BP. Extreme sedation should be avoided.

Box 46.3: Complications of SAH	
Neurological	**Systemic**
• Cerebral vasospasm	• Pulmonary oedema
• Raised ICT or hydrocephalus	• Cardiac failure
	• SIADH
• Intraventricular bleeding	• Diabetes insipidus
• Intracerebral haematoma	• Infection
• Hypothalamic lesions	• Venous thromboembolism
• Cranial nerve palsies	
• Cerebral oedema	

- General nursing and medical care as discussed in management "acute ischaemic stroke".
- Blood pressure must be controlled and monitored.
- *Seizures are not uncommon in SAH and can be catastrophic.* Prophylactic anticonvulsants (phenytoin in a loading dose of 15-20 mg/kg given over one hour period followed by maintenance of 300 mg/day) are recommended in all cases of SAH.
- To control severe headache, analgesics may be used.
- In stuporous or comatosed patients, the general measures for unconscious patients may be applied (oxygen therapy, patent airway, maintain adequate oxygenation, if need assisted ventilation, monitoring for vital signs and prevention of bed sores).
- Raised intracranial pressure or tension (ICT) controlled by mannitol in I.V. boluses (0.5 to 1.0 g/kg). Dexamethasone 4 mg I.V. every 6 hourly helps to reduce pressure. Adequate hydration be maintained by use of fluids.
- *Monitoring:* Blood pressure, heart rate, temperature, intake and output balance, arterial blood gases and electrolytes must be monitored.

2. Prevention of Rebleeding

The main complication of SAH is rebleeding which is often disabling or fatal. Blood pressure should be adequately controlled. Microsurgical clipping is the gold standard in the management of intracranial aneurysms. Though surgical clipping of an aneurysm can be attempted during first 48 hours but usually undertaken after about 10-14 days of SAH to prevent symptomatic vasospasm in postoperative period. Recently introduced endovascular treatment is an alternative for aneurysms not amenable to surgery.

Antifibrinolytic agents (Epsilon amino-caproic acid 30-60 mg/day I.V. in half dextrose saline is infused over 24 hours with the help of micro-drip apparatus or 4 gm orally after every 3 hours for a period of 4-6 weeks) can be given if surgery is not feasible, but their efficacy is not proved, and chances of cerebral infarction common. It is not recommended now-a-days because it may worsen the vasospasm.

3. Control of Vasospasm

Vasospams is an important complication of SAH and its severity is directly proportional to the amount of blood present in the subarachnoid space. The complication is diagnosed by clinical examination, CT scan, doppler study and digital substraction angiography. Intravenous nimodipine infusion is started as 1 mg/hour and if there is no precipitous fall in BP, then it is increased to 2 mg/hour infusion for few days followed by oral dose of 60 mg every 4-6 hourly for 2-3 weeks. The use of I.V. isoproterenol or nitroglycerine in an attempt to dilate the cerebral vessels has not proved beneficial. However vasospasm responds best to an increase in cerebral perfusion pressure by plasma volume expansion by I.V. albumin or plasma expanders or by vasopressor e.g. phenylephrine or dopamine and keeping the CVP between 8-12 mm of Hg. This treatment is contraindicated in cardiac patients.

4. Symptomatic Hydrocephalus

It can develop acutely which needs a ventriculostomy (ventricular drainage). Chronic hydrocephalus is best treated by ventricular CSF shunting which is its definite treatment if symptomatic.

Chapter 47

Status Epilepticus

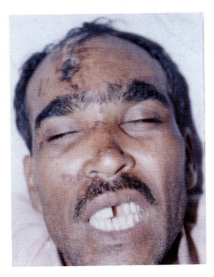

Fig. 47.1: A patient with status epilepticus. Note the injury on the head sustained during convulsions along with a fall of incisor during clenching of teeth

STATUS EPILEPTICUS

Definition

It is defined as continuous seizural motor activity for more than 30 minutes or recurrent seizures without recovery of consciousness between seizures. During seizures, patient may hurt himself/herself (Fig. 47.1) and there may be soiling of clothes with urine and faeces. Status epilepticus is a medical emergency as it has potential for neural damage and brain death, therefore, prompt and

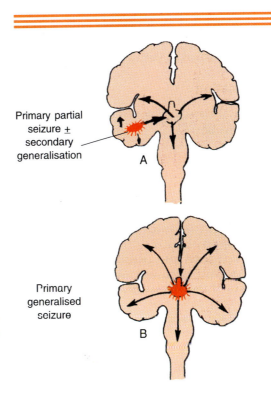

Fig. 47.2A and B: Types of seizure associated with status epilepticus (A) A partial seizure originates from a paroxysmal discharge in a focal area of the cerebral cortex and then subsequently spreads to rest of the brain through diencephalon—called secondary generalisation (B) In primary generalised seizure, the focus of excitation or discharge originates from the midline (diencephalic activating system) and then spreads bilaterally in symmetric fashion simultaneously (indicated by arrows)

appropriate treatment is essential. Most commonly, this condition refers to recurrent tonic clonic seizures (major status). Partial motor status is obvious clinically but complex partial status and absence status may be difficult to diagnose because the patient may just present in a dazed and confused state.

Note: There can be essentially as many types of status as there are types of epileptic seizures—See the classification

Nonconvulsive status epilepticus: The term is still evolving, but most patients with seizural activity on EEG without convulsive motor activity can be grouped under this category.

Classification

The clinical classification of status epilepticus is given in the Box 47.1:

Box 47.1: Clinical classification of status epilepticus

1. **Convulsive status epilepticus (Fig. 47.2)**
   A. Primary generalised major motor status
      - Tonic-clonic status
      - Myoclonic status
   B. Simple partial status epilepticus
   C. Generalised major motor status with partial onset
2. **Nonconvulsive status epilepticus**
   - Complex partial status
   - Absence status epilepticus (typical or atypical)

Aetiology

It is most common in children, the mentally handicapped individuals and in those with organic disease of the brain. In established epilepsy, status can be precipitated by factors given in the Box 47.2.

In children infection with fever is by far the most common cause of status.

Diagnosis

Diagnosis of overt tonic-clonic status epilepticus is not difficult when two or more convulsions occur

Box 47.2: Precipitants for status epilepticus

- Withdrawal of antiepileptic drugs or inadequate drug treatment. It is the most common identifiable precipitating factor for generalised convulsive status epilepticus.
- Intercurrent illness/infections
- Alcohol use
- Acute stroke
- Hypoxia/Anoxia
- Metabolic abnormalities
- Progression of underlying disease
- Trauma to the brain
- Tumours of brain

consecutively without regaining of consciousness between seizures in the absence of intake of benzodiazepines. However, after 30 to 45 minutes of uninterrupted seizures, the signs may become subtle. Patient may have mild clonic jerks of only fingers, or fine, rapid movements of eyes. There may be paroxysmal episodes of tachycardia, hypertension, pupillary dilatation. In such cases, EEG is the only method to establish the diagnosis. Thus, if the patient stops having overt seizures, yet remains comatosed, an EEG should be performed to rule out ongoing status epilepticus.

The diagnosis of *nonconvulsive status epilepticus* is often difficult because partial depression of consciousness or abnormal behaviour or confusion may mimic a psychiatric disorder. The diagnosis is confirmed by demonstration of ictal activity on EEG, therefore EEG also helps to differentiate nonconvulsive status epilepticus from hysterical behaviour or a psychiatric disorder.

Investigations

1. *The EEG:* All cases of status epilepticus should ideally be managed using simultaneous recording of EEG. It is also essential for diagnosis of status when convulsive movements have stopped and the patient has not recovered consciousness or when patient having a single convulsion fails to regain consciousness. It is actually indispensable investigation for nonconvulsive status.

2. *Biochemical profile* e.g. blood urea, blood sugar, serum creatinine, liver function tests, serum electrolytes, Ca^+ and phosphorous. These are done to find out any metabolic disorder as the cause of epilepsy.
3. Complete blood counts (TLC and DLC). C-Reactive protein, chest X-ray for evidence of any infection or aspiration.
4. Toxicological screening of blood and urine samples.
5. Antiepileptic drug levels.
6. *CT and MRI scan:* These imaging techniques help to find out the cause. The indications of brain imaging are given in the box 47.3. These are done to find out any structural lesion.

> **Box 47.3: Imaging of brain in epilepsy**
> **Indications**
> - Epilepsy starts after the age of 20
> - Focal seizures
> - Abnormal EEG with focal seizure source
> - Refractory or resistant seizure

7. *Lumbar puncture:* It is indicated when either an infective cerebral or meningeal disease is being suspected and there is no evidence of raised intracranial pressure or CT/MRI scans are noncontributory towards its cause. The CSF should be sent for biochemistry, cytology and culture.
8. Serology for syphilis, HIV, collagen vascular disease.

Management

Aims

1. Termination of status epilepticus.
2. Prevention of recurrence.
3. Treatment of potential precipitating cause(s).
4. Treatment of complications and underlying conditions.

Termination of Status Epilepticus

The measures are:

A. General
i. *Immediate as well s first-aid*
   - Move the patient away from danger (fire, water, machinery etc.).
   - After convulsions, put the patient in semi-prone position. In hospital, put the patient on railing bed.
   - Ensure clear airway.
   - Do not insert anything in mouth (tongue biting occurs at seizure onset and cannot be prevented by observer).
   - Secure intravenous access.
   - Blood samples should be drawn for haematology, serum biochemistry and antiepileptic drug concentration studies.
   - Give diazepam 10 mg I.V. (or rectally), repeat once only after 15 min, if necessary or lorazepam 4 mg I.V. stat.
   - Transfer the patient to intensive care area for monitoring neurological condition, blood pressure, respiration and blood gases.
   - Person may be drowsy and confused for 30-60 minutes after an epileptic attack hence, should not be left alone.

B. Pharmacological treatment:
i. If seizures continue after 30 minutes:
   - Give intravenous infusion (with cardiac monitoring) with one of the following:
     Phenytoin I.V. infusion of 15 mg/kg at a rate of 50 mg/min.
     Fosphenytoin I.V. infusion of 15 mg/kg at a rate of 100 mg/min.
     Phenobaribitone I.V. infusion of 10 mg/kg at a rate of 100 mg/min.
ii. If seizures still continue after 30-60 minutes (refractory status):
   - Start treatment with intubation and ventilation.
   - General anaesthesia using propofol or thiopental.
     Note: The treatment is continued for 12-24 hours after last seizure, then withdrawn slowly.

Prevention of Recurrence

Although seizures may stop after above therapy. Once status is controlled, patient may be put on long-term antiepileptic treatment with one of the followings:
- Sodium valporate 100 mg/kg I.V. over 3-5 mins, then 800-1200 mg/day orally.
- Phenytoin is given in a loading dose I.V. if already not given, then 300 mg/day.
- Carbamazepine 400 mg by nasogastric tube, then 400-1200 mg/day orally.
- Often, patients with severe brain injury require more than one antiepileptic drug at higher doses.
- Find out the cause and treat it accordingly.

Treatment of Complications

Status epilepticus, if unattended can lead to profound life-threatening systemic, metabolic and physiological disturbances (see Box 47.4). The mortality rate in status epilepticus has decreased tremendously because of better therapeutic maneuvers. The cause of death include: the underlying disorder, medical complications and status epilepticus itself. There is increased risk of intellectual impairment following repeated occurrence of status epilepticus.

Box 47.4: Complications of status epilepticus
- Sudden death
- Hyperpyrexia
- Peripheral circulatory failure
- Aspiration pneumonia
- Hypoxia, acidosis, hyperkalaemia, renal failure

Advise after Discharge and Follow Up

Until good control of seizure has been obtained, the epileptics have not to do certain activities (Don't) and has to adhere to certain things (Do's). These are given in the box 47.5.

Box 47.5: Advise to epilepticus

Don't
- Not to operate dangerous machinery
- Not to sit near open fires
- Not to swim in pools
- Not to lock the bath room during bathing
- Avoid mountaineering
- Driving and even cycling should be discouraged during first 6 months of treatment and then during period of withdrawl from antiepileptic drugs

Do's
- Take the antiepileptics regularly
- Continue treatment for at least 2-4 years.
- Withdraw the drug slowly over a period of 6-12 months

Epilepsy and Pregnancy

Guidelines of therapy:
- Epilepsy worsens during pregnancy especially in the last trimester as levels of anticonvulsants tend to fall, therefore, monitoring of drug levels is mandatory during pregnancy.
- All antiepileptic drugs are associated with foetal abnormalities except newer ones e.g. lamotrigine and gabapentine.
- To prevent neural tube defect during antiepileptic therapy, folic acid 5 mg daily should be started 2 months before conception. To reduce the incidence of haemorrhagic disease of newborn by antiepileptic treatment especially by enzyme-inducer drugs, maternal vitamin K supplement (20 mg orally/day) in the last month of pregnancy and intramuscular injection of Vitamin K (1 mg) at birth for infant are advised.
- Breast feeding as usual should be encouraged.

Chapter 48

Acute Meningitis

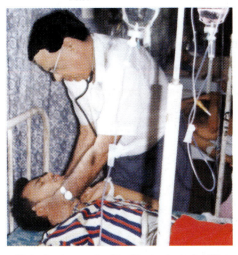

Fig. 48.1: Acute meningitis. Marked neck stiffness is present. Kernig's sign was positive in this patient

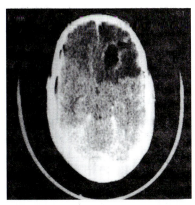

Fig. 48.2: Frontal lobe abscess. CT scan shows frontal lobe abscess in a patient with lung abscess who presented with pyogenic meningitis

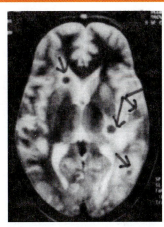

Fig. 48.3: CT scan showing multiple tuberculomas (arrows) in a patient with tubercular meningitis

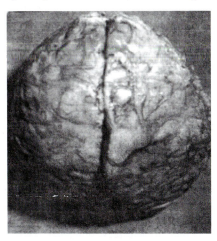

Fig. 48.4: MRI findings in a patient of acute fulminant bacterial meningitis (diffuse pus collection over the surface of brain) who later on died due to septic shock

ACUTE MENINGITIS (Fig. 48.1)

Acute meningitis is an inflammatory response to infection of leptomeninges (pia-arachnoid matter) with exudation into the cerebrospinal fluid (CSF) in the subarachnoid space. Acute meningitis may be bacterial (septic or pyogenic and tubercular), viral or fungal etc.

BACTERIAL MENINGITIS

It occurs due to bacterial invasion and subsequent inflammation of leptomeninges with CSF pleocytosis.

Pathogenesis

The common pathogens are given in the Table 48.1.

Table 48.1: Pathogens for acute pyogenic meningitis	
Common (> 80% cases)	**Less common**
• Haemophilus influenzae • Streptococcus pneumoniae • Neisseria meningitidis	• Listeria monocytogenes. It causes meningitis in neonates, elderly, alcoholics, immuno-compromised state etc. • Aerobic gram-negative bacilli (E. coli, Klebsiella, Pseudomonas aeruginosa, B. proteus). They produce meningitis at extremes of life

- **Note:** In developed nations, the *H. influenzae* used to be the most common cause of meningitis but now *S. pneumoniae* is the most common pathogens in children and adults in USA and other developed nations. In India, meningococcal meningitidis is the most common cause of bacterial meningitis

S. Pneumoniae, N. meningitidis and *H. influenzae* are transmitted by air-borne route by droplets or exchange of saliva. These bacteria initially colonise the nasopharynx, attach to the mucosal epithelial cells, secrete IgA protease enzymes that breakdown the protective mucosal layer to enter into the blood stream producing bacteremia. From the blood they reach to CSF by breaching the blood-brain barrier. Once the bacteria reach the CSF, they have an excellent chance of survival and multiplication because humoral defense mechanism depending on the immunoglobulins and complement activity, is absent.

However, bacterial meningitis can occur by hematogenous spread (Fig. 48.2), or through congenital neuroectodermal defects, craniotomy sites, middle ear, dental and sinus infection, and skull fractures.

Rarely, intracerebral abscess may rupture into the ventricle or subarachnoid space producing meningitis.

Precipitating Factors

These are given in Box 48.1.

Box 48.1: Predisposing factors/conditions for bacterial meningitis	
• Pneumonia • Otitis media, sinusitis, mastoiditis • Bacterial endocarditis • Splenectomy or asplenic state	• Hypogammaglobulinaemia • Alcoholism • Cirrhosis of liver • Multiple myeloma

Clinical Features

These include:
1. ***Symptoms and signs of infection:*** Fever, malaise, headache, aches and pains, vomiting, tachycardia, tachypnoea, convulsions in children.
2. ***Symptoms and signs of meningeal irritation:*** Pain in the neck, neck stiffness (Fig. 48.1), positive Kernig's and Brudzinski's signs.
3. ***Symptoms and signs due to raised intracranial pressure.*** Headache, projectile vomiting, blurring of vision, false localising signs (bilateral 6th nerve palsy, unilateral or bilateral fixed and dilated pupils, Cheyne-Stokes breathing, bilateral plantar extensor response etc.) may be present. In addition to this there may be coma,

decorticate and decerebrate rigidity. All these are ominous prognostic signs. Papilloedema is rare.
4. *Focal neurological signs:* These are common in pneumococcal meningitis and complicate 15-25% of patients. Focal neurological signs (unilateral cranial nerve palsies, hemiplegia, monoplegia, etc.) are due to cortical vein thrombosis, cerebral artery spasm, subdural empyema or rarely brain abscess. The seizures are also common in these patients.
5. *Symptoms and signs due to infecting organisms:*
   - Morbilliform/purpuric/petechial skin rash, ecchymoses and lividity of skin in meningococcal meningitis. DIC is common complication of meningococcal meningitis.
   - Associated lung, ear, sinus infection in pneumocoal meningitis.
   - Upper respiratory and ear infection in children associated with meningitis due to H. influenzae.
6. *The alteration of symptoms and signs in elderly and immunocompromised states:* The symptoms and signs in these two categories of patients are minimal in the form of fever, confusion and behavioral changes. The tonic-clonic seizure may occur.

Investigations

1. *Total and differential leukocytes count* may reveal polymorphonuclear leucocytosis.
2. *Blood culture* may be positive is some cases.
3. *CSF examination:* It is an essential procedure for confirmation of the diagnosis. Fundus examination should be done before to exclude papilloedema. It is not essential to perform CT or MRI before lumbar puncture if patient is not comatosed or does not have focal neurological signs. The CSF changes include:
   i. The CSF pressure is raised.
   ii. Fluid may be turbid and contains many neurophils (> 1000 cells/mm^3). It may be clear if patient is already taking antibiotics
   iii. The protein content is elevated (may be upto 500 mg/dl).
   iv. The sugar content is markedly low, may be less than 30 mg% (sugar is lower than tubercular meningitis). The value of CSF glucose is best determined by the ratio of CSF and serum glucose. The normal CSF to serum glucose ratio is 0.6. In majority of patients with pyogenic meningitis this ratio is < 0.3.
   v. *Gram's staining of CSF sediment* is extremely helpful as it allows rapid and accurate identification of micro-organisms and forms the basis for empirical antibiotic therapy.
   vi. *CSF culture:* The CSF culture is positive in 70-80% case of bacterial meningitis. The possibility of negative CSF culture increases if patients has already received antimicrobial therapy.
   vii. *Immunoelectrophoresis and other serological tests* to detect capsular antigen in CSF and are especially useful if CSF microscopy is negative or patient has already received antibiotics.
4. *X-ray chest:* It may show a patch of consolidation in pneumococcal meningitis.
5. *CT scan/MRI (Fig. 48.2 and 48.4 see front page):* It is helpful to diagnose hydrocephalus and brain abscess as a complication of meningitis (Fig. 48.2). Neuroimaging of brain should also be considered if the patient is comatosed or there are focal neurological signs or focal seizures and before lumbar puncture if treatment is delayed.

Management

Acute bacterial meningitis is a grave medical emergency, needs early diagnosis and early institution of antibiotic therapy to prevent significant mortality and morbidity associated with the disease. Any patient with suspected meningitis needs hospitalization.

1. **Antibiotic therapy:** Antibiotic therapy should be started soon after the diagnosis is suspected or confirmed with characteristic CSF findings without waiting for the isolation or identification of the causative pathogen.
   A. *Empirical therapy:* The choice of antibiotic depends on the age, underlying health status of the patient and its penetration into the CSF. In most patients, third generation cephalosporins (cefotaxime or ceftriaxone) are recommended. In young infants < 3 months of age), and elderly patients (> 50 years), a combination of third generation cephalosporin with broad spectrum penicillin (ampicillin) is recommended. Patients with head trauma and immunocompromised hosts need broader antibiotic coverage such as a combination of ceftazidime plus vancomycin (Table 48.2). The antibiotic therapy should be modified as soon as the result of CSF culture and antibiotic-sensitivity report become available.

   In recent years, an increasing number of penicillin-resistant strains of S. pneumoniae have been reported, adult patients with pneumococcal infection should receive ceftriaxone *plus* vancomycin unless proved otherwise.

   The antibiotic regimen depending on the pathogens isolated is depicted in the Table 48.3.
   B. *Duration of antibiotic therapy:* The antibiotic therapy for bacterial meningitis is variable depending on the organism isolated and antibiotic sensitivity. The duration of antibiotic therapy for the three common pathogens (S. penumoniae, N. meningitidis and H. influenzae) is one to two weeks; and for L. monocytogenes and gram-negative bacilli, it is 2-3 weeks (see the Table 48.3). It is essential that antibiotic therapy is continued in full dosage throughout this period because the penetration of these antibiotics is better with meninges inflamed, declines with improvement.
   C. *Response to treatment:* In responsive patient, the CSF becomes sterile 1 to 3 days after antibiotic therapy. The fever disappears within few days but may persist for several weeks. Dead bacteria may be seen on Gram's staining of CSF for several days.

   Repeat CSF should not be done if clinical recovery is satisfactory. It is warranted only in meningitis caused by gram-negative bacilli or when therapeutic response is inadequate or when complications arise.

Table 48.2: Empirical antibiotic theapy in acute bacterial meningitis		
Age and clinical setting	*Likely pathogen*	*Choice of antibiotic*
A. Immunocompetent		
• < 3 months	• Streptococcus • E. coli • Listeria	Ampicillin (100 mg/kg 8 hourly) plus ceftriaxone (50-100 mg/kg 12 hourly)
• 3 months to < 18 years	• N. meningitidis • S. pneumoniae • H. influenzae	Ceftriaxone (50-100 mg/kg 12 hourly) or Cefotaxime (50 mg/kg every 6 hours)
• 18 to 50 years	S. Pneumoniae	—As above—
B. Immunocompromised adults	• L. monocytogenes • Gram-negative bacilli	Ampicillin (2g I.V. 6 hourly) *plus* Ceftazidime (2g I.V. 8 hourly)
C. Penetrating head trauma and ventricular shunt in adults	• L. monocytogenes • Gram-negative bacilli • S. pneumoniae • Staphylococcus	Vancomycin (2 g every 12 hourly) *plus* Ceftazidime (2 g every 8 hourly)

Acute Meningitis

Table 48.3: Antibiotic regimen based on isolation of organism in bacterial meningitis

Organism	Antibiotic	CSF penetration	Dose	Duration
S. pneumoniae	• Penicillin G or	3 +	4 million units i.v. every 4 hourly	10-14 days
	• Ceftriaxone or	3 +	2 g I.V. 12 hourly	
	• Ceftriaxone plus vancomycin	3 +	2 g I.V. 12 hourly plus 500 mg I.V. 6 hourly	
N. Meningitidis	Penicillin G or	3 +	4 million units I.V. 4 hourly	7 days
	Ceftriaxone	3 +	2 g I.V. 12 hourly	
H. influenzae	Ceftriaxone or	3 +	2 g I.V. 12 hourly or	7 days
	Cefotaxime	3 +	2 g I.V. 6 hourly	
L. Monocytogenes	Ampicillin plus	3 +	2 g I.V. 4 hourly plus	14-21 days
	Gentamicin	1 +	1 mg/kg/8 hourly	
Gram-negative bacilli	Ceftriaxone or cefotaxime	3 +	As for H. influenzae	21 days
P. Aeruginosa	Ceftazidime plus	3 +	2 g 8 hourly	21 days
	intraventricular gentamicin	1 +		

2. *Adjuvant steroids therapy:* Corticosteroids have been shown to have some benefit in children, particularly, in diminishing the incidence of hearing loss in meningitis caused by *H. influenzae*. Adjunctive dexamethasone therapy (0.15 mg/kg I.V. every 6 hourly for 4 days) is often recommended in children and the first dose should be administered before antibiotic therapy is started. Corticosteroids have no role in adults.
3. *Supportive therapy:* It is symptomatic treatment and include:
   - Analgesic for headache and backache.
   - Careful nursing in a dark room if photophobia present.
   - I.V. fluids to maintain hydration. Electrolytes to be monitored and appropriately corrected.
   - In patients with signs of raised intracranial pressure, 20% mannitol or glycerol may be used to reduce the pressure.
   - In some patients, treatment of shock/DIC may be required (N. meningitidis).
   - Steps of treatment of unconscious patients are same as for any other unconscious (coma) patient.

Prophylaxis: The measures used for prophylaxis of meningococcal meningitis include:
1. *Drug* e.g.
   A. Rifampicin
      - Adults 600 mg bid × 2 days
      - Children 10 mg/kg for a day
      - Infants 5 mg/kg for a day.
   B. Ciprofloaxcin
      - 500 mg daily for 2 days.
2. *Vaccination:* Vaccine is not available.

Complications

1. Cerebral arteritis producing hemiplegia.
2. Venous sinus thrombosis.

3. Cerebritis and ventriculitis.
4. Subdural effusions/empyema.
5. Hydrocephalus.
6. Brain abscess (rare).

VIRAL MENINGITIS

Infection of the meninges and subarachnoid space by viruses is called *viral meningitis*. Viruses are the most common cause of aseptic meningitis—a generic term used for cases of meningitis in which bacteria cannot be isolated from the CSF. Viral meningitis is an acute, benign, self-limiting illness without any sequela or residual deficit. Less commonly, virus may produce recurrent or chronic meningitis.

Viruses causing aseptic meningitis: Under the modern diagnostic techniques, it can be shown that upto 85% of cases of acute aseptic meningitis are caused by entero-viruses (echo 3-7, 9, 11, 21, 30 and Coxsackie Ag and B 1-5). The remainder, are caused by other viruses (California encephalitis virus, St. Louis encephalitis virus, Western and Eastern equine encephalitis viruses), herpes viruses; HIV and mumps viruses (see Box 48.2).

Box 48.2: Virus causing aseptic meningitis

Common	Less common	Rare
• Enteroviruses	• HSV_1	• Adenoviruses
• Arboviruses	• Lymphocytic choriomeningitis virus	• Cytomegalo virus
• HIV		• Epstein-Bar virus
• HSV_2	• Mumps virus	• Influenzae A, B
		• Measles
		• Parainfluenzae,
		• Rubella etc.

Clinical Features

The cardinal features of viral meningitis include fever, headache and neck rigidity. The associated symptoms such as nausea, vomiting, abdominal pain, malaise are common. The symptomatology of aseptic (viral) meningitis is less marked than bacterial meningitis. The presence of altered mental status, seizures and focal neurological deficits indicate parenchymal involvement rather than meningitis alone. The disease is self-limiting and symptoms resolve within a period of 10 days.

Investigations

1. ***CSF examination:*** The CSF in viral meningitis shows (i) lymphocytic pleocytosis, (ii) slightly elevated proteins level and (iii) normal glucose content except in certain situations as discussed below: (i) Polymorphonuclear response in CSF may be seen in first 48 hours of illness especially in enteroviral, echovirus 9 or Eastern Equine virus infection. Repeat CSF after 12 hours may differentiate whether polymorphonuclear leucocytosis is due to viral or bacterial meningitis. A shift to mononuclearcytosis indicates viral; while persistent CSF polymorphonuclear cytosis indicates bacterial meningitis. The total cell count in CSF is less than 1000 cell/ml (ii) The glucose content is normal, may be decreased in meningitis due to mumps, lymphocytic choriomeningitis virus (LCMV); echo virus and other enteroviruses, and herpes simplex virus 2. (iii) The conditions producing CSF pleocytosis with low sugar content are given in Box 48.3.

Box 48.3: Causes of lymphocytic pleocytosis with low sugar content in CSF

- Fungal meningitis
- Listerial meningitis
- Tubercular meningitis
- Some groups of viral meningitis
- Sarcoid and neoplastic meningitis

2. ***CSF culture:*** The overall results of CSF are disappointing in viral meningitis. Similarly culture of other specimens such as urine, stool, blood yield negative results.
3. ***Polymerase chain reaction (PCR):*** Amplification of viral specific DNA or RNA from CSF using PCR amplification is an important method of diagnosing viral meningitis. Studies using CSF-PCR suggest that most cases of benign

recurrent lymphocytic meningitis are caused by HSV-2.

4. *Serological test:* The diagnosis is retrospectively made by viral antibody titre in CSF during acute and convalescent phase. The rise in CSF of viral antibody titre index in paired sera of serum and CSF more than 1.5 indicates CSF infection.

> *CSF/Serum antibody index > 1.5 is suggestive of viral CSF infection.*

5. *Other tests:*
   - Total and differential leucocyte count and ESR.
   - Platelets count.
   - Liver function tests.
   - Blood biochemistry (urea, electrolytes, glucose, creatinine, enzymes, etc.).

Management

- Symptomatic treatment with analgesics and antipyretics.
- Bed rest.
- Acute viral meningitis caused by HSV_1 or 2 may be treated with intravenous or oral acyclovir, oral famciclovir or oral valacyclovir although data supporting their efficacy is anecdotal.
- Acute HIV meningitis may respond to combined anti-retroviral therapy with zidovudine, a reverse transcriptase inhibitor and a protease inhibitor. Patient with deficient humoral immunity should receive a trial of I.V. gammaglobulin.

Most cases recover within 7-10 days. Resolution of CSF findings takes several weeks.

Tubercular Meningitis

Tubercular infection of the meninges (TBM) usually has a subacute or chronic onset, but occasionally presents in acute form similar to pyogenic meningitis. Most often the diagnosis is delayed until the patient develops impairment of consciousness or develops focal neurological signs/deficit. At this stage, patient's condition warrants an emergency management.

TBM is generally considered a disease of childhood, however, in recent years an increasing incidence has been observed in adults which account for about 50% of cases, develops commonly in those who are infected with HIV.

Tubercular meningitis results from the hematogenous spread of primary or post primary pulmonary disease, as a part of miliary tuberculosis or from the rupture of subependymal tubercular focus into subarachnoid space. In more than 50% of cases, there may be an evidence of a pulmonary lesion or miliary tuberculosis on X-ray chest.

Pathogenesis

Tubercular bacilli spread from the lungs to the brain via blood stream during the stage of primary complex formation and settle in different areas of the brain to form small subarachnoid or subependymal tubercles, the socalled *Rich's foci*. Most common site of tubercle formation is choroid plexus. One or more of such tubercles may rupture into subarachnoid space discharging *M. tuberculosis* leading to tubercular meningitis. The development of meningitis depends on the virulence and number of the bacilli and the immune response of the host.

Pathology

The disease commonly involves the basal meninges. Secondary involvement of vessels (vasculopathy) and parenchymal lesions of the brain are equally characteristic and are important clinically.

1. Basal meningeal exudate involves the *cranial nerves* (palsy) at the base of brain (II, III, IV, VI, VII, VIII) to a varying degree.
2. *Underlying encephalitis:* In the region of meningeal exudate, there is underlying encephalitis. TBM is thus pathologically a meningoencephalitis rather than meningitis.
3. *Vasculopathy:* Blood vessels of all types (artery, capillary and veins) are involved in vasculopathy associated with meningitis. The brunt is more on the arteries, and the lesions include periarteritis, fibrinoid necrosis, panarteritis (panvas-

culitis with intimal proliferation and luminal narrowing). Focal and diffuse ischemic brain changes develop due to occlusion of both small and medium-sized cerebral arteries.
4. *Tuberculoma formation:* The site of tuberculoma is commonly the cerebellum in children and cerebral hemispheres in adults (Fig. 48.3 on front page).
5. *Hydrocephalus:* A communicating hydrocephalus is common, develops due to blockage of basal cisterns in interpeduncular fossa by dense exudate or granulation tissue. At times, the obstruction may develop at the level of interventricular foramine, aqueduct of sylvius or foramina of *Luschka* and *Magendie*.
6. *Tuberculous encephalopathy* has been described in children where there is diffuse brain involvement due to perivascular demyelination with extensive oedema in the absence of above-mentioned pathological phenomenon to tuberculoprotein.

Clinical Features

The diseases has an insidious onset, evolves slowly over a period of 1-2 weeks—a course longer than that of bacterial meningitis. The initial symptoms are vague till the symptoms of meningeal irritation develop. They include listlessness, apathy, irritability, anorexia, nausea, vomiting and abdominal pain. There may be low grade fever. In about 10-15% in children and 25% adults, there is no history of fever. Acute onset of illness can occur in 50% of children but uncommon in adults. When meningeal irritation sets in, then there will be headache, vomiting becomes severe and signs of meningitis (neck rigidity, Kernig's sign) appear. Even meningeal signs may develop late in the disease or even may not appear.

The disease if untreated passes through three clinical stages:

Stage I (early disease): Patients presenting purely with meningitis with no disturbance in consciousness and without any neurological signs.

Stage II (moderate disease): Patients have signs of meningitis *plus* consciousness is disturbed and focal neurological signs are apparent. The focal neurological signs include; hemiparesis, cranial nerve palsies (II, III, IV, VI, VII, VIII) and involuntary movements. Raised intracranial pressure may occur secondary to hydrocephalus (hypertensive hydrocephalus). In infants, there is bulging of fontanellae and the enlargement of head; while in adults papilloedema develops.

Stage III (advanced disease): The patient is deeply comatosed with signs of brainstem dysfunction i.e.,decorticate and decerebrate rigidity, fixed dilated pupils, Cheyne-Stoke respiration with slow pulse rate or bradycardia.

Other modes of presentation of TBM include: acute meningitis, behavioral and intellectual changes, covulsions, visual failure due to (optochiasmatic arachnoiditis), isolated cranial nerve palsy, stroke and raised intracranial pressure.

Atypical or modified clinical picture occurs in vaccinated children. Clinical manifestations of TBM in HIV-infected individuals are same as for TBM otherwise, though picture develops more rapidly. Involuntary movements (fine resting tremors, dystonic posturing of limbs and choreiform movements) are common in children and usually subside after 4-6 weeks. Epileptic seizures may be present at any stage, more common in children than adults.

Investigations

1. **CSF examination:** The typical CSF findings in TBM are:
   - Clear or straw coloured fluid (when allowed to stand, forms a cob-web)
   - Raised proteins (100-500 mg/dl). Marked rise in CSF protein > 1g/dl indicates spinal block.
   - Low sugar (< 40 mg/dl or 50% of blood sugar at that time). The sugar in CSF starts rising with antitubercular treatment (ATT), indicates response to treatment.
   - Raised cell count (mononuclear leucocytosis < 500 cell/µL, but in acute stage there can be polymorphonuclear leukocytosis).

2. **Demonstration of tubercular bacilli** in smear or culture of CSF is the only method for establishing the diagnosis of TBM. Detection rate of AFB is poor in these specimens, even after centrifugation of CSF or staining the cob-web. Because of difficulties in isolating the organism, there is need for some simple, specific and rapid diagnostic test for accurate diagnosis. Numerous tests given in Box 48.4 have been devised but none is acceptable in clinical practice.
3. **Other tests**: Brain imaging may show hydrocephalus, brisk meningeal enhancement on enhanced CT/MRI and/or intracranial tuberculomas (Fig. 48.3).

Management

As soon as the diagnosis is made or strongly suspected, antitubercular drug therapy should be started to prevent death and permanent neurological sequelae. Treatment is usually started with the four first line drugs because they are well absorbed orally giving peak serum concentration at 2 to 4 hours, have bactericidal and sterilizing activity, low rate of induction of drug resistance and better penetration into CSF. The drugs, their dosage and side-effects are given in the Table 48.4. The four drugs to be given for 2 months followed by two drugs (isoniazide plus rifampicin) for one to one and half years.

Drugs should be given as a single daily dose before breakfast. In general, tuberculosis is treated for longer period in patients with concurrent HIV infection (i.e. for 2 years or more).

Response to treatment: It is monitored by repeated CSF examinations. With effective ATT, the following changes occur:
i. The CSF glucose rises.
ii. The elevated proteins fall.
iii. The CSF cell count fluctuates considerably, but over a period of weeks, it declines (unlike acute pyogenic or viral meningitis where it declines rapidly within days or a week).

In some cases, there may be relapse after satisfactory remission following treatment. The relapse is often due to stoppage of drugs, may develop even when adequate therapy is continuing. This may occasionally be due to development of drug resistance. It must be remembered that response to treatment may also cause deterioration of neurological signs due to healing process of

Box 48.4: Tests for diagnosis of TBM

A. Indirect tests	B. Direct tests (detection of chemical components or antigens of AFB)
• Adenosine deaminase (ADA) level in CSF	• CSF tuberculostearic acid (Gas chromotography or mass spectroscopy)
• Bromide partition test	• M tuberculosis antigen in CSF (ELISA)
• Antibody to AFB in CSF	• M. tuberculosis DNA (PCR)

Table 48.4: First line antitubercular drugs for TBM

	Isoniazide	Rifampicin	Pyrazinamide	Streptomycin	Ethambutol
Mode of action	Cell wall synthesis inhibitor	DNA transcription inhibitor	Unknown	Protein synthesis inhibitor	Cell wall synthesis inhibitor
Dose	4-6 mg/kg/day (usual 300 mg/day for an adult)	10-12 mg/kg/day (usual 450-600 mg/day for an adult)	30 mg/kg/day (usual 1-1.5 g/day for an adult)	20 mg/kg/day (usual 0.75 g/day for an adult)	15 mg/kg/day (usual 800 mg/day for an adult)
Major adverse effects	• Peripheral neuropathy • Hepatitis • Rash	• Febrile reactions • Hepatitis • Rash • GI disturbance	• Hepatitis • GI disturbance • Hyperuricaemia	• Deafness • Rash	• Retrobulbar neuritis • Arthralgia
Less common side-effects	• Lupoid reactions • Seizures • Psychosis	• Interstitial nephritis • Thrombocytopenia • Haemolytic anaemia	• Rash • Photosensitivity • Gout	• Nephrotoxicity • Agranulocytosis	• Rash • Peripheral neuropathy

tuberculosis (fibrosis) itself. Thus, progressively increasing hydrocephalus or spinal cord compression may be as result of adhesive arachnoiditis. If drug resistance is suspected, the four drug regime should be continued with addition of two new drugs (e.g. cycloserine and ciprofloxacin).

Role of corticosteroids: There is lot of controversy regarding their use routinely in TBM, but, however there is some agreement on their use under specific clinical situations:
   i. Evidence of rising intracranial pressure.
  ii. Progressive hydrocephalus.
 iii. Tuberculous encephalopathy in children.
  iv. Development of focal neurological deficit.
   v. Evidence of arachnoiditis on neuroimaging.

The dose of prednisolone is 1 mg/kg daily for 4 to 6 weeks. Some authorities use steroids in stage II and III disease in all patients.

Surgery

Surgery is indicated for prompt drainage of hydrocephalus. Deterioration of consciousness level plus suspicion of an enlarging obstructive hydrocephalus are indications for surgical drainage.

Chapter 49

Acute Viral Encephalitis

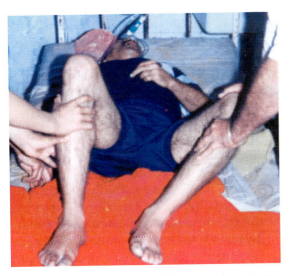

Fig. 49.1: Acute viral encephalitis being treated in the hospital. Patient is violent and has convulsions

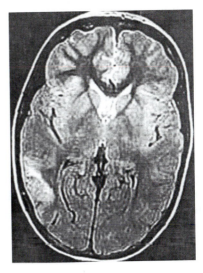

Fig. 49.2: Viral encephalitis. On MRI the single T2 weighted image of the brain shows abnormal asymmetric increased signals at the right temporo-parietal grey matter. There was little enhancement of the abnormal area after intravenous gadolinium contrast administration (not shown). This appearance of edema involving the temporal lobe was suggestive of viral encephalitis. The patient promptly received a course of antiviral therapy and recovered strength in her left upper extremity. Herpes simplex virus (HSV) was later confirmed as the causative agent by a rise in the cerebrospinal fluid antibody titer.

ACUTE VIRAL ENCEPHALITIS

Definition

Viral invasion and inflammation of the brain parenchyma is called *viral encephalitis*. It is an acute febrile illness with some evidence of meningeal involvement and symptoms and signs of diffuse and/or local brain substance involvement. If spinal cord is involved along with, then it is termed *encephalomyelitis*. It is far more serious than viral meningitis.

Causes

The causes are enumerated in Box 49.1.

Neurology

> **Box 49.1: Causes of viral encephalitis**
>
> **A. Immunocompetent individuals**
>
> *Common*
> - Arboviruses (Japanese, St. Louis, Western Equine, California)
> - Herpes simplex virus I (HSV-I) and HSV-II
> - Mumps
>
> *Less common*
> - Cytomegalovirus (CMV)
> - Ebstein-barr virus (EBV)
> - Human immuno-deficiency virus (HIV)
> - Measles virus
>
> *Rare*
> - Adenovirus
> - Influenza and para-influenza
> - Lymphocytic choriomeningitis virus (LCMV)
> - Rabies, rubella
>
> **B. Immunocompromised individuals** e.g. HSV, VZV, CMV, EBV, human herpes virus-6

Pathogenesis and Pathology

The viral entry and replication of the virus at extra neural locations leads to an interaction between the virus and host cells. Various host factors such as pH, mucosal integrity and local immunoglobulins influence the ability of viruses to invade the host and replicate efficiently. Most of the viruses follow blood route to reach the CNS. Neural route of transmission is applicable to rabies, neonatal HSV encephalitis and poliomyelitis. Upon reaching the CNS, the replication of the virus within nerve cells leads to cellular dysfunction and may lead to cell death. Certain viruses produce mild cellular dysfunction such as mumps virus; while others such as HSV-1 often leads to widespread damage to nerve cells. Immunosuppression is associated with an increased risk of reactivation of latent HSV infection in CNS.

Microscopic examination reveals perivascular and parenchymal infiltration with mononuclear cells and glial proliferation with nodules formation. Inclusion bodies may be seen in the cytoplasm or nucleus of brain cells. *Negri bodies* are inclusion bodies specifically seen in rabies.

Clinical Features

It includes:

1. *A prodromal phase of systemic symptoms and signs which may or may not precede the encephalitic phase.* This phase lasts for few days; includes nonspecific symptoms such as mild fever, bodyache, headache and malaise. In addition, there may be specific symptoms and signs indicating the specific virus infection such as skin rashes of coxsackie and echoviruses, upper respiratory symptoms (cough, coryza) are common with respiratory viruses (influenza, parainfluenza). Mumps may present with acute abdominal colic (pancreatitis) or parotid swelling (parotitis). The characteristic skin lesions of chicken pox, rubella and measles are evident before the encephalitis develops due to these viruses.

2. *After prodromal phase*: There is a short period of a febrile illness followed by encephalitic phase. This biphasic pattern is characteristically seen in arboviral encephalitis.

3. *The encephalitic phase:* The onset of encephalitis starts with fever, headache, photophobia, nausea, vomiting, signs of meningeal irritation. There is altered state of consciousness ranging from confusion, disorientation, stupor and coma. Convulsions are common (Fig. 49.1 on front page). Focal neurological deficits include; aphasia, hemiplegia, sensory deficits, visual field defects and cranial nerve palsies (see Box 49.2).

> **Box 49.2: Clinical presentations of viral encephalitis**
>
> - Alteration in consciousness
> - Headache
> - Aphasia
> - Ataxia
> - Personality changes
> - Seizures (focal, complex partial or generalised)
> - Hemiparesis
> - Cranial nerve palsies
> - Visual field defects
> - Papilloedema

Hypothalamic involvement can lead to diabetes insipidus and autonomic instability. SIADH (syndrome of inappropriate secretion of ADH) is a common manifestation. In severe cases, there can be cerebral oedema, signs of raised intracranial pressure and brainstem dysfunction.

Investigations

1. *Blood count* may show atypical lymphocytosis in EBV infection.
2. *CSF examination:* The characteristic findings include:
   - CSF lymphocytic pleocytosis.
   - Moderate rise in protein content.
   - Normal to mildly reduced sugar.
3. *Serological tests* using acute and convalescent serum may show 4-fold rise in specific antibody titres.
4. *Virus culture* from CSF and serum is some time possible.
5. *CSF-PCR:* Detection of herpes simplex virus (HSV) by a method of nucleic acid amplication using the polymerase chain reaction is sensitive (98%) and specific (100%) for diagnosis of herpes simplex encephalitis.
6. *Imaging studies:* CT scan may show temporal and frontal lobe changes in herpes simplex encephalitis (HSE) but MRI is preferred over CT scan for this purpose. Characteristic MRI findings in HSE include high-signal intensity T2 weighted images in the medial and inferior temporal lobes (Fig. 49.2 on front page). In Japanese encephalitis, MRI shows altered signal intensities in thalami, pons and basal ganglia region.
7. *EEG:* It may show bilateral slowing of background rhythm or diffuse/focal epileptiform discharge. In HSE, the EEG in addition to above changes, shows periodic lateralised epileptiform discharges localized to the temporal lobes.
8. *Brain biopsy:* Though it is the most definitive procedure to diagnose HSE but with the advent of CSF-PCR technology, its role is diminishing and is not routinely performed due to its invasive nature.

Management

Viral encephalitis is a medical emergency. Early diagnosis and early management is essential.
1. *General supportive management:* These include:
   - Airway should be cleared and an I.V. line established.
   - The general management of an unconscious patient should be applied here if patient is in coma.
   - Maintain fluid and electrolyte balance.
   - Seizures should be controlled with phenytoin or carbamazepine.
   - Cerebral oedema may be decreased by using mannitol in a dose of 0.5 g/kg of 20% solution I.V. over 20 minutes every 4-6 hours. Steroids may also be used to reduce cerebral oedema. Glycerol is also effective in reducing cerebral oedema.
2. *Specific antiviral treatment:* The details of chemotherapy available for some viral encephalitis is given in Box 49.3. The recommended empirical treatment of suspected herpes simplex encephalitis (HSE) is intravenous acyclovir in a dose of 10 mg/kg infused slowly over one hour after every 8 hours for 2-3 weeks. Adequate hydration must be maintained. The complications of the therapy include: (i) rise in blood urea, hence, its dose should be adjusted in renal insufficiency, (ii) thrombocytopenia, GI toxicity (lethargy, confusion, agitation, tremors, hallucinations, seizures). Both ganciclovir and foscarnet are also effective in CMV related CNS infection (See Box 49.3). Interferon-α has been

Box 49.3: Drug treatment of other viral encephalitis

Virus	Drug and dose	Toxic effects
Varicella zoster	Acyclovir; 10-15 mg/kg I.V. every 8 hourly for 10 days	• Renal toxicity • Thrombocytopenia • GI toxicity • Neurotoxicity
Cytomegalo virus (CMV)	Ganciclovir; 5 mg/kg after every 12 hours I.V. for 2-3 weeks Foscarnet (60 mg/kg I.V. 8 hourly) for 2-3 weeks, then maintenance dose	• Bone marrow suppression • CNS toxicity, Nausea, vomiting • Renal toxicity • Hypokalaemia and hypocalcaemia
Influenza	Amantadine (200 mg/day orally for 5-7 days)	• Depression • CHF • Nausea, vomiting • CNS toxicity

found effective in a trial on Japanese B encephalitis but is not a recommended treatment.

Response to acyclovir in HSE: According to recent reports, a diffusion-weighted MRI (DW-MRI) can be used to follow the effect of acyclovir. The increased signal intensities seen in HSE seem to disappear with effective treatment despite persistent abnormal signals detected on conventional T_2-weighted images.

Chapter 50

Acute Transverse Myelitis

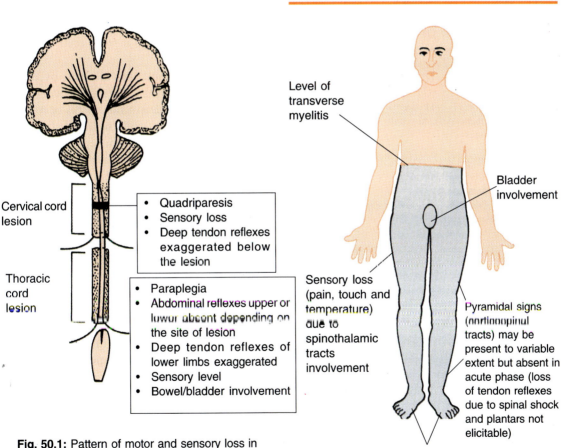

Fig. 50.1: Pattern of motor and sensory loss in transverse myelitis

Fig. 50.2: Clinical manifestations of acute transverse myelitis

ACUTE TRANSVERSE MYELITIS

Definition

Transverse myelitis is an acute or subacute monophasic inflammation of the spinal cord over a variable number of segments. It presents with acute onset paraplegia or quadriplegia with sensory deficit and sphincter paralysis.

Causes

It results from an autoimmune response triggered by infection and not from direct infection of the spinal cord. It can be due to demyelinating disorders. The causes are given in Box 50.1.

Box 50.1: Causes of acute transverse myelitis

A. Viral infection
- Poliomyelitis
- Postpoliomyelitis syndrome
- Acute encephalomyelitis (viral)
- Herpes zoster
- Rabies
- HTLV-1
- AIDS-related myelitis

B. Bacterial infection
- Acute suppurative myelitis with spinal abscess
- Tubercular myelitis
- Syphilitic myelitis

C. Fungal

D. Parasitic e.g. cysticercosis, schistosomiasis, malaria

E. Postinfectious (measles, mumps influenza, mycoplasma) and postvaccinal myelitis (tetanus, smallpox, rabies, poliomyelitis)

F. Demyelinating disorders
- Multiple sclerosis
- Neuromyelitis optica
- Acute dissemianted encephalomyelitis

G. Paraneoplastic (non-metastatic manifestation of malignancy)

H. Toxic
- Contrast media
- Intrathecal injections
- Triorthocresyl phosphate toxicity

Clinical Features

Patient may be of any age, presents with acute onset of neck or back pain followed by paraplegia or quadriplegia with a variable combinations of paraesthesias, sensory loss, motor weakness and sphincter disturbances, evolving within hours to several days. The sensory symptoms precede the motor symptoms. Sensory symptoms may be mild only or there may be a devastating functional transection of the cord. Paraesthesias may begin in one lower limb (starting from the foot) followed by other limb and ascend symmetrically or asymmetrically to the trunk where transverse involvement of the cord produces a sharp girdle like pain (a band of constriction around the abdomen or trunk) with a sharply defined spinal cord level indicating the myelopathic nature of the process— this feature differentiates it from acute Guillain-Barre syndrome.

Sensory symptoms are followed by motor system involvement with upper motor neuron signs. In severe cases, the deep tendon jerks or reflexes may be absent due to spinal neuronal shock, but persistence of areflexia over few segments of spinal cord indicates acute necrotic myelitis.

Physical signs (Figs 50.1 and 50.2): Cord lesion with a level produces following signs:

1. *Upper motor neuron type of paralysis* (paraplegia or quadriplegia) with hypertonia, hyper-reflexia and bilateral extensor plantar response below the level of lesion. This is due to interruption of descending corticospinal tracts. Areflexia with bilateral plantar extensor response indicate spinal shock, seen in severe cases.

2. *Sensory loss*: There will be a variable degree of sensory loss below the level of the lesion due to interruption of ascending spinothalamic and posterior column sensory tracts.

3. *Bladder and bowel disturbances:* Incomplete lesion of the spinal cord affects the inhibitory fibres of the sympathetic system leading to difficulty in holding the urine (*precipitate micturition*), can also interfere with the descending fibres for voluntary control of micturition from cerebral cortex causing retention of urine or *hesistancy of* micturition. Retention of urine can also occur due to spinal shock.

> *Hesitancy or retention of urine is a common bladder disturbance in acute transverse myelitis.*

4. *Impairment of sweating or vasomotor control* below the level of the lesion due to interruption of autonomic fibres.
5. *Root pain and root anaesthesia* at the level of the lesion due to nerve root irritation/compression.
6. *Segmental lower motor neuron* signs (a reflex level). There may be fasciculations, wasting or areflexia involving few segments due to interruption of reflex arc or damage to the anterior horn cells.

> **Note:** Acute transverse myelitis is an inflammatory lesion which is not uniformly distributed process, hence partial or incomplete cord lesions are common which tend to produce less severe or partial deficit depending on the tracts involved.

Spinal shock: It occurs due to acute neuronal injury leading to loss of reflex activity below the site of the lesion. It has to be differentiated from LMN type of paralysis. Flaccid paralysis below the level of the lesion along with sensory loss and urinary/fecal retention with bilateral plantar extensor response indicate spinal shock due to acute spinal cord injury rather than a LMN type of paralysis. Spinal shock may persist for 1-6 weeks, hence, acute paraplegia due to transverse myelitis may be misdiagnosed as Guillain-Barre syndrome or acute severe peripheral neuropathy but so extensive global sensory loss with bladder dysfunction are rare in a peripheral lesion.

Localisation of the lesion in transverse myelitis. It is tabulated (Table 50.1).

Investigations

The purpose of the investigations is to determine the site and the nature of the lesion.
1. ***TLC, DLC*** may show lymphocytosis. ESR may be raised.
2. ***X-ray*** chest to rule out tuberculosis or malignancy lung in patients suspected to be having tubercular myelitis or paraneoplastic syndrome.
3. ***X-ray spine*** (dorsal/lumbosacral) may show an evidence of tubercular osteitis if acute tubercular myelitis is suspected, otherwise X-ray spines are noncontributory.
4. ***MRI:*** It is an ideal investigation for detecting areas of demyelination, diagnosing myelitis or cord swelling due to inflammatory or toxic myelopathies. MRI distinguishes myelitis from other causes of compressive myelopathy.
5. ***CSF examination:*** Ideally an MRI scan should precede lumbar puncture to rule out compressive myelopathy (spinal cord compression). The CSF findings in myelitis may be normal or may show rise in CSF proteins with mononuclear cells. Initially there may be polymorphonuclear pleocytosis. The oligoclonal banding is a variable finding; when present, is associated with future evolution of multiple sclerosis.
6. ***Visual evoked potential:*** There may be accompanying optic neuritis if myelitis is suspected to be a part of demyelinating disease *(Devic's disease)*.

Management

1. **General measures:**
   - *Care of the skin*: Proper cleanliness and frequent change of position every 2-3 hourly is necessary to prevent bed-sores.
   - *Care of bowel and bladder:* Initially use a condom catheter drainage in man or a permanent indwelling catheter in either sex.
   - *Care of respiration:* High cervical cord lesions of acute ascending transverse myelitis may cause varied degree of respiratory failure requiring artificial ventilation. Patient should be daily followed for respiratory movements; if there is suspicion of impending respiratory paralysis, the patient may be shifted to respiratory intensive care unit. In the meantime, endotracheal intubation may be done. Continuous suction is necessary.

Neurology

Table 50.1: Localisation of spinal cord level in transverse myelitis (Fig. 50.1)

Cervical cord (Quadriplegia)

- High cervical cord lesion (C_1-C_4) are characterised by UMN type of quadriparesis with or with respiratory muscles or diaphragmatic paralysis. Patient may complain of suboccipital pain radiating to neck and shoulder.
- Lesions of C_4-C_5 produces UMN type of quadriparesis with preserved respiratory function.
- Lesion of C_5-C_6 causes quadriplegia with loss of biceps and supinator jerks while other jerks are exaggerated.
- Lesion of C_7 produces quadriparesis with loss of triceps jerks, normal biceps and supinators and exaggerated lower limb jerks.
- Lesions of C_8 causes loss of finger flexion with exaggeration of deep tenden jerks in the lower limbs. Other upper limb tendon reflexes are normal.

Thoracic cord (Paraplegia)

- Lesion above T_6 produces paraplegia with loss of abdominal reflexes. The upper most level of the lesion is decided by sensory loss over the chest
- Lesions of mid thoracic cord (C_6-C_9) produces loss of upper abdominal reflexes. The umbilicus is pulled downwards due to contraction of abdominal muscles. There is UMN type of paraplegia
- Lesions at T_9-T_{10} produces paraplegia with loss of lower abdominal reflexes with preserved upper abdominal reflexes. There is upward movement of umbilicus during contraction of abdominal muscles.

- Prevention of deep vein thrombosis by calf compression devices.
- Adequate fluid and hydration.
- Psychological support to keep up the morale of the patient by explaining the reversible nature of the disease.

2. **Specific therapy:**
   - Find out the cause and treat it accordingly. In a large number of cases, no cause is found out. For herpes zoster, HSV and EBV myelitis, use acyclovir (10 mg/kg tid for 10-14 days).
   - High-dose corticosteroids (1mg/kg/day) for two weeks then taper off the dose. High dose methylprednisolone is effective. The steroids are useful in postinfectious, postvaccinal and demyelinating type of acute transverse myelitis.

Chapter 51

Acute Spinal Cord Compression

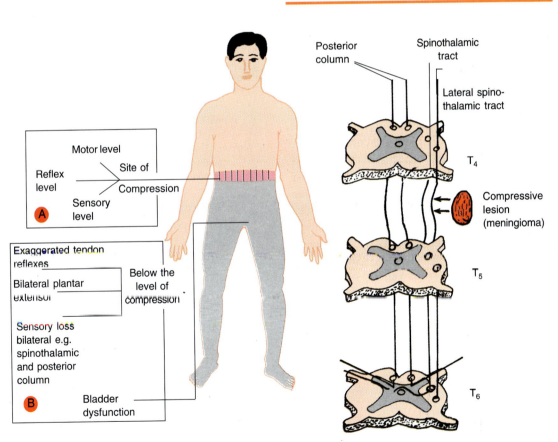

Fig. 51.1: Spinal cord compression showing signs (A) at the level and (B) below the level of compression. A level or demarcation is must between normal and abnormal signs in spinal cord compression

Fig. 51.2: Diagrammatic representation of the tracts compressed by meningioma (indicated by double arrows) in between T_4 and T_5 segments

ACUTE SPINAL CORD COMPRESSION (PARAPLEGIA/QUADRIPLEGIA)

Definition

The spinal cord is nothing but tubular extension of medulla oblongata starting at C_1 level (its junction with medulla) and ends at the vertebral body of L_1 (the conus medullaris) and is enclosed in a bony spinal canal. The spinal cord may be compressed antero-posteriorly from within (cord disease) or from without by the diseases of vertebral body and surrounding meninges. The clinical presentation is *paraplegia* or *quadriplegia*.

Acute spinal cord compression is one of the most common neurological emergencies encountered in clinical practice, is important to recognise it early clinically so as to plan emergency investigations and surgical intervention if needed.

Causes

The clinical expression of cervical cord compression is spastic quadriplegia and that of thoracic cord compression is spastic paraplegia. The causes of acute spinal cord compression (acute compressive myelopathy) are given Table 51.1. A space occupying lesion within the spinal canal may damage the nervous tissue either directly by pressure or indirectly by interfering with blood supply (vasculopathy); oedema from venous obstruction impairs neuronal function. The early stages of the spinal cord damage before neuronal death is reversible, hence early diagnosis and treatment is essential.

Clinical Features

History

A careful history and examination is essential for diagnosis of compressive myelopathy, to find out its possible cause and to differentiate it from non-compressive myelopathy of acute nature. Points to be noted on history are:
1. Age of the patient.

Table 51.1: Causes of spinal cord compression

1. *Extradural compression (involvement of vertebral bodies and intervetebral disc).* It comprises 80% cases of compression
   A. Vertebral bodies
      - Trauma (fracture dislocation)
      - Metastatic carcinoma (e.g. breast, bronchus, prostate, lymphoma, thyroid)
      - Myeloma
      - Tuberculosis
   B. Disc lesion:
      - Intervertebral disc prolapse (degenerative)
      - Trauma
   C. Inflammatory
      - Epidural abscess
      - Cold abscess
      - Granuloma
      - Arachnoiditis
   D. Epidural haemorrhage
2. *Intradural extramedullary compression:* It constitutes 15% cases of compression
   - Tumours e.g. meningioma, neurofibroma, ependymoma, metastasis, lymphoma, leukaemia.
   - Subdural abscess
3. *Intradural intramedullary:* It constitutes 5% of the cases
   - Tumours e.g. glioma, ependymoma, metastasis
   - Haematomyelia

2. Clinical setting in which signs and symptoms evolved. Spinal cord trauma (fracture dislocation, disc prolapse, haematomyelia) can lead to compressive myelopathy within hours of onset.
3. History of fever or associated systemic illness. This will favour the infective cause of myelopathy.
4. History of preceding viral infection or vaccination for post-infective or demyelinating myelopathy.
5. Initial symptoms and their progression.
6. Onset and evolution of motor weakness (i.e. rate of progression, symmetrical or asymmetrical, proximal or distal).
7. Nature, pattern and distribution of sensory loss.
8. Presence and distribution of radicular pain, if any.

Acute Spinal Cord Compression

9. Evidence and type of bowel/bladder involvement.
10. Presence of hiccups or paradoxical respiratory movements indicate phrenic nerve involvement.

Neurological Examination

- Higher functions.
- Cranial nerve examination.
- *Motor system examination:* This will differentiate between upper motor neuron and lower motor neurons signs which will narrow down the differential diagnosis.
- Sensory loss; type (root, tract, cord or peripheral neuropathy type), site if any.
- Examination of autonomic nervous system e.g. bowel, bladder and sexual dysfunction.
- Local examination of spine.
- Gait abnormalities.

Symptoms of Spinal Cord Compression

The onset of symptoms of spinal cord compression is usually slow but can be acute as a result of trauma or metastases, especially if there is associated arterial occlusion (ischaemic myelopathy). The symptoms are given in Box 51.1.

Pain and sensory symptoms appear early; while motor symptoms and sphincter disturbance appear late.

Box 51.1: Symptoms of spinal cord compression

1. *Pain:* It may be localised over the spine or may be in the form of radicular pain that increases with sneezing, coughing, bending and straining.
2. *Sensory:* Paraesthesias, numbness or cold extremities especially the lower limbs, which spread proximally towards the site of compression.
3. *Motor:* Weakness, heaviness or stiffness of limbs most commonly of the legs in paraplegia and all the four limbs in quadriplegia.
4. *Sphincters:* Urgency or hesitancy of micturition leading to acute retention of urine.

Signs of Cord Compression

The signs vary according to the site of compression and the structures involved. There may be tenderness over the spine if there is vertebral disease, and this may be associated with local kyphosis.

The signs of spinal cord compression are given in Box 51.2 and diagrammatically represented in Figs 51.1 and 51.2.

Box 51.2: Signs of spinal cord compression

1. **Signs at the site of compression.**
   Involvement of the roots at the level of compression produces:
   i. Dermatomal sensory loss due to nerve root compression.
   ii. Segmental lower motor neuron signs i.e. areflexia, fasciculations, and wasting due to interruption of reflex arc or damage to anterior horn cells.
2. **Signs below the level of compression.**
   A. **UMN type of motor paralysis (due to involvement of pyramidal tracts)**
      - Hypertonia (spastic paraplegia/quadriplegia)
      - Hyper-reflexia (deep tendon jerks are exaggerated)
      - Loss of superficial reflexes (abdominal, cremasteric)
      - Bilateral plantar extensor response
   B. **Sensory signs**
      - Loss of superficial sensations e.g. pain, touch and temperature due to interruption of spinothalamic tracts
      - Loss of posterior column sensations (e.g. position vibration and joint sense)
      - Bladder dysfunction e.g. distension of the urinary bladder

   Note: Partial or incomplete cord lesions tend to produce less severe or partial neurological deficit depending on the structures involved.

Spinal shock: Acute spinal cord injury may produce depression of the reflex activity resulting in areflexia—a state called spinal shock. It may last for 1 to 6 weeks, hence, may mimic LMN type of paralysis of Guillain-Barré syndrome from which it has to be differentiated. It is however rare for Guillain-Barré syndrome to produce a total and global loss of sensory function below a given level.

Any acute spinal cord involvement can lead to spinal shock in which there is flaccid paralysis with loss of all the tendon reflexes and plantars are either inelicitable or show extensor response

As stage of spinal shock passes off, the reflexes return to exaggerated level and plantars become bilateral extensors.

Compressive myelopathy due to intramedullary or extramedullary pathology produces different clinical syndromes (Table 51.2).

Specific Localisation of the Lesion

When there are UMN signs in the lower limbs or in all four limbs with sensory loss, then one has to decide about the site of the lesion (Table 51.3).

Investigations

The purpose of investigations is to establish the site and the nature of the lesion. These are:

1. **TLC and DLC for infective lesion:** The ESR is raised in infective pathology especially tuberculosis.

Table 51.2: Differences between extramedullary and intramedullary compression

Feature	Extramedullary compression	Intramedullary compression
Type of compression	Compression is from outside, symptoms arise due to pressure effects on roots and spinal cord	Compression is from within due to expansion of the lesion, symptoms arise due to compression of grey matter and white matter directly or by their destruction
Extent of involvement	Involves few segments, produces focal signs	Involve multiple segments and may even involve the whole cord producing widespread signs
Root pain	Root pain is a characteristic feature	• Central pain over lumbar spines in conus medullary lesion • Roots pain with cauda equina syndrome
Sacral sensory loss with spastic paralysis	Early	No sacral sensory loss (sacral sparing)
Bowel and bladder involvement	Late	Early
Dissociated sensory loss	Absent	Dissociated sensory loss present, characteristically seen in syringomyelia
Spinal deformity	Visible, palpable or radiographic evidence of vertebral destruction e.g. cold abscess or 'gibbus'	Bony changes are unusual
Radiological findings • Plain X-ray spine	• Erosion of the pedicles (an early sign of neurofibroma) • Reduction of intervertebral space is characteristic of Pott's disease • Preservation of intervertebral space is diagnostic of secondaries	No change in the bones
• CT myelogram	• A classic "meniscus sign" in intradural compression (tumours) • A "brush border sign" is characteristic of extradural compression (tumours)	"Expansion sign" is diagnostic of syringomyelia

Table 51.3: Specific sites of the lesion with corresponding signs and symptoms

Site	Motor Symptom/signs	Sensory Symptoms/signs	Horner's Syndrome
Above C_5 level	• UMNs signs in all four limbs (spastic quadriplegia) • Paradoxical respiratory movement if diaphgram (C_4) is involved	Sensory loss of all modalities in all four limbs	May be present
Mid-cervical (C_5-C_6)	• Loss of biceps and supinator jerks, LMN paralysis (muscle wasting) at the site of compression • UMN paralysis below the site of compression e.g. exaggerated triceps, finger flexion and other tendon jerks of lower limbs	• Segmental sensory loss over the arms	May be present
Lower cervical (C_7-C_8)	• Normal biceps and supinator jerks • Triceps jerk are lost • UMNs signs in lower limbs (spastic paraplegia)	Segmental sensory loss over arms and forearms	May be present
Thoracic cord (above T_6)	• Spastic paraplegia • Loss of abdominal reflexes	• Sensory level over the chest	Absent
Mid-thoracic (T_6-T_9)	• Spastic paraplegia • Loss of abdominal reflexes • Umbilicus may be pulled downwards	Sensory loss over abdomen below	Absent
Lower thoracic (T_9-T_{12})	• Spastic paraplegia • Preservation of upper abdominal and loss of lower abdominal reflexes	• Sensory loss over abdomen below umbilicus	Absent
Conus medularis lesion (Cord and cauda equina lesion)	• Only bilateral plantars extensor • LMN paraplegia	• Sacral loss of sensation	Absent

2. *X-ray chest:* It is done to rule out tuberculosis or bronchogenic carcinoma in patients suspected with Pott's disease or metastases.
3. *X-ray spine (AP and lateral):* X-rays of spines (cervical, thoracic, lumbosacral) are done to find out the vertebral fracture/collapse in patients with injury, disc prolapse (in old patients), bony erosions (seen in metastases) or evidence of tubercular osteitis.
4. *MRI spine:* It is a special tool to differentiate compressive from noncompressive myelopathy, defines the spinal lesion clearly and helps to plan emergency treatment if needed. It has replaced CT and myelography in the diagnosis of spinal cord masses and can differentiate malignant lesions from other masses.
5. *CT myelography:* It localises the lesion, helps to differentiate extramedullary and intramedullary compression and defines the extent of compression.
6. *CSF examination:* The CSF should be taken at the time of myelography. In cases of complete spinal block, CSF shows a normal cell count with a markedly elevated proteins producing yellow discoloration of the fluid (*Froin's syndrome*). Acute deterioration may develop after myelography for which it is essential to alert the neurosurgeon in advance.
7. *Needle biopsy of the tumour* may be required before radiotherapy to establish the histological diagnosis.

Differential Diagnosis

The conditions producing acute paraplegia are briefly discussed individually.

1. **Traumatic myelopathy.** Acute trauma may cause cord compression by fracture/dislocation of cervical or thoracic spine, is commonly associated with spinal neuronal shock. In less severe injury, signs and symptoms of extradural compression will appear. CT scan confirms the diagnosis of bony lesion; while MRI may be done for detecting damage to the discs, ligaments and pre or paravertebral tissue.
2. **Nontraumatic spinal cord compression:** It may include: infection of bone, subdural or epidural space, disc prolapse, neoplastic compression, epidural hematoma etc.
   i. *Infection:* Acute infection of subdural or epidural space results in an abscess formation, may or may not be associated with osteomyelitis. Pyogenic osteomyelitis (due to staphylococci, streptococci, E. coli, salmonella etc.) is common in the West while tubercular osteitis is common in Asia and Africa. Epidural abscess is characterised by fever, roots pain, spinal tenderness and other signs of infection followed by paraplegia or quadriplegia within few days. The abscess is common cause of compression in young. Tubercular osteitis on the other hand, has protracted illness with slow onset of paraplegia. X-ray spine will reveal an erosion, destruction of intervertebral disc and reduction of the disc space. MRI is investigation of choice. It will differentiate epidural from subdural abscess and will delineate the associated myelitis.
   ii. *Prolapse of intervertebral disc:* It is a common cause of acute spinal cord compression in old age. Acute disc prolapse due to degenerative disease of the spine is more common in lumbosacral region (L_{4-5} and L_5S_1) and may cause acute spinal cord compression but central disc protrusion at this site will compress cauda equina leading to cauda equina syndrome characterised by:
   - Roots pain in the legs.
   - Loss of sensation over sacral dermatomes (perineum and anal region).
   - Loss of bladder or anal sphincter control.
   iii. *Compression of cord by tumours or metastases:* Secondaries from bronchus, breast, GI tract, prostate, kidney etc. may metastasise in the vertebral body or spine leading to acute cord compression. The common site of involvement is thoracic region. The compression is acute or subacute in onset progresses over days to weeks. Acute cord compression occurs either due to sudden enlargement of tumour or haemorrhage into the tumour or due to sudden collapse of infiltrated vertebral body.

X-ray spine (AP and lateral) will show destruction of vertebral body or bodies with preservation of intervertebral space. CT Scan/MRI localise the lesion and define its extent. Other tests (chest X-ray, USG abdomen) may be done to find out the primary lesion.

The primary tumours i.e. meningioma or neurofibroma produces intradural extramedullary compression (read extramedullary compression).

Epidural hematoma: It is an uncommon but a recognised cause of extradural compression due to bleeding in the patients receiving anticoagulants or suffering from a bleeding disorder or arteriovenous malformations. Bleeding following lumbar puncture is rare cause of compression. The clinical picture is of radiculomyelopathy characterised by roots pain and paraparesis.

Management

1. **General measures:** All the general measures such as care of skin, bowel and bladder, prevention of deep vein thrombosis by leg exercises, psychological support discussed in the

management of transverse myelitis are applicable here also.
2. **Specific therapy:** Nature of specific treatment depends on the underlying cause:
   i. *Traumatic paraplegia:*
      - Spinal traction for vertebral dislocation
      - Surgery for spine.
      - Urgent surgical decompression.
      - High dose methylprednisone if given within 8 hours of injury improves motor-sensory function in the long run.
   ii. *Nontraumatic spinal cord compression:*
      - Appropriate or broad spectrum antibiotic therapy for pyogenic infection such as acute epidural abscess.
      - Laminectomy for decompression of cord
      - ATT for tuberculosis of the spine.
      - Vascular surgery (ligation of a feeding vessel, excision of AVM).
   iii. *For neoplastic extramedullary spinal cord compression*
      - Glucocorticoids are given in higher doses (dexamethasone 40 mg/day) to reduce cerebral oedema. The dose is reduced to 20 mg until radiotherapy is completed.
      - Local radiotherapy is initiated as early as possible.
      - If radiotherapy fails or not tolerated, then surgery (decompression or vertebral body compression) is indicated.
   iv. *Intradural tumours require surgical resection.*

Chapter 52

Acute Inflammatory Demyelinating Polyradiculoneuropathy

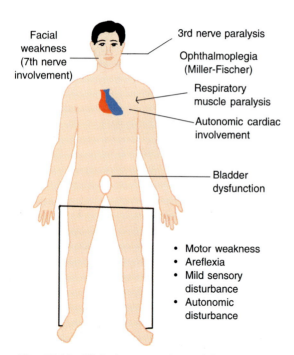

Fig. 52.1A: Clinical presentations of Guillain-Barré syndrome

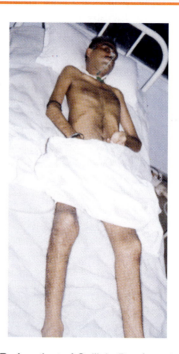

Fig. 52.1B: A patient of Guillain-Barré syndrome with LMN paralysis and bilateral foot drop (Feet are not shown)

ACUTE INFLAMMATORY DEMYELINATING POLYRADICULONEUROPATHY (AIDP)

Definition

Acute inflammatory demyelinating polyradiculoneuropathy (AIDP) is defined as an immune mediated demyelinating disorder with an acute onset characterised by a syndrome of rapidly developing flaccid paralysis, areflexia, paraesthesias with minimal sensory loss and albumino-cytological dissociation in the CSF (cerebrospinal fluid). It is also popularly known as *Guillain-Barré syndrome* after the name of French neurologist (1916).

Acute Inflammatory Demyelinating Polyradiculoneuropathy

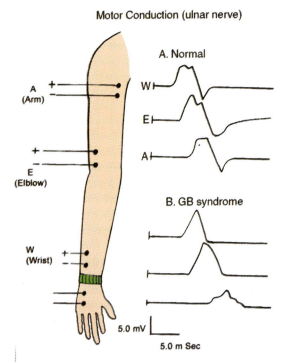

Fig. 52.2: Motor nerve conduction study in ulnar nerve. A. Normal B. GB syndrome (Read text)

Aetiopathogenesis

A history of preceding viral infection such as cytomegalovirus (CMV), Epstein-Barr virus (EBV), hepatitis virus (B and C), mumps and herpes virus is present in about 50-60% of cases. Other infections (campylobacter jejuni, typhoid, mycoplasma, filarial), vaccination (for rabies, small-pox, oral polio, tetanus toxoid) and events like bee sting, surgery, MI, idiopathic glomerulonephritis and bone marrow transplantation have been implicated.

Campylobacter jejuni shares an identical immunogenic region with the ganglioside GM-I in the human peripheral nerve, and causes more severe form of the disease with axonal degeneration with or without demyelination.

The *Miller-Fischer* syndrome, has close association with anti-GQ-1b antibody and, is specifically associated with ophthalmoplegia.

Three important pathological changes in AIDP are: (i) inflammation (ii) demyelination and (iii) remyelination. In a minority of cases, intense axonal damage and degeneration occurs which does not recover.

Macrophages, autoreactive T lymphocytes and interferon-gamma cause damage to myelin sheath by penetrating the Schwann cells. The remaining Schwann cells divide and remyelinate the bare axons.

Classification

A tentative classification of Guillain-Barré syndrome subtypes has been proposed based on the various clinical expressions and different electrophysiological and pathological findings, is given in Box 52.1.

> **Box 52.1: Classification of Guillain-Barre syndrome**
>
> - Acute inflammatory demyelinating polyradiculoneuropathy
> - Acute motor axonal neuropathy
> - Acute motorsensory axonal neuropathy
> - Miller-Fischer syndrome
> - Acute pandysautonomia

Clinical Features (Fig. 52.1A and B)

Guillain-Barré syndrome (GBS) or AIDP is a nonseasonal illness, affects persons of all age groups. About two thirds of patients report on a preceding illness or event such as upper respiratory or GI tract infection, vaccination, surgery 1-4 weeks before the onset of neurological manifestations. The agent responsible for prodromal symptoms remains unidentified. These agents have already been discussed in aetiopathogenesis.

Patients commonly present with acute onset minor sensory disturbances in the form of paraesthesias followed by weakness of limbs which may be ascending (common) or descending (rare). In some patients, there may be severe pain in extremities and back. The common presentation is symmetrical weakness of the lower limbs that ascends proximally over hours to several days to involve arms, facial and oropharyngeal muscles and in severe cases respiratory muscles. Less often, weakness may start in proximal groups of muscles of the limbs or cranial nerve muscles (Box 52.2) i.e. face (7th nerve), ocular (3rd nerve) and oropharyngeal (bulbar nerves). Its severity is variable from mild illness (patient is still able to walk unassisted) to quadriplegia. The diminution or loss of tendon reflexes (hyporeflexia or areflexia) is a characteristic and invariable feature. Sensory loss is uncommon, but occasional patient may develop glove and stocking distribution of sensory loss. Sphincter disturbance may occur. Papilloedema may be present in about 1% of cases.

Box 52.2: Cranial nerve involvement in GBS

- Facial—7th nerve (50%)
- Bulbar—9th, 10th, 12th, (30%).
- Ocular 3rd nerve (10%)

By definition, progression of AIDP or GBS ends by 1 to 4 weeks of acute illness, if progression continues longer for 4 to 10 weeks; the condition is termed as *subacute inflammatory demyelinating polyradiculoneuropathy* and if progression continues beyond 12 weeks or multiple relapses occur, then it is called *chronic inflammatory demyelinating polyradiculoneuropathy (CIDP)*.

The proportion of patients developing respiratory failure and requiring assisted ventilation is about 12-23%. Autonomic dysfunction may occur (See Box 52.3).

The ECG changes can occur due to autonomic dysfunction such as ST-T abnormalities, QRS widening, QT prolongation and various forms of heart blocks.

Clinical GBS Variants

- *Miller-Fischer syndrome* is characterised by ataxia, areflexia and ophthalmoplegia.
- *Acute pandysautonomia* is characterised by rapid onset sympathetic and parasympathetic failure without somatic sensory and motor involvement although reflexes are lost during the course of illness. These patients develop orthostatic hypotension, dry eyes, anhidrosis, fixed pupils, fixed heart rate and bladder and bowel disturbances.
- *A pure motor variant of GBS* characterised by acute flaccid paralysis without clinical and electrophysiological involvement of sensory nerves have been described.

The diagnostic criteria of AIDP or GBS syndrome are given in the Table 52.1.

Table 52.1: Diagnostic criteria of AIDP or GBS (Adapted from Asbury and Cornblath)

1. **Features essential for diagnosis**
   - Progressive weakness in both arms and both legs
   - Areflexia
2. **Features supportive of diagnosis**
   - Progression of clinical features over days to 4 weeks
   - Mild sensory symptoms or signs
   - Cranial nerve involvement (bilateral 7th nerve)
   - Recovery beginning 2-4 weeks after progression
   - Autonomic dysfunction
   - Absence of fever at the onset
   - Elevated CSF proteins with < 10 cells/m^3
   - Typically electrodiagnostic features
3. **Features making the diagnosis doubtful**
   - Sensory level
   - Asymmetry of signs and symptoms
   - Severe, persistent bowel and bladder disturbance
   - More than 50 cells/m^3 of CSF

Box 52.3: Autonomic dysfunciton in GBS

Sympathetic system		Parasympathetic system	
Decreased activity	*Increased activity*	*Decreased activity*	*Increased activity*
• Orthostatic hypotension	• Hypertension	• Urinary retention	• Bradycardia
• Anhidrosis	• Tachycardia	• G.I. atony	• Heart blocks
	• Tachyarrhythmias	• Iridoplegia	• Asystole
	• Diaphoresis		

Investigations

The cerebrospinal fluid (CSF) examination and serial electrophysiological studies are critical for confirming the diagnosis of GB syndrome. Other tests are inconsequential.

1. *CSF examination:* Initially in GBS, the CSF may be normal, then becomes abnormal on subsequent examinations and shows elevated proteins with normal cell count (albumino-cytological dissociation). If the cells count is greater than 20 mononuclear cells/m^3, one should think of HIV infection or Lyme's disease. Transient oligoclonal IgG bands and elevated myelin basic protein levels may be detected in CSF in some patients. In approximately 10% of patients, CSF proteins may remain normal throughout the period of GBS.

2. *Electrophysiological studies:* Abnormalities on electrophysiological studies have been documented in about 90% cases of GB syndrome and reflect multifocal demyelination associated with secondary axonal degeneration. The electrophysiological studies i.e. nerve conduction (Fig. 52.2 on front page) may reveal increased distal latency, conduction slowing, conduction block; F wave slowing and decreased nerve conduction velocities. The EMG shows decreased motor unit recruitment. Subsequently, if any amount of axonal degeneration occurs, fibrillation potentials appear 2 to 4 weeks after the onset.

Differential Diagnosis

Certain conditions that produce acute or subacute motor weakness simulating GB syndrome are given in Box 52.4.

Management

Ideally, all patients of GBS should be hospitalised for observation and subsequent management depending on the situation. Patients should preferably be treated in ICU.

Box 52.4: Clinical conditions simulating GBS

1. *Acute peripheral neuropathies*
   - Herpetic porphyrias
   - Diphtheria
   - Tick paralysis
   - Drug toxicity (arsenic, lead, OP compounds)
   - Vasculitis
   - Lyme's disease
2. *Disorders of neuromuscular junction*
   - Botulism
   - Myasthenia gravis
3. *Myopathies*
   - Hypokalaemic periodic paralysis
   - Rhabdomyolysis
4. *CNS disorder*
   - Poliomyelitis
   - Transverse myelitis
   - Basilar artery syndrome

---

1. *Supportive treatment:* Careful observation of cardiopulmonary function, prevention of complications (respiratory and autonomic) in ICU provides best chance for favourable outcome. Respiratory and bulbar functions, the ability to cough, heart rate and BP must be closely monitored in ICU. Look for the signs of respiratory muscle paralysis and impending respiratory failure given in Box 52.5. Monitor FVC and negative inspiratory pressure every 4 hourly while awake. Rapidly declining FVC, is an indication for intubation and ventilatory

---

Box 52.5: Sings of impending/respiratory paralysis

1. *Signs of respiratory muscle paralysis*
   - An increase in respiratory rate
   - Inability to count upto 20 in one breath
   - Use of accessory respiratory muscles
   - Suppressed cough
   - Paradoxical inwards movements of abdomen during inspirations
2. *Signs of impending respiratory paralysis*
   - Decreasing forced vital capacity
   - Declining maximal respiratory pressures
   - Hypoxaemia on ABG

support. Continuous suction may be done to remove the secretions to prevent atelectasis.
- BP monitoring and frequent ECGs may allow early detection of life-threatening situations that require prompt treatment.
- Nutritional support to be provided in the form of high caloric protein diet or by beginning enteral feeding as early as possible.
- Subcutaneous heparin or low molecular-weight heparin together with thromboembolic deterrent stockings may be advised routinely in patients immobilised for more than 2 weeks to lower the risk of thromboembolism.
- Culture of secretions, frequent blood and urine cultures must be done for early detection of infection and prompt treatment.
- Chest physiotherapy and frequent aspiration of the secretions to prevent chest infection and atelectasis.
- Care of skin, eyes, mouth, bowel and bladder is essential aspect of supportive therapy.
- Frequent change of posture to be done to prevent bed sores. Physical therapy is started early because it prevents contractures, joint immoblisation and venous stasis.

2. **Specific therapy:**
   i. *High dose corticosteroids:* Corticosteroids were recommended for their potent anti inflammatory and immunosuppressive effects. The London prednisolone Group using oral prednisolone for 2 weeks during acute phase of illness has shown no beneficial effect. Even high dose methyl prednisolone (500 mg/day for 5 days) also failed to show any benefit. Based on these observations, it is now advocated that steroids play no role in GBS management.
   ii. *Plasmapheresis:* It is a technique that permits separation of whole blood into plasma and cellular components using either a centrifugal cell separator or filtration across a semipermeable membrane. Three randomized trials have recommended the benefit of plasma exchange in GBS by shortening the recovery time and decreasing the chances of becoming ventilator-dependent. Therapeutic plasmapheresis is recommended for patients with moderate to severe GBS. The schedule entails a series of 5 exchanges (40-50 ml/kg) with a continuous flow machine on alternate days using saline and albumin as replacement fluid. Patients with mild disease may benefit from 2 exchanges.

   Plasmapheresis removes several factors such as antimyelin antibodies, cytokines, complement components and other inflammatory mediators of GBS.

   iii. *Liquorpheresis (CSF filtration):* It is a new technique developed to purify CSF from pathological factors responsible for GBS.
   iv. *Intravenous immunoglobulin:* Intravenous immunoglobulin (I.V.Ig) contains normal polyvalent immunoglobulin G derived from a large number of blood donors demonstrated an equivalent benefit similar to plasmapheresis in GBS. Both treatment modalities (plasmapheresis and I.V.Ig) being equally effective, hence, there is no added advantage to use them together.

   Indications of I.V.Ig in acute GBS
   Acute GBS with inability to walk 10 meters independently presenting within 2 weeks of diseases onset

There is no consensus to use I.V.Ig in patients who do not fulfill this criteria. The dose of I.V.Ig is 0.4 mg/kg/day for 5 days or 0.5 g/kg/day for 4 days (a total of 2 g/kg of body weight). The complications of both plasma exchange or plasmapheresis and I.V.Ig are given in Box 52.6.

Box 52.6: Complications of plasma exchange and I.V.Ig therapy	
Plasma exchange	**Intravenous Immunoglobulin**
A. *Cardiovascular* • Hypotension • Arrhythmias • MI • ARDS B. *Complications due to I.V. access* Septicaemia and thrombosis C. *Allergic reactions* D. *Transfusion hepatitis or HIV infection* E. *Bleeding, hemolysis and death*	• Headache, back pain, myalgias • Fever, tachycardia • Rash, alopecia, eczema • Neutropenia, haemolysis • Aseptic meningitis • Immune-complex arthritis • Thromboembolism, deep vein thrombosis • Transfusion hepatitis • Hypotension, acute renal failure (transient) • CHF • Anaphylaxis

Prognosis

About 3% of patients with GBS die, mostly due to complications of ventilatory support; but some may die suddenly due to autonomic failure. Those who survive recover remarkably but all cases do not recover fully. Several survivors fail to achieve the previous level of activity. About 10% of cases may have severe disability.

Chapter 53

Cortical Venous and Dual Sinus Thrombosis

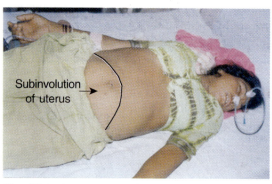

Fig. 53.1: A postpartum female with sagittal sinus thrombosis. She was unconscious, had seizures and plantars were extensors. The subinvolution of uterus is encircled

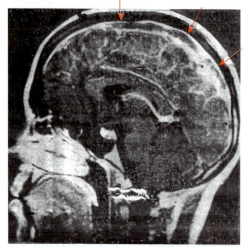

Fig. 53.2: MRI showing a sagittal sinus thrombus (indicated by arrows)

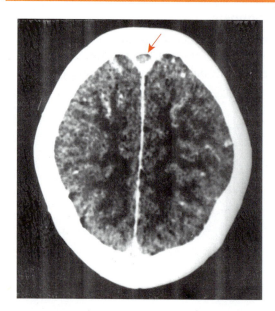

Fig. 53.3: CT scan showing a sagittal sinus thrombus (⇓). Note inverse lamda (λ) sign

CORTICAL VENOUS AND DUAL SINUS THROMBOSIS

Definition

A thrombosis of cerebral (cortical) veins or dual sinus is a common complication of hyper-coagulable state (following pregnancy or post partum period (Fig. 53.1)) or local infections (CNS, ear, nasal sinuses etc.) that leads to focal and/or generalised neurological manifestations.

Causes

The causes may be systemic (general) or local (see Box 53.1).

Clinical Features

Cerebral venous occlusion causes an increase in intracranial pressure and local ischaemia/infarction which is often haemorrhagic. The clinical features are divided into:

1. *Features due to cortical vein thrombosis:* These are focal features depending on the area involved. These include focal cortical deficits (aphasia, hemiplegia etc.), and seizures (focal or generalised). The deficit may increase if spreading thrombophlebitis occurs.
2. *Features of cerebral venous sinus thrombosis:* The clinical features depend on the dual sinus involved (see Box 53.2).

Investigation

1. TLC may show leucocytosis and there may be raised ESR.
2. CSF examination is not performed because it is commonly associated with raised intracranial pressure (ICP). Therefore CT scan should be done before CSF to rule out raised ICP. Otherwise, CSF may show nonspecific changes such as rise in proteins.
3. CT/MRI scan shows haemorrhagic infarction underlying the occluded veins and may show

---

Box 53.1: Causes of cerebral venous thrombus

General
- Pregnancy and postpartum state
- Sepsis or septic shock
- Prolonged dehydration or hypotension
- Oral contraceptive use
- Polycythaemia, sickle cell anaemia, leukaemia
- Hyperviscosity syndrome
- Antiphospholipid syndrome, deficiency of proteins C and S
- Debilitating states or malignancy
- Postoperative
- Cyanotic heart disease

Local
- Sinusitis, mastoiditis, otitis
- Pyogenic meningitis
- Subdural empyema
- Facial skin infection
- Trauma e.g. head injury
- Jugular vein catheterisation
- Skull fracture

Box 53.2: Clinical features of cerebral venous sinus thrombosis

Sinus Involved	Clinical features
1. Cavernous sinus thrombosis	• Chemosis, proptosis, ptosis, headache, ophthalmoplegia (internal and external), papilloedema, retinal haemorrhage and reduced sensation in trigeminal first division • Involvement is often bilateral, and patient is ill with fever and toxaemia
2. Superior sagittal sinus (Fig. 53.1)	• Headache, papilloedema, seizures, coma • May involve veins of both hemisphere producing weakness of both legs (paraplegia) or quadriplegia with predominant lower limbs involvement and sensory focal deficits • Fever, neck stiffness.
3. Transverse sinus	• Headache, hemiparesis, convulsions, papilloedema.
4. Jugular foramen or jugular vein	• Commonly transverse sinus thrombosis spreads to jugular vein; hence its features may be present • 9th, 10th and 11th cranial nerve palsies.

thrombosis in the involved veins and sinuses (Figs 53.2 and 53.3 on front page).
4. MR angiography confirms the diagnosis.

Management

1. *Supportive treatment:*
   - Correction of fluid and electrolyte balance to correction dehydration.
   - Care of unconscious patient (coma). The steps have been discussed in the chapter on coma management.
   - Decongestive therapy (mannitol, glycerol, steroids) may be used to lower raised intracranial pressure.
   - Antibiotic therapy for infection or sepsis.
   - Seizures should be controlled by anticonvulsants.
   - Ventilatory support may be needed.
   - *Gynaecological examination for sepsis and postpartum status:* Retained products of conception if detected should be removed.
2. *Specific therapy with anticoagulants:* Unless there are major contraindications (e.g. septic shock), anticoagulant therapy with low molecular heparin may prove helpful provided haemorrhage is not prominent feature of infarction.

Chapter 54

Raised Intracranial Pressure

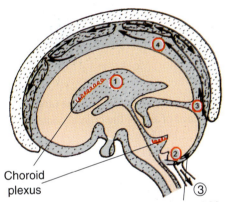

Fig. 54.1: Circulation of the CSF. (1) The CSF is synthesised in choroid plexes of the ventricles, and flows from the lateral and third ventricles through an aqueduct to 4th ventricle. (2) Through foramina of lushka and magendie, it exits the brain flowing over the hemispheres. (3) Down around the spinal cord and roots in the subarachnoid space in continuous with cerebral subarachnoid space. (4) It is absorbed into the dural venous sinuses via arachnoid villi

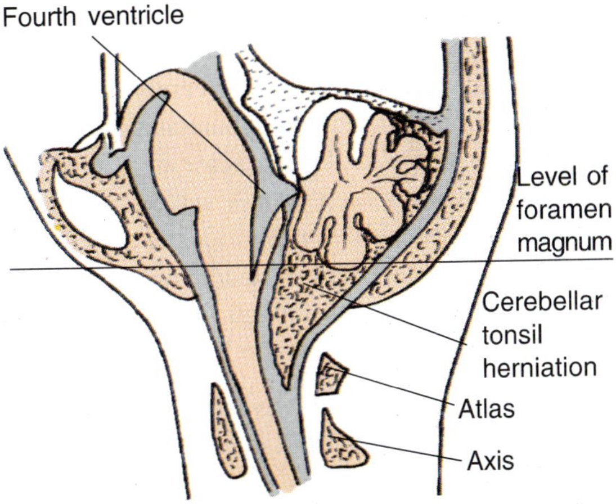

Fig. 54.3: Tonsillar cone (diagram). There is displacement of cerebellar tonsils below the level of foramen magnum due to raised intracranial pressure

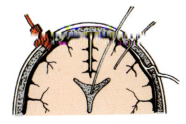

Fig. 54.4: Intracranial pressure monitoring

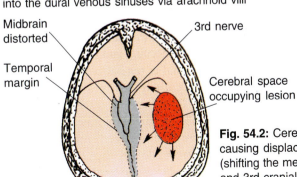

Fig. 54.2: Cerebral space occupying lesion causing displacement of midline structures (shifting the medial temporal lobe, midbrain and 3rd cranial nerve)

RAISED INTRACRANIAL PRESSURE

Definition

The normal CSF pressure measured through lumbar route with an individual in the lateral decubitus position, ranges from 50 to 200 mm of Hg. The normal circulation of CSF is depicted in Figure 54.1

Now-a-days a variety of intracranial pressure (ICP) recording devices implanted in the lateral ventricle, subdural space or extradurally are in use. More recently intraparenchymal placement devices have been introduced which record ICP through an electronic pressure transducer.

This is particularly useful in measuring ICP in severe head injuries with diffuse cerebral oedema and chinked ventricles and subarachnoid spaces. In addition to pulsatile character of ICP three pressure waves are seen. The A waves are pathological and appear only in significantly raised ICP (50-100 mm water). The B and C waves are not considered pathological though these occur with increasing frequency when the ICP is increasing.

> Normal intracranial pressure within the cranial cavity measured indirectly is 5-10 mmHg. Any ICP above 15 mmHg is taken as raised intracranial pressure.

Pathophysiology

The volume of the intracranial contents (brain + CSF + blood) is constant regardless of the pressure generated within it.

$$V\ intracranial = V_{brain} + V_{csf} + V_{blood} = Constant$$

Any changes in volume of one of its contents occurs at the cost of other two (Munro-Kelly principle). This is not applicable to the pliable skull of infants.

The brain being dependent mainly on oxygen, suffer during hypotension and hypoxia—the two major factors for secondary damage to the brain.

Initially when the volume of the intracranial contents increases, there is no increase in CSF pressure due to buffering mechanisms such as shift of CSF and then venous blood flow from the cranial cavity, followed by a minimal compression of the parenchyma. Once the buffering capacity is exhausted, the ICP starts rising. When the expansion of the mass lesion is slow e.g. a tumour, the compensatory mechanisms can mask the rise in ICP. Fast expanding mass lesions shift the midline structures to opposite side (Fig. 54.2).

The effects of raised ICP are:
  i. *Herniation syndromes* (Fig. 54.3—Read clinical features).
  ii. *Fall in cerebral perfusion pressure.*

Cushing's reflex is a protective mechanism that leads to increase in blood pressure and fall in the pulse rate in an effort to increase cerebral perfusion pressure in patients with raised ICP.

Causes

Any lesion which increases the volume (and consequently pressure) of any of the cranial contents will lead to raised ICP. They are:
  i. Cerebral oedema. (Increased brain parenchyma).
  ii. Space-occupying lesions (extra volume).
  iii. Hydrocephalus (increased CSF volume).

MRI can now differentiate between the two types of cerebral oedema i.e. vasogenic and cytopathic. The differences are given in Box 54.1. The causes of raised ICP are given in table 54.1.

Clinical Features

1. ***Symptoms and signs of raised pressure itself:***
   The classic triad i.e. headache, projectile vomiting and papilloedema is seen in majority of the cases with raised ICP. The headache is severe, occurs in early morning and disturbs the sleep of the patient and is generalized. This is due to decreased venous return in supine position leading to CO_2 retention, vasodilatation and increased ICP. Headache is relieved in sitting position due to improved venous return. Vomiting is projectile and often associated with nausea and it relieves the headache. The rising

Table 54.1: Causes of raised intracranial pressure

1. **Congenital (obstructive)**
   - Arnold-Chiari malformations
   - Aqueductal stenosis
   - Dandy-Walker syndrome
   - Agenesis of arachnoid villi
2. **Head injury (traumatic)**
3. **Infections**
   - Meningitis (pyogenic, tubercular)
   - Encephalitis
   - Cerebellar abscess
4. **Space-occupying lesions**
   - Brain tumours (craniopharyngioma, medulloblastoma, astrocytoma, ependymoma, metastases)
   - Colloid cyst of third ventricle
   - Neurocysticercosis
5. **Intracranial haemorrhage**
   - Cerebral haemorrhage
   - Subarachnoid haemorrhage
   - Hypertensive encephalopathy
6. **Venous obstruction**
   - Cortical thrombophlebitis
   - Dural sinus thrombosis
7. **Idiopathic**
   - Otitic hydrocephalus
   - Polycythaemia vera
   - Addison's disease
   - Hypoparathyroidism
   - Oral contraceptives
   - Drugs induced e.g. tetracycline, penicillin, sulpha-methoxazole, nalidixic acid
   - Hypervitaminosis A
   - Galactosaemia
   - Hypophosphatasia

pressure results in papilloedema which may result in blurring of the vision, secondary optic atrophy and blindness. Severely raised ICP results in apathy, clouding of consciousness progressing to stupor and coma.

2. *Localising symptoms and signs depending on the cause and site of involvement:* Convulsions, paresis/paralysis of the limbs, cranial nerve involvement may occur due to expanding mass lesion which is the cause of raised ICP.
3. *False localising signs:* These signs occur in raised ICP but do not have any localizing value such as:
   i. Bilateral plantar extensor response.
   ii. Pupillary changes.
   iii. Bilateral 6th nerve palsy.
   iv. Bilateral mild cerebellar dysfunction.
4. *Herniation syndromes:* Two types of herniation syndrome have been described:
   i. *Central herniation syndrome* includes herniation of central structures (diencephalon and brain-stem). When central herniation supervenes, there may be occipital headache with neck stiffness. Respiratory irregularities (Cheyne-Stokes respiration to tachypnoea, to irregular slow respiration), pupillary changes, decorticate posturing and bilateral extensor plantar response, bradycardia and hypertension may follow. Eventually, apnoea appears and the pupils become dilated and fixed. Hypotension appears and brain death follows shortly after that

Box 54.1: Differences between two types of cerebral oedema

Vasogenic	Cytopathic
Produces focal signs and symptoms due to oedema	The clinical signs are generalised, non-localising i.e. convulsions, coma
Blood brain barrier remains open	Blood brain barrier is closed
Activated diffusion coefficeint is increased	Activated diffusion coefficient is reduced
MRI shows increased interstitial fluid	MRI shows swollen cells
Responds to steroids	Does not respond
It is associated with tumours, haemorrhage, abscess, meningitis, cerebral infarction	Seen in haemodialysis and ketoacidosis

ii. *Uncus's transtentorial herniation* leads to "Kernohan's notch" phenomenon and often produces the clinical triad of coma, contralateral decerebration and a dilated ipsilateral pupil. Occasionally posturing or hemiparesis occurs ipsilateral to the side of the herniation, due to pressure on the contralateral cerebral peduncle from the edge of tentorium cereberi. Progression of uncal syndrome caudally leads to central syndrome.

Investigations

1. *X-ray skull* may reveal sutural diastasis (separation of sutures) in infants, thinning and increased convolutional markings (silver-beaten appearance), erosion of anterior clinoid processes, widened and deep sella-turcica.
2. *CT scan of brain* shows dilatation of ventricular system (dilatation of temporal horn is an early sign), effacement of cisterns, an underlying lesion and periventricular lucency and compression of the ventricle(s).
3. *MRI scan:* It can differentiate between vasogenic and cytopathic cerebral oedema, predicts response to shunts.
4. *Intracranial pressure monitoring (Fig. 54.4).*

Management

1. *Treatment of the underlying cause:* The ideal treatment of raised ICP is to find out the cause and treat it accordingly, for example CSF diversion for hydrocephalus, drainage of an abscess, removal of a clot or a tumour.
2. *Measures to reduce the ICP:* There are some medical and surgical measures to reduce the ICP, which may prove life-saving. Generally any ICP above 25 mg Hg needs treatment.
   A. *General:*
      - Airway patency to be ensured and maintained. Elevate the head by 30-45°. Avoid neck flexion.
      - Symptomatic treatment with antipyretic, analgesics and anticonvulsants (if convulsions occur).

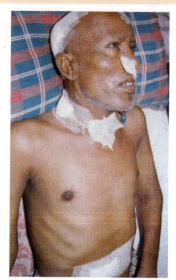

Fig. 54.5: Surgical drainage of hydrocephalus with ventriculoperitoneal shunt

- Adequate hydration by fluids.
- Catheterisation of bladder to avoid straining.
- The role of moderate hypothermia is controversial.

B. *Medical treatment:* The drugs that reduce the ICP are given in Box 54.2. Intubation and short-period hyperventilation have been used to reduce raised ICP.

Box 54.2: Drugs used to reduce ICP

1. Mannitol (20%) e.g. 100 ml I.V. 4-6 hourly
2. Glycerol (10%) e.g. 1.2 g/kg over 4 hours
3. Dexamethasone. It is used in vasogenic ICP. Dose is 10-20 mg/24 hour in divided doses.
4. Frusemide e.g. 20-40 mg I.V.

C. *Surgical methods:*
   i. *Ventricular drainage:* Lumbar drainage is indicated as an emergency procedure only in benign raised intracranial hypertension.
   ii. Long-term measures for reduction of elevated ICP involve shunting procedures i.e. ventriculo-peritoneal shunt (Fig. 54.5), lumbar peritoneal shunt, endoscopic third ventriculostomy and endoscopic stent placement in cerebral aqueduct.

Part Six

Haematology

Chapter 55

Acute Haemolytic Anaemia

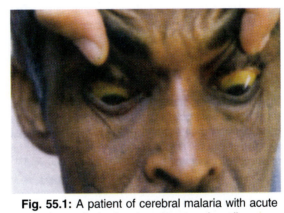

Fig. 55.1: A patient of cerebral malaria with acute haemolysis developed severe jaundice

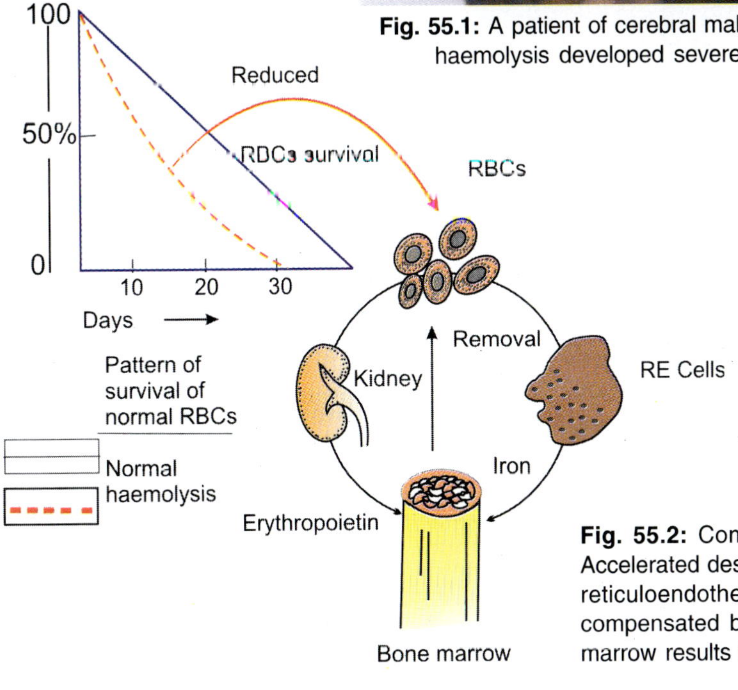

Fig. 55.2: Components of normal erythropoiesis. Accelerated destruction of red blood cells (RBCs) by reticuloendothelial system (RE cells) which is not compensated by erythroid hyperplasia in the bone marrow results in haemolytic anaemia

Haematology

ACUTE HAEMOLYTIC ANAEMIA

Normal life span of RBCs is 120 days, after which they are removed from circulation by macrophages of reticuloendothelial system (RES) present in liver, spleen and bone marrow. Normal destruction of RBCs results in release of haemoglobin which splits into *heme (iron)* and *globin* fractions. Iron of heme is recycled via transferrin to the marrow for reutilisation; while protoporphyrin is broken down to bilirubin, gets conjugated in the liver and excreted in the gut, where it is converted into stercobilinogen and stercobilin. Most of the stercobilinogen is excreted in the faeces (normal stool colour is due to this pigment) but some of it is partially reabsorbed and excreted as urobilinogen and urobilin in urine (present normally in urine in 1:10 concentration). Normal serum bilirubin levels are maintained by regular destruction and synthesis of RBCs.

Globin chains are broken down and converted into aminoacids which are reutilized for protein synthesis in the body.

Normally, there is no intravascular hemolysis

Definition

Anaemia resulting from rapid increased red cell destruction is known as *haemolytic anaemia* which may be congenital or acquired. Haemolytic anemias are characterised by features of accelerated red cell destruction and a compensatory erythroid hyperplasia (reticulocytosis is the hallmark). As such the increased red cell production requires an extra amount of folic acid and vit. B_{12}, hence, their deficiency may prove disastrous.

Aetiological Classification

Haemolytic anaemias may be due to intracorpuscular defect (usually congenital) or extracorpuscular defect (usually acquired). Depending on the clinical presentation, haemolytic anaemia may be acute (usually acquired haemolytic anaemia or congenital G6PD deficiency precipitated by drugs) or chronic (usually congenital). The classification is given in the Table 55.1.

Consequences of Haemolysis

Shortening of RBCs survival does not always cause anaemia as there is a compensatory increase in

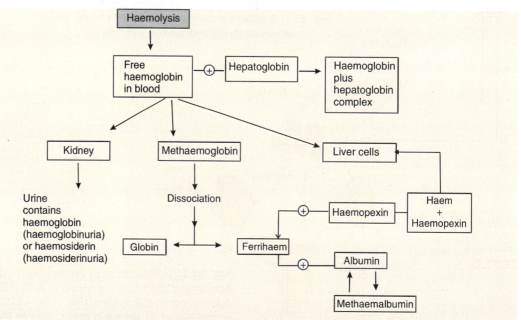

Fig. 55.3: The fate of haemoglobin in plasma during haemolysis

Sites of Haemolysis

1. **Intravascular haemolysis (Fig. 55.3):** When RBCs are rapidly destroyed within circulation, free haemoglobin is released into the plasma. Free haemoglobin is toxic to cells and the body has evolved a binding mechanism so as to minimise its toxicity. Haptoglobin, an alpha globulin produced by the liver is first to bind free haemoglobin to form *haptoglobin-haemoglobin complex* which is too large to be excreted by the kidneys, hence, is degraded by the liver (RE cells). Haptoglobin is used for binding to Hb, hence, its levels are reduced in intravascular haemolysis. Once haptoglobins are saturated, free haemoglobin is oxidised to form *methaemalbumin* which is detected on spectrophotometry of the plasma (Schumm's test). Methaemalbumin is degraded and free haem formed which binds to a second binding protein called *haemopexin*.

   When all the protective mechanisms are overloaded, free haemoglobin appear in the urine called *hemoglobinuria* a characteristic feature of intravascular haemolysis. When haemolytic process is fulminant as seen in malaria, this give rise to black urine. In smaller amounts renal tubular cells absorb the haemoglobin, degrade it and store the iron as hemosiderin. When the renal tubular cells containing hemosiderin are shed off into the urine, *haemosiderinuria* results which is always indicative of intravascular haemolysis.

2. **Extravascular haemolysis:** In most haemolytic conditions, red cells destruction is extravascular and little or no depletion of haptoglobin occurs—a differentiating feature from intravascular haemolysis. The red cells are removed from the circulation by macrophages in RE system of liver and spleen.

Evidences for Haemolysis

1. **Increased red cell destruction:** It leads to:
   - Elevated serum bilirubin predominantly indirect (unconjugated hyperbilirubinaemia)

Table 55.1: Aetiological classification of haemolytic anaemia

Intracorpuscular defects
1. Abnormalities of RBC interior
   a. Enzymatic defect
      - Associated with pentose-phosphate pathway deficiency i.e. G6PD deficiency and others.
      - Associated with Embeden-Meyerhof pathway deficiencies i.e. pyruvate kinase deficiency and others.
   b. Haemoglobinopathies
      - Thalassaemia syndrome
      - Sickle cell anaemia (Hb-S)
      - Other abnormal haemoglobin (Hb-C, Hb-E, Hb-D)
      - Unstable haemoglobin disease
2. Membrane defect
   - Hereditary spherocytosis
   - Hereditary elliptocytosis
   - Paroxysmal nocturnal haemoglobinuria
   - Spur cell anaemia

Extracorpuscular defects
1. Antibody-mediated (*immune haemolysis*)
   - Autoimmune haemolytic anaemia
   - Other immune-mediated haemolysis
2. Infections
   - Malaria (falciparum)
   - Bartonella
   - Clostridium
3. Mechanical
   - Microangiopathic haemolytic anaemia e.g. DIC, disseminated malignancies, vasculitis, TTP etc.
   - Mechanical valve (traumatic)
   - March haemoglobinuria
4. Chemical and physical agents
   - Snake bite, bee sting, spider bite etc.
   - Arsenicals
5. Hypersplenism

RBCs production in the marrow. Normal marrow has tremendous capacity to become hyperplastic and compensate for haemolysis, hence, anaemia occurs only when this compensation becomes inadequate (Fig. 55.2). The erythroid hyperplasia in the bone marrow is reflected by expansion of active marrow resulting in reticulocytosis (immature red cells) in the peripheral blood, thus, *reticulocytosis* is a hallmark of haemolysis. The reticulocytes are larger than red cells and stain light blue on a peripheral blood film.

- Excessive urinary urobilinogen.
- Reduced levels of haptoglobins.
- Raised serum lactic dehydrogenase (LDH).

2. ***Increased red cell production:*** It leads to:
   - Reticulocytosis.
   - Macrocytosis if folic acid and vit B_{12} insufficient.
   - Erythroid hyperplasia of the marrow.
   - Radiological changes in the bone (skull and tubular bones).

3. ***Morphological change in RBCs:*** These occur in some haemolytic anaemias:
   - Spherocytosis (hereditary spherocytosis).
   - Sickle cell (sickle cell disease).
   - Elliptocytes (Elliptocytosis).
   - Red cells fragments.
   - *Acanthocytes* (Spur cell anaemias or severe liver disease).
   - Agglutinated cells (cold agglutinin disease due to cold IgM antibodies).
   - Heinz bodies (unstable Hb disease, oxidant stress).

4. ***Altered osmotic fragility and Coomb's test*** (direct test detects anti-IgG and anti-C_3 on RBC surface while indirect test detects IgG antibody in serum in autoimmune haemolytic anaemia).

5. ***Demonstration of shortened red cell survival***
   - Red cell survival studies using 51Cr-labelled. RBCs. The dominant site of destruction can be shown with external body counting over the liver and spleen.

6. ***Evidences of intravascular haemolysis:*** These are in addition to stated above if haemolysis is intravascular and differentiates it from extra-vascular haemolysis. These are:
   - Raised levels of plasma haemoglobin (hemoglobinaemia).
   - Very low or absent haptoglobins.
   - Haemoglobinuria and haemosiderinuria.
   - Presence of methaemalbumin (positive Schumm's test).

Clinical Presentations

1. ***Hereditary haemolytic anaemias*** may be asymptomatic or may present with anaemia, jaundice and splenomegaly or may present with complications (chronic) such as haemolytic facies, ankle ulcers, pigment gallstones, growth retardation in children, pathological fractures. They may present *acutely* with crises i.e. aplastic crisis due to B_{19} parvo virus, megaloblastic crisis due to folic acid deficiency and acute haemolytic crisis due to accelerated haemolysis.

2. ***Acquired haemolytic anaemia:*** In most patients with acquired haemolytic anaemia, red cells are made normally but are prematurely destroyed because of damage acquired in circulation. The damage is extracorpuscular, is mediated by antibodies or toxins that predispose the cells for premature destruction (haemolysis). Therefore, these anaemias are episodic, occur after some challenge, present actually with manifestations of intravascular haemolysis (antibodies or toxin mediated) or extravascular haemolysis (hypersplenism). Malaria is common cause of acute acquired haemolytic anaemia (Fig. 55.1 on front page).

Therefore acute haemolytic anaemia may present as a crisis such as:
1. Aplastic crisis.
2. Haemolytic crisis.
3. Megaloblastic crisis.
4. Hypersplenism (sequestration crisis).

1. ***Aplastic crisis:*** It is frequently seen in congenital haemolytic anaemia such as sickle cell anaemia, β-thalassaemia, hereditary spherocytosis and pyruvate kinase deficiency. The infection by B_{19} *parvo virus* is the most common precipitating cause. It may be sporadic or endemic. Transmission of virus is via faeco-oral route or droplets infection.

The symptom and signs of infection such as fever, malaise, chills, upper respiratory or gastrointestinal symptoms precede the episode of aplastic crisis. The investigations reveal very low haemoglobin and hypoplasia of the bone marrow (low reticulocyte count, erythroblastopenia). Diagnosis is mainly clinical. Serology for presence of specific IgM antiviral antibodies or demonstration of parvo virus B_{19} particles in the blood on electron microscopy is confirmatory. Erythropoiesis ceases for 48-72 hours, though crisis may last for 1-2 weeks. Treatment is immediate red cell infusion to raise the haemoglobin. Supportive care should be instituted. The crisis is self-limiting. A single attack of parvo virus confers life-long immunity.

2. *Haemolytic crisis:* It is rather infrequent but early recognition is necessary to save life. The patients of unstable haemoglobin disease or enzymes deficiency (G6PD, pyruvate kinase) may develop sudden fall in haemoglobin under the effect of oxidant stress due to febrile/infective illness. The haemoglobin breaks down and gets precipitated as *Heinz bodies*—a characteristic feature. The inheritance of G6PD deficiency is sex-linked and affects approximately 1% of the Indian males. It is common in Parsees (15%), Bhansoli (11%), Khatri (9%), Punjabi (3%), Kutchi (3%) and Muslims (25%). The list of drugs that cause haemolysis in G6PD deficiency and unstable haemoglobins are listed in Box 55.1.

> **Box 55.1: Drugs and chemicals responsible for haemolysis in G6PD deficiency and unstable haemoglobin disease**
>
> - *Antimalarials* e.g. primaquine, pamaquin, quinine, chloroquine
> - *Sulphonamides* e.g. sulphamethoxazole, sulphapyridine, sulphasalazine, sulphanilamide
> - *Fluoroquinolones* e.g. nitrofurantoin, nalidixic acid, norfloxacin, ciprofloxacin
> - *Sulphones* e.g. dapsone
> - *Analgesic* e.g. acetanilide
> - *Miscellaneous* e.g. Vit K, doxorubicin, methylene blue, niridazole, toludene blue, furazolidine, naphthalene (moth-balls)

Autoimmune haemolytic anaemia in which the haemolysis is mainly extravascular in the spleen due to antibodies may present with fulminant haemolytic picture sometimes. The malarial parasite (falciparum) causes acute haemolytic anaemia or crisis (See Fig. 55.2 on front page) due to the reduced RBC survivals in normal healthy persons.

The clinical features of acute haeolytic crisis are given in Box 55.2.

3. *Megaloblastic crisis:* Hacmolytic anaemia of any cause increases the demand of folic acid, therefore, concomitant folic acid deficiency may result in megaloblastic crisis. The folic acid deficiency may be precipitated by rapid growth or pregnancy or diminished intake (anorexia) or alcoholism. The clinical features are same. In this condition, there will be macrocytosis in

> **Box 55.2: Characteristics of acute haemolytic crisis**
>
> 1. **History**
>   - Fever
>   - Infection
>   - Systemic illness or predisposing illness
>   - Drugs
>   - Family history
> 2. **Clinical features**
>   *Symptoms*
>   - Pallor, weakness, dyspnoea, tachycardia, fatigue, abdominal pain
>   - Jaundice (yellowness of eyes)
>   - Dark colour of urine and feces
>   - Splenomegaly (recent appearance or sudden increase in pre-existing splenomegaly)
>   - Hepatomegaly (mild)
>
>   *Signs*
>   - Anaemia
>   - Jaundice
> 3. **Investigations**
>   i. *Investigations to confirm haemolysis have already been discussed*
>   ii. *Investigations to find out the cause*
>   - PBF for malarial parasite, Heinz bodies
>   - Serology for parvovirus B_{19} and other viruses
>   - Coomb's antiglobin tests (direct and indirect)
>   - Tests for underlying disorders especially the neoplasms of immune system (CLL, Hodgkin's and non-Hodgkin's lymphoma), collagen vascular disease or immunodeficiency disease

the peripheral blood film instead of normocytic normochromic picture of haemolytic anaemia. The bone marrow shows megaloblastosis.

4. **Splenic sequestration crisis** is usually seen in children under the age of two years. It results from sudden trapping of blood in spleen leading to sudden fall in haemoglobin > 2g/dl or more. This type of crisis is common in sickle cell anaemia and its variants Hb SC disease or Hb-Sβ-thalassaemia wherein splenomegaly is a characteristic feature. The precipitous fall in haemoglobin if not managed promptly, death may result. Over 10% deaths occur during first decade in children with sickle cell disease. In severe cases, splenectomy is indicated, therefore, the mothers of the child with sickle cell disease can be taught to detect the enlarging spleen in the child during acute illness and bring him to emergency.

Management

It is essentially supportive during the attack. Most of the attacks of haemolytic crisis are self-limiting.

Aims of Treatment

- To identify haemolytic process, its nature and measures to arrest it.
- To identify the type of crisis.
- Any red cell inclusions (Heinz bodies) or infection (malarial parasite, bacterial or viral).
- Any other leucocytes and platelets abnormalities.

Steps

1. Arrangement be made for blood transfusions, therefore, immediate blood grouping and cross-matching should be ordered.
2. Send the blood for:
   - Complete blood count, red cell indices, reticulocyte count and PBF for type of anaemia or for malarial parasite.
   - Serum bilirubin (total and differential).
   - LDH and folate.
   - Urea and electrolyte.
   - Bone marrow examination.
   - Serology for viral infection (parvovirus B_{19}).
3. Carry out the followings:
   - Rest, treatment of fever and pain if present.
   - O_2 through mask.
   - Adequate hydration by fluids.
   - *Transfusions*: Packed RBCs transfusion is needed at the earliest. Each unit to be transfused within 2-4 hours. The total requirement varies depending on the haemoglobin/haematocrit, hence, reassessment should be made after two blood transfusions.
   Note: Blood or red cell transfusion may be hazardous in acquired haemolytic anaemia (having antibodies in plasma) as it may induce further haemolysis. However, it does not deter the transfusion if emergency demands it.
   - Supplement folic acid 5 mg daily followed by life-long replacement of 1 mg daily.
   - No iron supplementation is warranted unless there is concomitant iron deficiency.
   - Corticosteroids for autoimmune haemolytic anaemia (1 mg/kg/day) for 4-6 weeks followed by gradual reduction of the dose). Immunosuppressive drugs (cyclo phosphamide, azathioprine) are other alternative to steroids.
   - *Treatment of infection:* Antimalarial for falciparum infection, use artesunate/artemether for this purpose as quinine may precipitate haemolysis. Antibiotic for bacterial infection.
   - Treatment of underlying primary disease responsible for haemolysis.
   - Consider splenectomy on an individual basis weighing its hazards and benefits.

Chapter 56

Thrombocytopenia

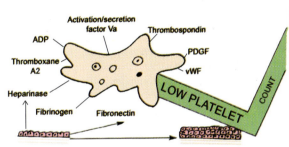

1. Adhesion → 2. Activation → 3. Aggregation of platelet

Fig. 56.1: Events in primary hemostasis. (1) First event is platelet adhesion and its interactions with vascular endothelium (2) This is followed by platelet activation and secretion. Some of the products elaborated by the platelets are depicted (3) Final event is binding of activated platelets to vascular endothelium in the process of platelet aggregation
Abbreviation: ADP= Adenosine diphosphate, PDGF = Platelet derived growth factor vWF = von Willebrand's factor

THROMBOCYTOPENIA

The platelets are one of the formed elements of blood and take part in hemostasis (Fig. 56.1). Platelets also play a role in fibrinolysis and clot retraction. Disorders of platelets manifest as bleeding disorders. Hemostatic process requires an adequate number of platelets that are functioning normally, failing which primary hemostatic process is compromised.

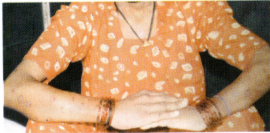

Fig. 56.2: A patient with thrombocytopenic purpura. Note the purpuric spots over the upper extremities

Definition

Thrombocytopenia is defined as a decrease in platelet count to below $150 \times 10^9/L$ ($< 1,50,000/mm^3$). A normal platelet count is $150-350 \times 10^9/L$.

Causes

Platelets arise from the fragmentation of megakaryocytes which are very large, polypoidal bone marrow cells produced by the process of endomitosis. They undergo 3-5 cycles of chromosomal duplication without cytoplasmic division. After leaving the bone marrow, one-third of the platelets are sequestrated in the spleen. While the other two thirds circulate for platelet functions and remain for 7-10 days (normal life span of platelets). Normally, only a small mass of platelets is consumed in process of hemostasis; so most of the platelets circulate until they become old or senescent and are removed by phagocytic cells.

The process of thrombocytosis (platelets production) is regulated by thrombopoietin (TPO) binding to its megakaryocyte receptors. A reduction in platelet mass increases the level of TPO and thereby stimulates megakaryocytes and platelets production. Recombinant TPO is being tested for clinical use for prevention and treatment of thrombocytopenia in patients receiving cytotoxic therapy.

The causes of thrombocytopenia are given in Table 56.1. The thrombocytopenia is caused by one of the three mechanisms, i.e. decreased bone marrow production, increased splenic sequestration, and accelerated destruction of platelets.

Autoimmune thrombocytopenia is the most common (acquired) cause in young subjects. Exposure to drugs, toxins, venom (snake bite), infections (malaria, dengue), gram-negative septicaemia and DIC are other common causes of thrombocytopenia encountered in clinical practice. Splenomegaly due to any cause and/or hypersplenism leads to thrombocytopenia by increasing platelets destruction, also diminishes the effectiveness of platelets transfusion in these conditions and splenectomy is the answer to these problems. The drugs causing thrombocytopenia are given in Box 56.1.

Table 56.1: Causes of thrombocytopenia

1. *Impaired production*
    A. *Generalised bone marrow failure*
     - Aplastic anaemia
     - Megaloblastic anaemia
     - Leukaemia
     - Myeloma
     - Myelofibrosis
     - Marrow infiltration by solid tumours or others (myelophthisic process)
     - Thrombopoietin deficiency
    B. *Selective reduction of platelets*
     - Drugs, physical agents
     - Chemicals
     - Viral infections
2. *Excessive destruction/consumption*
    A. *Immune*
     - Autoimmune thrombocytopenic purpura
     - Secondary immune thrombocytopenia (SLE, CLL, viral infection, drugs)
     - Alloimmune neonatal thrombocytopenia
    B. *Coagulation*
     - Disseminated intravascular coagulation
     - Thrombotic-thrombocytopenic purpura
     - Haemolytic-uraemic syndrome
    C. *Microangiopathy*
     - Valvular disorders
    D. *Increased sequestration by spleen*
     - Splenomegaly due to any cause, e.g. infective, congestive, infiltrative, neoplastic, etc.
    E. *Hypersplenism*, e.g. portal hypertension, myeloproliferative disease, lymphoma
    F. *Dilutional loss*
    G. *Massive transfusions of stored blood*

Box 56.1: Drugs causing thrombocytopenia

1. *Suppression of platelets production*
    - Myelosuppressive drugs, e.g. cytosine arabinoside, daunorubicin, cyclophosphamide, busulfan, methotrexate, 6-mercaptopurine, vinca alkaloids
    - Thiazide diuretics
    - Ethanol (binge drinker)
    - Oestrogens
2. *Immunologic platelet destruction*
    - Antibiotics, e.g. sulphonamide, tetracyclines, novobiocin, PAS, rifampicin, chloramphenicol
    - Cinchona alkaloids, e.g. quinine, quinidine
    - Sedatives, hypnotics, anticonvulsants (carbamazepine)
    - Digoxin
    - Alpha methyldopa
    - Anti-inflammatory, e.g. aspirin, phenylbutazone
    - Chloroquine, gold salts, arsenicals
    - Insecticides

Clinical Features

Thrombocytopenia is a common clinical disorder in clinical practice, but thrombocytopenia with bleeding is a medical emergency and is associated with high morbidity and mortality if bleeding is intracranial and/or intra-abdominal.

The clinical manifestations of thrombocytopenia vary from asymptomatic or mild disease to life-threatening visceral bleeding. The common sites of bleeding are:

- Skin e.g. petechiae, purpura (Fig. 56.2) ecchymosis.
- Mucous membrane and gum bleeding.
- Nasal bleeding (epistaxis).
- Genitourinary tract bleeding (haematuria, menorrhagia).
- Intracranial and intra-abdominal bleeding.

The severity of bleeding correlates with the degree of thrombocytopenia:

i. As long as count is between $100-140 \times 10^9/L$ (1,00,000-1,40,000/mm^3), the patients are asymptomatic and bleeding time remains normal. These are mild cases of thrombocytopenia just detected on platelet count.

ii. Counts between 50,000 to 1,00,000 per cubic millimeter (moderate thrombocytopenia) prolong the BT and bleeding occurs only during trauma, surgery or administration of drugs.

iii. Count below 50,000 (severe thrombocytopenia) leads to easy bruising, manifesting as purpura or bleeding with minimal trauma.

iv. A platelet count less than 20,000 mm^3 (very severe thrombocytopenia) leads to spontaneous bleeding such as petechiae, ecchymosis and internal bleeding (brain or GI tract).

Clinical Evaluation of a Case with Thrombocytopenia

It depends on:
1. History.
2. Clinical examination.
3. Investigations.

History

Certain elements on the history are important to determine whether bleeding is caused by underlying hemostatic disorder or by a local anatomic defect. The profuse bleeding during dental extraction, following trauma, child-birth or minor cuts or surgery indicate hemostatic defect. Following points are to be recorded on history in a patient with bleeding:

1. History suggestive of petechial spots, ecchymosis, epistaxis, gum bleeding, haematuria, menorrhagia, etc.
2. Ask for any recent drug intake or chemotherapy.
3. Antecedent viral infection (e.g. dengue fever/ Arbo virus).
4. Connective tissue disorders—skin rash, photosensitivity, joint and/or renal involvement.
5. Similar episode(s) in the past.
6. Family history of similar illness.
7. Pregnancy.

Certain clinical manifestations that are characteristic of primary hemostatic disorder (platelet defects) are given in Box 56.2. These features also differentiate it from secondary hemostatic failure (coagulation disorders).

Physical Findings on Examination

Look for the following:

Box 56.2: Clinical manifestations of primary and secondary hemostatic failure

Feature	Platelet disorder (defect of primary hemostasis)	Coagulation disorders (defect of secondary haemostasis)
1. Onset of bleeding following trauma	Immediate	Delayed (hours or days)
2. Site of bleeding	Superficial, e.g. skin, mucous membrane, gums, nose, GI tract, genitourinary tract	Deep, e.g. joints, muscles, retroperitoneal
3. Physical findings	Purpura, ecchymosis	Hematomas, haemarthrosis
4. Family history	Autosomal dominant	Autosomal or X-linked recessive
5. Response to therapy	Immediately stops with local pressure	Requires sustained systemic therapy

304 Haematology

- Petechiae, purpura, ecchymosis, nasal or gum bleeding.
- Facial puffiness.
- Record BP.
- Lymphadenopathy, rash, joint involvement.
- Splenomegaly.
- CNS involvement.

Investigations

They are done to confirm the diagnosis, to exclude other conditions and to determine the cause of thrombocytopenia.

  i. *Bleeding time* is prolonged
 ii. *The blood count* should include WBC, RBC and platelets. Peripheral blood film for any abnormality of platelets. Reticulocyte count to be done for bone marrow response. The reduced platelet count determines the severity of thrombocytopenia and serves as a guide for blood transfusion.
iii. *Bone marrow study:* Normal or increased number of megakaryocytes are found in the bone marrow, which is otherwise normal.
 iv. *Blood biochemistry and other investigations* to find out the underlying cause or primary disease.
  v. *Coagulation profile* to rule out coagulation disorders as a cause of bleeding. Assay of von Willebrand's factor is also done for platelet dysfunction.
 vi. *Serology* for viral and connective tissue disorders.
vii. *Detection of platelet antibodies* not only confirms the diagnosis but also rules out other causes of excessive destruction of platelets.
viii. *Imaging studies:* Ultrasonography for splenomegaly and CT scan for any intracranial bleed.

Management

It includes: General measures, hemostatic measures including platelet transfusions and measures directed against the underlying cause or primary disease.

1. ***General measures:*** It includes precautionary measures (Do's and Don'ts) in thrombocytopenia (see Box 56.3).
2. ***Measures to stop bleeding:*** The hemostatic measures may be local or systemic:
   A. Local measures
   - Compression bandages.
   - Nasal packing for epistaxis.
   - Application of thrombin or other hemostatic agents.

   B. *Systemic*
   - Procure I.V. line immediately in case of bleeding.
   - Platelet transfusions.
   - Treat other hemostatic abnormalities.

In the meantime, the patient is being assessed, following investigations must be ordered in order to save life-threatening complications:
- Complete blood count including platelet count, reticulocyte count and blood smear.
- Blood group.
- Blood biochemistry.
- Urine for hematuria.
- Fundus examination.
- Others (screening for DIC, autoantibodies).
- Bone marrow.

Box 56.3: Precautionary measures in thrombocytopenia

Do's	Don't (Avoid)
• Apply firm pressure on venupuncture site while collecting samples or I.V. administration for 10 minutes • Stop drugs known to induce thrombocytopenia or bone marrow suppression	• Avoid trauma • Stop use of hard tooth brushes or metal razors • Avoid intramuscular injection • Avoid use of NSAIDs • Avoid rectal examination, catheterization, suppositories and enemas

Platelets Transfusions

Platelet transfusions are life-saving in patients with severe thrombocytopenia (count < 20,000 mm^3) or when there is excessive bleeding. Platelet transfusions should be given to maintain a count above 100×10^9/L (1,00,000/mm^3) or else a target platelet count of 50×10^9/L is adequate.

Platelet transfusions are not much of value in states of accelerated destruction such as ITP; and not used in thrombotic states like hemolytic, uremic syndrome or thrombotic thrombocytopenia purpura as they are likely to be consumed.

Platelets for transfusion are derived either from random donor blood or apheresis from a single donor. It is best to use single-donor platelet apheresis in autoimmune states so as to minimize transfusion-related risks. The apheresed single-donor platelet pack raises the platelet count by 50×10^9/L.

Certain points to be borne in mind while transfusing platelets are summarized in Box 56.4.

3. **Treatment of underlying cause/primary disease:**
   - Withdrawal of an *offending drug/toxin*. Use antisnake venom in case of snake bite poisoning.
   - *ITP:* It is treated by steroids, intravenous immunoglobulin, anti-RhD, danazol, colchicine, immunosuppression and/or splenectomy.
   - *Hemolytic uremic syndrome/thrombotic thrombocytopenia purpura* (Read the respective emergency).
   - *Infections:* Use appropriate antibiotics.
   - *Malignancies* by appropriate chemotherapy or radiotherapy.

4. *Newer agents:*
   - Interleukins and recombinant thrombopoietin are being tried to prevent or reduce thrombocytopenia in patients receiving cytotoxic chemotherapy. Rituximab (anti-CD20 monoclonal antibody) has been proved effective on long-term basis as an alternative to steroids in ITP.

> **Box 56.4: Points to be remembered for platelet transfusion**
> - Platelets have short life span (about 5 days), therefore, fresh platelets should be transfused.
> - Platelets should be transfused rapidly within 10 minutes.
> - Platelets awaiting transfusions are stored at room temperature (20°-40°C) in a gently agitated state.
> - Platelet transfusion does not require cross-matching. Group-compatibilty of donor platelets/plasma may be ideal.
> - Unnecessary platelet transfusion generate alloimmunization reducing the efficacy of further transfusions, hence, should be avoided.

Chapter 57
Thrombotic Thrombocytopenic Purpura (TTP)

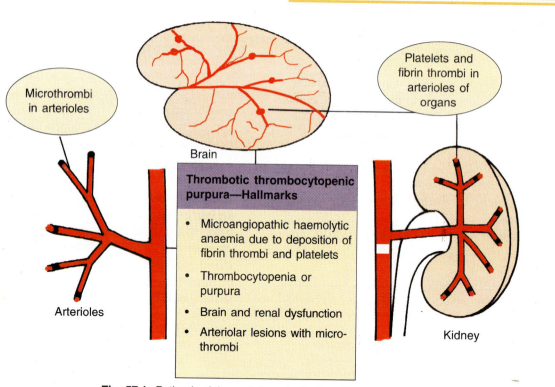

Fig. 57.1: Pathophysiology of thrombotic thrombocytopenic purpura

THROMBOTIC THROMBOCYTOPENIC PURPURA (TTP)

Definition

It is a disorder of intravascular coagulation in which platelets and fibrin are deposited at the site of arteriolar lesions in various organs (Fig. 57.1). This results in thrombocytopenia and haemolytic anaemia due to fragmentation of the red cells (traumatic haemolysis).

Pathogenesis

The pathogenesis of TTP is unknown. The manifestations are as a result of localised platelet thrombi and fibrin deposition in microvasculature. Arterioles are filled with hyaline material (fibrin and platelets) and similar material may also be seen beneath the endothelium of involved vessels. Immunofluorescence studies have shown deposition of immunoglobulins and complement in arterioles indicating an immunologic origin. Microaneurysm of arterioles may also be seen.

Causes

No specific cause is known. It is considered to be an immunological in origin. It is commonly associated with pregnancy, AIDS, scleroderma and Sjogren's syndrome.

Clinical Features

It is common in all age groups, primarily in young adults more common in females. TTP may be acute in onset but its course spans over days to weeks in most of the patients and occasionally may continue for months.

The **symptoms** and **signs** vary depending on the number and sites of arteriolar lesions. The classic *pentad* of TTP consists of:
1. Microangiopathic haemolytic anaemia with fragmentation of RBCs.
2. Signs of intravascular haemolysis.
3. Thrombocytopenia.
4. Neurological findings.
5. Impaired renal function.

The anaemia is mild to very severe, normocytic and normochromic. The thrombocytopenia may also be mild to severe producing bleeding tendencies. The neurological and renal abnormalities appear only when platelet count is markedly reduced (< 20 to $30 \times 10^3/\mu L$). Fever is often an accompaniment. The organ involvement is due to occlusion of microcirculation as a result of fibrin thrombi and platelets leading to tissue hypoxia.

Proteinuria and mild rise in blood urea may be the presenting feature of renal involvement followed by continued rise in urea and a fall in urine output if renal failure develops.

Neurological manifestations appear in more than 90% of cases and may be a cause of death in some patients. Altered state of consciousness, confusion, delirium occur initially followed by focal neurological signs and symptoms such as seizures, hemiparesis, aphasia and visual field defects. These neurological manifestations may fluctuate and terminate in coma.

Investigations

1. *Haemoglobin* is low.
2. *Platelet count* is low.
3. *PBF* shows fragmented RBCs—a pathognomonic finding.
4. *Tests for haemolysis.* Serum LDH levels are raised due to intravascular haemolysis. Hemoglobinuria may be present. Hepatoglobin levels are reduced. Direct Coomb's test is negative.
5. *Tests for coagulation* such as PT, PTT, fibrinogen level and fibrin split products are usually normal or only mildly abnormal.
6. *Tissue biopsy:* Biopsies of skin, muscles, gingiva, lymphnode may demonstrate fibrin thrombi within arterioles.
7. *Bone marrow* may be hypocellular.

Diagnosis and Differential Diagnosis

The diagnosis is based on clinical features (hemolytic anaemia with fragmented RBCs, thrombocytopenia, fever, neurologic and renal manifestations) and investigations listed above.

It has to be differentiated from a similar disorder known as *haemolytic-uraemic syndrome* which is characterised by the same arteriolar lesions which are only confined to kidneys. This disorder is common in children. Often the patient has a prodrome of a bloody diarrhoea caused by *E. coli* 0157-H7 and the lesions are thought to be due to the elaboration of *shiga-like verotoxins* that bind to renal vascular endothelium. Patients usually infants or children present with acute haemolytic anaemia, thrombocytopenia, acute intravascular haemolysis and oliguric renal failure. There is no neurologic symptom. The peripheral blood findings and coagulation tests are usually indistinguishable from TTP.

Management

1. *Plasmapheresis coupled swith fresh-frozen plasma infusion:* Until recently, the disease was considered to be universally fatal but now with the availability of plasmapheresis, more than 90% of cases can survive if therapy is immediately instituted. The plasmapheresis can be done daily or even twice daily with plasma replacement. The response is judged by an increase in platelet count, fall in LDH levels and fragmented red cells. If response is obtained, plasmapheresis is continued but less frequently for several weeks to months.
2. *Role of corticosteroids and antiplatelet agents:* The efficacy of this treatment is not known.
3. *Immunosuppression with vincristine or cyclophosphamide and splenectomy* have been used in patients refractory to plasmapheresis.
4. *Platelet transfusions* should not be given because they will act as '*fuel to fire*' and can precipitate thrombotic events.
5. *Care of comatose patient:* Some patients may develop deep coma. The management of coma is same as discussed in respective chapter.
6. *General supportive measures* with I.V. fluids and oxygen must be given to treat hypoxia.

Chapter 58

Haemophilia

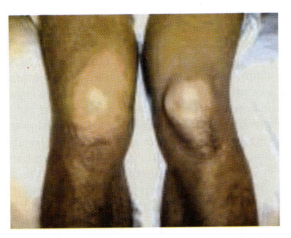

Fig. 58.1: Haemarthrosis of the right knee of a boy with haemophilia

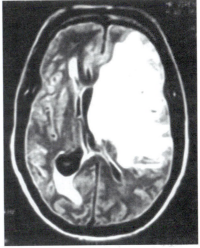

Fig. 58.2: CT scan showing a major intracranial bleed in a haemophilic patient

Coagulation disorders arise either due to congenital deficiency of a single factor e.g. factor VIII resulting in haemophilia A and factor IX resulting in haemophilia B, or due to acquired multiple factors deficiencies secondary to liver disease or anticoagulant therapy. Both haemophilia A and B are uncommon congenital disorders of coagulation, affect primarily the males and are transmitted by females. Both are X-linked recessive disorders, almost exclusively arise as a result of an abnormality in the gene-coding for that coagulation factor.

HAEMOPHILIA A

Definition

It is a congenital disorder of coagulation resulting from deficiency of factor VIII (antihaemophilic factor). It is most frequently encountered disorder of coagulation in clinical practice. It occurs in about 1 of 10,000 males. It is an X-linked disorder where the males are sufferers and females are the carriers. About two thirds of all patients have positive family history; while in other one-third mutation occurs *de novo*. A haemophilic person will have all his sons as normal, and all his daughters as carriers. A carrier woman has a 50% chance of having a carrier daughter or a haemophilic son in each pregnancy.

Haemophilia 'breeds true' within a family due to transmission of the same abnormality of the factor VIII gene; thus, if one individual has severe haemophilia, all others affected will have a severe form of the disease. Female carriers of haemophilia may also have reduced factor VIII levels because of random activation of the X-chromosomes in the developing fetus (lyonisation). A reduced factor VIII level in a carrier will result in mild bleeding disorder, therefore, all known or suspected carriers of haemophilia should have their factor VIII level measured.

Clinical Features

As already discussed, it being a X-linked disorder, manifests clinically in males. Superficial bruising or bleeding into soft tissue (hematomas) or joints (haemarthrosis) are the hallmarks of haemophilia A. Though a congenital disorder, bleeding is not noticed until babies are about 6 months old (e.g. a period of inactivity), occurs after that period because now the baby is up and about and is prone to trauma. Subcutaneous haematomas may be the earliest manifestation noted in a child as he begins to crawl; followed by bleeding into joints as he starts walking. These bleeding episodes continue throughout life.

The normal factor VIII level is 50-150% and is usually measured by a clotting assay. The severity of manifestations correlates with the degree of deficiency of factor VIII (Table 58.1).

Bleeding can occur at any site and may give rise to symptoms and signs related to pressure on adjacent organs or exsanguination. The sites of bleeding are:

1. **Spontaneous mucosal bleeding** is uncommon and is visible as small swellings (haematomas)
2. **Bleeding into tight compartments** of thighs, forearms and legs lead to respective compartmental syndromes due to compression of the neighbouring and underlying structures.

Table 58.1: Severity of haemophilia and clinical features (UK criteria)

Degree of severity	Factor VIII or IX level	Clinical features
Severe	< 20%	Spontaneous haemarthrosis and muscle haematomas, severeal times in a month
Moderate	2-10%	Minor trauma or surgery induces bleeding
Mild	10-50%	Major trauma or surgery results in excessive bleeding

3. **Bleeding into pharynx** leads to airway obstruction.
4. **Bleeding into joints (haemarthrosis Fig. 58.1)**, occurs spontaneously in severe haemophilia and after trauma in moderate haemophilia. The joints affected are large, i.e., knees, elbows, ankles and hips. A typical patient may have joint bleeding one or two in numbers every week. Patients become aware of joint bleeding because they feel an abnormal unusual sensation in the joint warranting immediate steps to arrest the bleedings otherwise it will continue resulting in a hot, swollen and very painful joint. Without these symptoms, bleeding continues for days before subsiding. Recurrent haemarthrosis may lead to synovial hypertrophy, cartilage destruction and secondary osteoarthritis, and ultimately resulting in limitation of movements and making walking difficult.
5. **Bleeding into muscles (haematomas)** is a characteristic feature of haemophilia. It can occur in any muscle but calf and psoas muscles are commonly affected. A large psoas bleed may press on the femoral nerve. Calf haematomas are serious because calf being a tight compartment leads to compression of soleus and gastrocnemius muscles. Untreated haemorrhage causes rise in pressure within compartment with eventual ischaemia, necrosis, fibrosis and subsequent contraction and shortening of Achilles tendon.
6. **Bleeding into CNS (Fig. 58.2)** though uncommon may cause stroke and unless treated promptly may be fatal. This is an emergency situation.

7. **Intra-abdominal bleeding** (intra or retroperitoneal) is uncommon and difficult to quantify and can be large producing hypotension or shock. It should be taken seriously as an emergency situation.

Diagnosis

The diagnosis is made on:
   i. Clinical features consisting of history of joint and soft tissue bleeding.
   ii. X-linked inheritance pattern. Males suffer from the disease.
   iii. Long history of bleeding with recurrent episodes leading to arthropathy in large joints.
   iv. Laboratory tests or investigations which not only confirm the diagnosis, but help to determine severity and planning of future management.

Investigations

1. *A normal prothrombin time and an abnormal activated partial thromboplastin time* indicate coagulation disorder.
2. *Correction of abnormal partial thromboplastin time (APTT) fully by pooled normal plasma.* In patients with factor VIII deficiency, APTT should also get corrected with plasma from a patient with factor IX deficiency. In a patient with factor IX deficiency (haemophilia B) it gets corrected with normal plasma or plasma from a patient with factor VIII deficiency.
3. *Specific factor VIII coagulation assay* will confirm the diagnosis. It is also important to screen for the presence of inhibitors to factor VIII or IX at diagnosis and thereafter.

Management

It is an incurable disease and the males being the sufferers are likely to have bleeding in day-to-day life activities due to mild trauma (moderate disease) or spontaneously (severe disease). Recurrent bleeding into the joints or muscles may lead to contractures and crippling deformities, hence, preventive measures should be taken not to allow these complications to occur. This is only possible by making the child/adolescent and his family members understand the implications and the management of the condition. They should be able to recognise the bleeding early and be familiar with its management. It is also necessary for them to understand the genetics and mode of inheritance of haemophilia so that preventive measures can be taken if they desire so.

Patients with mild haemophilia (factor level > 30%) do not have symptoms unless challenged by trauma or surgery. Moderate disease can produce bleeding with minor trauma and severe haemophilia may lead to spontaneous bleeding, which at times, may be fatal, therefore moderate to severe disease needs immediate attention and management.

The goal of therapy is to make the life of the child comfortable and normal as he grows up. This requires the family and the patient understand the treatment plans.

Treatment Plans

It includes:
1. Management of acute bleed.
2. Management of chronic complications.
3. Physical therapy and rehabilitation
4. Management before and during minor or major surgery.
5. Carrier detection and prevention.

Management of Acute Bleed or Bleeding Episodes

Bleeding episodes should be treated early by raising the factor VIII level by replacement, additional red cell infusion if indicated (if severe anaemia) and other non-factor replacement measures to control the bleed. The quantity and duration of factor VIII replacement depend on the site and severity of bleeding as discussed below:

> *1 IU/kg of factor VIII raises the plasma levels by 2% with a half-life of 8-12 hours. The aim is to achieve plasma concentration of factor VIII above 50%, hence, a large amount of factor VIII concentrate may be needed to stop active bleeding. The rough estimate to achieve 50% level (0.5 units/ml of plasma) in the expected plasma volume of 40 ml/kg in a 60 kg man, the dose of factor VIII will be 0.5 × 40 × 60 = 1200 IU.*

Factor IX in haemophilia B is needed more than factor VIII in haemophilia A to achieve the same level. This should be born in mind while treating haemophilia B episode.

The target level of factor VIII to be achieved with duration of factor VIII replacement to control bleeding at different sites is given in Box 58.1. Epistaxis often stops with local measures.

Box 58.1: Target factor VIII level for control of acute bleed

Site	Level to be achieved	Duration
CNS	About 50%	7-14 days
Muscles, soft tissues	10-20%	2-3 days
GI bleed		

The bleeding in haemophilia is controlled with factor VIII concentrates or by other methods.

1. *Factor VIII concentrates:* Factor VIII concentrates are freeze-dried and stable at 4°C and can therefore be stored in domestic refrigerators. This facility allows the patient to treat themselves at home, thus, has revolutionized haemophilia care. Ideally plasma derived virus-inactivated factor VIII concentrates or recombinant factor concentrate may be employed because of their good safety record and low risk of viral carriage e.g. HIV. When factor VIII concentrates are not available, the cryoprecipitates, fresh frozen plasma or a fresh whole blood may be used. When fresh frozen plasma is thawed at 4°C, certain products remain as a precipitate—cryoprecipitate. One bag of cryoprecipitate usually contains 80-100 IU of factor VIII activity and one international unit of factor VIII/IX activity is defined *"as the quantity present in one milliliter of fresh pooled plasma."* These products are cheaper and are widely available than lyophilized factor VIII concentrate. The greatest drawback of cryoprecipitate or other blood bank products is transmission of virus infection (Hepatitis B and C) as they are not subjected to virus inactivation process.

   The other serious consequence of factor VIII infusion is the development of anti-factor VIII antibodies, which arise in about 20-30% of severe haemophilics. Such antibodies neutralise rapidly the therapeutic infusion and making the treatment relatively ineffective. Such individuals may be treated with porcine factor VIII because antibody may have lower activity against animal factor VIII than against the human type. Alternatively, infusion of activated clotting factors e.g. VIII or Feiba (factor eight inhibitor bypassing activity—an activated concentrate of factors II, IX and X) may stop bleeding.

   In addition to factor VIII concentrate therapy, the bleeding site should be immobilized either by splinting or bed rest.

2. *Other pharmacological agents:*
   - Desmopressin (DDAVP) is used in patients with mild to moderate haemophilia (Factor VIII level 10% or more) to raise its level by three to five fold. It is given intravenously or intranasally. This is often sufficient to treat a mild bleed or cover minor surgery such as dental extraction. It has no role in management of severe haemophilia.
   - Antifibrinolytic agents (e.g. epsilon aminocaproic acid or tranexamic acid) are useful in management of mucosal bleeds. They are also used as an adjunct to cryoprecipitate or factor VIII concentrate for dental procedures

or extraction. A single infusion of cryoprecipitate or factor VIII concentrate coupled with the administration of 4 to 6 g of epsilon-aminocaproic acid four times daily for 72 to 96 hours is used for filling a carious tooth or dental extraction. Epsilon-aminocaproic acid is also effective when used as mouth wash.

Surgery or procedure in haemophilics
For major oral and periodontal surgery and extractions of permanent teeth, patient should be hospitalised and treated with factor VIII concentrate. Therapy should begin just before surgery and continued for a minimum of 48-72 hours.

Management of Chronic Orthopedic Complications

The musculoskeletal complications such as chronic synovitis, deforming arthropathy, pseudotumours, muscles wasting or debilitation can be managed by physiotherapy and minimal factor support. The consultation of orthopedic surgeon and a physiotherapist or hematologist is necessary for management of such cases.

Physiotherapy and Rehabilitation

Once bleeding has settled, the patient should be mobilised and given physiotherapy to restore strength to the surrounding muscles. Regular physiotherapy under proper guidance can prevent and significantly reduce the morbidity due to deforming arthropathy. Importance of physiotherapy should be explained to all patients with haemophilia.

Carrier Detection Antenatal Diagnosis and Prevention

Carriers have reduced or low normal factor VIII/IX coagulant activity. This information is utilized to assign carrier status. In families with haemophilia A, the ratio of factor VIIIc to the von Willebrand factor, which is normal in carriers, can be used with about 90% accuracy in assigning carrier status.

The use of molecular genetic techniques has revolutionised the ability to identify carriers and the antenatal diagnosis of haemophilia. Antenatal diagnosis can be undertaken in a female who has a high probability of being a carrier. This is determined by chorionic villous sampling usually around 10 to 11 weeks of gestation, sexing the fetus and using informative factor VIII probes. Alternatively, fetus can be sexed at 16 weeks of gestation by aminocentesis and, if male, a fetal blood sample obtained at about (19-20 weeks).

HAEMOPHILIA B (CHRISMAS DISEASE)

Haemophilia B is due to deficiency of factor IX. It is also X-linked recessive disorder. This disorder is clinically indistinguishable from haemophilia A but is less common. The frequency of bleeding episodes depends on the severity of the deficiency of factor IX level.

Treatment is with factor IX concentrate i.e. it is used in the same way as factor VIII is used for haemophilia A. Carrier detection and antenatal diagnosis can be accomplished if the specific mutation is known.

Chapter 59

Disseminated Intravascular Coagulation (DIC)

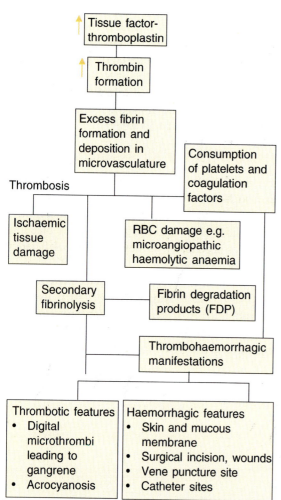

Fig. 59.1: Pathogenesis of DIC and its thrombohaemorrhagic manifestations

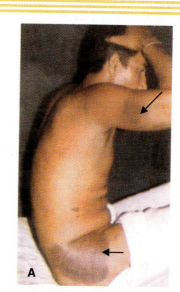

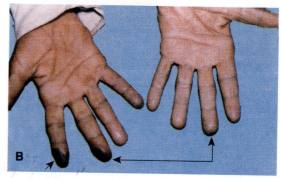

Fig. 59.2: Disseminated intravascular coagulation (DIC). Note the haemorrhagic manifestations in **A** (arrows) and thrombotic features i.e. gangrene of fingers in **B** (arrows)

DISSEMINATED INTRAVASCULAR COAGULATION (DIC)

Definition

It is an acquired coagulation disorder in which there is widespread generation of fibrin due to activation of the extrinsic pathway by release of tissue factor (thromboplastin), activation of intrinsic pathway by diffuse endothelial damage or generalised platelet aggregation.

There is consumption of coagulation factors and platelets (consumption coagulopathy) and secondary activation of fibrinolysis leading to production of FDPs which may further contribute to coagulation defect by inhibiting fibrin polymerization.

DIC can be either an explosive and life threatening bleeding disorder or a relatively mild or subclinical disorder diagnosed on laboratory parameters.

Pathophysiology (Fig. 59.1)

The following are the steps in pathogenesis of DIC:

1. *Thrombin generation that overpowers its controlling mechanism:* In most forms of DIC, the tissue factor—TF (thromboplastin) is released which activates the extrinsic pathway of coagulation by interacting with factor VII thereby initiating coagulation. The sepsis, cytokines, endotoxin, trauma, ischaemia, tumor cells can initiate DIC by release of TF. In DIC, thrombin formation is excessive, uncontrolled and overcomes the factors (antithrombin III, activated protein C) which normally inhibit thrombin formation.

2. *Fibrin deposition in microcirculation:* Large amounts of thrombin generated leads to fibrin formation from fibrinogen leading to its deposition in the microvasculature. Widespread microvascular thrombosis produces tissue ischaemia and organ damage. Microangiopathic haemolytic anaemia is a consequence of DIC as RBCs are sheared by the intravascular fibrin strands.

3. *Consumption of platelets and coagulation factors:* As DIC continues, the platelets and coagulation factors are trapped and consumed beyond the capacity of the body to compensate. This contributes to bleeding.

4. *Secondary fibrinolysis and production of fibrinogen degradation products (FDPs):* In response to thrombosis, endothelial cells secrete plasminogen activators to initiate fibrinolysis (secondary fibrinolysis). Plasmin formed from activation of plasminogen degrades both the fibrinogen and fibrin leading to the formation of FDPs, thus, dissolves clots thereby increasing the risk of bleeding. FDPs interfere with fibrin polymerisation, thrombin activity and platelet function that further aggravate bleeding tendency.

5. *Role of cytokines:* DIC in different diseases result from release of various cytokines that act through activation of coagulation pathway. DIC occurs as mediators are released from macrophages, monocytes and endothelial cells. Tissue necrosis factor (TNF) and IL-1 can cause production of TF which initiates DIC. Many of the effects of DIC such as hypotension or acute lung injury may be due to the effects of these cytokines *per se*.

Causes

The causes are given in Box 59.1.

Clinical Features

The relative rates of formation and breakdown of fibrin determine if the patient is asymptomatic, has features of bleeding or thrombosis or both (Fig. 59.2).

The clinical presentation varies with the stage and severity of the syndrome. It may be asymptomatic (laboratory parameters provide the diagnosis) or may present with florid thrombo haemorrhagic manifestations and shock.

> **Box 59.1: Causes of DIC**
>
> 1. **Infections**
>   - Viral infections e.g. arboviruses, varicella, rubella.
>   - Gram negative septicaemia
>   - Meningococcaemia
>   - Malaria (falciparum)
>   - Rocky mountain spotted fever
> 2. **Malignancy**
>   - Acute promyelocytic leukaemia
>   - Adenocarcinomas e.g. lung, prostate, pancreas
> 3. **Obstetric conditions**
>   - Abruptio placentae
>   - Retained dead fetus
>   - Pre-eclampsia
>   - Aminiotic fluid embolism
> 4. **Haemolytic transfusion reactions** eg. ABO incompatible blood transfusion.
> 5. **Snake venom.**

Haemorrhage is the most common presentation characterised by spontaneous bruising (Fig. 59.2A), mucosal bleeding/oozing, bleeding from open wound and vene puncture or catheter sites. Usually bleeding is associated with varying degree of shock which is out of proportion to the degree of blood loss. Shock is probably due to cytokines. Evidence of major organ dysfunction is common syndrome of MOF usually involving the pulmonary, renal, hepatic and CNS systems.

Less often, patients present with thrombotic manifestations i.e. acrocyanosis, thrombosis, and pregangrenous changes in digits (Fig. 59.2B) genitalia, and nose—areas where blood flow is markedly reduces by vasospasm or microthromi.

DIC may be acute or chronic. Acute DIC is commonly seen in clinical practice, manifests with bleeding that can be rapidly progressive. Acrocyanosis is common during acute DIC due to microthrombi or vasospasms of digital vessels. On the other hand, chronic DIC occurs from a weak or intermittent activating stimulus. In this type, the production and destruction of clotting factors and platelets is balanced called compensated DIC. Patients may have episodes of mild bleeding or ecchymosis. *Trousseau's syndrome* is a chronic form of DIC. Chronic DIC is seen in patients with intrauterine fetal death, adenocarcinomas of various organs, vasculitis and giant haemangioma.

Investigations

The pathogenesis of laboratory findings is depicted in Figure 59.3.

1. ***Peripheral blood film examination:*** It may show low platelets count, and schistocytes or fragmented RBCs that arise from cell trapping and damage within fibrin thrombi/polymerisation.
2. ***Platelet count*** is reduced due to consumption of platelets.
3. ***PT and PTT and TT*** (thrombin time) are prolonged due to consumption coagulopathy (Fig. 59.3).
4. ***Fibrinogen levels*** are reduced due to depletion of coagulation proteins.
5. ***Fibrin degradation products*** (FDPs). They are increased due to intense secondary fibrinolysis.

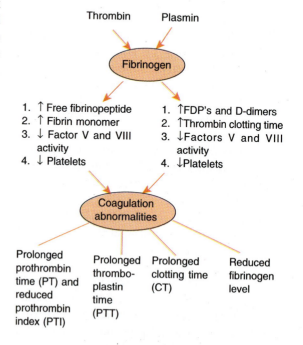

Fig. 59.3: Pathogenesis of laboratory changes in DIC. ↑ means increase ↓ means decrease

6. **D-dimers are increased.** It is done by immunoassay and is more specific FDP assay. It is both specific and sensitive test.

Management

Acute DIC is a life-threatening emergency, requires urgent treatment.
1. *General supportive care:* It means to support the circulation.
   - Tissue perfusion must be maintained by replacing intravenous fluids.
   - Oxygen therapy to correct hypoxia.
2. *Correction of precipitating/underlying cause:* Specific measures to stop DIC will depend on its cause;
   - Appropriate antibiotic for sepsis along with supportive measures.
   - Termination of pregnancy for obstetric complications causing DIC is often necessary.
   - Anti-snake venom and other measure for snake bite.
3. *Replacement therapy (haemostatic support):* In DIC, there are low levels of platelets, coagulation factors and fibrinogen leading to thrombocytopenia, prolonged PT, APTT and TT. Replacement therapy in acute DIC aims to arrest bleeding by haemostatic support till the underlying/precipitating cause is corrected whenever possible. Replacement therapy is also indicated where some invasive procedure is required like insertion of a central line. The blood components to be transfused include:
   - *Fresh frozen plasma (FFP).* It contains all the clotting factors including fibrinogen, antithrombin III and protein C. The FFP is administered in the dose of 15-20 ml/kg and the coagulation times are checked. If correction is not adequate, repeat doses may be needed after 6-12 hours.
   - *Cryoprecipitate:* If FFP is not sufficient to replace fibrinogen and the fibrinogen levels are below 100 mg%, cryoprecipitate may be given in addition to FFP. Each unit of cryoprecipitate contains about 250 mg of fibrinogen. For an adult to 60-70 kg, with fibrinogen level < 50 mg/dl, administration of 1.5 g fibrinogen (6 units of cryoprecipitate) should raise fibrinogen level to 100 mg/dl.
   - *Platelet concentrates:* 4 to 6 units (1 unit/10 kg of body weight) of platelet concentrates may be infused if platelet count is < 50,000/mm^3. Coagulation time and platelet counts need to be monitored every 6-12 hours and further replacement given till there is clinical response (bleeding stops), and the haemostatic parameters (platelet count, fibrinogen levels, PT, APTT and TT) are maintained without replacement indicating recovery from DIC.

Monitor platelet count, PT, APTT, fibrinogen level and FDPs after every few hours throughout the period of replacement therapy.

Patients with asymptomatic DIC do not require replacement therapy unless a surgical procedure is planned.

4. *Role of heparin:* Heparin being an anticoagulant, its use appear theoretically attractive to stop formation of thrombin in DIC, but actually it is not. For a patient who is actively bleeding, heparin would aggravate the bleeding before any potential benefits. In most of the typical situations of DIC (i.e. 95% of patients) heparin therapy has not been found useful in many controlled trials. The limited indications of heparin therapy in DIC are:
   - Chronic DIC of malignancy (Trousseau's syndrome).
   - Hypofibrinogenaemia with retained dead fetus prior to induction of labor.
   - In AML-M3 prior to initiation of chemotherapy.
   - When patient does not demonstrate rise in platelet count and coagulation factor following replacement therapy and continues to bleed implying ongoing consumption.

The dose of heparin, if indicated, is 15 units/kg/hour by continuous infusion or 300-500 U/hr. Low molecular heparin has been tried in chronic and acute DIC with beneficial effects.

5. ***Role of antithrombin III:*** In DIC, low levels of antithrombin III predict poor prognosis. High doses of antithrombin III (120-250 units/kg/day) for 2-3 days have been shown to have reversed DIC in one study; while most other studies have demonstrated improvement in coagulation profile and a shortened duration of DIC with the use of antithrombin III.

6. ***Other therapies:***
   - Epsilon-amino caproic acid (EACA) and tranexamic acid are antifibrinolytic agents, are not used routinely as they may lead to serious thromboembolic complications. Occasionally, they are given along with replacement therapy in patients who continue to bleed to reduce fibrinolytic activity.
   - Protein C infusion have prevented DIC in animals but its result has not been established in humans.
   - Gabexate mesylate (an inhibitor of serine proteases including thrombin and plasmin) has been tried in Japan with clinical and hematological improvement in DIC, but its clear advantage is yet to be reported.
   - An inhibitor of tissue factor activity i.e. recombinant nematode anticoagulation protein C2 is being tried.

Chapter 60

Agranulocytosis or Severe Neutropenia

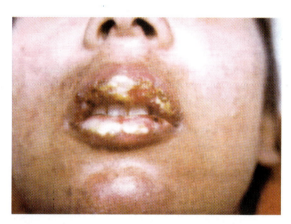

Fig. 60.1: A patient of agranulocytosis induced by drug; developed severe infection of the oral cavity with difficulty in swallowing and opening the mouth. Note redness, swelling and excoriation of lips and mucous membrane of oral cavity

AGRANULOCYTOSIS OR SEVERE NEUTROPENIA

Definition

Neutropenia is defined as circulatory neutrophil count below 1.5×10^9/L. (< 1500 cells/mm^3). The term *agranulocytosis* means a virtual absence of neutrophils, is used when neutropenia occurs as a reaction (immunologic) to drugs. This is an acute medical emergency characterised by high grade fever, sore throat and oral and/or perianal ulcers. Recovery is the rule if the offending drug is withdrawn and infection is prevented.

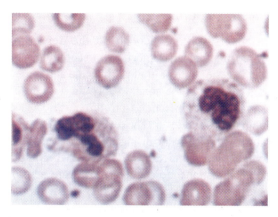

Fig. 60.2: In infection or toxic states, neutrophils have azurophilic granules (see the dark staining cytoplastic granules—toxic granules)

Consequences of Neutropenia

1. Neutropenia is mild when the count is between 1000-1500 cells/mm^3 and may have no consequence.
2. When neutrophil count falls below 1000 cells/mm^3 or µL, the susceptibility to infections increases.
3. When the count is less than 500 cell/µL or mm^3, control of endogenous microflora (mouth, gut) is impaired and opportunistic infections become common.
4. When absolute count of neutrophils (band forms and mature neutrophils combined) falls below 200 cells/µL, the inflammatory process is absent.

Causes

The causes of neutropenia are related to (i) *decreased production* (ii) *ineffective granulocytopoiesis* (iii) *increased destruction* or (iv) *excessive peripheral pooling*. The causes are given in the Table 60.1. Hereditary neutropenias are rare; for example *Kostmann's syndrome* (count < 100 neutrophils/µL) is severe and often fatal. The *Schwachman's syndrome* is more benign associated with pancreatic insufficiency. The most common neutropenias are iatrogenic i.e. autoimmune or drug induced (see Box 60.1).

Clinical Features

The manifestations depend on the degree of neutropenia. Bacterial infections are common. The onset may be acute or gradual. In acute and severe cases (Fig. 60.1) the conditions begin with upper respiratory tract infection, sore throat, throat and mouth ulcers and fever. The fever may be the only feature without any localising sign. Bacterial pneumonias, fungal infection of throat, erythroderma and GI infections are common. In severe neutropenia, septicaemia and shock may occur due to infection if immediate antibiotic therapy is not started.

Evaluation of a Case with Neutropenia

- Patients with neutrophil count > 1000 cells/µL are mild cases without any significant abnormality on examination or laboratory testing, often recovers spontaneously within 2 weeks after stopping the offending agent and may not need further evaluation.

Table 60.1: Causes of neutropenia

1. *Decreased production*
   A. Congenital
      - Kostmann's syndrome
      - Schwachmann-Diamond syndrome
   B. Acquired
      - Drug induced (see Box 60.1)
      - Chemicals e.g. benzene
      - Infections (see Box 60.2)
      - Acquired aplastic anaemia
      - Myelodysplastic syndrome
      - Acute leukaemia, hairy cell leukaemia
      - Malignant infiltration of marrow
2. *Impaired or ineffective granulocytopoiesis*
   - Deficiency of folic acid and vitamin B_{12}
   - Drugs
   - Paroxysmal nocturnal haemoglobinuria
3. *Peripheral destruction*
   - Antineutrophilic antibodies and/or splenic trapping
   - Autoimmune disorders e.g. Felty's syndrome, rheumatoid arthritis, SLE
   - Drugs as hapten (incomplete antigen)
   - Hypersplenism
4. *Miscellaneous*
   - Overwhelming bacterial infections
   - Haemodialysis
   - Cardiopulmonary bypass
   - Cyclic neutropenia

Box 60.1: Drug induced neutropenia

Group	Examples
Anti-inflammatory agents	Phenylbutazone, gold, indomethacin, pencillamine, naproxen
Antithyroid drugs	Carbimazole, propylthiouracil
Antiarrhythmics	Quinidine, procainamide
Antihypertensives	Captopril, enalapril, nifedipine
Antidepressants/psychotropics	Chlorpromazine, amitriptyline, dothiepin, mianserin
Antimalarials	Pyrimethamine, chloroquine
Anticonvulsants	Phenytoin, sodium valproate, carbamazepine
Antibiotics	Sulphonamide, penicillins, cephalosporins, chloramphenicol
Cytotoxic drugs:	• Alkylating agents (nitrogen mustard, busulfan, chlorambucil, cyclophosphamide) • Antimetabolites (6-MP, methotrexate, 5-flucytosine)

Agranulocytosis or Severe Neutropenia

- Patients with neutrophil count < 1000 cell/µL should be investigated and treated urgently. In patients presenting with fever, sepsis, neutropenia, it is not always easy to decide whether the neutropenia is the result or the cause of infection. In such cases, a PBF examination revealing more than 20% "band forms" indicates active bone marrow and neutropenia is the result of infection.
- History of fever, anaemia, mouth ulcers, lymphadenopathy, hepatosplenomegaly suggest acute leukaemia, could be confirmed on PBF examination.
- Cyclic neutropenia characterised by malaise, fatigue, mouth ulcers occur in cyclic manner after every 2-3 weeks, can be diagnosed easily.
- History of exposure to drugs and chemicals (given in Box 60.1) must be asked. Look for evidence of infection causing neutropenia (See Box 60.2).

> **Box 60.2: Infections causing neutropenia**
> 1. Viruses
>   - HIV
>   - Infectious mononucleosis
>   - Hepatitis
> 2. Rickettsiae
> 3. Gram-negative septicaemia, typhoid fever
> 4. Chronic infections
>   - Malaria
>   - Kala-azar
>   - Disseminated tuberculosis
>   - Visceral leishmaniasis

- Systemic examination for systemic disorders such as SLE, rheumatoid arthritis and Felty's syndrome must be carried out.

Investigations

The investigations are done to confirm the diagnosis, to assess its severity, to find out the cause and to differentiate *true* from pseudoneutropenia.

1. **Peripheral blood film examination** (i.e. absolute neutrophils count) will confirm the diagnosis and determine the severity. Toxic granulation of neutrophils may be seen in neutropenia with septicaemia (Fig. 60.2).
2. **Bone marrow examination:** To see the bone marrow activity in patients with severe neutropenia without any cause e.g. viral fever or drugs.
3. **Other investigations** are cause-specific:
   - Antinuclear antibodies.
   - Rheumatoid factor.
   - Serum immunoelectrophoresis.
   - Serum vitamin B_{12} and folic acid levels.
   - Antineutrophil antibodies.
   - Epinephrine mobilisation test (increase in absolute neutrophil count (ANC) after 30 minutes of 0.3 ml of 1:1000 epinephrine subcutaneously) is useful to assess the risk of infection. It also helps to differentiate true from pseudoneutropenia. Increase in ANC to > 2000 cells/µL is an indicator of good neutrophil reserve.

Management

1. **General measures:** Severely neutropenic patients are highly prone to endogenous and hospital-acquired infections. The patients with severe neutropenia need hospitalisation with following supportive measures to be adopted to prevent infection:
   i. Good hand-washing practices by hospital personnel, attendants and relatives.
   ii. Isolation of patient. No attendant or personnel with an evidence of infection should be allowed to visit such patients.
   iii. Skin cleansing properly especially at orifices. Clean oral cavity and teeth frequently to avoid infection.
   iv. Avoid intramuscular injection. Aseptic technique to be adopted for I.V. access.
   v. Avoid fruits, uncooked vegetable and salads. Sterile food (irradiated or pressure cooked) should be given.
2. **Treatment of infection:** Antibiotic should not be used prophylactically because of emergence of resistant strains. Attempts should be made to localise the infection and to identify the causative organism. Therefore, culture of throat

secretions, urine, sputum and blood should be sent immediately. X-ray chest may also be got done. These patients should be given a combination of 2 or 3 broad-spectrum bactericidal antibiotics such as an aminoglycoside *plus* broad spectrum penicillin *plus* cephalosporine in case there is an evidence of infection or fever. If fever does not subside despite adequate antibiotic cover, amphotericin B or fluconazole is given on empirical basis. Antibiotic therapy in such patients is guided by culture and sensitivity reports. Antibiotics should be continued at least 5 days after the patient becomes afebrile.

3. *Treatment of neutropenia:* The final outcome of neutropenic patients depends on the effective management of underlying cause. The use of recombinant hematopoietic colony-stimulating factor (CSF) such as granulocyte colony-stimulating factor (GM-CSF) 5 mg/kg/day have been successfully used to correct neutropenia associated with massive chemotherapy or radiotherapy. They may also be useful for other hypoplastic neutropenias. Other cytokines such as interleukin 3 (IL-3) and stem cell factor have been reported to act synergistically with G-CSF/GM-CSF.

Androgens are not effective in raising neutrophil counts. Prednisolone may be useful in raising the neutrophil count in autoimmune neutropenia.

4. *Treatment of underlying cause:* Transient neutropenia or agranulocytosis as a reaction to drugs is reversible if offending drug or chemical is withdrawn. If neutropenia is associated with systemic disorder, the treatment of systemic illness/disorder must be given simultaneously.

Chapter 61

Aplastic Anaemia

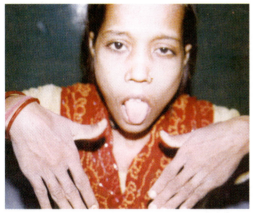

Fig. 61.1: Aplastic anaemia. The patient complained of tachycardia, fatigue and dyspnoea. Note the generalised pallor

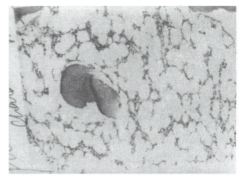

Fig. 61.3: Bone marrow examination showing only few cells and increased fat spaces (hypocellular marrow)

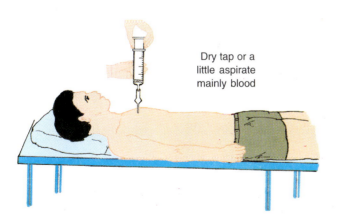

Fig. 61.2: Bone marrow aspiraiton may show dry tap

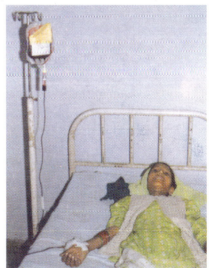

Fig. 61.4: Blood transfusion is being given to a patient with aplatic anaemia

APLASTIC ANAEMIA

Definition

Aplastic anaemia is defined as pancytopenia with hypocellularity (aplasia) of the bone marrow. In some conditions, only one or two cell lines may be affected. Aplastic anaemia due to bone marrow failure implies peripheral cytopenia arising primarily as a result of a specific defect in bone marrow precursor cells to produce mature cells. This distinguishes true bone marrow failure (aplastic anaemia) from myelodysplastic syndromes where peripheral cytopenia is associated with hypercellular marrow with dysplastic changes.

It is an uncommon condition that may be inherited but is more commonly acquired.

Mechanisms

Aplastic anaemia is due to a reduction in the number of pleuripotential stem cells together with a fault in those remaining cells, or is acquired due to an immune reaction against them so that they are unable to repopulate the bone marrow. Failure of one cell line may occur resulting in isolated deficiency such as the absence of red cell precursors in pure red cell aplasia.

Causes

The cause of aplastic anaemia are given in Box 61.1. The exact way by which aplastic anaemia is produced by various agents is unknown. Genetic factors play a role. Immunological mechanisms play a dominant role.

Damage to haemopoietic stem cell occurs in two ways:
1. Damage to DNA (irradiation, busulphan, benzene and chloramphenicol).
2. Damage to cell membrane affecting metabolic machinery (viruses, most drugs, immune mediated). Most cases of acquired haemolytic anaemia belong to this group.

Box 61.1: Causes of aplastic anaemia

1. **Inherited**
   - Fanconi syndrome
   - Schwachman-Diamond syndrome
   - Reticular dysgenesis
2. **Acquired**
   A. *Idiopathic (primary)*
   B. *Secondary*
      i. *Drugs*
         - Cytotoxic drugs, idiosyncratic reactions
         - Antibiotics e.g. sulphonamides, chloramphenicol
         - Antirheumatic drugs e.g. pencillamine, gold, phenylbutazone, indomethacin
         - Antithyroid drugs
         - Anticonvulsants
         - Immunosuppressants e.g. azathioprine, busulphan, cyclophosphamide, chlorambucil, vinblastine, 6-mercaptopurine
      ii. *Chemicals*
         - Industrial solvents
         - Benzene-containing solvents e.g. kerosene, carbon tetrachloride
         - Insecticide e.g. organophosphorus, carbamates, DDT (chlorinated hydrocarbon)
      iii. *Irradiation*
         - Ionising radiation (radiodiagnosis, radiotherapy, nuclear power station)
      iv. *Viruses*
         - Hepatitis viruses
         - Epstein-Barr viruses
         - HIV
      v. *Pregnancy*
      vi. *Paroxysmal nocturnal haemoglobinuria*

Clinical Features

The onset of aplastic anaemia is usually insidious. The most common presenting features are due to:
- Anaemia.
- Thrombocytopenia.
- Neutropenia.

1. ***Symptoms and signs of anaemia:*** Symptomatic anaemia is seen in all cases. The symptoms include weakness, fatigue, breathlessness on

Aplastic Anaemia

exertion. There is generalised pallor (Fig. 61.1). If anaemia is severe, tachycardia and murmurs associated with high flow rates (haemic murmurs) may be present. It is hereby stressed that in spite of severe anaemia, hepatosplenomegaly and lymphadenopathy are notably absent.

2. **Symptoms and signs of thrombocytopenia:** Thrombocytopenia produces bleeding from the skin (petechiae, ecchymosis), nose (epistaxis), gums (gum bleeding), vagina (menorrhagia) or gastrointestinal (haemetemesis or malena). There may be conjunctival haemorrhages.

3. **Symptoms and signs due to neutropenia:** Neutropenia predisposes to severe bacterial infection. Sometimes, infection may be presenting feature and fever may be the only symptom without any localising sign. Bacterial and fungal infections of the throat, pneumonias, erythroderma and gastrointestinal infections occur commonly.

Investigations

The laboratory diagnosis is made on the basis of:
  i. Pancytopenia with normocytic normochromic blood picture. Often, there may be macrocytosis.
  ii. Reticulocytopenia or virtual absence of reticulocytes.
  iii. Bone marrow examination (Fig. 61.2). There is hypocellular or aplastic bone marrow with increased fat spaces (Fig. 61.3). Sometimes, bone marrow tap may be dry.
  iv. Marrow cytogenic studies distinguish aplastic anaemia from myelodysplastic syndrome and Fanconi's anaemia. In acquired aplastic anaemia, no cytogenic abnormalities are seen.
  v. Screening for paroxysmal nocturnal haemoglobinuria (haem test, sucrose lysis test and urinary hemosiderin) should be done at the time of diagnosis and periodically during therapy and follow up as many cases develop PNH specially after immunosuppressive therapy.
  vi. Screen for hepatitis virus (A, B and C) and HLA typing for prospective bone marrow transplantation.

Differential Diagnosis

Aplastic anaemia should be differentiated from other conditions producing pancytopenia such as:
1. Subacute or aleukaemic leukaemia.
2. Myelodysplastic syndrome.
3. Hypersplenism (e.g. portal hypertension, infiltrative splenomegaly).
4. Bone marrow infiltration (carcinoma, myelofibrosis).
5. Megaloblastic anaemia.
6. Osteopetrosis (Marble bone disease).
7. Systemic lupus erythematosus.
8. Paroxysmal noctural haemoglobinuria (PNH).
9. Disseminated tuberculosis.
10. Overwhelming infection.

Management

The aim of treatment is to restore normal bone marrow function. To achieve this, withdrawal of the aetiologic agent, good supportive care followed by definite therapy are essential.

1. **Withdrawal of the aetiologic agent** or treatment of underlying condition is the most direct approach to the management of aplastic anaemia. Discontinuation of a suspected drug, thymectomy in patients with thymoma, or delivery or therapeutic abortion in patients with pregnancy associated aplastic anaemia may result in recovery of the blood counts. Unfortunately, these cases are very small in number.

2. **Supportive therapy:** Once the diagnosis of aplastic anaemia is made, blood transfusions (Fig. 61.4) are necessary to raise the haemoglobin and blood counts. Transfusions of blood products from family members should be avoided in prospective transplant candidates to prevent sensitization to minor histocompatibility antigens which increase the risk of graft

rejection after transplantation. Wherever possible, only CMV negative blood products should be given to CMV—seronegative potential transplant candidates to reduce incidence of CMV infection in post-transplant period.

Platelet transfusions should be given only when the platelet count is < 10,000/mL or if there is active bleeding. If feasible single donor platelet with HLA matched platelets are preferred to minimise the risk of sensitization especially in prospective bone marrow transplant candidates.

Packed red cells also should be transfused when the haemoglobin level is < 7 g/dl. Packed red cells should be filtered to remove leukocytes and platelets to reduce sensitization. Chronic administration of red cell transfusions results in secondary haemochromatosis, as each unit has approximately 200 to 250 mg of iron. Serum ferritin levels should be monitored, and chelation therapy with desferoxamine should be given to reduce iron overload.

Patients with aplastic anaemia who develop sepsis or any other severe bacterial infections require intensive parenteral antibiotic therapy. Hence in febrile neutropenia (absolute neutrophil count < 0.5 per 10^9/L), prompt institution of appropriate antibiotic cover is of paramount importance. Usually, a third generation cephalosporins or a newer penicillin along with an aminoglycoside is the initial therapy. However, if fever persists, antifungals are added as aspergillosis and candidiasis are common in these patients. Herpetic lesions need intravenous acyclovir. Prophylactic use of antibiotics in a febrile neutropenic patients has no benefit and predisposes to the emergence of resistant strains.

3. **Immunosuppressive agents:** In most of the cases of aplastic anaemia, the exact cause remains unknown, but one of the possible aetiological mechanisms could be autoimmune origin. In the absence of a compatible donor, immunosuppressive therapy offers a 50 to 75% chance of long-term survival. Two important drugs used in combination or sequentially are anti-lymphocyte globulin (ALG) or antithymocyte globulin (ATG) and cyclosporine. It is preferred mode of therapy in patients of severe aplastic anaemia (i.e. pancytopenia with neutrophils < 0.5 per 10^9/L, platelets < 20 per 10^9/L) who are older than 20 years of age and also in patients with very severe aplastic anaemia (neutrophil count < 0.2 per/10^9/L) and who are less than 20 years of age but have no bone marrow donor.

The basis for the effects of ALG/ATG is unclear, but immunosuppression is the possible mechanism which manifests within 2-3 months after administration. The dose of ALG is 10-20 mg/kg daily as I.V. infusion over 10 hours for 8-10 days. Oral steroids are given for 7-10 days along with ALG as prophylaxis for serum sickness. Platelet transfusions are required during ALG or ATG infusion as they can produce thrombocytopenia with bleeding. Side-effects of ALG therapy include, anaphylaxis, serum sickness, haemolysis, thrombocytopenia, leucopenia, infections, etc.

The experience with cyclosporine is not much. Cyclosporine and ALG/ATG induce similar response rate. Combined therapy with ATG and cyclosporine induces higher and earlier response as compared to ALG/ATG alone, particularly in patients with very severe aplastic anaemia. Two dose regimens i.e. low dose (5 mg/kg/day in divided doses) and high dose (10-15 mg/kg/day in two divided doses) are used but response rates with higher dose regimen is better. Side-effects include hypertension, gum hypertrophy, hepatic dysfunction, hyperkalaemia, hypertrichosis, seizures, infections and malignancies. There is no role of *glucocorticoids* and *androgens* as primary form of therapy in aplastic anaemia. However in mild aplastic anaemia, androgens may be useful in improving cytopenias. However short causes of steroids are employed as a prophylaxis against serum sickness during ALG therapy.

4. ***Haematopoietic growth factors (HGF):*** Recombinant haematopoietic growth factors i.e. erythropoietin, granulocyte-colony stimulating factor (G-CSF), granulocyte macrophage-colony stimulating factor (GM-CSF), interleukins (ILS) 1, 3 and 6 and stem cell factor can improve the blood counts, particularly the neutrophil count, in only a small number of patients. In patients who respond, blood count drops to pretreatment values following discontinuation of growth factors. Therefore, their use particularly G-CSF following intensive immunosuppression with ATG and cyclosporine has resulted not only in a reduced frequency of infection because of correction of neutropenia but also increase the response rate.

5. ***Bone marrow transplantation:*** Transplantation from an HLA compatible sibling is a definite and curative treatment for aplastic anaemia. The recommendations for bone marrow transplantation are clear for children, adolescents and young. The first line treatment in these patients is bone marrow transplantation (BMT). However, opinion is divided regarding BMT in older adults even if a sibling donot is available as results of immunosuppressive therapy (IST) and BMT are comparable. Current survival rates achievable with BMT (70-90%) reflect improvement in post-transplant management. High dose cyclophosphamide with ATG for pretransplant immunosuppression and cyclosporine prophylaxis for graft versus host disease (GVHD) after transplantation has markedly reduced the incidence of graft failure and GVHD and has significantly improved long-term survival (90% at 2 years after transplantation).

Chapter 62

Acute Leukaemias

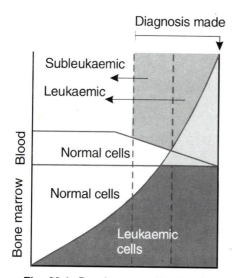

Fig. 62.1: Development of leukaemia

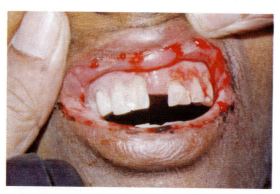

Fig. 62.2: Gum bleeding due to acute leukaemia

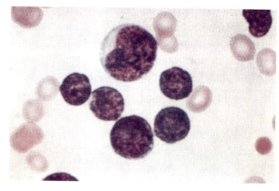

Fig. 62.3: Leukaemic cells in acute lymphoblastic leukaemia characterised by round or convoluted nuclei, high nuclear/cytoplasmic ratio and absence of cytoplasmic granules in peripheral blood

ACUTE LEUKAEMIAS

Definition

Acute leukaemias are malignant proliferation of lymphoid or myeloid precursor cells resulting in accumulation of blast cells (> 25% of the marrow cells are blast cells) in the bone marrow with subsequent replacement of normal haematopoiesis (Fig. 62.1). Extra-marrow infiltration involves lymphnodes (lymphadenopathy), spleen (splenomegaly), liver (hepatomegaly) or other organs. Acute lymphoblastic leukaemia is a disease of childhood whereas acute myeloid leukaemia (AML) is most frequently seen in adults.

Aetiology

The exact aetiology is unknown. No single cause can be pinpointed in acute leukaemia. The factors that predispose to leukaemias are given in the Box 62.1.

Box 62.1: Factors associated with leukaemias
1. Genetic predisposition
   - Increased incidence of leukaemia in identical twins of patients with leukaemia
   - Increased incidence occurs in Down's syndrome, Bloom's syndrome, ataxia telengiectasia and others.
2. Retrovirus
   - Adults T cell leukaemia/lymphoma (HTLV-1)
3. Cytotoxic drugs
   - Chlorambucil
   - Procarbazine
4. Ionising radiation
   - A significant exposure to atomic radiation
   - Following therapeutic radiotherapy and diagnostic radiographs of the fetus in pregnancy
5. Exposure to benzene and aromatic hydrocarbons in industry
6. Immune deficiency states
   - Hypogammaglobulinaemia

Terminology and Classification

The terms 'acute' and 'chronic' reflect the speed of evolution of the disease. In acute leukaemia, the history is usually short and life expectancy without treatment is also short. In chronic leukaemia, the patient remains unwell for months and survival usually extends over years.

Acute leukaemias are classified into:
1. Acute lymphoblastic leukaemia (ALL).
2. Acute myeloblastic leukaemia (AML).

Subclassification of acute lymphoblastic and acute myeloblastic leukaemia is given in Tables 62.1 and 62.2. The WHO has modified FAB classification of acute myeloid leukaemia by reducing the number of blasts required for diagnosis from 30% to 20% and incorporated molecular, morphologic and clinical features (Table 62.3).

Table 62.1: Subclassification of acute lymphoblastic leukaemia

Immunological subtype	% of cases	FAB subtype
Pre-B ALL	75 (most common)	L1, L2
T cell ALL	20 (Uncommon)	L1, L2
B cell ALL	5 (Rare)	L3

Clinical Features

Acute leukaemia presents with symptoms and signs of short duration (days to months). The symptoms and signs result from:

1. *Expansion of leukaemic cells at the expense of normal haematopoietic cells* leading to anaemia; thrombocytopenia and granulocytopenia in various combinations.
2. *Infiltration of leukaemic cells* into other organs i.e. liver, spleen, mediastinum, CNS, soft tissue and testis.
3. *Expansion of the leukaemic mass within marrow* of bones leads to bone pain and sternal tenderness.
4. *DIC* may occur with acute promyelocytic leukaemia (AML-M3).
5. *Gum hypertrophy* and *leukaemia cutis* are characteristic of acute monocytic leukaemia (AML-M_4/M_5).

The symptoms and signs of acute leukaemia are depicted in Box 62.2.

Investigations

1. *Total WBC* count is elevated, can be as high as 1,00,000/mm^3 or more. It can be normal or low in about 50% of cases. The peripheral blood film shows blast cells and other primitive cells (Fig. 62.3).
2. *The haemoglobin is low (anaemia)* and the platelet count is decreased (thrombocytopenia).
3. *Bone marrow* aspiration is done to confirm the diagnosis. The marrow is hypercellular with replacement of marrow elements by

Table 62.2: FAB classification of acute myeloid leukaemia (AML)

Subtype	FAB type	Frequency (%)	Morphology	Cytochemistry (staining)		
				MPO	SB	NSE
AML minimally differentiated	M0	3-5	No azurophil granules	(−)	(−)	(−)
AML without maturation	M1	15-20	A few azurophilic granules or Auer rods	(±)	(±)	(−)
AML with maturation	M2	25-30	Azurophilic granules, Auer rods are often present	(++)	(++)	(−)
Acute premyelocytic leukaemia	M3	5	Hypergranular promyelocytes, Auer rods	(+++)	(+++)	(−)
Acute myelomonocytic leukaemia	M4	20-25	≥ 20% monocytic blasts and granulocytic blasts	(++)	(++)	(++)
Acute monocytic leukaemia	M5	5	• Monoblastic (M5A) • Promonocytic (M5B)	(±)	(−)	(++)
Acute erythroleukaemia	M6	5	Erythroblasts > 50% of nucleated cells Myeloblasts > 30% of non-erythroid cells	(±)	(−)	(−)
Acute megakaryocytic leukaemia	M7	10	Megakaryoblasts > 30% of all nucleated cells 'Dry' aspirate; biopsy is done	(−)	(−)	(−)

Table 62.3: WHO classification of AML

i. AML with recurrent cytogenetic translocations
   AML with t(8;21) (q22;q22); *AML1 (CBFα)/ETO*
   Acute promyelocytic leukemia [AML with t(15;17)(q22;q12) and variants; *PML/RARα*)
   AML with abnormal bone marrow eosinophils [inv(16) (p13;q22) or t(16;16) (p13;q22) *CBFβ/MYH1*]
   AML with 11q23 *(MLL)* abnormalities
ii. AML with multilineage dysplasia
   With prior myelodysplastic syndrome
   Without prior myelodysplastic syndrome
iii. AML and myelodysplastic syndrome, therapy-related
   Alkylating agent-related
   Epipodophyllotoxin-related
   Other types
iv. AML not otherwise categorized
   AML minimally differentiated
   AML without maturation
   AML with maturation
   Acute myelomonocyt leukemia
   Acute monocytic leukemia
   Acute erythroid leukemia
   Acute megakaryocytic leukemia
   Acute basophilic leukemia
   Acute panmyelosis with myelofibrosis

leukaemic blast cells in varying numbers. For diagnosis of acute leukaemia, bone marrow must show 25 to 30% blasts cells (> 25%). It is also essential to confirm the complete remission and relapse following treatment. In addition to morphological evaluation, the cells are also subjected to cytochemistry, electron microscopy, immunophenotyping, cytogenetics and molecular studies. In general, ALL blasts cells are smaller, have a thin rim of cytoplasm and are Tdt-positive. AML blast cells are larger, have discrete chromatin granules, multiple nucleoli and auer rods. They are Sudan black and myeloperoxidase positive.

4. **Immunophenotyping:** The recent development of monoclonal antibodies as well as advances in flow cytometry has made immunophenotyping readily available (Table 62.4). It is useful in:
   • Definite lineage (B cell versus T cell) and stages of differentiation of ALL and identifying characteristic features of AML.

Acute Leukaemias

Box 62.2: Symptoms and signs of acute leukaemia

Presentation	Symptoms	Signs
Anaemia	Tiredness, weakness, exertional dyspnoea	Pallor, tachycardia, tachypnoea, murmurs, good volume pulse
Thrombocytopenia	Easy bruising, gum bleeding (Fig. 62.2) epistaxis, malena (GI haemorrhage), visual disturbance	Ecchymosis, purpura, mucosal bleeding, gum hypertrophy, retinal haemorrhage
Granulocytopenia	Fever, sore throat, respiratory infection (pneumonia)	• Signs of infection (sore throat or mouth ulcers) • Signs of respiratory infection (pneumonia) • Peri-rectal abscess
Leukaemic infiltration	• Dragging pain in abdomen due to masses • Infiltration in skin, soft tissue	• Lymphnode enlargement • Liver and/or spleen enlargement • Sternal tenderness • The mass lesion present as a tumour of leukaemic cells (granulocytic sarcoma or chloromas)
CNS involvement	Headache, vomiting, convulsions	• Papilloedema • Intracranial bleed with localising or diffuse signs

Table 62.4: Immunophenotyping in acute leukaemia

Subtype	Flow cytometry/monoclonal antibodies
ALL	
T cell	CD4 (helper)/CD8 (suppressor)
B cell	CD 19 (B4)/CD 20 (B1)/CD 22 (Surface)
Pre-B	CD9
CALLA	CD 10
AML	
M1, M2, M3	CD 13 or CD 33
M4, M5	CD 11 or 13 or 14 or 15 or CD 33
M6	Glycoprotein, spectrin
M7	CD 41 (Glycoprotein 11b/111a)/CD 43

Table 62.5: Chromosomal abnormalities and oncogenes in acute leukaemia

Type	Chromosomal aberration	Involved
1. ALL		
• Early B type	t (4: 11)	? MLL
• Common ALL type	t (4: 19)	BCR-ABL
• Pre-B	t (1: 19)	IGH-IL3
• B-ALL	t (8:14)	IGH-MYC
2. AML		
• M2	t (8:21)	
• M3	t (15:17)	PML RAR α
• M4	inv 16	
• M5	t (9:11), 11q 23	
• M6	del (7q) and del (5q)	
• M7	t (12.21), trisomy 21	

- Aiding in lineage determination of acute leukaemias that are morphologically undifferentiated.
- In differentiating acute leukaemia from other non-hematological disorders.
- Recognizing mixed lineage/biphenotypic acute leukaemia (ALL with myeloid markers or AML with lymphoid markers).

5. *Chromosomal abnormalities:* Three major techniques of molecular analysis such as southern blot analysis (commonly used), the PCR and fluorescent in situ hybridization demonstrate chromosomal abnormalities inherent in leukaemic cells (Table 62.5).

6. *LDH, uric acid and alkaline phosphatase:* Levels in the blood are elevated in acute leukaemia due to rapid turnover of the cells.
7. *Coagulation profile* may show features of DIC in AML-M3.
8. *CSF examination:* It is mandatory in all patients of ALL to evaluate CNS involvement at presentation and during follow-up.

9. *X-ray chest:* It may show a mediastinal mass in T-cell ALL.
10. *Renal function* e.g. urea and creatinine.

Management

I. Specific chemotherapy.
II. Supportive therapy.

The first decision in management of acute leukaemia must be whether or not to give specific therapy because it is generally aggressive and has many side-effects. It may not be appropriate for the very elderly or patients with other disorders to use aggressive chemotherapy. In these patients, only supportive therapy is sufficient. The general strategy for acute leukaemia is given in the Fig. 62.4.

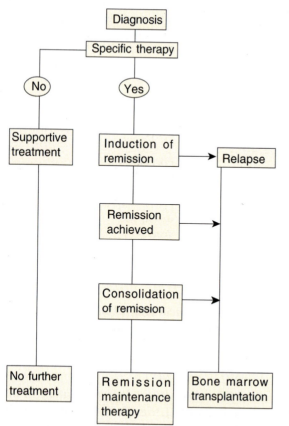

Fig. 62.4: Treatment plan in acute leukaemia

I. Specific Chemotherapy

The aim of treatment is to destroy the leukaemic clone of cells without destroying the residual normal stem cell components from which repopulation of hemopoietic tissues will occur to restore normal hemopoiesis.

Once decision to give it has been taken, the patient should be prepared for it as follows:
1. Existing infections identified and treated such as UTI, oral candidiasis, dental, gingival and skin infections.
2. Anaemia corrected by blood transfusions or red cells concentrate infusions.
3. Thrombocytopenia controlled with platelet transfusions.
4. If possible, insert central venous line for delivery of chemotherapy.
5. Therapeutic regimen should be explained to the patient for compliance.

Steps of Therapy

1. *Remission induction phase:* It means to reduce the leukaemic cells below the level of morphologic detection. This is achieved by combination chemotherapy. During this phase, patient goes through a period of severe bone marrow hypoplasia requiring intensive support, and in-hospital care.
2. *Remission consolidation phase:* If remission has been achieved by induction therapy, residual leukaemic tissue is destroyed by therapy during the consolidation phase. This consists of a number of courses of chemotherapy again resulting in periods of marrow hypoplasia.
3. *Remission maintenance phase:* Maintenance therapy generally not indicated in AML. If the patient of ALL remains in remission after consolidation phase, then low dose oral therapy is given for 18 months to 2 years as maintenance therapy. If relapse does not occur, then it is discontinued thereafter and patient is observed.

Cranial irradiation and intrathecal methotrexate is necessary for CNS prophylaxis in ALL to prevent CNS relapse. The drugs most commonly employed

Table 62.6: MCP-841 protocol for ALL in children

Drug	Dose	Days
Induction phase I (month 1 and 3)		
L-asparaginase	6000 U/m^2	2, 4, 6, 8, 10, 12, 14, 16, 18, 20 (alternate day therapy)
Vincristine	1.4 mg/m^2	1, 8, 15, 22, 28 (weekly therapy)
Daunomycin (daunorubicin)	30 mg/m^2	8, 15, 28
Prednisolone	40 mg/m^2	1 to 28 (daily)
Intrathecal methotrexate	12 mg	1, 8, 15, 22, 28
Induction-2 (month 2)		
Cyclophosphamide	750 mg/m^2	1, 15
6-mercaptopurine	75 mg/m^2	Days 1 to 7, 15 to 22
Intrathecal methotrexate	12 mg	1, 8, 15, 22
Cranial radiotherapy	1200 cGy	Days 5 to 15
Consolidation phase (month 4)		
Vincristine	1.4 mg/m^2	1, 15
Cyclophosphamide	750 mg/m^2	1
Daunomycin (Daunorubicin)	30 mg/m^2	15
Cytosar (cytosine-arabinoside)	100 mg/m^2	1, 2, 3 and 15, 16, 17
6-mercaptopurine	750 mg/m^2	1 to 8 and 15 to 22
Maintenance phase		
(3 monthly cyclic therapy for 6 cycles)		
L-asparaginase	6000 U/m^2	1, 3, 5, 7
Vincristine	1.4 mg/m^2	1
Daunorubicin (Daunomycin)	30 mg/m^2	1
Prednisolone	40 mg/m^2	Day 1 to 7
6-mercaptopurine	75 mg/m^2	Days 15 to 90 (5 days a week)
Methotrexate	15 mg/m^2	Days 15, 22, 29 i.e. weekly therapy upto 90 days

for two main varieties of acute leukaemia are listed in Box 62.3

If a patient fails to go into remission with induction treatment, alternative drug combinations can be tried but outlook of such patients is poor unless they undergo allogeneic stem cell transplant.

The most commonly used intensive treatment protocol (MCP-841) for ALL in children is given in Table 62.6.

II. Supportive Therapy

Adequate supportive therapy is needed during or following aggressive chemotherapy:
  i. **Anaemia** is treated with red cell concentrate to raise haemoglobin above 10 g/dl.
  ii. **Thrombocytopenia:** Bleeding due to thrombocytopenia is treated by platelet transfusions

Box 62.3: Drugs regimens in different phases of acute leukaemias

Phase	ALL	AML
Induction	• Vincristine (I.V.) • Prednisolone (oral) • L-asparaginase (I.V.) • Daunorubicin (I.V.) • Methotrexate (intrathecal)	Daunorubicin (I.V) Cytarabin (I.V) Etoposide (I.V. or oral) Thioguanine (oral)
Consolidation	Daunorubicin (I.V.) Cytarabin (I.V.) Etoposide (I.V.) Methotrexhate (I.V.)	Cytarabin (I.V.) Amsacrine (I.V.) Mitozantrone (I.V.)
Maintenance	Prednisolone (oral) Vincristine (I.V.) Mercaptopurine (oral) Methotrexate (oral)	Not recommended

to maintain the count above $10 \times 10^9/L$. Coagulation abnormalities, if occur, should be appropriately treated.

iii. *Infection:* Fever (> 38 °C) lasting over 1 hour in a neutropenic patient (neutrophil count < $1 \times 10^9/L$) indicates possible septicaemia. Parenteral antibiotic (broad-spectrum) therapy including a combination of an aminoglycoside (e.g. gentamicin) with a broad spectrum penicillin (e.g. piperacillin/tazobactum) is used on empirical basis. This combination is best bactericidal and should be continued for 5 days after fever has subsided. This therapy covers both gram-positive (*Staph. aureus* and *staph. epidermidis*) and gram-negative (*E. coli, Pseudomonas, Klebsiella*) organisms that are likely to be involved in infection in a neutropenic patient. Patients with lymphoblastic leukaemia are prone to develop pneumonia due to *pneumocystis carinii* which responds to co-trimoxazole.

Fluconazole is used for both prophylaxis and treatment of oral and pharyngeal monolial infection.

For systemic fungal infection (candidiasis or aspergillosis), intravenous amphotericin is used (0.5-1 mg/day for 3 weeks). Amphotericin is hepatic and renal toxic, hence, renal and hepatic functions should be monitored during therapy.

Herpes simplex infection is treated with acyclovir.

iv. **Adequate hydration** with oral or intravenous fluids must be maintained because most of these patients are severely anorexic.

v. *Administration of allopurinol* (a xanthine oxidase inhibitor) to treat and prevent hyperuricaemia.

vi. **Metabolic abnormalities:** In certain types of leukaemias where the rate of cell division is rapid e.g. B type ALL, T type ALL, patients may develop "*tumour lysis syndrome* characterised by *hypercalcaemia*, high level of *phosphates* and *hyperkalaemia* resulting from a high rate of cellular breakdown. This is a potential life-threatening situation and difficult to treat once it develops. It can be prevented by adequate hydration during chemotherapy if uric acid levels are high. Dialysis may be required in certain cases. Therefore, during chemotherapy to leukaemia, electrolytes and uric acid should be monitored.

vii. **Psychological support:** Patient's morale should be kept up by answering his/her questions from time to time. Fear must be allayed as far as possible.

Bone Marrow Transplant (BMT)

The bone marrow or stem cell transplantation is done with a hope of 'cure' in acute leukaemia.

1. *Allogeneic bone marrow transplantation:* Bone marrow transplantation from a suitable syngeneic (identical twin) or allogeneic (non-identical) donor (HLA and mixed lymphocyte culture matched) is increasingly being tried as the only therapeutic measure with the hope of 'cure' in young leukaemic patients (< 20 years of age). The basic principle of marrow transplantation is to reconstitute the patient's haemopoietic system after total body irradiation and intensive chemotherapy (called conditioning therapy) to aplate the recipient's haemopoietic and immunological tissue. The indications of bone marrow transplantation in acute leukaemia are given in Box 62.4.

> **Box 62.4: Indications of bone marrow transplantation in acute leukaemia**
>
> - AML in first remission
> - ALL (common pre-B type) in second remission
> - T and B cell lymphoblastic leukaemia in first remission

After conditioning, healthy marrow (matched for HLA) from a suitable donor is injected intravenously. The injected cells 'home' to the marrow start haemopoiesis (production of RBCs, WBCs and platelets) within 3-4 weeks. It takes longer time (1-2 years) to have good lymphocyte function. Therefore, during this period after

> **Box 62.5: Complications of allogeneic BMT**
> - Mucositis
> - Infection (viral, bacterial and fungal)
> - Acute graft versus host disease
> - Pneumonitis
> - Cataract formation
> - Chronic graft versus host disease
> - Secondary malignant disease
> - Infertility

transplantation, patients are at increased risk of infections.

The main complications of allogeneic BMT are given in Box 62.5. The long-term survival for patients undergoing allogeneic BMT in acute leukaemia is around 50%. Upto 30% succumb to procedure-related morbidity (e.g. graft versus host disease etc.) and in rest 20%, the disease relapses.

Graft versus host disease (GVHD): The GVHD and interstitial pneumonitis are causes of concern in BMT because they may cause serious morbidity and mortality. GVHD is due to cytotoxic activity of donor T lymphocytes which become sensitized to their new host considering it as foreign. The GVHD may be acute or chronic.

Acute GVHD: It occurs usually after 2-3 weeks of transplantation but may be delayed (upto 60 days). It may involve skin, liver and gut, may vary from mild to lethal disease. It appears to be associated with infection, but the cause of association is unknown. Various agents used to prevent it includes methotrexate, cyclosporine, ATG, high doses of steroids and T cell depletion of donor marrow. The more severe disease is very difficult to control but high doses of corticosteroids may be useful.

Chronic GVHD: This may occur independently or may follow acute disease described above. It has late onset (few weeks to few months). Its manifestations resemble a connective tissue disorder, although in mild cases, a rash may be the only presenting feature. Chronic GVHD is treated with *steriods*. Cyclosporine can be used in association with steriods.

2. **Autologous bone marrow transplantation—peripheral blood stem cell transplantation:**
   In autologous bone marrow transplantation, the patient's own marrow is harvested and frozen, to be given back again after achieving a good remission with intensive chemotherapy. It is indicated in patients of acute leukaemia in whom good or complete remission has been achieved with chemotherapy and acceptable HLA-matched donor is not available for allogeneic BMT. This procedure carries a lower-mortality rate than the allogeneic BMT but the greatest disadvantage of this procedure is high relapse rate (50%). Autologous bone marrow transplantation in acute leukaemia is better than chemotherpay alone.

Stem cells for transplantation were originally obtained by harvesting them from the bone marrow. Recently, they have been collected from the peripheral blood during recovery phase following a period of chemotherapy induced marrow hypoplasia. The dose of stem cell collected from the peripheral blood is much greater than that of harvested from the marrow, hence, making *stem cell transplantation* easier and a reduction in transplant-related mortality to less than 10% in patients under 55 years of age.

Prognosis: Without treatment, the median survival rate of patients with acute leukaemia is about 3 weeks. Median survival for ALL patients is about 2 years and for AML patients about one year if remission is achieved. The poor prognostic features in acute leukaemia are given in Box 62.6.

> **Box 62.6: Poor prognostic factors in acute leukaemia**
> - Increasing age
> - High leucocyte count at the time of diagnosis
> - CNS involvement in ALL at diagnosis
> - Male sex
> - Cytogenetic abnormalities
> - Presence of Philadelphia chromosome in ALL

Chapter 63

Blood Transfusion Related Complications

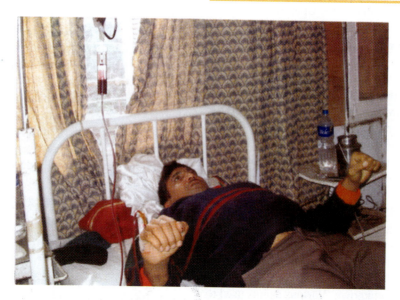

Fig. 63.1: Blood transfusion reaction. Patient developed chills and rigors following blood transfusion

BLOOD TRANSFUSION RELATED COMPLICATIONS

The study of red cells (RBCs) antigens and antibodies directed against them forms the basis of transfusion medicine. The cells and proteins in the blood express antigens which are controlled by polymorphic genes i.e. a specific antigen may be present in one individual but not in others. A blood transfusion may immunise the recipient against the donor antigens as the recipient does not have that antigen called *alloimmunisation* and antibodies produced in recipient are called *alloantibodies*. Repeated blood transfusions increase the risk of alloimmunisation.

Antibodies directed against RBCs antigens may result from natural exposure (food and bacteria), called autoantibodies; are of IgM type. These antibodies are often insignificant clinically due to the low affinity for antigens at body temperature. However, these IgM antibodies can activate complement cascade and result in haemolysis. On the other hand, antibodies that result from allogenic exposure such as transfusion or pregnancy are

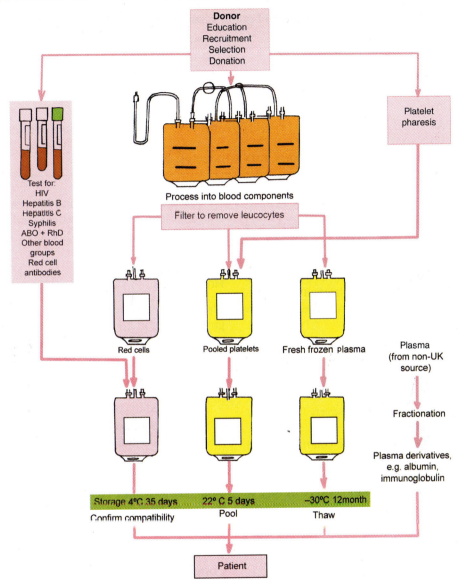

Fig. 63.2: Blood donation (collection), processing and storage

usually of IgG type. The IgG antibodies commonly bind to antigens at warmer temperature and may haemolyse RBCs. Unlike IgM, the IgG antibodies can cross placenta and bind fetal RBCs having the corresponding antigen, resulting in *haemolytic disease of the newborn or hydrops fetalis.*

Alloimmunisation to leucocytes, platelets and plasma proteins may also result in transfusion complications such as fever and urticaria but generally do not cause haemolysis.

Therefore complications resulting from the blood transfusions may be immunological (alloimmunisation, incompatibility) and nonimmunological such as transmission of infection, volume overload, iron overload, bleeding, electrolyte changes, thrombophlebitis and air embolism.

Haematology

Box 63.1: RBC blood group systems and alloantigens

Group	Anigens	Alloantibody	Reactions
Rh (D, C/c, E/e)	RBC protein	IgG	HTR, HDN
Lweis (Le^a, Le^b)	Oligosacharride	IgM/IgG	Rare HTR
Kell (K/k)	RBC protein	IgG	HTR, HDN
Duffy	-do-	-do-	-do-
Kidd	-do-	-do-	HTR (often delayed) HDN (mild)

HTR = Haemolytic transfusion reaction, HDN = Haemolytic disease of new-born

Blood Groups

The blood groups are determined by antigens on the surface of RBCs. The ABO and Rh systems are important blood groups but incompatibilities involving many other blood groups (such as Lewis, Kell, Duffy, Kidd), may cause haemolytic transfusion reactions and/or haemolytic disease of new born (see Box 63.1).

ABO System

This is most important system because naturally occurring IgM anti-A and anti-B antibodies are capable of producing rapid and severe haemolysis of incompatible RBCs.

The ABO system is under the control of a pair of allelic genes H and h, and also three allelic genes, A, B and O, producing the genotype and phenotypes given in the Table 63.1. The A, B and H antigens are very similar in structure. The H gene codes for enzyme H which attaches fructose to the basic glycoprotein backbone to form H substance which is precursor for A and B antigens.

The A and B genes control specific enzymes responsible for the addition of H substance for group A and B. The O gene is amorphic and does not transform H substance and therefore O is not antigenic. The A, B and H antigens are present on most body cells, tissue fluids (saliva and gastric juice).

Rh System

The Rh system is the second most important blood group system in pretransfusion setting because of the high frequency of development of IgG RhD antibodies in Rh-negative individuals after exposure to RhD-positive red cells following blood transfusions or during pregnancy

The antibodies (anti-D alloantibody) formed are of major importance in causing HDN and HTR. About 85% people are Rh-positive in a population. The system is coded by two allelic antigen pairs E/e and C/c while the third pair is D (called RhD positive) and no D (RhD-negative). The three Rh genes E/e, D and C/c are arranged in tendem on chromosome I and inherited as a halotype cDE or Cde.

Complications of Blood Transfusion

The adverse effects of blood transfusion or complications of blood transfusion are tabulated

Table 63.1: Antigen and antibodies in ABO system in order of frequency

Phenotype	Genotype	Antigens	Antibodies
O (46%)	OO	None	Anti-A and Anti-B
A (42%)	AA or AO	A	Anti-B
B (90%)	BB or BO	B	Anti-A
AB (3%)	AB	A and B	None

Blood Transfusion Related Complications

Table 63.2: Complications of blood transfusion

1. *Immunological*
   i. Alloimmunisation
   ii. Incompatibility
      a. Red cells
         - Immediate haemolytic transfusion reactions (HTR)
         - Delayed haemolytic transfusion reactions
      b. Leucocytes and platelets
         - Nonhaemolytic (fibrile) transfusion reactions
         - Post-transfusion purpura
         - Poor survival of transfused platelets and granulocytes
         - Graft vs host disease
      c. Plasma proteins
         - Urticaria and anaphylactic reactions
2. *Nonimmunological*
   i. Transmission of infection
      - Transmisson of infection e.g. hepatitis (B, C, D), HIV, other viruses (CMV, EBV, HTLV-1)
      - Parasites e.g. malaria, trypanosomiasis, toxoplasmosis
      - Transfusion of blood contaminated with bacteria
   ii. Volume overload (hypervolaemia)
   iii. Iron overload due to multiple transfusions
   iv. Bleeding and electrolyte changes: Massive transfusion of stored blood may cause bleeding and electrolyte changes
   v. Thrombophlebitis
   vi. Air embolism

(Table 63.2). These reactions though rare but can be fatal. About 50% of the fatalities associated with blood transfusion are due to immediate haemolytic transfusion reactions; the remainder are mainly due to post-transfusion hepatitis.

Diagnosis and Management

I. Immunological

Transfusion reactions may result from immune and nonimmune mechanisms. Immune reactions (immediate or delayed) are often due to preformed donor or recipients antibodies. However, cellular elements (RBC, platelets and leucocytes) and plasma proteins may also cause adverse reactions. These are:

A. ***Alloimmunisation:*** All transfusions carry a risk of immunisation to the many antigens present on RBCs, leucocytes, platelets and plasma proteins. Alloimmunisation does not cause clinical problems with first transfusion, but subsequent transfusions may result in transfusion reactions such as HDN and rejection of tissue transplants (graft vs host disease).

B. ***Acute haemolytic transfusion reactions:*** These occur when the recipient has preformed antibodies that lyse the donor RBCs. These are due to incompatible blood transfusions (ABO system) that result in poor survival of RBCs. This is most serious acute complication of blood transfusion. There is complement activation by antigen and antibody reaction usually due to IgM antibodies.

Clinical Features
- Rigors, chills, fever (Fig. 63.1 on front page).
- Acute lumbar pain or chest pain.
- Tachypnoea, tachycardia, hypotension.
- Haemoglobinuria.
- Acute renal failure.
- Activation of coagulation may occur; bleeding due to DIC is bad prognostic sign.

Diagnosis

The diagnosis is confirmed by finding an evidence of haemolysis (e.g. haemoglobinuria) and incompatibility between donor and recipient. All documentations should be checked to locate the error such as:
- Sample taken from a wrong patient.
- Mislabelling of the blood sample (patient's name on the sample is not correct).
- Labelling or handling error in the laboratory
- Failure to perform proper identity checks before the blood is transfused i.e. blood transfused to a wrong patient. The blood grouping of the patient's sample (sent for compatibility test), a new sample taken from the patient after reaction and the donor units should be checked to confirm whether error has taken

place. This is a serious matter, needs meticulous checks at all stages in the procedure of blood transfusion. The laboratory tests for haemolysis are raised indirect bilirubin, LDH levels and low serum hepatoglobin and haemoglobinuria.

Treatment
- At the first instance of any suspicion, the transfusion should be stopped and the donor unit returned to the blood bank laboratory with a new blood sample from the patient to exclude a haemolytic transfusion reaction (HTR).
- The immune complexes that result in RBCs lysis can precipitate acute renal failure. Diuresis should be induced using frusemide or mannitol with intravenous fluids.
- Tissue factor released from the lysed erythrocytes can initiate DIC. Coagulation profile such as PT, APTT, fibrinogen and platelet count should be monitored in patients with haemolytic reaction, if develops, treated accordingly (Read chapter on DIC).
- Monitoring the patient's vital signs before and during transfusion reaction is important to identify these reactions properly.
- Additional RBCs transfusion may be necessary to treat falling hematocrit.

C. *Delayed haemolytic reactions*
This may occur in patients alloimmunised by previous transfusion or pregnancies. The antibody level is too low to be detected by pre-transfusion compatibility testing but a secondary immune response occurs after transfusion, resulting in delayed haemolysis usually by IgG antibody.

Clinical Features
- Patient develops anaemia and jaundice about a week after transfusion due to an extravascular haemolysis.
- Most patients are clinically silent.
- The blood film shows spherocytosis and reticulocytosis.
- Direct antiglobulin test is positive.

Treatment
- No specific therapy is usually required, although additional RBCs transfusion may be necessary to treat falling haematocrit.
- A good transfusion history by the clinician can lower the risk. If the patient has had past transfusion or cross matching difficulties, the blood bank may be able to locate the problem.

D. *Febrile nonhaemolytic transfusion reaction*
Febrile reactions are a common complication of blood transfusion in patients who have previously been transfused or pregnant. The usual cause is the presence of leucocytes antibodies in the recipient against the transfused leucocytes leading to release of pyrogens. These reactions are characterised by mild fever (> 38°C), chills and rigors, flushing and tachycardia. Analgesic may be needed to reduce fever, and blood transfusion should be stopped. Febrile reactions may be prevented further by the use of leucocyte-depleted blood in such patients.

E. *Transfusion-related acute lung injury:* Potent leucocyte antibody in the plasma of donors who are usually multiparous women, may cause severe pulmonary reactions called *transfusion-related acute lung injury* characterised by fever, cough, dyspnoea, haemoptysis and shadowing in perihilar and lower lung fields on the chest X-ray. Treatment is supportive. Patient usually recover without sequelae. Testing the donor's plasma for anti-HLA antibodies can support the diagnosis.

Allergic (Urticaria) and Anaphylactic (Systemic Anaphylaxis) Reactions

a. *Urticarial (allergic) reactions* characterised by pruritic rash, oedema, headache, dizziness are often attributed to plasma proteins incompatibility, but in most cases, they are unexplained. They are common but rarely severe.

Mild reactions may be treated symptomatically by temporarily stopping the transfusion and administration of chlorpheniramine 10 mg I.V. The transfusion may be completed after the signs and/or symptoms resolve. Patients with history of allergic reactions to blood should be premedicated with an antihistamine. Cellular components can be washed to remove residual plasma for extremely sensitized patient.

b. *Anaphylaxis* is a severe reaction, presents after transfusion of only a few milliliters of blood component. Symptoms and signs include difficulty in breathing, acute bronchospasm (wheezing), hypotension, shock, loss of consciousness and respiratory arrest.

Treatment of anaphylaxis include:
- The transfusion should be stopped.
- Adrenaline (0.5 mg I.M. or S.C. 1:1000 dilution) with chlorpheniramine 10 mg I.V. stat. Steriods may be used in severe cases.
- Endotracheal intubation and maintain vascular access in severe cases.

Prevention: Prevention of allergic reactions, include: Patients who are IgA deficient may be sensitized to this Ig class and are at risk of developing this reaction associated with plasma transfusion. Individuals with severe IgA-deficient should receive only IgA deficient plasma and washed cellular blood components. Therefore, patients who have anaphylactic or repeated allergic reactions to blood components should be tested for IgA-deficiency.

Post-transfusion purpura: This reaction presents as thrombocytopenia 7 to 10 days after platelet transfusion and occurs predominantly in females and is related to presence of platelet-specific antibody in the recipient's serum, and the most frequently recognised antigen in HPA-Ia found on the glucoprotein IIIa receptor. This delayed thrombocytopenia is due to production of antibodies that react to both donor and recipient platelets. Additional platelet transfusions may worsen the thrombocytopenia and should be avoided. Treatment with I.V. immunoglobulin may neutralise the offending antibodies, or plasmapheresis can be used to remove the antibodies if needed.

II. Non-immunological Reactions

a. *Volume overload:* Blood components are volume expanders, can lead to volume overload on rapid transfusion. Monitoring the rate and volume of transfusion along with the administration of a diuretic can reduce this complication.

b. *Iron overload*: Each unit of RBC contain 200-250 mg of iron. Iron overloading is rare, affects various organ systems i.e. endocrine, hepatic and heart commonly after 100 units of transfusion. Alternative therapy to blood transfusion i.e. erythropoietin is preferable if large amount is needed to be transfused.

c. *Hypothermia:* Blood components stored in refrigeration (4°C) or frozen (-18°C or below) can result in hypothermia when rapidly transfused. Cardiac arrhythmias can result due to exposure of SA node to cold fluid. Use of an in line warmer will prevent this complication.

d. *Hyperkalaemia and hypocalcaemia:* RBCs leakage during storage increases the plasma concentration of K+ in the unit. Neonates and patients of renal failure are at high risk of hyperkalaemia. Citrated blood transfusions can lead to hypocalcaemia because citrate chelates the calcium.

e. *Infections:* Include transmission of hepatitis, HIV, syphilis, malaria etc.

Part Seven

Endocrinology and Metabolism

Chapter 64

Diabetic Ketoacidosis (Diabetic Coma)

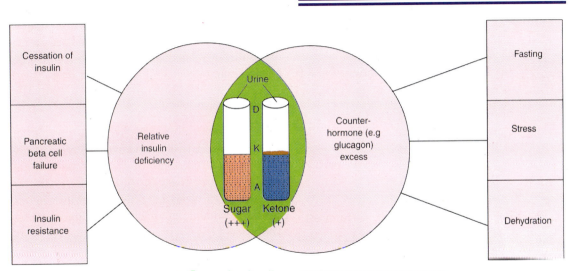

Fig. 64.1: Concepts of pathogenesis of diabetic ketoacidosis

DIABETIC KETOACIDOSIS (ACUTE DIABETIC COMA)

Definition

It is a metabolic complication of diabetes in which hyperglycaemia is associated with metabolic acidosis due to markedly raised (>5 mmol/L) ketone levels. It is a dire medical emergency and remains a serious cause of morbidity and mortality if left untreated principally in type I diabetics. It can occur in both types of diabetes mellitus but commoner in type I and rare in type II.

Pathophysiology (Figs 64.1 and 64.2)

The concept of pathogenesis of diabetic ketoacidosis is depicted in Figure 64.1.

It is often caused by cessation of insulin intake or inadequate insulin dosage in established type I diabetics, but it may result from physical (infection, surgery) or emotional stress despite continued insulin therapy. In the former case, there is rise of glucagon due to insulin insufficiency/withdrawal; while in stress, the stimulus for glucagon release is epinephrine. These hormonal changes have following effects:

346 Endocrinology and Metabolism

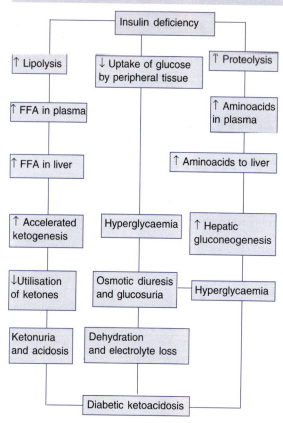

Fig. 64.2: Pathophysiology of diabetic ketoacidosis

Box 64.1: Precipitating factors for diabetic ketoacidosis

- Infections (pneumonia, UTI, gastroenteritis, sepsis)
- Alcohol intake
- Acute vascular episodes (cerebral, coronary, peripheral)
- Acute MI
- Trauma
- Drugs e.g. steriods, thiazides
- Surgery
- Emotional stress
- Pancreatitis
- Ignorance about the disease
- Poverty, unemployment

1. They induce neoglucogenesis and impair peripheral utilisation of glucose leading to severe hyperglycaemia (Fig. 64.2).
2. They activate the ketogenic process and thus initiate the development of metabolic ketoacidosis. For ketosis to occur, there is increased levels of free fatty acids in the plasma which are transported to liver for oxidation and conversion to ketones bodies (Fig. 64.2).

The overproduction of ketones by the liver is the primary event of ketoacidosis in addition to hyperglycaemia in diabetic ketoacidosis. Dehydration results due to osmotic diuresis.

Precipitating Factors

As diabetic ketoacidosis results primarily due to deficiency of insulin, hence, patient may present with diabetic ketoacidosis straightway without any knowledge of being diabetic. Otherwise, in patients of type I diabetics, it results either due to cessation of insulin or inadequate dosage of insulin. The precipitating factors are given in Box 64.1.

Clinical Features

Diabetic ketoacidosis (DKA) is the presenting feature in about 10% of undiagnosed cases. They are brought in the state of coma to the hospital where the diagnosis is confirmed. A similar proportion of cases may also develop it spontaneously without any precipitating illness/cause. The onset of DKA is insidious occurring over hours or days. *The triad of type I diabetes "polyuria, polydipsia, polyphagia"* is characteristic due to hyperglycaemia and osmotic diuresis. Unique feature of DKA is that patient is dehydrated in the presence of excessive thirst. Weakness, lethargy, headache, myalgia are nonspecific symptoms. About 25% of patients of DKA present with *GI symptoms* such as vomiting (coffee ground in appearance) and abdominal pain which may be mistaken for *acute abdomen (acute appendicitis)* and even operated upon. No patient is to be subjected to surgery without urine examination. The pain in abdomen is related to acidosis, is due to pooling of fluid in the intestinal tract. Ileus is due to temporary autonomic neuropathy, electrolyte disturbance and hyperglucagonaemia. Vomiting in DKA is an ominous sign. The respiratory symptoms include dyspnoea and deep rapid respiration. The *CNS* symptoms include weakness, altered mental status, drowsiness and eventually coma. This is due to dehydration, hypotension and increased plasma osmolarity.

Physical Signs

1. There is *tachypnoea, tachycardia* and *low body temperature (hypothermia)*. These are due to acidosis which stimulates the respiratory centre (tachypnoea) and causes vasodilatation (tachycardia) and hypothermia (low body temperature).
2. *Signs of dehydration* (e.g. dry tongue, mucous membrane and skin, soft eyeballs, sunken cheeks) and hypotension or shock (cold clammy skin, oliguria and obtunded consciousness).
3. *Kussmaul breathing*, a deep and rapid respiration is due to metabolic acidosis.
4. *Acetone smell* (like 'pear drops' or nail varnish remover) is due to hyperketonaemia.
5. There may be *hypotonia, hyperreflexia* and *incoordinated ocular movements*.
6. *Obtunded consciousness, stupor or coma*. The deterioration of consciousness is proportional to plasma osmolarity which is calculated as = 2 (Na + k) + glucose / 18 plus urea ÷ 6

The normal osmolality is 280–300 mOsm/kg

Consciousness is disturbed when it is high as follows:

- 314 mOsm/kg produces drowsiness
- 340 mOsm/kg produces semicoma
- 370 mOsm/kg produces coma

Investigations

The characteristic metabolic abnormalities diagnostic of DKA are depicted in Box 64.2.

Diagnosis and Differential Diagnosis

The diagnosis of DKA in a patient known to have type I diabetes is not difficult, but has to be differentiated in a patient who is not known to be diabetic.

Box 64.2: Biochemical features of DKA

Increased (↑)	Decreased (↓)
• Blood glucose	• Serum sodium
• Plasma ketone	• Serum potassium but can be normal
• Plasma osmolality	• Serum magnesium
• Haematocrit	• Bicarbonate
• WBC count	• PCO_2
• Blood urea	
• Serum FFA and triglycerides	

The DKA has to be differentiated from CVA, hypoglycaemia and hyperosmolar coma due to altered mental status (coma). Uraemia and alcohol poisoning have to be differentiated because of presence of metabolic acidosis.

Gastroenteritis has to be differentiated because of nausea, vomiting and signs of dehydration in DKA.

The first step in diagnosis is to test the urine for glucose and ketones (Fig. 64.1). If urine is negative for ketone, another cause for the acidosis is likely. If it is positive, plasma glucose examination is required to be certain. Hyperglycaemia and ketonuria confirm the diagnosis of DKA (a strongly positive urine dipstick for glucose and ketone—Fig. 64.1).

The ketones may be tested by semiquantitative methods (by using a reagent strip in serial dilutions of the plasma. Undiluted plasma may give a strongly positive result when starvation alone is the problem while a strong reaction in dilution exceeding 1:1 is a presumptive evidence of ketoacidosis. The causes and diagnosis of ketonuria are given in Box 64.3.

Complications of DKA

1. Cerebral oedema.
2. Acute respiratory distress syndrome.

Endocrinology and Metabolism

Box 64.3: Differential diagnosis of ketonuria

Causes of ketonuria	Diagnosis
• Diabetic ketoacidosis	Hyperglycaemia with ketonaemia/ketonuria
• Starvation	Low glucose, normal bicarbonate
• Alcoholic ketoacidosis	Normal blood glucose or mildly elevated glucose, history of alcoholism
• Salicylate poisoning	Elevated serum salicylate levels

Box 64.4: Average loss of fluid and electrolyte in adult DKA of moderate severity

- Water 6L. About half of the deficit (3L) is in intracellular volume and remaining half is in extracellular volume
- Sodium 500 mmol
- Potassium 350 mmol
- Chloride 400 mmol

3. Thromboembolism.
4. Disseminated intravascular coagulation.
5. Acute circulatory failure.

Management

Principles of Treatment

1. Replacement of fluid loss to correct dehydration and hyperosmolality.
2. Correction of electrolytes especially Na^+ and K^+.
3. Identification and correction of a precipitating cause.
4. Correction of hyperglycaemia with insulin and fluid replacement.
5. Close monitoring of the patient by laboratory parameters (e.g. plasma glucose, urea, electrolytes, arterial pH and bicarbonate) at an interval of 1-2 hours initially until the patient's condition stabilizes.

A. Management of DKA in Adults

Fluids and Electrolyte

The average loss of fluid and electrolyte in moderately severe diabetic ketoacidosis in an adult in shown in Box 64.4.

Adequate tissue perfusion is necessary for insulin to act. An intravenous infusion of isotonic (0.9%) saline should be started after taking blood sample for laboratory analysis. The treatment schedule is given in the Table 64.1.

Insulin

Rapid acting (soluble) insulin is used either intravenously or intramuscularly (see the Table 64.1). An initial bolus dose of 0.15 unit/kg of insulin is given I.V. followed by 0.1 unit/kg/hour infusion. If used intramuscular, then given 20 U insulin stat than 6 U/hour.

Other Considerations

- Continuous gastric aspiration if patient is in coma.
- If no urine is passed within 4 hours, then catheterize.
- Give an antibiotic early in case of infection or if an invasive procedure is used.
- Give oxygen if PaO_2 is < 80 mmHg.
- Start glucose replacing normal saline when blood glucose drops to < 250 mg/dl.
- Potassium replacement is done depending on the serum concentration of K^+ and monitoring is done by the ECG (Table 64.1).
- The controversy of bicarbonate therapy in DKA is resolved and HCO_3 is given depending on the pH. A blood pH < 7.0 is an indication for bicarbonate administration.

Response to Treatment

Two points must be emphasised while monitoring the response to treatment:

1. The plasma glucose level invariably falls more rapidly than the plasma ketone level; it may be possible that plasma glucose is approaching normal but ketone bodies are still present. Therefore, insulin administration should not be

Diabetic Ketoacidosis (Diabetic Coma)

Table 64.1: Diabetic ketoacidosis management in an adult

Treatment		Hours of therapy					Comment
		I	II	III	IV	V	
1. Fluid							250-500 ml over next 4 hours. If Na+ is > 145 mEq/L, and the patient is not hypotensive, half normal saline (0.45%) should be given
• Normal saline (0.9%)		1000 ml	1000 ml	500 to 1000 ml	500 to 1000 ml	250 to 500 ml	
2. Rapid acting regular insulin (soluble)	I.V. infusion	10 units stat, 5-10 units/hour					Double the dose of insulin 1-2 hourly if < 10% drop (e.g. 60-70 mg%) in glucose or no improvement in anion gap or pH
	I.M. dose	20 units stat	6U	6U	6U	6 U	Reduce when glucose is < 250 mg% and progressive improvement in anion gap or pH
3. Start of 5% dextrose		Start only when blood glucose drops to < 250 mg/dl (replacing normal saline)					Run 5% dextrose, 150-250 ml/hr with adequate insulin (5-10 U/hourly I.V. or I.M.) to keep glucose between 150-200 mg/dl until metabolic control is achieved (pH = 7.3 and $HCO_3 > 15$ mEq/L)
4. Potassium infusion		• 40 mEq over an hour if K+ < 3.0 mEq/L • 30 mEq over an hour if K+ is 3-4 mEq/L • 20 mEq over an hour if K+ is 4-5 mEq/L • Stop infusion if K+ is > 5 mEq/L N.B. to be given in 500 ml of normal saline over 1 hour					• Use ECG monitoring throughout as a guide to K+ therapy • Keep K+ between 4-5 mEq/L • Ensure the patient has good urine output
5. Bicarbonate administration		• If pH > 7.0. No bicarbonate • If pH 6.9-7.0, 46 mmol (one ampoule) in 200 ml water for injection • If pH < 6.9, then 89 mmol/2 ampoule in 400 ml of water for injection					• Infuse at 200 ml/hr, repeated with 15 mEq KCl every 2 hours until pH is >7.0
6. Phosphate therapy		If serum phosphate < 1.0 mg/dl, give phosphate otherwise not indicated					• Give 20-30 mEq/L of potassium phosphate in replacement fluid

stopped because glucose concentration is approaching normal, rather, as mentioned above, glucose should be started with insulin replacing normal saline until the ketosis has disappeared which may take few days.

2. As discussed above, plasma ketone values are not very helpful in assessing clinical response.
3. The key parameters of accurate assessment to response is the pH and the calculated anion gap.

All patients should be followed by maintaining a chart outlining the amount and timing of insulin and fluids together with a record of vital signs, urine output and blood biochemistry. Without such a record, therapy tends to become chaotic.

Continue with regimen until fluid deficit replaced, ketonuria abolished and adequate oral intake of carbohydrate feasible. Now the patient can be shifted to his old regimen of insulin again by monitoring of glucose and adjustment of meals.

Treatment of Precipitating Factors

Precipitating causes of DKA should be searched for in each and every case and appropriate measures taken to treat them. Education of the patient is an important aspect for insulin therapy. Since infection is the most common precipitating cause, routine antibiotic therapy is sufficient. Treatment of underlying or precipitating illness such as CVA, AMI, trauma or stress, if present.

Endocrinology and Metabolism

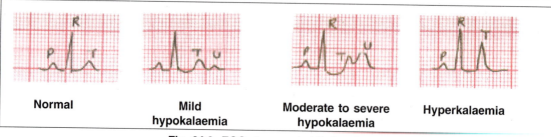

Fig. 64.3: ECG changes in K+ disturbance

Table 64.2: DKA management in children

Treatment	Hours of therapy						Comments
		I	II	III	IV	V	
Normal saline (0.9%)			As required based on the degree of dehydration and required speed of rehydration				
Rapid acting insulin	I.V. infusion	0.1 U/kg/hr					Reduce when glucose is < 250 mg/dl and progressive improvement in anion gap/pH
	I.M if no I.V. access	0.1 U/kg	0.1 U/kg	0.1 U/kg	0.1 U/kg		
5% dextrose		Start only when blood glucose drops to < 250 mg/dl replacing normal saline					Change to 5% dextrose with 0.45% NaCl at a rate to complete rehydration in 48 hours and maintain plasma glucose between 150-250 mg/dl (10% dextrose with electrolytes may be required)
Potassium infusion		• K+ < 2.5 mEq/L					• Administer 10 mEq/L of KCl I.V. over one hour
		• K+ 2.5 - 3.5 mEq/L					• Administer KCl (40-60 mEq/L I.V. solution until K is > 3.5 mEq)
		• K+ 3.5-5.5 mEq/L					• Administer KCl (30-40 mEq/L) in I.V. solution to maintain serum K+ at 3.5-5.5 mEq/L
		• K+ > 5.5 mEq/L					• Do not give I.V. potassium. Monitor K+ hourly until K+ is < 5.5 mEq/L
Bicarbonate		• pH < 7.0					• Repeat pH after initial rehydration. Bolus dose of NaHCO$_3$ (2mEq/Kg) added to 0.45% NaCl over one hour
		• pH > 7.0					• No HCO$_3$ therapy is indicated

Treatment of Complications

In children, cerebral oedema is common cause of death, can be treated by bolus infusion of 1g mannitol/kg of body weight in the form of 20% solution or intravenous dexamethasone 8 to 12 mg initially, then 4 mg every 6 hours.

B. Management of DKA in Children (Table 64.2)

Use ECG (Fig. 64.3) as a guide to therapy. Check glucose and electrolytes every 2-4 hourly until they become stable.

Prevention

Diabetic ketoacidosis can be an initial presentation in a child, therefore, physician should be alert if a child presents with dehydration, fever, hyperventilation or drowsiness or polyuria and polydypsia.

- Type I diabetic during sick period should be managed properly with periodic review of glucose and ketones.
- Use supplemental short-acting insulin during stress.
- Treat infection with antibiotic cover. Adjust the dose of the insulin during infection as insulin requirement rises during infection.
- Insulin should not be stopped even if the child refuses to take usual diet. A palatable liquid diet containing carbohydrates and salt may be given along with insulin and adequate fluid intake. If child does not retain fluid, it is advisable to shift the child to a hospital.
- Check urine ketone whenever blood glucose is > 300 mg/dl.

Hyperosmolar Hyperglycaemic Non-Ketotic Coma (HHNKC)

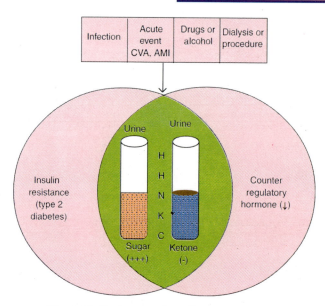

Fig. 65.1: Pathogenesis and diagnosis of HHNKC

HYPEROSMOLAR HYPERGLYCAEMIC NON-KETOTIC COMA (HHNKC)

Definition

Hyperosmolar hyperglycaemic non-ketotic coma is an acute metabolic decompensation of the diabetic state in **type 2 diabetic**s, characterised by extreme hyperglycaemia (blood glucose > 600 mg/dl) and increased osmolality (> 320 mOsm/kg) without significant ketosis or acidosis.

Aetiology: The patients of type 2 DM prone to develop it include:

1. Type 2 diabetes detected for the first time (undiagnosed diabetics).
2. Middle aged or older diabetics (> 50 years of age).
3. Those living alone.
4. Those with no access to medical treatment.
5. Those with associated infection or stroke.

Hyperosmolar Hyperglycaemic Non-Ketotic Coma (HHNKC)

Precipitating illness/factors: Certain illnesses/factors precipitating HHNKC in known type 2 diabetics are:

- Acute infections, burns, trauma.
- Vascular episode (CVA or AMI).
- Alcohol excess or excessive consumption of beverages.
- Hyperalimentation.
- Drugs e.g. thiazides, steroids, phenytoin, chlorpromazine, diazoxide, immunosuppressive, sympathomimetics, beta-blockers, calcium channel blockers etc.
- Recurrent vomiting.
- Dialysis (peritoneal or haemodialysis) in a patient with uraemia.
- Use of osmotic agents (e.g. mannitol).

Pathogenesis (Fig. 65.1)

Hyperosmolar hyperglycaemic nonketotic coma (HHNKC) is a known and dreadful complication of type 2 diabetes. It is a syndrome of profound dehydration produced by persistent sustained hyperglycaemia which is more than DKA, results in profuse osmotic diuresis (fluid loss or dehydration) which the patient is not able to compensate by drinking enough water to keep up with urinary fluid losses. The dehydration results in further rise in blood sugar. The patients who are prone to develop the syndrome are elderly diabetics living either alone or in a nursing home or develop a stroke or infection that worsens further hyperglycaemia and prevents adequate water intake. The full blown picture usually develops when urine output falls considerably. Loss of total body water relative to total body sodium is greater resulting in hyperosmolality.

Absence of ketosis is due to higher levels of endogenous insulin reserve (type 2 diabetics have insulin resistance with some insulin reserve), inhibition of lipolysis by the hyperosmolar state, lower levels of counter-regulatory hormones and free fatty acids than in DKA and there is an associated glucagon resistance.

Coma is due to hyperosmolar state induced by severe dehydration and hyperglycaemia. Plasma osmolality > 340 mOsm/kg is associated with obtunded consciousness progressing to coma.

Clinical Features

The features of HHNKC evolves over several days to weeks. The patient may have polyuria, polydipsia and polyphagia for days and weeks with vomiting, dehydration and weakness prior to development of drowsiness or coma. As the syndrome progresses, the important protective measure i.e. thirst is impaired due to depression of thirst centre in hypothalamus by hyperosmolality or hyperglycaemia. Other CNS features include seizural activity—some time Jacksonian in type, myoclonic jerks, transient hemiplegia and transient visual symptoms (hemianopia). Infections, particularly pneumonia and gram-negative septicaemia are common and indicative of grave prognosis. Bleeding probably caused by disseminated intravascular coagulation (DIC) and acute pancreatitis may occur.

The physical findings include, tachycardia, signs of dehydration, rapid shallow respiration (in contrast to deep laboured breathing in DKA), hypotension or shock, altered mental status (drowsiness or coma).

Investigations

They are given in Box 65.1.

Box 65.1: Laboratory parameters in hyperosmolar hyperglycaemic nonketotic coma

Plasma glucose (mg/dl)	> 600
Arterial pH	> 7.30
Serum bicarbonate (mEq/L)	> 15
Effective serum osmolarity (mOsm/kg)	>320
Note: The effective serum osmolarity is calculated by = 2 × Na (mEq/L) + glucose divided by 18 (mg/dl)	
Anion gap ($Na^+ + K^+$) - ($Cl^- - HCO_3^-$)	20
Urine or serum ketone	Small or absent
Blood urea/creatinine	May be high
Serum sodium	Normal or high

Diagnosis and Differential Diagnosis

The diagnosis of HHNKC should be suspected in any elderly diabetic who presents with acute or subacute deterioration of CNS functions with profound dehydration. There may be an evidence of infection. Diagnosis is made by hyperglycaemia, hyperosmolality and mild acidosis without ketonuria or ketonaemia (Fig. 65.1). Prerenal azotaemia is present. The acidosis is mild without ketosis, is due to a combination of starvation, retention of inorganic acids secondary to renal hypoperfusion and elevation of plasma lactate (due to hypotension or shock).

The differences between two common types of coma i.e. DKA and HHNKC are tabulated (Table 65.1).

Management

As mortality rate in HHNKC is high (> 50%), hence immediate treatment is necessary.

Principles

1. Fluid replacement to correct dehydration.
2. Low or small doses of insulin to correct hyperglycaemia.
3. Correction of electrolytes (e.g. Na^+ and K^+).
4. Identification and correction of precipitating cause. Above all, frequent monitoring for glucose, pH, electrolytes, urea, creatinine is necessary.

1. ***Correction of dehydration by intravenous fluids:*** The most important measure is rapid infusion of large amounts of intravenous fluids to reestablish circulation and urine flow. The average fluid deficit is more (10-11L) as compared to DKA (6L only). While free water is ultimately needed because of hyperosmolar state, initial therapy still should be with isotonic (0.9%) saline and 2 to 3 litres should be given during first one to two hours. Subsequently, half-strength (0.45%) saline should be used. As the glucose level approaches normal, 5% dextrose can be given as a vehicle for free water. Hydration alone will often result in reversal of hyperosmolar coma and decreases plasma glucose. Fluid replacement should correct estimated deficits within first 24 hours. In patients with renal or cardiac compromise, monitoring of serum osmolality, and CVP monitoring must be performed during fluid replacement and to avoid unnecessary fluid overload.

Table 65.1 Differentiating features between DKA (diabetic ketoacidosis) and HHNKC (hyperosmolar hyperglycaemic nonketotic coma)

Feature	DKA	HHNKC
Age	Younger patients	Older patients
Type of DM	Common in type I	Common in type 2
Dehydration	Mild to moderate	Marked
Respiration	Kussmaul breathing	Shallow, rapid respiration
Consciousness	Diminished	Comatosed
Temperature	Normal or low	May be high
Blood glucose	> 250 mg/dl	> 600 mg/dl
Blood urea	Normal or slightly raised	Markedly raised
Sodium	Low to normal (125-140 mmol/L)	Normal to high (130-160 mmol/L)
Potassium	Low to normal (3-5.0 mEq/L)	Normal to high (4-6.0 mEq/L)
Bicarbonate	< 15 mmol/L	16-30 mmol/L
Ketones in blood	Marked (++ to +++)	Absent to minimal (+)
Osmolarity	High (300-380 mOsm/kg)	Very high (350-450 mOsm/kg)
Anion gap	40	20

2. ***Insulin therapy:*** Many authors recommend small doses of insulin as many patients are extremely hypersensitive to insulin and the glucose concentration may fall suddenly. However, insulin administration is similar to management of DKA. Regular insulin by continuous intravenous infusion is the treatment of choice. Once hypokalemia is excluded, an intravenous bolus dose of regular insulin (0.15 U/Kg) may be given followed by 0.1U/Kg/hour in adults until blood glucose comes to 300 mg%). When glucose concentration approaches 300 mg%, the dose of insulin is reduced to 0.05 to 0.1 U/kg/hour and dextrose (5%) may be added to the intravenous fluids. Thereafter maintenance state of glucose (around 250 mg%) is achieved by neutralization of glucose with insulin until patient become conscious and starts accepting orally.

3. ***Potassium replacement:*** Despite total body potassium deficit, mild to moderate hyperkalaemia is not uncommon in HHNKC. Insulin therapy and volume expansion decrease the K^+ concentration, hence, K^+ replacement is required early in the management than DKA. Once renal function is assured, K^+ may be given to prevent hypokalaemia. Potassium supplementation (20-30 mEq/L) may be initiated after serum levels fall below 5.0 mEq/L and urine output is good. This potassium supplementation is sufficient to maintain serum K^+ of 4-5 mEq/L.

4. ***Other supportive measures:*** These are similar to DKA (Read DKA). Seizures in HHNKC syndrome should not be taken as a manifestation of primary cortical pathology and unnecessary phenytoin may not be given. Treatment with phenytoin not only fails to relieve seizures which are due to hyperosmolality but worsen hyperglycaemia by impairing endogenous insulin release.

5. ***Identify the precipitating factors*** and efforts should be made to correct them to avoid future episodes.

6. ***Complications:*** All the complications are preventable.
   - *Hypoglycaemia.* This is most common complication of HHNKC due to overzealous administration of insulin as well as hypersensitivity to insulin.
   - *Hypokalaemia:* Potassium levels fall rapidly with fluid replacement and initiation of insulin; if not prevented or corrected early, may result in hypokalaemia which may induce cardiac arrhythmias.
   - *Hyperglycaemia.* It occurs secondary to interruption/discontinuance of intravenous insulin therapy after recovery without subsequent coverage with subcutaneous insulin.
   - *Cerebral oedema:* It is rare but frequently fatal. The exact pathogenesis is unknown but is attributed to sudden movement of water into CNS when plasma osmolality declines too rapidly with treatment. It is, therefore, necessary to replace Na+ and water deficits gradually and to add dextrose to infusion fluid as soon as blood glucose reaches between 250-300 mg%. These measures reduce the incidence of cerebral oedema.

Chapter 66

Hypoglycaemia

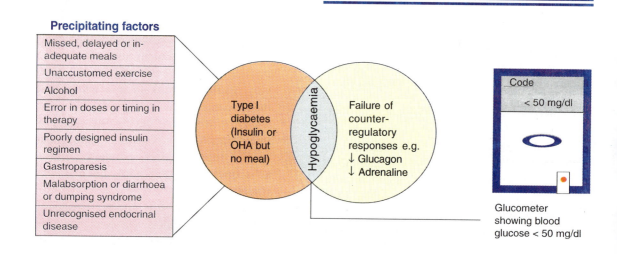

Fig. 66.1: Aetiopathogenesis and diagnosis of hypoglycaemia

HYPOGLYCAEMIA

Definition

It is defined as low blood sugar (< 50 mg%) or relatively low plasma glucose usually associated with symptoms of sympatetic overactivity and neuroglycopenia. According to DCCT (Diabetic Control and Complication Trial), hypoglycaemia is defined as an event or state resulting in seizures, confusion, coma and other neurological symptoms consistent with hypoglycaemia (e.g. sweating, palpitation, hunger or blurred vision) and fingerprick blood glucose less than 50 mg% and its amelioration by treatment that raises the blood glucose.

Hypoglycaemia is major hazard of insulin treatment and is also common with oral hypoglycaemia agents (OHA) especially in elderly. Neonatal hypoglycaemia in infants born to diabetic mothers is well-known.

Hypoglycaemia is a medical emergency requiring urgent management. Today, with advances in the management of diabetes and its complications, cases of hypoglycaemia progressing to coma and death are being seen rarely.

Occasionally, hypoglycaemia may be the presenting feature of an illness and is called spontaneous hypoglycaemia.

Hypoglycaemia

Aetiology

The most common cause of hypoglycaemia in diabetes is iatrogenic e.g. drug-induced; whereas spontaneous hypoglycaemia in non-diabetic population is due to multiple causes. The causes of hypoglycaemia in diabetics are summarized in Box 66.1 and illustrated in Fig. 66.1.

Box 66.1: Causes of iatrogenic hypoglycaemia in diabetics

- Missed or delayed meals
- Excess of insulin
- Sudden reduction in diet or more fasts
- Unaccustomed exercise
- Alcohol use
- Alimentary causes e.g. diarrhoea, malabsorption, diabetic gastroparesis
- Renal failure
- Change in drug therapy or insulin
- Error in doses and its timing
- Poorly planned treatment regimen
- Endocrinal causes e.g. Addison's disease, hypothyroidism
- Patient's causes e.g. unintelligent, uncooperative, poor, uneducated etc.

Spontaneous hypoglycaemia Spontaneous hypoglycaemia occurring in nondiabetic population is classified into (i) fasting and (ii) postprandial (reactive). The differences are summarised in Box 66.2.

The causes of fasting as well as postprandial hypoglycaemia are given in the Table 66.1.

Box 66.2: Differential diagnosis of spontaneous hypoglycaemia

Fasting	Postprandial (reactive)
• Low blood sugar occurs after hours of fasting	• Low blood sugar occurs in response to meals hence, called reactive
• It occurs usually in the presence of a disease (see the long list of causes)	• It usually occurs in the absence of disease i.e. normal population or associated with anxiety
• It occurs due to an imbalance between glucose production and utilisation in peripheral tissue	• The most common cause is alimentary hyperinsulinism

Table 66.1: Causes of fasting and postprandial hypoglycaemia

Fasting hypoglycaemia

I. *Primarily due to underproduction of glucose*
   A. Hormones deficiencies
      - Hypopituitarism
      - Adrenal insufficiency
      - Glucagon insufficiency
      - Catecholamine insufficiency
   B. Enzymatic defect
      - Glucose-6-phosphatase
      - Liver phosphorylase
      - Pyruvate carboxylase
      - Fructose 1-6 biphosphatase
   C. Substrate deficiency
      - Ketotic hypoglycaemia of infancy
      - Severe malnutrition
      - Late pregnancy
   D. Liver disesae
      - Severe hepatitis or cirrhosis
      - Hepatic congestion
   E. Drugs
      - Alcohol
      - Propranolol, salicylates

II. *Primarily due to overutilisation of glucose*
   A. Hyperinsulinism
      - Insulinoma
      - Exogenous insulin or sulphonylureas
      - Insulin-autoimmunity
   B. Inappropriate insulin levels
      - Extrapancreatic tumours
      - Systemic carnitine deficiency
      - Cachexia with fat depletion e.g. cancer

Postprandial hypoglycaemia

   A. Alimentary hyperinsulinism
      - Post gastrectomy
      - Post-gastrojejunostomy
      - Post-pyloroplasty
      - Post-vagotomy
   B. Hereditary fructose intolerance. It is a cause in children
   C. Galactosaemia—a cause in children.
   D. Leucine sensitivity—a cause in infants.
   E. Idiopathic
      - True
      - Pseudohypoglycaemia—occurs during stress or anxiety. It is also seen in certain chronic leukaemias when leucocytes count are markedly elevated, which utilise the glucose. This is usually asymptomatic

Counter-regulatory mechanisms: In response to a falling blood sugar, there is normally increased secretion of counter-regulatory hormones which antagonize the blood-glucose lowering effects of insulin. *Glucagon* and *adrenaline* are the most potent of these, hypoglycaemia-induced secretion of glucagon becomes impaired within 5 years of developing type I diabetes. Similarly after several years, the adrenaline response to hypoglycaemia also becomes defective; so that if hypoglycaemia develops, glucose recovery may be seriously compromised. Autonomic neuropathy may also contribute to defective adrenaline response. Those who develop deficient counter-regulatory responses may also have impaired central activation of neuroendocrine secretion. Failure of counter-regulatory mechanisms with impaired awareness of hypoglycaemia alter the glycaemic threshold for the onset of hormone secretion and symptoms in the affected patients i.e. blood glucose has to fall to a critical lower level to trigger these responses.

Clinical Features

The symptoms and signs of hypoglycaemia are given in Box 66.3, occurs due to:
1. *Autonomic overactivity* (sympathetic overactivity).
2. *Neuroglycopenia* as brain being the main utilizer of glucose.

In most instances, the patient has no difficulty in recognizing the symptoms of hypoglycaemia and can take appropriate timely measures. However, in certain circumstances (e.g. during sleep or during periods of strict glycaemic control) and in certain types of patients (e.g. patients with long duration of diabetes), warning symptoms are not always perceived by the patient even when awake, so that appropriate action is not taken and neuroglycopenia with reduced consciousness ensues. Occasionally, sudden death occurs during sleep in an otherwise healthy young type I diabetic ("dead-in-bed" syndrome), hypoglycaemia-induced cardiac arrhythmias or acute respiratory arrest with impaired baroreflex sensitivity has been proposed as the cause.

When blood sugar falls rapidly, adrenergic (sympathetic) symptoms predominate, but if the fall of blood sugar is gradual neuroglycopenic symptoms dominate.

Patients who have frequent episodes of hypoglycaemia may not experience the symptoms of hypoglycaemia until blood glucose is well below the 50 mg/dl level and they may usually present with serious neurological deficits. This phenomenon is termed as *hypoglycaemic unawareness*, seen in type I diabetics with long duration of diabetes, is reversible in the initial stages.

Reactive spontaneous hypoglycaemia as discussed earlier occurs in response to food (3-5 hours ingestion of food). True reactive hypoglycaemia occurs in non-diabetic patients who have undergone some sort of gastrointestinal surgery or suffer from some gastrointestinal disorders. Rapid gastric emptying with inappropriate insulin release is the proposed mechanism of hypoglycaemia in such patients.

Fasting hypoglycaemia e.g. during fasting state, indicates some underlying disease which results in either underproduction or overutilisation of glucose under the effect of insulin.

Diagnosis

If a person with diabetes mellitus presents with symptoms of hypoglycaemia, it is usually safe to conclude that no special diagnostic tests are needed to confirm it because such a hypoglycaemia is almost

Box 66.3: Symptoms and signs of hypoglycaemia

Sympathetic overactivity	Neuroglycopenia
• Palpitation	• Headache
• Sweating	• Fatigue
• Anxiety	• Impaired consciousness
• Tremors	• Dizziness
• Shivering	• Inappropriate behaviour
• Pallor	• Difficulty in speech
• Vomiting	• Confusion, drowsiness
	• Seizures
	• Focal neurological signs such as hemiplegia, amnesia
	• Coma

always therapy-induced (insulin or OHA induced). The only unequivocal test is demonstration of low blood sugar (< 50 mg %) during the episode.

If a nondiabetic develops similar symptoms particularly confusion, loss of consciousness or convulsions, then a diagnostic work-up is required as follows:

1. *Document hypoglycaemia* from finger-prick by glucometer or dextrostix and draw samples for glucose, insulin levels, C-peptide, ketones, liver function tests etc.
2. *Tests for spontaneous hypoglycaemia* (post-prandial): The only unequivocal diagnostic test is to document hypoglycaemia (< 50 mg%) during spontaneously developed symptoms.
   - A 5-hour oral glucose tolerance test showing a plasma glucose of 50 mg % or less is suggestive.
3. *Diagnostic tests for insulinoma:*
   - An insulin level of 20 µU/ml or more in the presence of blood glucose value below 40 mg/dl.
   - Elevated circulating proinsulin levels (C-peptide) differentiates between insulinoma and factitious hyperinsulinism (See Box 66.4).

> **Box 66.4: Diagnostic clues to factitious hypoglycaemia**
> - Low blood sugar
> - High immunoreactive insulin levels } This triad is pathognomonic
> - Low C-peptide level

   - C-peptide suppression test: Absence of suppression of C-peptide during hypoglycaemia induced by 0.1 ml of insulin/kg/hr is diagnostic. A normal person would suppress the peptide level to 50% or more during hypoglycaemia.
   - Insulin/glucose ratio > 0.4 suggest insulinoma. Normally this ratio is less than 0.4.

After recovery from the emergency situation, appropriate tests such as ultrasound, CT scan and MRI are done to arrive at the diagnosis and to locate the tumour (insulinoma) preoperatively.

Differential Diagnosis

The differences between hypoglycaemic coma and hyperglycaemic coma are tabulated in Table 66.2.

Table 66.2: Salient features of hypoglycaemic and hyperglycaemic coma

Feature	Hypoglycaemic coma	Hyperglycaemic coma
Pulse rate	Increased	Increased
Pulse volume	Good	Weak (low)
Temperature	May be low or normal	May be low
Respiration	Shallow or normal	Rapid and deep
BP	Normal, may be increased	Decreased
Skin and tongue	Moist	Dry
Breath	No acetone smell	Acetone smell may be present
Reflexes	Brisk	Diminished
Urine glucose	Negative	Positive
Plasma glucose	< 50 mg/dl	> 200 mg/dl
Plasma acetone	Negative	Usually present
Plasma HCO_3	Normal	< 20 mEq/L
PCO_2	Normal	Diminished
Blood pH	Normal	< 7.3

Management

Severe hypoglycaemia means as "hypoglycaemia requiring the assistance of another person for recovery", can result in serious morbidity and has a recognised mortality of 2-4% in insulin-treated patients. The unrecognized mortality may be still higher. Therefore, hypoglycaemia associated with unconsciousness or stupor should be treated on emergency basis. The treatment should not be withheld for want of a biochemical confirmation of diagnosis. The steps of treatment include:

1. Intravenous administration of 25-50 ml of 50% glucose through a big vein over a period of 2-3 minutes followed by an infusion of 5 to 10% glucose. An unconscious patient may improve within 15-20 minutes to permit ingestion of sugar. In case of conscious patient, 20 g of sugar, honey or dextrose tablets may be used. Sulphonylurea-induced hypoglycaemia lasts longer (> 48 hours), hence, requires continuous

monitoring and prolonged infusion of glucose. In patients who do not regain consciousness within 1-2 hours, cerebral oedema should be suspected for which I.V. dexamethasone may be administered along with mannitol.
2. Glucagon (1 mg I.M.) is preferable where peripheral veins are collapsed.
3. Treatment of the underlying cause of hypoglycaemia would be essential to prevent relapses:
   - The treatment of postprandial hypoglycaemia is just alteration in dietary habits. Frequent small feeds are advised in nonspecific reactive hypoglycaemia, the diet should contain some slowly absorbable carbohydrates and more proteins.
   - Anticholinergics may be useful in reducing rapid gastric emptying.
   - Avoidance of lucine containing diet in leucine sensitivity.
   - Avoid use of alcohol.
   - Avoid food containing sugar or fructose, if there is hereditary fructose intolerance.

Chapter 67

Thyroid Crisis or Storm

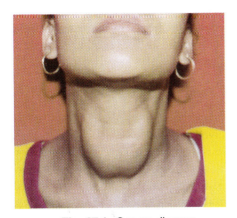

Fig. 67.1: Graves disease

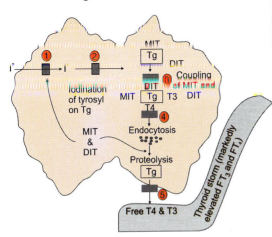

Steps in hormone synthesis
(1) Iodine uptake (2) Iodination of tyrosyl on thyroglobulin (Tg) (3) Coupling reaction (4) Endocytosis (5) Release of free T_4 and T_3

CLINICAL FEATURES

- Staring look or frightening face
- Wide palpebral fissures
- Exophthalmos
- Lid lag or lid retraction
- Excessive watering of eyes
- Diplopia

- Tachycardia
- Good volume or water-hammer pulse
- Exertional dyspnoea
- CHF
- Hypotension instead of hypertension
- Cardiac arrhythmias (AF is common)

- Diarrhoea or steatorrhoea
- Vomiting
- Weight loss

- Nervousness, irritability
- Restlessness, psychosis
- Tremors
- Muscular weakness (proximal myopathy)
- Exaggerated tendon reflexes
- Confusion, stupor, coma

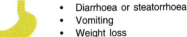

- Perspiration
- Loss of hairs
- Pretibial myxoedema
- Redness of palms
- Hot skin (hyperpyrexia)

- Menstrual irregularity
- Abortions
- Infertility
- Loss of libido or impotence

Miscellaneous
- Hyperpyrexia (> 104°F)
- Excessive thirst
- Dehydration
- Undue excitability/anger

Fig 67.2: Features of thyroid storm (markedly elevated FT_3 and FT_4 hormones)

THYROID CRISIS OR STORM

Definition

Thyrotoxic crisis or storm is a life-threatening situation due to fulminant increase in the signs and symptoms of thyrotoxicosis. This rare condition with a mortality of about 10% is rapid deterioration of thyrotoxicosis with hyperpyrexia (> 104°F), severe tachycardia (or new onset arrhythmia) and altered mental status with extreme restlessness.

Causes

The causes of thyrotoxicosis and thyrotoxic crisis are same because the latter condition just presents with an exaggerated form of the former. The most common cause of thyroid storm is Graves' disease. The other causes are listed in Box 67.1.

> **Box 67.1: Causes of thyrotoxicosis and thyroid crisis**
>
> - Graves' disease (Fig. 67.1)
> - Multinodular toxic goitre
> - Solitary toxic adenoma
> - Factitious thyrotoxicosis (self administration of excessive thyroid hormone)
> - Iodine-induced hyperthyroidism (*Jodbasedow's disease*)
>
> *Note:* precipitation of underlying thyrotoxicosis due to the causes mentioned above lead to thyroid crisis, hence, they are the primary events.

Precipitating Factors

The primary event is thyrotoxicosis. The secondary events leading to thyroid storm are not quite clear. The basic precipitating event is either an increase in free hormone level due to a shift from protein-bound state to free-hormone state secondary to circulating inhibitors to binding, or there is an exaggerated response to a given level of thyroid hormones or both. The exaggerated sympathetic response or hyperadrenergic response seen in thyroid storm is due to increase in the number of baroreceptors on the target cells and post-receptor events. A large number of factors both thyroidal and non-thyroidal can precipitate thyroid crisis in a patient with thyrotoxicosis (see Box 67.2).

> **Box 67.2: Precipitating factors responsible for thyroid storm/crisis**
>
> | Thyroidal factors (acute rise in thyroid hormone) | Nonthyroidal illness |
> |---|---|
> | • Surgery on thyroid | • Surgery of any type |
> | • Withdrawal of antithyroidal drugs | • CVA, sepsis |
> | • Radio-iodine therapy | • Diabetic ketoacidosis |
> | • Iodinated contrast media use | • Trauma |
> | • Vigorous thyroid palpation | • Stress e.g. emotional |
> | | • Pulmonary embolism |

In the past, this syndrome occurred postoperatively in patients poorly prepared for surgery, but now it is less common. Now, so called *medical storm* occurs commonly in untreated or inadequately treated patients. It is precipitated by surgery or a complicating illness usually sepsis.

Clinical Features (Fig. 67.2)

Most patients presenting with thyroid storm/crisis have received either under-treatment (inadequately treated) or no treatment or have recently developed the disease (fresh case). However, thyrotoxic crisis may occur in a patient previously unrecognised to have thyrotoxicosis especially in an elderly with a nodular goitre.

There are no specific diagnostic criteria but high grade fever (> 104°F) out of proportion than infection, severe tachycardia and CNS symptoms (irritability, restlessness, delirium or coma) with hypotension in setting of thyrotoxicosis should raise the possibility of thyroid crisis (Fig. 67.2). The elderly usually go into congestive heart failure and develop cardiac arrhythmias (atrial fibrillation). Atypical presentation (apathetic thyrotoxicosis with thyroid storm characterised by apathy, prostration and coma but with minimal elevation of temperature) can occur in elderly. A scoring system used for diagnosis of thyroid storm is given in the Table 67.1.

Investigations

1. *Thyroid hormones:* The FT_3 and FT_4 are markedly elevated and TSH is markedly

Table 67.1: Scoring system for diagnosis of thyroid storm (Burch et al.) in a patient with thyrotoxicosis

Dysfunction	Score
1. Thermoregulatory dysfunction	
• 99°—99.9°F	5
• 100°—100.9°F	10
• 101°—101.9°F	15
• 102°—102.9°F	20
• 103°—103.9°F	25
• > 104°	30
2. CNS effects	
Agitation (mild)	10
Delirium, lethargy, psychosis	20
Severe seizure, coma	30
3. GI tract and hepatic dysfunction	
• No dysfunction	0
• Moderate dysfunction (vomiting, diarrhoea, pain abdomen)	10
• Jaundice (severe)	20
4. CVS dysfunction	
Heart rate 90-109/min	5
110-119/min	10
120-129/min	15
130-139/min	20
> 140/min	25
5. Others	
• Atrial fibrillation	10
• Congestive heart failure	
Mild—pedal oedema	5
Moderate—Basal crepts	10
Severe—Pulmonary oedema	15
• History of precipitating cause	10

- With total score > 45, thyroid storm is highly likely
- Score between 25-44 suggest impending storm
- Score < 25, thyroid storm is unlikely

depressed. The levels of the hormones can not differentiate a patient with thyrotoxicosis from thyroid storm because there is no cut off limit of elevated hormones in the two conditions and secondly hormone levels are not directly related to the clinical picture. The diagnosis of thyrotoxicosis is purely clinical.

2. Renal, hepatic profile to see their dysfunction under the effect of thyroid hormones.

3. *Blood sugar:* Both hyperglycaemia and hypoglycaemia can occur in thyroid storm.
4. *Serum calcium:* There may be hypercalcaemia under the effects of thyroid hormones.
5. *X-ray chest (PA view)* may show enlargement of cardiac silhouette.
6. *ECG*: This may show good voltage of QRS complexes, severe tachycardia, cardiac arrhythmias (AF is common).

Management

Since the diagnosis of thyroid crisis/storm is made clinically, therefore, treatment should begin after sending the samples for thyroid hormones assay.

Aims of treatment

- Supportive therapy.
- To undertake measures to alleviate thyrotoxicosis as early as possible.

1. **Supportive measures:**
   A. *Correction of dehydration:*
   - Adequate amount of fluids (glucose and saline) to correct dehydration as early as possible. Vitamins should be supplemented.
   - Glucocorticoids: They are indicated because of increased glucocorticoid requirements in thyrotoxicosis, and because adrenal reserve may be reduced. It also inhibits peripheral conversion of T_4 to T_3 as discussed below.

   B. *Treatment of pyrexia:*
   - Patient should be preferably placed in a cooled, humified, oxygen tent, if possible.
   - To bring down fever with external cooling and acetaminophen. Avoid salicylates as they increase free thyroid hormone levels.

   C. *Treatment of congestive heart failure or tachyarrhythmias.*
   - Digitalisation is required to control ventricular rate in those with atrial fibrillation.

- Diuretics are added to digoxin for treatment of CHF.

2. *Specific therapy:*
   It is aimed at to bring down the elevated thyroid hormones and to block their systemic effects. The measures include:
   i. *Inhibition of thyroid hormone synthesis by antithyroid drugs:* As injectable preparation of antithyroid drugs is not available, therefore, oral therapy with neomercazole (60-120 mg/day) or propylthiouracil (1000-1500 mg/day) is started orally followed by a maintenance dose of 60 mg neomercazole or 600 mg of propylthiouracil (PTU). PTU has an added effect of reducing conversion of T_4 to T_3.
   ii. *Inhibition of hormone release:* Large doses of iodine e.g. Lugol's iodine (20 drops t.d.s.), saturated solution of KI (8 drops t.d.s.) or sodium iodide 1g I.V. or sod. iopodate 1-3 g oral prevents the release of preformed hormone in circulation. Iodine should be given only after about an hour of antithyroid drug therapy otherwise iodine will facilitate hormone biosynthesis. Improvement is seen within 24 hours and hormones level come down to normal or near normal within 5 to 7 days. After this, iodine can be withdrawn and antithyroid drugs therapy continued for thyrotoxicosis.
   iii. *Blockade of conversion of T_4 to T_3.* Dexamethasone 4 mg every 6-8 hourly inhibits peripheral conversion of T_4 to T_3, then it is gradually tapered off. It also provides protection against relative deficiency of steroids during thyroid storm as discussed under supportive measures.
   PTU, beta blockers and sodium iopodate also decrease peripheral conversion of T_4 to T_3.
   iv. *Removal of thyroid hormone from circulation:* Plasmapheresis has been used for this purpose in few studies. This mode of therapy is routinely not available.
   v. *Blockade of peripheral effects of hormones:* Propranolol in dose of 20-80 mg every 6 hourly is drug of choice to counter the peripheral effects of thyroid hormones especially on CVS and CNS. Treatment can be given initially with I.V. propranolol (0.5—1 mg). Esmolol—an ultrashort acting beta-blocker is preferred in patients with CHF in dose of 250-500 mg/kg I.V. stat followed by infusion at a rate of 50-100 mg/kg/min.
   vi. The *precipitating cause* should be found out and treated simultaneously.

Chapter 68

Myxoedema Coma

MYXOEDEMA COMA

Definition

It is an advanced stage of long-standing hypothyroidism (Fig. 68.1) characterised by florid symptoms and signs of hypothyroidism with hypothermia and stuporous or comatose state provoked by a precipitating factor.

Myxoedema coma is a medical emergency, seen in older persons, occurs commonly during winter months and carries a high mortality rates (about 50%) if left untreated.

Precipitating Factors

The factors that push the patient of hypothyroidism into myxoedema coma are given in Box 68.1.

> **Box 68.1: Precipitating factors for myxoedema coma**
> - Infection e.g., pneumonia
> - Exposure to cold
> - Trauma
> - GI bleeding
> - Stroke
> - CNS depressants e.g. tranquillisers and sedatives
> - Cardiovascular disease (e.g. CHF)
> - Respiratory disease (infection, COPD)

Clinical Features

1. *Altered mental status or coma:* The mental deterioration is gradual. To start with, patient may have confusion or disorientation before lapsing into coma.
2. *Altered thermoregulation:* Myxoedema coma is usually but not always accompanied by a subnormal body temperature (as low as 25°C). Because the ordinary clinical thermometers do not record such low temperatures as they are not graduated below 33° or 35°C, the true severity of hypothermia may not be appreciated. The body is cold and dry. Hypothermia may precede the development of coma.

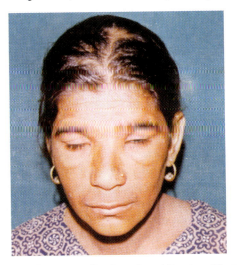

Fig. 68.1: Long-standing hypothyroidism in a 65 years female. Note the gross features of hypothyroidism (e.g. periorbital oedema, thick lips, wrinkles, swollen face, dry skin). Such a patient is prone to develop myxoedema coma under the effect of a precipitating factor but it is a rare phenomenon

3. ***Other features:*** In addition to characteristic features of hypothyroidism such as weight gain, cold intolerance, hoarseness of voice, bradycardia, dry toad skin, sparse hair, nonpitting oedema, menstrual irregularity, impotence and constipation etc. there may be some other features or some altered features:
   - The patient may display areflexia (loss of tendon reflexes) instead of delayed tendon jerks.
   - Patient may have hypotension instead of hypertension of hypothyroidism.
   - Seizures may accompany the comatose state.
   - Hypoventilation (hypoxaemia, hypercapnia) with depressed shallow respiration may be caused by respiratory muscle weakness, upper airway obstruction by large tongue (macroglossia) or depression of respiratory centre.
   - Hypoglycaemia may occur due to hypothyroidism combined with cortisol deficiency.

Investigations

They are done to confirm the diagnosis and to find out the precipitating cause.
1. ***T_3, T_4, TSH:*** The T_3 and T_4 levels are low and TSH levels are high.
2. ***Plasma cortisol:*** This is done to find out cortisol insufficiency which is commonly associated with it.
3. ***Random blood sugar:*** Hypoglycaemia can occur.
4. ***Blood gas analysis*** to find out hypoxaemia and hypercapnia.
5. ***Serum sodium and plasma osmolarity:*** Dilutional hyponatremia is common in 50% of patients due to inappropriate secretion of ADH.
6. ***EKG:*** For low voltage graph or cardiac involvement (conduct defects, pericardial effusion).
7. ***Chest X-ray:*** May show cardiomegaly due to pericardial effusion or features of congestive cardiac failure.

Differential Diagnosis

The conditions which are associated with coma and hypothermia may mimic myxoedema coma. These include:
1. ***Brain stem infarction*** in older persons may lead to both coma and hypothermia.
2. ***Hypothermia*** due to any cause and renal failure may itself induce physiological changes simulating myxoedema such as delayed relaxation of deep tendon reflexes. Coma is due to hypothermia and renal failure.

Management

Myxoedema coma is an medical emergency, carries a high mortality, hence, treatment must begin before the biochemical confirmation of the diagnosis.
1. ***Replacement thyroxine therapy:*** The treatment ideally recommended is intravenous thyroxine 500-600 μg stat then 100 μg I.V. daily till patient comes out of coma but intravenous preparation of thyroxine is not available in India, therefore, oral therapy with 500 μg is begun followed by 100 μg 6 hourly through Ryle's tube.
2. ***Concomitant hydrocortisone therapy:*** As there is associated adrenal insufficiency or reduced adrenal reserve, hydrocortisone intravenous infusion (5-10 mg/hour) may be administered after collecting the blood sample for basal cortisol level. If plasma cortisol is normal, this can be stopped.
3. ***Supportive therapy:***
   - *Endotracheal intubation and ventilatory support* if respiratory depression present and needs ventilation.
   - *Fluid replacement:*
     - Avoid hypotonic fluids because of risk of water intoxication due to SIADH.
     - Fluid restriction (< one litre) for severe dilutional hyponatremia, if present.
     - Glucose infusion for hypoglycaemia.
   - *Gradual rewarming of the body with blankets* to prevent heat loss. Avoid active rewarming

as this may lead to vascular collapse due to vasodilatation.
- *In case of hypoglycaemia*, 25-50% glucose solution may be given.
- *General care of coma patient.* It consists of frequent turning or change of posture, prevention of aspiration by suction, care of bowel and bladder etc.
- *Vitals should be monitored.*
- *Treatment of coexisting diseases* such as infection by antibiotics. Management of other associated disease appropriately.

Mortality

The mortality is very high (60-70%): Severe hypothermia, delay in initiating therapy, inadequate doses of thyroxine, failure to recognize and treat the precipitating factors are responsible for it.

Chapter 69

Acute Adrenal Crisis/Insufficiency

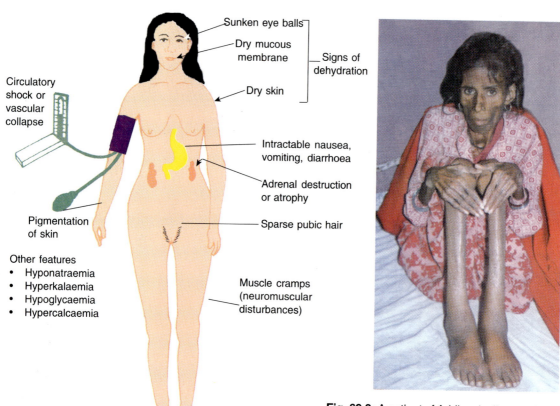

Fig. 69.1: Clinical features of acute adrenal insufficiency (acute precipitation of Addison's disease)

Fig. 69.2: A patient of Addison's disease. Note sunken cheeks and eyeballs, dry pigmented skin and mucous membrane. Patient had long duration of diarrhoea and developed pedal oedema. Such a patient is likely to develop acute crisis during sepsis or surgery

ACUTE ADRENAL CRISIS OR INSUFFICIENCY

Definition

Acute adrenal crisis or insufficiency is sudden deterioration of adrenocortical functions due to several processes. On one hand, it may be due to rapid and overwhelming intensification of chronic adrenal insufficiency (Addison's disease), on the other hand, there may be acute adrenal destruction secondary to haemorrhage, sepsis or sudden withdrawal of steroids etc.

Adrenal crisis is a medical emergency, needs immediate attention and treatment. If diagnosis is missed, the patient will probably die of it.

Causes

They are given in the Table 69.1.
1. *Precipitation of chronic adrenal insufficiency* by sepsis, surgical stress or intercurrent disease.
2. *Acute bilateral destruction of adrenal glands* by haemorrhage (anticoagulation or a coagulation disorder), embolisation or sepsis in previously healthy subjects.
3. *In children, it may be associated with septicaemia* (pseudomonas infection or meningococaemia—called *Waterhouse-Friederichsen syndrome*).
4. *Sudden withdrawal of steroids* from patients with adrenal atrophy due to chronic steroid use.
5. It may occur in patients with *congenital adrenal hyperplasia or those with poor adrenal reserve* when they receive drugs causing further suppression of steroid synthesis such as phenytoin, rifampicin and ketoconazole etc.

Clinical Features

Features of acute adrenal insufficiency are shown in Fig. 69.1 on front page of chapter. The features result from glucocorticoids and mineralocorticoids and androgens deficiency with ACTH excess (see Box 69.1). In fact acute adrenal crisis include: overwhelming symptoms and signs of Addison's disease (Fig. 69.2) such as acute circulatory failure or shock with severe hypotension, dehydration, hyponatraemia, hyperkalaemia and in some instances hypoglycaemia and hypercalcaemia. Muscle cramps, intractable nausea, vomiting and diarrhoea, and unexplained fever may be present. The crisis is often precipitated by surgery or sepsis.

Investigations

1. *Plasma cortisol (morning and evening):* It will be low. A plasma cortisol in normal range in acutely ill patient does not rule out adrenal insufficiency.
2. *One hour ACTH stimulation test*: In adrenal insufficiency, serum cortisol does not rise in response to ACTH.
3. *ACTH levels* will help to diagnos whether adrenal insufficiency is primary (high level) or secondary (low level).
4. *Serum Na^+ and K^+ level.* Serum Na^+ is normal to low and K^+ is high
5. *CT scan* of adrenal glands may reveal the underlying cause.

Management

Aims

- Rapid elevation of glucocorticoids levels.
- Replacement of sodium and water deficits. The

Table 69.1: Aetiology of adrenal crisis/acute adrenal insufficiency	
Adrenal causes	*Pituitary causes*
• Sudden precipitation of Addison's disease of adrenal origin	• Postpartum pituitary necrosis (Sheehan's syndrome)
• Bilateral adrenal haemorrhage (anticoagulant therapy or a coagulation disorder)	• Necrosis or bleeding into pituitary microadenoma
• Bilateral adrenal thrombosis e.g. antiphospholipid syndrome	• Head trauma
	• Lesions of pituitary stalk
• Adrenal necrosis due to sepsis or septicaemia (Waterhouse-Friederichsen syndrome)	• Pituitary or adrenal surgery for Cushing's syndrome

370 Endocrinology and Metabolism

> **Box 69.1: Symptoms and signs of adrenal Insufficiency**
>
> *Glucocorticoid deficiency*
> - Weight loss, weakness
> - Anorexia, nausea, vomiting
> - Diarrhoea or constipation
> - Postural hypotension
> - Shock
> - Hypoglycaemia, hyponatraemia and hypercalcaemia
>
> *ACTH excess*
> - Pigmentation on sun-exposed ares, pressure sores e.g. elbow, knee and mucous membrane, conjunctivae, palmar creases and recent scars
>
> *Mineralocorticoid insufficiency*
> - Hypotension
> - Shock
> - Hyponatraemia
> - Hyperkalaemia
>
> *Adrenal androgen insufficiency*
> - Decreased body hair (e.g. pubic, axillary) and loss of libido especially in females

hyponatraemia (Na+ < 120 mmol/L) is in itself an emergency. This may lead to delirium, coma and seizures.

- There is little time to consider specific laboratory confirmation of the diagnosis in an adrenal crisis which is a life-threatening emergency, hence, the management is often instituted immediately when the diagnosis is made.

Treatment

1. *Fluid replacement:* Large volume of 5% dextrose in saline or 0.9% normal saline (2-3 L) should be infused immediately.
2. *Steroid replacement therapy:* Intravenous hydrocortisone 100 mg I.V. as a bolus or dexamethasone 4 mg I.V. stat, followed by a continuous infusion of hydrocortisone at a rate of 10 mg/hour. An alternative approach is to give 100 mg I.V. hydrocortisone as a bolus, then 100 mg I.V. after every 6 hours until gastrointestinal symptoms abate and patient starts accepting orally.

   Dexamethasone is preferred because its effect lasts for 12-24 hours and it does not interfere with measurement of plasma or urinary steroids during subsequent ACTH stimulation test.
3. *Treatment of hypotension or shock:* Effective treatment of hypotension or shock requires glucocorticoid replacement and repletion of sodium and water deficits. Vasoactive agents (e.g. dopamine) may be indicated in severe hypotension as an adjuvant to fluid therapy.
4. *No need for mineralocorticoid replacement:* With large doses of steroids e.g. 100 to 200 mg hydrocortisone, the patient receives a maximal mineralocorticoid effect, hence, supplementation of mineralocorticoid will be superfluous.
5. *Identification of precipitating cause and its treatment:* After initial treatment, the precipitating cause of acute adrenal insufficiency (e.g. bacterial infection, viral gastroenteritis) should be looked for and appropriately treated.

Following improvement, the steroid dosage is tapered over next few days to maintenance levels, and mineralocorticosteroid therapy is reinstituted. Most patients who present with acute adrenal insufficiency have deficiency of both glucocorticoids and mineralocorticoids, hence, in addition to maintenance dose of glucocorticoids (7.5 to 10 mg/day), a life-long replacement of mineralocorticoid (fludrocortisone 0.05 to 0.1 mg/day) can be started as soon as saline drip is stopped and patient accepts orally.

Prevention

1. *Concurrent illness:*
   The patient is advised to add salt to the diet during the period of excessive exercise with sweating, hot weather/season and during vomiting or diarrhoea. During an episode of febrile illness, patient should double the dose of steroids for 3-5 days and consult his/her physician if the illness persists longer. Acute

gastroenteritis needs immediate hospitalization for fluid and steroids therapy to prevent dehydration and shock.

2. **Surgery:**
   Minor procedures under local anaesthesia (e.g. dental extraction) do not need any change in steroid regimen. *Moderate stressful procedures* (e.g. endoscopy, bronchoscopy, arteriography), need to be covered with an additional dose of 100 mg of hydrocortisone I.V. just before surgery, another 100 mg is given just before anaesthesia and then 100 mg I.V. every 8 hourly till the patient stabilizes. The steroid dose is then tapered rapidly to maintenance dosage.

Chapter 70

Pituitary Apoplexy

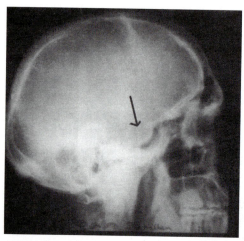

Fig. 70.1: X-ray skull (lateral view) There is widening and deepening of pituitary fossa (↓) with destruction of clinoid processes suggestive of a pituitary tumour

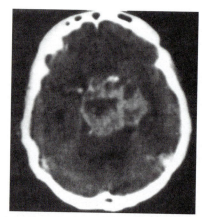

Fig. 70.2: CT scan showing a pituitary tumour with haemorrhage (hyperdense area)

PITUITARY APOPLEXY

Definition

Pituitary apoplexy—A rare endocrinopathy characterised clinically by sudden headache, visual disturbances, ophthalmoplegia, signs of meningeal irritation and altered mental status caused by sudden or abrupt haemorrhage or infarction of the pituitary gland.

Although haemorrhage occurs in 10-15% cases of pituitary adenomas but most of them are clinically silent. Pituitary apoplexy may be diagnosed only in 2-10% of adenomas on development of typical features or on resolution of hypersecretory states. Pituitary apoplexy may be a presenting feature of a pituitary tumour (Figs 70.1 and 70.2). It has also been observed that pituitary apoplexy (upto 65%) occurs in patients with undiagnosed pituitary adenoma.

Pathophysiology

Haemorrhage and necrosis of the pituitary adenoma are the cardinal pathological features of pituitary apoplexy and occur due to:
i. Pituitary adenomas are more vulnerable to bleeding than other tumours.

ii. A rapidly growing adenoma outstripes its blood supply and produces ischaemia followed by necrosis and secondary haemorrhage.
iii. Compression of a large pituitary stalk carrying blood vessels by an expanding tumour mass may render the entire anterior lobe ischaemic followed by secondary haemorrhage.
iv. Fragility of the tumour blood vessels predispose to bleeding.

Causes and Predisposing Factors

The predisposing factors are given in Box 70.1.

Clinical Features

The clinical features are due to tumour mass and its pressure effects within sella turcica and outside sella turcica (Table 70.1).

Presentation can be acute characterised by rapid onset of neurological symptoms and coma. Death can occur. In subacute presentation, symptoms evolve over days to weeks and may present with evidence of hormone deficiency at a later date.

Course

The clinical course of pituitary apoplexy varies hence, difficult to predict the outcome. In mild *benign form*, the symptoms (headache and visual disturbances) develop slowly and persist over days to weeks and then improve; *in fulminant form*, the sudden onset of blindness, coma and hemodynamic disturbances (respiratory and cardiac) may lead to death.

Recovery of functions may occur with or without surgical intervention. Residual endocrine disturbance is the rule and panhypopituitarism invariably persists in most of cases. In some cases, there may be selective loss of one or two trophic hormones.

Differential Diagnosis

Because of its diverse clinical presentation, pituitary apoplexy has to be differentiated on clinical and investigative grounds from the following conditions:
1. Subarachnoid haemorrhage.
2. Bacterial meningitis.

Box 70.1: Predisposing factors for pituitary apoplexy

- Radiation
- Drugs e.g. bromocryptine, anticoagulants and oestrogens
- Following cardiac surgery
- Following procedures e.g. angiography
- Following severe coughing and sneezing
- Head trauma
- Pregnancy
- Diabetes
- Following dynamic tests for pituitary function e.g. pituitary stimulation tests

Table 70.1: Clinical presentations of pituitary apoplexy

Structure involved/compressed	Symptoms and signs
• Sudden enlargement of tumour mass	• Headache, sudden and severe retro-orbital and frontal pain
• Optic nerve	• Decreased visual acuity and visual field defects
• The III, IV and VI cranial nerve compression	• Ophthalmoplegia, ptosis and pupillary defects
• Meningeal irritation (disruption of dura or leakage of blood into subarachnoid space)	• Nausea, vomiting, headache, alteration in the level of consciousness e.g. lethargy, stupor and coma
• Internal carotid artery	• Hemiplegia
• Compression of corticotrophs (loss of ACTH)	• Acute adrenal insufficiency
• Compression of gonadotrophs (loss of LH, FSH)	• Gonadal dysfunction
• Compression of pituitary stalk	• Diabetes insipidus
• Compression of thyrotrophs	• Hypofunction of thyroid
• Nonspecific, noncompressive	• Fever, anosmia, CSF rhinorrhoea and facial pain. Respiratory and cardiac rhythm disturbances

Investigations

- *Plain X-ray skull:* It may show enlargement of sella turcica and destruction of clinoid processes (Fig. 70.1 on front page). It can be normal also.
- *Lumbar puncture and CSF* examination is carried out only if pituitary apoplexy has presentation like bacterial meningitis. The CSF may show pleocytosis, raised proteins but sugar is normal. RBCs may or may not be present.
- *CT/MRI scan:* The CT scan of the head may show a high density or inhomogenous gland with or without evidence of blood in subarachnoid space and MRI scan is more useful than CT scan in identifying pituitary haemorrhage or haemorrhage in a tumour (Fig. 70.2).
- *Angiography:* It is done to differentiate pituitary apoplexy from subarachnoid haemorrhage due to aneurysmal rupture.
- *Other hormone levels:* Initially they may be normal except cortisol whose deficiency may develop acutely. Thyroid hormones (T_3, T_4, TSH) and gonadal hormone fall over weeks.

Management

1. *Medical treatment of hypopituitarism:* It invariably relieves pituitary apoplexy. Hydrocortisone 100 mg I.V. initially, then every 6 to 8 hourly until surgery is done. Acute adrenal insufficiency is common and an early finding in pituitary apoplexy. Electrolytes and fluids should be administered carefully to correct hydration and electrolyte balance. Patient should be watched closely for diabetes insipidus. In acute setting, other hormone replacement may not be required but subsequently steroids, thyroid hormone and gonadal hormones (testosterone in males, oestrogen and progesterone in females) may be required as replacement therapy on long-term basis.

2. *Surgical treatment:* Neurosurgical decompression via trans-sphenoidal approach is definite therapy for pituitary apoplexy. Rapid down-hill course and severe visual loss are indications for surgery. Recent evidence suggests that early decompression may partially or completely restore the pituitary functions and lessen the need for hormonal replacement therapy.

Chapter 71

Hypocalcaemia

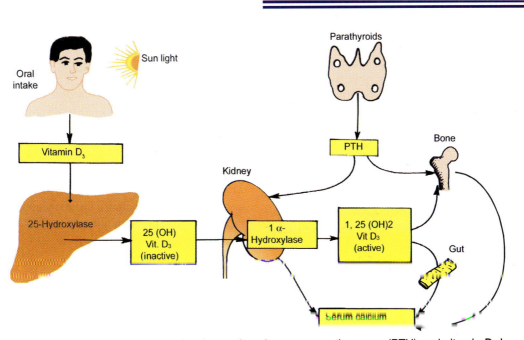

Fig. 71.1: Calcium homeostasis showing interactions between paratharmone (PTH) and vitamin D. Low calcium level leads to tetany (See Fig. 71.2)

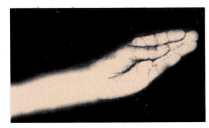

Fig. 71.2: Manifest tetany characterised by spontaneous carpel spasms (main d' accoucheur hand)

HYPOCALCAEMIA

Normal calcium homeostasis is maintained within normal range (8.5 to 10.5 mg/dl or 2.1 to 2.5 mmol/dl) by parathyroid hormone (PTH), vitamin D and calcitonin (Fig. 71.1). About 50% of calcium is unbound and is responsible for physiological actions. Rest 50% is bound to albumin (40%) and anions (10%). Changes in pH influence the binding of calcium. Alkalosis produces hypocalcaemia by increasing the binding of calcium to albumin while acidosis has the reverse effect.

Definition

Hypocalcaemia is defined as a state in which calcium concentration in serum falls below the lower limit of normal i.e. 8.5 mg/dl after correction for serum albumin

> *Correction formula: Add 0.8 mg/dl to serum calcium level with every 1g/dl fall in serum albumin level below 4g/dl.*

Causes

Hypocalcaemia may occur in acute, subacute and chronic forms. Acute hypocalcaemia is usually transient and asymptomatic, occurs in intensive care setting and severe sepsis, burns, acute renal failure and following extensive blood transfusions with citrated blood (see Box 71.1). Acute hypocalcaemia with certain illness or medications (protamine, heparin and glucagon) is also transient, does not produce tetany and resolves with treatment of medical conditions or stoppage of drug. Acute pancreatitis also causes hypocalcaemia by precipitation of Ca^{++}, does not require treatment except the underlying cause.

Box 71.1: Causes of acute hypocalcaemia

- Sepsis
- Burns
- Acute pancreatitis
- Acute renal failure
- Alkalosis
- Drugs e.g. diuretics, protamine, heparin and glucagon
- Toxic-shock syndrome
- Hypomagnesaemia
- Extensive transfusions
- Plasmapheresis
- Malignancy
- Alcohol excess
- Parathyroid surgery

Chronic hypocalcaemia, however, is usually symptomatic and requires treatment. The most common cause of chronic hypocalcaemia is hypoparathyroidism (PTH deficiency). Vitamin D deficiency leads to hypocalcaemia in children than in adults. In advanced osteomalacia, adults may also manifest with hypocalcaemia. The classification of chronic hypocalcaemia is tabulated (Table 71.1), is based on the PTH level and its ineffectiveness due to the fact that PTH is responsible for minute to minute regulation in serum calcium concentration.

Table 71.1: Functional classification of chronic hypocalcaemia

I. **PTH deficient** (*hypoparathyroidism*)
   - Hereditary hypoparathyroidism
   - Acquired hypoparathyroidism (e.g. autoimmune, irradiation, postsurgical, infiltrative)
   - Hypomagnesaemia

II. **PTH ineffective**
   A. Vitamin-D deficiency
      - Lack of sun exposure
      - Dietary deficiency
      - Malabsorption
   B. Defective vit. D metabolism
      - Anticonvulsants (e.g. phenytoin)
      - Vitamin D dependent ricket (type I)
   C. Vitamin D resistance
      - Pseudohypoparathyroidism
      - Vitamin D dependent type II rickets
      - Vitamin D resistant rickets

III. **PTH overwhelmed**
   A. Severe, acute hyperphosphataemia
      - Tumour lysis
      - Acute renal failure
      - Rhabdomyolysis
   B. Osteitis fibrosa after parathyroidectomy

Clinical Features

The clinical manifestations vary from asymptomatic state to life-threatening features like convulsions, tetany (Fig. 71.2), laryngeal spasm, depending on the level of ionized calcium. The neuromuscular and neurological manifestations of hypocalcaemia are due to enhanced neuromuscular excitability due to lowered threshold; and common features include tetany, perioral paraesthesias, numbness, muscle cramps and fasciculations. The symptoms and sign of hypocalcaemia and tetany are given in Boxes 71.2 and 71.3.

Severe hypocalcaemia can cause mental features (irritability, depression, psychosis), seizures, myopathy and heart failure. The QT interval is prolonged on ECG and arrhythmia can occur. In

Hypocalcaemia

Box 71.2: Clinical features of hypocalcaemia

Mental:	Irritability, depression, psychosis, convulsions
Neurological:	Tetany (the features are given in box 71.3), paraesthesias, seizures.
Cardiac:	Precipitation of CHF by betablockers, arrhythmias, prolonged QTc on ECG.
Eye:	Cataracts, optic neuritis, papilloedema

Box 71.3: Symptoms and signs of tetany

Children

A characteristic triad of carpopedal spasm, stridor and convulsions may occur in various combinations. The hands in carpopedal spasm, carpel spasm adopt a peculiar posture in which there is flexion at metacarpophalangeal joint and extension at the interphalangcal joints and there is apposition of thumb (*main d'accoucheur hand*) as depicted in the Fig. 71.2. Pedal spasms are less frequent. The stridor (loud sound) is produced by closure of the glottis.

Adults

Tingling sensations in the peripheral parts of limbs or around the mouth. Less often painful carpopedeal spasms, muscle cramps, facial grimacing may occur. Stridor and convulsions are rare.

some cases, there may be increased intracranial pressure including papilloedema. Respiratory arrest can occur.

Latent tetany (absence of signs and symptoms of tetany) is diagnosed by provocative tests:

1. *Trousseau's sign (Fig. 71.3 on next page):* Raising the BP above systolic level by inflating the sphygmomanometer cuff, produces typical carpopedal spasms within 3-5 minutes.
2. *Chvostek's sign:* A tap at the facial nerve in front of tragus at the angle of jaw produces facial twitchings within 3 minutes.

Diagnosis and Differential Diagnosis

Hypocalcaemia is suspected in a patient with tetany and other features described above. Tetany can occur due to alkalosis and magnesium deficiency. The differential diagnosis of hypocalcaemias is given in the Table 71.2.

Table 71.2: Differential diagnosis of hypocalcaemia

Condition	Total serum calcium concentration	Ionised serum calcium concentration	Serum phosphate concentration	Serum PTH concentration	Comment
1. Hypoalbuminaemia	↓	N	N	N	Adjust calcium by correction formula
2. Alkalosis • Respiratory (e.g. hyperventilation) • Metabolic (e.g. Conn's syndrome)	N	↓	N	N or ↑	Read the textbook
3. Vit. D deficiency	↓	↓	↓	↑	Read text
4. Chronic renal failure	↓	↓	↑	↑	It is due to depressed hydroxylation
5. Hypoparathyroidism • Post-surgical • Idiopathic • Infants	↓	↓	↑	↓	Read textbook
6. Pseudohypoparathyroidism	↓	↓	↑	↑	Characteristic phenotype
7. Acute pancreatitis	↓	↓	N or ↓	↑	• Usually clinically evident • Serum amylase ↑

↑ - Increase   ↓ - Decrease   N-Normal

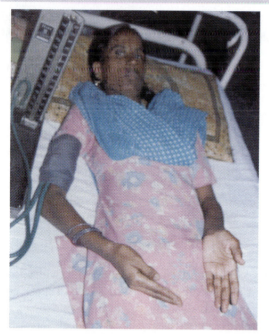

Fig. 71.3: Latent tetany converted into manifest tetany by Trousseau's sign

Management

Treatment for hypocalcaemia depends on severity and its progression. *Mild* hypocalcaemia needs only observation and oral supplementation of calcium and vitamin D. *Severe* symptomatic hypocalcaemia should be treated as an emergency with 10% calcium gluconate (90 mg elemental calcium in 10 ml); 2 ampoules (20 ml) infused I.V. over 10 minutes followed by infusion of 60 ml in 500 ml of glucose (1 mg/ml) at a rate of 0.5—2.0 mg/kg/hour. Serum calcium should be monitored every 4-6 hours and infusion rate adjusted to keep the serum calcium between 8-9 mg/dl. This is followed by oral calcium and vitamin D supplementation. Hypomagnesemia, if present, may be corrected by magnesium administration simultaneously. If tetany is not relieved by giving calcium, magnesium may be tried.

Hypocalcaemia due to hyperventilation (alkalosis) can be overcome by rebreathing expired air in a paper bag or administering 5% CO_2 in oxygen.

Treatment of *chronic* hypocalcaemia due to hypoparathyroidism is with oral calcium (2-4 g of elemental calcium every day) and vitamin D (0.5-2 µg calcitrol/day) for life-long. Commercial preparations of PTH for hypoparathyroidism are unsatisfactory as its administration needs frequent injections and hormone therapy becomes ineffective due to antibody formation.

Chapter 72

Hypercalcaemia (Hypercalcaemic Crisis)

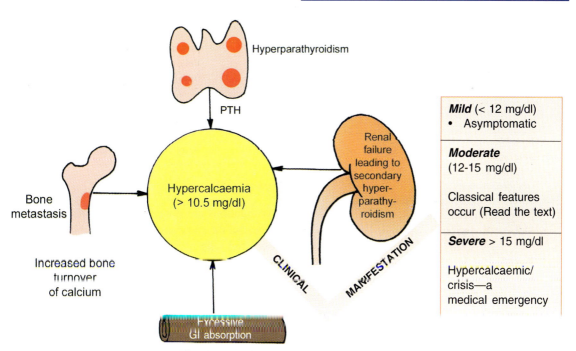

Fig. 72.1: Pathogenesis of hypercalcaemia

HYPERCALCAEMIA

Definition

It is defined as a state in which serum calcium level is above the upper limit of the normal i.e. above 10.5 mg/dl in the presence of normal serum protein.

It is detected most frequently during routine biochemical analysis in asymptomatic patients. However, it presents with chronic symptoms in most of cases; occasionally, patient presents as an acute emergency with hypercalcaemic crisis (severe hypercalcaemia with dehydration).

Causes

Hypercalcaemia results either from an increased entry of calcium into the extracellular fluid (from bone resorption or intestinal absorption) or a decreased renal calcium clearance (Fig. 72.1).

380 Endocrinology and Metabolism

More than 90% of cases are due to hyperparathyroidism or associated with malignancy. The common causes of hypercalcaemia are given in the Table 72.1.

Table 72.1: Causes of hypercalcaemia

I. *Parathyroid related (e.g. normal or high PTH)*
  - Primary hyperparathyroidism (solitary adenoma, MEN type I) or tertiary hyperparathyroidism
  - Lithium therapy
  - Familial hypocalciuric hypercalcaemia

II. **Nonparathyroidal (e.g. low PTH)**
  i. *Malignancy associated*
     - Solid tumour with metastases
     - Solid tumour with release of PTH related protein
     - Haematological malignancies (e.g. multiple myeloma, leukaemia, lymphoma)
  ii. *Vitamin D related*
     - Vitamin D intoxication
     - Increased 1, 25 (OH)2 D; sarcoidosis and other granulomatous diseases
  iii. *Associated with high bone turnover*
     - Hyperthyroidism
     - Immobilisation
     - Thiazides
     - Vitamin A intoxication
  iv. *Associated with renal failure*
     - Severe secondary hyperparathyroidism
     - Aluminium intoxication
     - Milk-alkali syndrome
  v. *Artifactual*
     - Venous stasis
     - Glassware contamination

Clinical Features

The clinical features depend on the severity of hypercalcaemia. Its presentation varies from asymptomatic state to severe symptomatic hypercalcaemia associated with altered sensorium and coma. Generally symptoms appear when serum calcium is more than 12.0 mg/dl, but some patients even at this level are asymptomatic. When calcium exceeds 13 mg/dl (3.2 mmol/L), calcification in kidneys, skin, vessels, lungs, heart and stomach and renal insufficiency may develop, particularly if blood phosphate levels are normal or elevated due to impaired renal function. Severe hypercalcaemia is usually defined as serum calcium levels of 15 mg/dl (3.7 mmol/L) or above, is a medical emergency. When serum calcium is in-between 15 to 18 mg/dl, coma and cardiac arrest can occur.

Fluid loss secondary to hypercalcaemia induced polyuria and vomiting produces dehydration and reduction in GFR. This leads to a further rise in serum calcium setting up a vicious cycle and ends in a hypercalcaemic crisis. The symptoms and signs of hypercalcaemia are given in Box 72.1.

Box 72.1: Symptoms and signs of hypercalcaemia

CNS:	Mental confusion, depression, lethargy, inability to concentration, fatigue, stupor and coma
GIT:	Nausea, vomiting, anorexia, constipation, peptic ulcer disease
Renal:	Polyuria, nocturia, polydipsia due to tubular defects, dehydration, renal stones, nephrocalcinosis
Cardiac:	Bradycardia, AV blocks, arrhythmias, hypertension, short QTc interval on ECG.
Eye:	Band keratopathy, calcification of lens

Investigations

Investigations are done to confirm the diagnosis, to find out the cause and to exclude other disorders associated with hypercalcaemia.

1. **Raised serum calcium on initial estimation:** It must be confirmed on two or three occasions along with phosphorus and serum alkaline phosphatase. Urinary calcium excretion also helps in the diagnosis.

   Clue: A patient with raised serum calcium, low phosphorous and normal to increased urinary calcium is likely to have hyperparathyroidism because of increased PTH or PTH reactive protein secretion.

2. **Measure PTH levels**. Elevated PTH (parathormone) levels in the presence of hypercalcaemia suggest:
   - Hyperparathyroidism.
   - Ectopic PTH from a neoplasm.
   - Familial hypocalciuric hypercalcaemia.

3. **Localisation of parathyroid adenoma if hyperparathyroidism is the** cause. Ultrasonography, CT scan, thallium technetium substraction scan in isolation or in combination help in the diagnosis (Fig. 72.2).

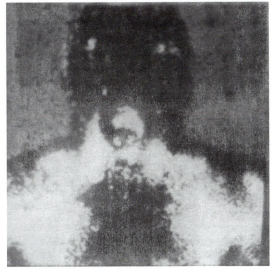

Fig. 72.2: Thallium-technetium substraction scan revealed a parathyroid adenoma in a patient with hyper parathyroidism

4. **If PTH levels are low**, then it indicates non-parathyroidal hypercalcaemia and should be investigated accordingly:
   - Increased Ca^{++} and increased phosphate with high urinary calcium indicate vitamin D Intoxication, excessive absorption of Ca^{++} from GI tract, excessive release of phosphate from bones in malignancy, renal diseases and granulomatous disease.
5. **Investigations for malignancy and multiple myeloma** in older people should be carried out.

Diagnosis and Differential Diagnosis

The diagnosis of hypercalcaemia is based on clinical features with raised serum calcium on two to three occasions. Further investigations are done to find out the cause. Differential diagnosis rests between its differential causes.

Hypercalcaemia in an adult who is asymptomatic is usually due to primary hyperparathyroidism.

In malignancy—associated hypercalcaemia, symptoms of malignancy bring the patient to the clinician and hypercalcaemia is detected on biochemical investigations. In such patients, the interval between detection of hypercalcaemia and death is often less than 6 months.

Long duration of symptoms of hypercalcaemia (i.e. one to 2 years) along with renal stones, primary hyperparathyroidisms is likely the cause rather than malignancy.

Management

The type of treatment is based on the severity of hypercalcaemia and nature of associated symptoms. Except in malignancy-associated hypercalcaemia, acute management of hypercalcaemia is usually successful prior to definite therapy. The serum calcium can be decreased significantly (3 to 9 mg/dl) within first 24-48 hours to relieve acute symptoms, prevent death from hypercalcaemic crisis and permit further investigations to find out the cause. Treatment of chronic hypercalcaemia by medical therapies is less satisfactory unless underlying cause can be corrected. The various therapies for hypercalcaemia are given in the Table 72.2.

Although many agents are available, but bisphosphonates and hydration with or without forced diuresis (saline infusion *plus* a loop diuretic) are the most useful therapies for hypercalcaemia as an acute emergency. In selected cases, calcitonin, steroids and/or dialysis may be useful. Other therapies like gallium nitrate, plicamycin, oral phosphate are rarely used.

The most effective way to reduce calcium in emergency situation (hypercalcaemic crisis) is rehydration with isotonic saline (except cardiac patients or patients with CRF). Intravenous bisphosphonates should be given to patients with severe hypercalcaemia along with saline. The onset

382 Endocrinology and Metabolism

Table 72.2: Therapies for severe hypercalcaemia

Therapy	Dose and route	Onset of action	Comments/monitor
A. *Most useful therapies*			
• Hydration with saline	250-1000 ml/hour	Hours during infusion	Look for fluid overload
• Forced diuresis (Saline + frusemide)	20-80 mg of frusemide, 4-6 hourly I.V.	Hour during treatment	Look for electrolytes, monitor K+
B. *Bisphosphonates*			
• First generation e.g. etidronate	7.5 mg/kg/day I.V.	1-2 days	• Infuse over 4-24 hours, half the dose in renal failure • Hyperphosphataemia may occur
• Second generation e.g. Pamidronate	30-90 mg/week as I.V.		• Infuse over 4-24 hours, half the dose in renal failure • May casue fever (20%), hypo-phosphataemia, hypocalcaemia
C. *Calcitonin*	4-8 U/kg every 6-12 hourly I.M. or S.C.	Within few hours	• Allergic reactions, give test dose • Tachyphylaxis
D. *Other therapies*			
Plicamycin	25 mg/kg/day I.V.	Days	Monitor blood count, LFT
Prednisolone	20 mg bid or tid orally		• Useful in certain malignancies • Produces glucocorticoids side-effects
EDTA	50 mg/kg/day I.V.	During use	• Hypercalcaemic crisis • Avoid in renal failure
Dialysis	Low or no calcium dialysate haemodialysis/ peritoneal dialysis)	Days	• Useful in hypercalcaemic crisis in renal failure

of action of bisphosphonates is delayed by 24-48 hours. *Pamidronate* having a long duration of action (weeks to months) is a preferred drug; is given in a dose of 30-90 mg as an I.V. infusion. It normalizes the calcium in most of the patients. *Calcitonin* is another drug which has a short duration of action, can bring down the calcium rapidly in few cases. Tachyphylaxis is a problem with calcitonin, hence, simultaneous use of bisphosphonates is **needed. Steroids** are used for treatment of hypercalcaemia due to sarcoidosis. vitamin D intoxication, lymphoma and hematological malignancies. Intravenous phosphate has calcium lowering effect but there is associated risk of precipitation of calcium as calcium phosphate complex with its use. Fatal hypotension and ARF have been reported with its use. Dialysis removes the calcium rapidly and dramatically and is used to lower calcium in presence of renal failure or volume overload.

Part Eight

Nephrology

Chapter 73

Acute Nephritic Syndrome

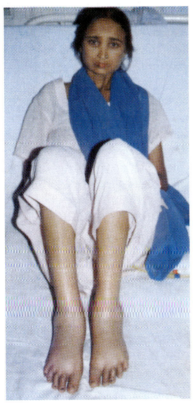

Fig. 73.1: An 18-year-old female presented with hypertension, oedema, puffiness of face with haematuria—acute nephritic syndrome

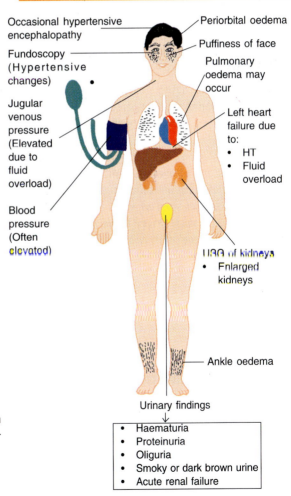

Fig. 73.2: Clinical manifestations of acute nephritic syndrome

ACUTE NEPHRITIC SYNDROME

Definition

The acute nephritic syndrome (Fig. 73.1) is the clinical correlate of acute glomerulonephritis and is characterised by:

- *Haematuria* (macroscopic or microscopic-red cell casts are typically present in urine).
- *Proteinuria* (<3.5 g/day—not in nephrotic range; usual is 1-2 g/day).
- *Hypertension and oedema:* Owing to salt and H_2O retention.
- *Oliguria* (urine output < 400 ml/day). It is due to depressed GFR.
- *Uraemia*—acute renal failure.

Pathology

The hallmark of acute nephritic syndrome is glomerular inflammation (hypercellularity) and the classic pathologic correlate of the nephritic syndrome is *proliferative glomerulonephritis*. The proliferation of glomerular cells is due initially to infiltration of the glomerular tuft by neutrophils and monocytes with subsequent proliferation of *endothelial* and *mesangial* cells (endocapillary proliferation). In **most severe form,** nephritic syndrome is associated with acute inflammation of most of glomeruli e.g. *acute diffuse proliferative glomerulonephritis.* In **less severe form,** fewer than 50% of the glomeruli may be involved i.e. focal proliferative glomerulonephritis. **In its mildest form,** cellular proliferation is just confined to the measangium i.e. mesangioproliferative *glomerulonephritis.*

Rapidly Progressive Glomerulonephritis (RPGN)

It is a clinical correlate of nephritic syndrome but is of subacute onset characterised by development of renal failure over weeks to months, in association with a nephritic urinary sediments, subnephrotic proteinuria, oliguria, hypervolaemia, oedema and hypertension. The classic pathologic finding is severe extracapillary proliferation leading to crescents formation in more than 50% of glomeruli (crescentic glomerulonephritis). In practice, the clinical term rapidly proliferative glomerulonephritis (RPGN) and the pathological term crescentic glomerulonephritis are interchangeably used.

Both acute nephritic syndrome and RPGN are part of a spectrum of presentation of immunologically mediated proliferative glomerulonephritis. In acute nephritic syndrome, the immune response is acute; while it is subacute in RPGN.

Causes of Acute Nephritic Syndrome

The causes of acute nephritic syndrome and RPGN are more or less same and both can result from renal-limited primary glomerulonephritis or secondary glomerulopathy complicating systemic disease.

Most common causes include; post-streptococcal glomerulonephritis, bacterial endocarditis, immune-complex nephritis as in SLE and effect of circulating autoantibodies against glomerular basement membrane (GBM) in Goodpasture's syndrome. The causes are given in Box 73.1.

Clinical Features (Fig. 73.2)

1. **Oedema or puffiness of face** in the early hours of the morning with or without oedema feet. It is due to proteinuria, salt and water retention, hypertension and reduced GFR.
2. **Oliguria:** Urine output is less than 400 ml/day. It is due to depressed GFR.
3. **Subnephrotic proteinuria < 3.5 g/day:** It leads to oedema, occurs due to leakage of proteins into Bowman's capsule due to glomerular injury and subsequently into the urine.
4. **Smoky or brown coloured urine:** Oliguria with smoky urine is a characteristic feature of acute nephritic syndrome. The change in colour of the urine is due to gross or microscopic haematuria.
5. **Hypertension:** The headache, giddiness, malaise and weakness in acute nephritic syndrome is associated with hypertension which is due to salt and water retention. Occasionally

Acute Nephritic Syndrome

> **Box 73.1: Diseases associated with acute nephritic syndrome**
>
> **A. Primary glomerular diseases**
> - Membranoproliferative glomerulonephritis (GN)
> - Mesangial proliferative GN
> - Pauci-immune GN (rapidly progressive crescentic)
>
> **B. Secondary to systemic diseases**
> - *Post-infectious GN*
>   – Bacterial e.g. post-streptococcal
>   – Viral e.g. HBV
>   – Parasitic e.g. malaria
> - *Systemic collagen vascular diseases*
>   – Systemic lupus erythematosus
>   – Systemic vasculitis e.g. PAN, Wegner's granulomatosis
> - *Haematological diseases*
>   – Henoch-Schonlein purpura
>   – Haemolytic-uraemic syndrome
>   – Thrombotic thrombocytopenic purpura
>   – Cryoglobulinaemia
>   – Serum sickness
> - *Glomerular basement membrane (GBM) diseases*
>   – Goodpasture's syndrome
>
> **C. Miscellaneous**
> - Guillian Barré syndrome
> - DPT vaccination IgA nephropathy

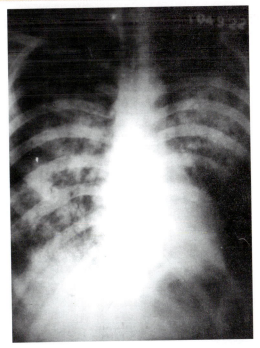

Fig. 73.3: Pulmonary oedema in a patient with acute nephritic syndrome

hypertension may be associated with mental features called *hypertensive encephalopathy*.

6. **Circulatory congestion or left heart failure:** It occurs due to capillaritis, increased cardiac output, and shortened circulation time, complicated further by acute left heart failure (pulmonary oedema Fig. 73.3.) due to salt and water retention and hypertension, producing cough, breathlessness, end-inspiratory crackles and rales. Haemoptysis may occur.

7. **Associated features:** In classical post-streptococcal GN causing acute nephritic syndrome, the patient is usually a child, will have history of sore throat 1-3 weeks prior to the onset of syndrome. Streptococcal tonsillitis or pharyngitis, otitis media, or cellulitis may be responsible. The latent period of 1-3 weeks is for formation of immune complexes and their deposition into glomeruli. The features of underlying cause or systemic illness, or causative agent may be present at the time of acute nephritic syndrome.

Investigations

A list of investigations is given in the Table 73.1. If the clinical diagnosis of acute nephritic syndrome is clear cut e.g., in post-streptococcal glomerulonephritis, renal imaging or renal biopsy are usually unnecessary. A biopsy is required if the diagnosis is uncertain; i.e. clinical features are unusual, or if renal failure is rapidly progressive suggesting the diagnosis of RPGN (crescentic glomerulonephritis).

Differential Diagnosis

The differential diagnosis is depicted in Fig. 73.4.

Management

The management is directed to control the symptoms and signs till the illness is resolved in post-streptococcal GN which is usually a self-limiting illness; otherwise cause has to be found out and properly treated.

Nephrology

Table 73.1: Investigations of acute nephritic syndrome

Investigations	Positive findings
• Complete urine examination	Proteinuria and high specific gravity
• Microscopic urine examination	RBCs (dysmorphic) and red cells casts
• Blood urea and serum creatinine	May be elevated
• Culture (throat swab, ear discharge swab or swab, from inflamed skin)	Nephrogenic strains of group A β-haemolyticus streptococci not always
• ASO-titre	Elevated in poststreptococcal nephritis
• C_3 level	May be reduced
• Antinuclear antibody	Present in significant titre in SLE
• Creatinine clearance	Reduced
• 24 hours urinary protein	Subnephrotic proteinuria (< 3.5 g/day)
• Chest X-ray	Cardiomegaly, pulmonary oedema—not always
• Renal imaging	Usually normal
• USG of kidneys	May show mildly enlarged kidneys with normal echogenicity
• Renal biopsy	Glomerulonephritis

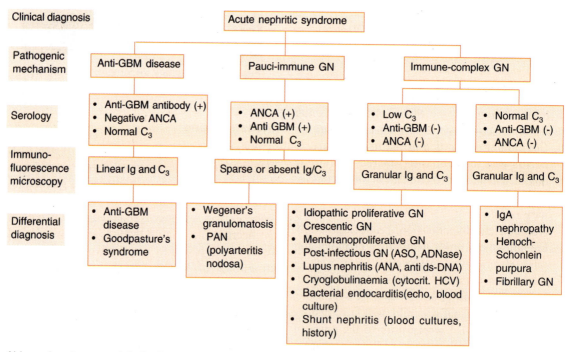

Abbrev: Ig = Immunoglobulin C_3 = third component of complement; ANA = Antinuclear anitbody; Anti-ds DNA = Anti-double stranded DNA antibody; HCV = Hepatitis C virus; Echo = Echocardiogram; ASO = Anti streptolysin-O antibody titre; ADNase = Anti-deoxyribonuclease antibody titre

Fig. 73.4: Flow chart depicting the differential diagnosis of acute nephritic syndrome based on complement (C_3), anti-glomerular basement membrane (Anti-GBM) antibody and ANCA (antineutrophil cytoplasmic antibody)

1. *Rest:* Hospitalization of the patient for observation and assessment is necessary. Strict bed rest is advised to patients with severe hypertension or pulmonary oedema.
2. *Monitoring:* Most patients require daily recording of fluid intake and output, daily weighing and measurement of BP.
3. *Infection:* Antibiotics are used to eradicate the infection in case of post-streptococcal GN. Sore throat may be treated with penicillins. Long-term prophylaxis after the development of streptococcal glomerulonephritis is not recommended.
4. *Diet, salt and fluid control:* Salt restricted diet is necessary. Proteins are restricted only if severe uraemia is present. In oliguric patients, fluid restriction is necessary to maintain body weight and to avoid fluid overload. During diuretic phase, liberal fluids with salt and potassium become necessary. Sodium and potassium are to be monitored.
5. *Diuretics:* They are used to control oedema, fluid overload and hypertension. Frusemide 40 mg I.V. daily for few days may be necessary initially because of renal failure, followed by oral substitution.
6. *Hypertension:* It is controlled by diuretics, salt restriction, fluid adjustment and anti-hypertensive drugs such as angiotensin converting enzyme inhibitors (ACE inhibitors) i.e. enalapril 2.5-10 mg daily or angiotensin receptors antagonists e.g. losarten 25-50 mg/day either alone or in combination may be used depending on the severity of hypertension.
7. *Immunosuppression:* Glucocorticoids and immunosuppressive drugs are mainstay of treatment for anti-GBM disease, Pauci-immune GN and immune-complex GN complicating SLE and RPGN.
8. *Plasmapheresis:* It is useful adjunct to immunosuppression in patients with severe immune-complex nephritis.
9. *Dialysis:* Peritoneal dialysis, hemodialysis or haemofiltration will be required in cases with severe renal failure.
10. *Treatment of complications:* Such as hypertensive encephalopathy and pulmonary oedema is on the same lines as discussed individually in respective sections as full chapters.

Chapter 74

Acute Renal Failure

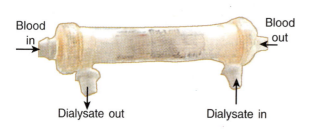

Fig. 74.1A: Hollow fibre dialyser

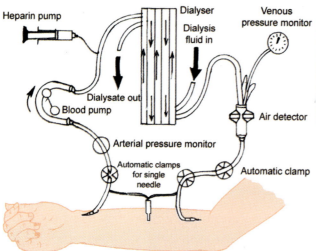

Fig. 74.1B: Diagrammatic representation of haemodialysis

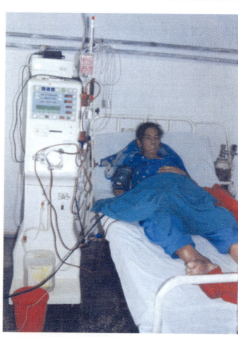

Fig. 74.2: A patient of acute renal failure being dialysed in haemodialysis section

ACUTE RENAL FAILURE

Definition

Acute renal failure (ARF) is defined as sudden and most often reversible loss of renal functions, which develops over a period of day or weeks, leads to retention of waste products of metabolism such as urea and creatinine. An increase in plasma creatinine concentration to > 200 µmol/L (> 2 mg%) is often taken as the biochemical definition of renal failure. A reduction in urine output (oliguria) occurs usually but not always.

Acute on chronic renal failure: Sudden deterioration of renal functions with rapid rise in blood urea and creatinine with fall in GFR (urine output) in a patient of established chronic renal failure is called acute on chronic renal failure.

Causes

Depending on the cause, acute renal failure is classified into three groups:
1. **Pre-renal:** Cause lies outside the kidney, is commonly due to contraction of blood volume.
2. **Renal:** Cause lies inside the kidney (intrinsic renal disease).
3. **Post-renal:** Cause lies below the kidney in its excretory passage i.e., pelvis, ureter, bladder and urethra

The causes are given in the Table 74.1.

The most common causes of ARF are: blood loss, fluid and electrolyte depletion, diarrhoea, non-diarrhoeal G.I. infections, glomerulonephritis, poisoning (drugs, snake venom, heavy metals) and G6PD deficiency associated with intravascular hemolysis. Fluid depletion is the major cause of ARF in tropics due to infectious diarrhoea leading to hypovolaemia. Heat stroke is another cause in tropics. Infectious diarrhoea is also a common cause in children. Acute glomerulonephritis and RPGN together account for large number of cases of ARF in children.

Malaria is a common cause of ARF in tropical countries. Falciparum infection causes most of these cases due to intravascular haemolysis or heavy parasitaemia. Intravascular haemolysis in malaria could also be drug-induced in patients with G6PD deficiency. Leptospirosis can also lead to ARF but is rare in India.

Acute interstitial nephritis due to drugs (β-lactams, sulfonamides, NSAIDs, rifampicin), herbal indigenous medicine and certain bacterial and viral infections are emerging as important causes of ARF.

Septic abortions, pre-eclampsia, abruptio placentae, placenta previa and postpartum ARF are important obstetric causes of ARF.

Table 74.1: Aetiological classification of acute renal failure

1. **Pre-renal**
   Renal hypoperfusion/underperfusion
   - Fluid loss (vomiting, diarrhoea)
   - Blood loss (haemorrhage)
   - Diuretics
   - Sepsis (decreased vascular resistance)
   - Anaphylaxis (vasodilation and blood pooling)
   - Burns (loss of fluid, plasma, blood etc.)
   - Cardiac failure (low cardiac output)
   - Heat stroke (perspiration)
   - Hypoproteinaemia (retention of extracellular fluid)
   - Renal vascular disease e.g. renal artery stenosis/occlusion, vasculitis
   - Hepatorenal syndrome
2. **Renal**
   - Acute glomerulonephritis
   - Interstitial nephritis e.g. due to drugs, pyelonephritis (infection), and idiopathic
   - Acute tubular necrosis e.g. ischaemic, toxic (radio-contrast media, antibiotics), rhabdomyolysis, haemoglobinuria
   - Renovascular hypertension, pre-eclampsia
   - Diseases of renal microvasculature e.g. disseminated intravascular coagulation, thrombotic thrombocytopenic purpura, haemolytic-uraemic syndrome.
3. **Post-renal**
   i. Ureteric e.g. calculi, blood clot
   ii. Bladder neck obstruction e.g. benign prostatic hypertrophy, calculi, cancer
   iii. Urethra e.g. stricture, congenital valves

Obstructive uropathy (stone, tumour retroperitoneal fibrosis) is also an important group leading to ARF. Benign hypertrophy of prostate is another important cause of reversible ARF.

Pathogenesis

In pre-renal reversible ARF, renal hypoperfusion is the most important underlying mechanism, systemic hypotension is present in most of these cases. When perfusion pressure falls as in shock, hypovolaemia, heart failure or narrowing of the renal arteries; two compensatory mechanisms come into action i.e. vasodilatation under the effect of prostaglandins and vasoconstriction under the effect of catecholamines, angiotensin and/or vasopressin; the net effect being vasoconstriction resulting in fall in GFR.

In post-renal reversible failure, the intratubular and ureteral pressure rises with progression of disease and this leads to rise in intravascular resistance and fall in GFR subsequently. Intratubular obstruction due to uric acid and oxalate crystals, calcium and myeloma proteins leads to ARF.

Acute renal failure due to intrinsic renal disease is complex in pathogenesis. There may be one or more of the following abnormalities i.e. haemodynamic changes, tubular back-leakage of filtrate or decrease in glomerular permeability.

Pathology

The pathological changes in ARF may be seen in glomeruli, interstitium, tubules and small vessels of the kidney and these are variable. Acute tubular necrosis (ATN) is probably the most common pathological lesion in established ARF. ATN may result from ischaemia or nephrotoxicity caused by chemicals and bacterial toxins and frequent use of nephrotoxic antibiotics. Renal ischaemia is due to sepsis, hypovolaemia, haemorrhage and shock.

The ischaemic insult causes lipid peroxidation of cell membrane lipids, influx of Ca^{++}, cell swelling, mitochondrial dysfunction, denaturation of proteins and death of tubular cells. Loss of adhesion between tubular cells and the basement membrane leads to shedding of cells into tubular lumen, where they cause obstruction. Break in the tubular basement membrane allows tubular contents to leak into the interstitial tissue and cause interstitial oedema.

In nephrotoxic ATN, a similar sequence is observed as described above, but it is initiated by direct toxicity to tubular cells. It is due to oxygen free radicals leading to lipid peroxidation of membrane lipids, binding of toxins or drugs to target proteins to interfere with cellular respiration and inhibition of cell protein synthesis. Examples are aminoglycosides (gentamicin) cytotoxic agent (cisplatin) and the antifungal drug (amphotericin). The common exogenous nephrotoxins causing ATN and ARF and given in Box 74.1.

Box 74.1: Common nephrotoxins causing ATN and ARF

1. *Antimicrobial*
   - Aminoglycosides (gentamicin)
   - Amphotericin B
   - Vancomycin
   - Sulphonamides
2. *Anti-inflammatory drugs*
   - NSAIDs
3. *Cytotoxic drugs/agents*
   - Cyclosporine
   - Cisplatin
4. *Organic solvents*
   - Ethylene glycol
5. *Bacterial toxins*
6. *Herbomineral indigenous drugs*

Fortunately, tubular cells can regenerate and reform the basement membrane. If the patient is supported during the regeneration phase, kidney functions return.

ARF may be caused by acute glomerulonephritis (post-streptococcal) and RPGN. The changes in the kidneys are different. These are characterized by marked proliferation of glomerular cells and frequently epithelial crescents formation (crescentic GN). Similarly in acute interstitial nephritis causing ARF, the pathological changes include peritubular and interstitial infiltration with polymorphs and eosinophils.

Acute Renal Failure

Table 74.2: Clinical features based on cause of ARF

Cause	Clinical features	Urinalysis
I. Pre-renal azotaemia	• Symptoms and signs of dehydration (e.g. thirst, postural hypotension, tachycardia, low JVP, dryness of mouth, skin, mucous membrane, weight loss and oliguria). • Decreased 'effective' circulatory volume e.g. heart failure, cardiac tamponade, hepato-renal syndrome • Treatment with NSAIDs or ACE inhibitors	• Hyaline casts • High specific gavity > 1018 • FeNa < 1% • U_{Na+} < 10 mmol/L
II. Intrinsic renal azotaemia		
A. Renal vessel disease		
• Renal artery thrombosis embolism	• History of atrial fibrillation or recent MI • Flank or abdominal pain • Haematuria and/or oliguria	• Proteinuria • RBCs in urine (occasional)
• Renal vein thrombosis	• Evidence of nephrotic syndrome or pulmonary embolism • Flank pain, oedema feet	• Proteinuria, haematuria
B. Glomerular disease		
• Glomerulonephritis/ vasculitis	• Compatible clinical history (e.g. recent sore throat, skin infection), sinusitis, lung haemorrhage, skin rash, or ulcers, arthralgias, new cardiac murmurs, history of hepatitis B or C infection)	• Red cell and granular casts • Mild proteinuria • RBCs, WBCs in urine
• Haemolytic uraemic syndrome or thrombotic thrombocytopenic purpura	Compatible clinical history (e.g. recent GI infection, cyclosporine), fever, pallor, ecchymoses, neurological abnormalities	• May be normal • Mild proteinuria • Red cells/granular casts
• Malignant hypertension	Severe hypertension with headache, cardiac failure, retinopathy, neurologic dysfunction, papilloedema	• Proteinuria and/or haematuria may be present
C. Acute tubular necrosis		
• Ischaemic ATN	Recent haemorrhage, hypotension e.g. cardiac arrest, surgery	• Muddy brown granular or tubular epithelial casts • FeNa > 1% • U_{Na+} > 20 mmol/L • Specific gravity < 1.015
• Toxins-induced ATN —Exogenous	Recent radiocontrast study, nephrotoxic antibiotics or cytotoxic drugs, sepsis, chronic renal failure (acute on chronic renal failure)	Same as above
—Endogenous	History suggestive of rhabdomyolysis (seizures, coma, ethanol abuse, trauma) • History suggestive of haemolysis (malarial infection, G6PD deficiency, blood transfusion) • History suggestive of tumour lysis (chemotherapy), myeloma (bone pain) or ethylene glycol ingestion	Urine supernatant positive for heme Urine supernatant pink and positive for heme Urate crystals, dipstick negative, proteinuria, oxalate crystal respectively
D. Acute tubulointerstitial renal diseases		
• Allergic interstitial nephritis	• Recent ingestion of drug, fever, rash or arthralgias	• WBCs and RBCs casts • Urine contains RBCs, WBCs
• Acute pyelonephritis	Fever, dysuria, flank pain and tenderness, pyuria, toxic look	• Leucocytes, red cells • Proteinuria • Bacteria in urine-culture may be positive
III. Post-renal azotaemia	• Abdominal or flank pain, haematuria palpable distended bladder	• Usually normal, haematuria if renal stone disease is suspected

Clinical Features

The clinical features depend on the type of ARF and the causative factor (Table 74.2). ARF is usually asymptomatic and is diagnosed by biochemical parameters such as recent rise in blood urea or serum creatinine. Oliguria (urine output < 400 ml/day) is frequent but not an invariable feature because nonoliguric acute renal failure is also known and clinically recognised entity. Patients of pre-renal azotaemia complain of thirst, and have postural hypotension and tachycardia. There will be signs of dehydration.

The patients of renal azotaemia present with symptoms and signs of the underlying disease/cause (see the Table 74.1). Oedema feet and hypertension may occur due to salt and water retention.

Occurrence of gross haematuria with or without flank pain and a distended bladder points to post-renal cause such as benign prostate hypertrophy in > 50 years old male.

Investigations

1. *Urinalysis:*
   A. *Specific gravity and osmolarity:* Volume depletion in pre-renal azotaemia stimulates sodium and water reabsorption producing urine of high specific gravity > 1.018. Measurement of urine osmolarity and ratio of urine to plasma osmolarity are other renal indices of diagnostic value. The great majority of patients with oliguric pre-renal ARF have urine osmolarity above 350 mOsm. The ratio of urine to plasma osmolarity less than 1.1 suggest ATN (Table 74.3).
   B. *Chemical composition:* Mild proteinuria is consistent with pre-renal and obstructive disorders, but can also be seen in most cases of acute interstitial nephritis. Massive proteinuria occurs in renal vein thrombosis. Positive reaction for blood indicates heme pigment, may be seen in conditions associated with microscopic or gross haematuria, hemoglobinuria and myoglobinuria.
   C. *Urinary sediment:* The urinary sediment is scanty in pre-renal and post-renal ARF. Presence of crystals and RBCs in urine point towards post-renal ARF. In ATN, epithelial cells, casts and coarse granular pigment casts are seen. The urine sediments in pre-renal and renal azotaemia are given in Table 74.3.
   D. *Urinary sodium:* The assessment of urinary sodium in oliguric patients differentiates pre-renal and renal ARF (Table 74.3). Urinary concentration of sodium below 20 mEq/L in oliguric renal failure suggests pre-renal ARF.
   E. *Creatinine and urea:* The ratio of urinary to plasma creatinine is a useful parameter for classifying ARF. Ratios greater than 40 strongly suggests pre-renal ARF; while

Table 74.3: Urinary abnormalities in pre-renal and renal azotaemia

Abnormality	*Pre-renal*	*Renal (ATN)*
Specific gravity	> 1.020	< 1.010
Urinary osmolarity (mOsm/kg)	> 500	< 350
Urine to plasma osmolarity (ratio)	> 1.1	< 1.1
Urine Na+ (mEq/L)	< 20	> 20
FeNa (%)	< 1	> 1
Urine to plasma creatinine ratio	> 40	< 40 (may be even < 20)
Renal failure index	< 1	> 2
Urinary sediment	Scanty	Active
Urinary proteins	Minimal	Moderate to severe

$$FeNa\ (\%) = \frac{U_{Na}/P_{cr}}{P_{Na} \times U_{cr}} \times 100 \qquad \text{Renal failure index} = \frac{U_{Na}}{U_{cr}/P_{cr}}$$

values less than 40 (even < 20) can occur in both renal and post-renal ARF.

2. **Blood biochemistry:** In ARF, the urinary waste products excretion is inadequate, hence, both the blood urea and serum creatinine rise in ARF depending on its severity. Serial measurements of urea and creatinine in blood are helpful in planning the management of ARF as these parameters do not differentiate between various causes of renal failure. In severe ARF, blood urea may rise by 20-40 mg% and serum creatinine by 1-2 mg% daily.

Hyponatremia and hyperkalemia are important electrolyte disturbance in ARF. Patients with moderate to severe ARF may show evidence of metabolic acidosis (low plasma bicarbonate concentration).

3. **Radiological examination:**
   - *Ultrasound of kidneys:* It is most commonly employed investigation, determines the size and echogenicity of the kidneys, helps to differentiate between acute and chronic renal failure and Doppler ultrasound helps to assess the patency of renal artery and veins. Presence of normal sized or slightly enlarged kidneys points towards intrinsic ARF. Small contracted kidneys (< 9 cm) raise the possibility of chronic renal failure. Dilated pelvicalyceal system indicates obstructive uropathy.
   - *Plain X-ray abdomen:* It is used to determine kidney size, shape and to identify radiopaque calculi.
   - *Intravenous pyelography:* It is best avoided in ARF because of contrast induced deterioration of renal function. USG and CT scan provide more valuable informations.
   - *Contrast enhanced CT scan:* It provides reliable information regarding size of the kidneys and presence of hydronephrosis. It is also required to confirm acute bilateral cortical necrosis if patient remains oliguric for more than 3 weeks.
   - *Arteriography and venography:* Renal arteriography has a role in ARF secondary to sudden interruption of renal blood flow as occurs in renal artery thrombosis/embolism. Venography is useful for confirming renal vein thrombosis.
   - *Renal biopsy:* Renal biopsy may be considered in those patients in whom the cause of ARF is uncertain or in cases where disease specific therapy is needed, for examples; glomerulonephritis, vasculitis or acute interstitial nephritis.

Management

1. *General principles:* The initial treatment of ARF is focussed on reversing the underlying cause and correcting fluid and electrolyte balance. By definition, pre-renal azotaemia is rapidly reversible upon correction of the primary haemodynamic abnormality and post-renal azotaemia resolves upon relief of obstruction. Therefore, every effort should be made to prevent further injury and provide supportive measures until recovery of renal functions has occurred. Renal functions recover spontaneously in patients with ATN, but other causes of ARF require specific therapies.

The decision to give fluid or to remove fluid is most difficult, requires careful physical examination and CVP monitoring. Fluid challenge (Fig. 74.2) is of value in patients suspected to have pre-renal azotaemia or early ATN and should be tried in patients without clinical evidence of fluid overload. Restoration of renal blood flow with intravenous volume expansion is ineffective in restoring renal functions once ATN is established.

Management of Acute Tubular Necrosis (Established Renal Failure)

Established ARF develops following severe and prolonged pre-renal ARF. In such cases, the histological pattern of acute tubular necrosis is usually seen. Alternatively, patients may present *de novo* with established ARF due to intrinsic disease of the kidneys e.g. RPGN or obstructive uropathy.

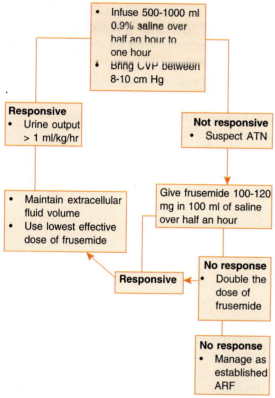

Fig. 74.2: Fluid challenge as a guide for differentiation and management of the pre-renal azotaemia and ATN

Aims of emergency resuscitation:
- Treatment of hyperkalaemia ($K^+ > 6$ mEq/L).
- Control of hypertension, left heart failure or volume overload, if associated.
- Correction of metabolic acidosis.
- To find out the underlying cause and treat it accordingly.
- Measure urine output, weight, BP, blood urea and creatinine daily.
- In case of deterioration of clinical condition, falling GFR (persistent oliguria), rising urea, creatinine, an emergency dialysis may be instituted (Fig. 74.2).

The steps of management are:
1. *Fluid therapy:* In patients with established ARF, the fluid intake should be restricted to sum of previous day urine output *plus* 500 ml for insensible loss. Replace other fluid losses (gastric aspirate, diarrhoea etc). with equal amounts of saline. In febrile patients, add 100-150 ml/day of fluid for each degree rise in body temperature over 37°C.
2. *Diuretic therapy:* Diuretics have been tried in patients with ATN to decrease its severity. They are useful in early course of ATN (e.g. immediately after hypotension, mismatch transfusion, crush injury, burns etc.), can convert oliguric state to non-oliguric state. Although nonoliguric state has better outcome than oliguric state, but there is no convincing evidence till date that conversion from an oliguric to nonoliguric state decreases either the mortality or the need for dialysis. At present, there is no convincing evidence to confirm usefulness of diuretics in prevention of ischaemic ATN. Diuretics are used as continuous infusion (frusemide 200-400 mg) in normal saline rather than intermittent infusion. Diuretics are detrimental in ARF induced by radio-contrast agent and rhabomyolysis.
3. *Low-dose dopamine:* Low dose dopamine (1-3 µg/kg/min) was used earlier as renovasodilator and considered as renoprotective. Most clinical trials have failed to demonstrate its effectiveness either in prevention or treatment of established ARF. It is best avoided. Use of higher doses of dopamine may however be required in hypotensive patients to maintain the BP.
4. *Nutrition:* Protein intake needs to be restricted in patients with ARF. In mild to moderate cases, about 30 g of proteins can be given per day. Adequate calories should be given with vitamins and mineral supplementation. In critically ill patients, nutrition is provided through nasogastric tube or parenterally. Patient should be advised to restrict intake of potassium containing foodstuffs i.e. fruits, and dry fruits to avoid hyperkalaemia.

Acute Renal Failure

5. *Potassium balance:* Hyperkalaemia (serum K^+ > 5.5 mEq/L) is a serious biochemical abnormality and is the leading cause of death in ARF. Acidosis, uraemia and hypercatabolic state contribute to hyperkalaemia. Several modes of therapy for hyperkalaemia are available. Mild to moderate hyperkalaemia can be treated by medical means (e.g. insulin with glucose, use of calcium gluconate and cation exchange resins), but in severe hyperkalaemia (serum K+ > 7 mEq/L) dialysis is desirable. For treatment (read chapter on hyperkalaemia).
6. *Acid-base balance*: Mild to moderate metabolic acidosis is common in ARF, does not require treatment. However, the advanced cases of ARF need 50-100 ml of 7.5% $NaHCO_3$ every 8 to 12 hourly to maintain serum bicarbonate > 15 mEq/L. Avoid sodium bicarbonate in patients with fluid overload.
7. *Nephrotoxic drugs:* They should be discontinued or avoided. The doses of medications that require kidneys for their elimination should be adjusted.
8. *Platelet dysfunction:* Platelet dysfunctions (aggregation, adhesiveness) occur in uraemia *per se* and predispose to bleeding. Patients with prolonged bleeding time or with active bleeding can be treated by cryoprecipitate or desmopressin. H_2 receptor antagonists can be given prophylactically to prevent an upper GI bleeding.
9. *Treatment of infection:* Sepsis is most common cause of death in ARF. The rate of infectious complications is very high (80%). Infections can occur via indwelling catheter or venous catheters. Pulmonary, urinary and wound infections occur frequently in post-traumatic and post-operative cases, need energetic treatment. Prophylactic antibiotics have no role. If infection is suspected clinically and patient's condition is deteriorating, antibiotics (gentamicin or amikacin *plus* a third generation cephalosporin) should be started pending cultures reports. Full doses may be given initially followed by adjustment doses subsequently.
10. *Dialysis (Fig.74.1 and 74.2):* This should be considered as an adjunct to the conservative therapy for ARF. Indications for dialysis in ARF are not specific but have to be individualized. Some guidelines for dialysis are:
    1. *Biochemical:*
        - Blood urea > 200mg/dl.
        - Serum creatinine > 10 mg/dl.
        - Serum K+ > 6 mEq/L (an evidence of hyperkalaemia).
        - Serum HCO_3 < 10 mEq/L (metabolic acidosis)
        - pH < 7.2 (metabolic acidosis).
    2. *Clinical:*
        - Oliguria < 400 ml/day for 5 days
        - Anuria (urine output < 50 ml/day) for 3 days
        - Fluid overload or pulmonary oedema
        - Symptomatic uraemia i.e. uraemic encephalopathy, uraemic pericarditis, uraemic bleeding diathesis, resistant heart failure.

    A review of experience with early and daily dialysis in hypercatabolic states reveals marked improvement in patient's survival. Good dialytic therapy simplifies management of ARF. Diet and fluid can be liberalized and most uraemic symptoms are ameliorated.

Modes of Dialysis
1. *Intermittent hemodialyses:* It is standard form of renal replacement therapy for patients with ARF.
2. *Intermittent peritoneal dialysis:* It is preferred over hemodialysis in patients who are either hemodynamically unstable or have active bleeding. It is not to be used in patients with peritonitis or who have undergone abdominal surgery.

3. *Continuous renal replacement therapy:* It includes continuous arterio-venous or veno-venous haemofiltration, dialysis or haemodiafiltration. In critically ill patients, the continuously administered therapies are preferred now-a-days. Their advantages over intermittent dialysis include more strict fluid and metabolic control, decreased haemodynamic instability and an enhanced possibility of removing cytokines in patients with sepsis or multiorgan failure. Another advantage is to administer unlimited nutritional support parenterally. The disadvantage of this therapy is that it needs prolonged anticoagulation and constant monitoring.

11. *Newer therapies:*
    i. Atrial natriuretic peptide has been tried to attenuate the severity of renal failure, but was not found useful in ARF in controlled human trials.
    ii. Calcium channels blockers: They have received considerable attention in prevention and treatment of ATN, but as these drugs produce hypotension and thereby decrease renal perfusion, their use is not justified.
    iii. Acetylcysteine in dose of 600 mg twice a day has been found effective in preventing radiocontrast induced renal failure.
    iv. Insulin-like growth factors: A trial of insulin-like growth factor in ischaemic ATN in humans did not reveal any beneficial effect.
12. *Specific treatment of intrinsic renal disease:* i.e. acute GN, vasculitis by steroids, alkylating agents and/or plasmapheresis depending on primary pathology.

Recovery Phase (Diuretic Phase of ATN)

Recovery in ARF is usually associated with diuresis. There is step-wise increase in urine flow, but, sometimes a large amount of urine (5-8 L) may be passed, which should be taken care of. Excessive loss of water, sodium, potassium occurs. Fluid losses are better managed with half-isotonic saline. Patients should be encouraged to drink water *ad lib* to satisfy their thirst; remaining fluid deficit is corrected by parenteral fluid therapy. Electrolytes should be monitored during this period and appropriate replacement done whenever needed.

Prevention of ARF

Because there are no specific therapies for treatment of ischaemic or nephrotoxic ARF, hence, prevention is of utmost importance. Many cases of ischaemic ARF can be avoided by monitoring cardiovascular functions and intravascular volume in high risk patients. Some guidelines are:

1. Aggressive restoration of intravenous volume has been shown to reduce incidence of ARF dramatically after major surgery, trauma, burn or cholera.
2. The incidence of nephrotoxic ARF can be reduced by tailoring the dose of nephrotoxins (aminoglycosides, cyclosporine) according to body size and GFR in patients with pre-existing renal impairment. Hypovolaemia should be avoided in patients receiving nephrotoxic medications.
3. Allopurinol and forced diuresis are useful in patients at high risk for acute urate nephropathy (e.g cancer chemotherapy in leukaemias) Forced alkaline diuresis may also prevent or attenuate ARF in patients receiving high-dose methotrexate or suffering from rhabdomyolysis.
4. N-acetylcysteine limits acetaminophen-induced renal injury if given within 24 hours of ingestion.
5. Dimercaprol—a chelating agent may prevent heavy-metal nephrotoxicity.
6. Ethanol inhibits ethylene glycol metabolism to oxalic acid and other toxic metabolites, hence, useful in ethylene glycol intoxication as an adjuvant to haemodialysis..

Part Nine

Poisonings

Chapter 75

Management of a Case with Poisoning

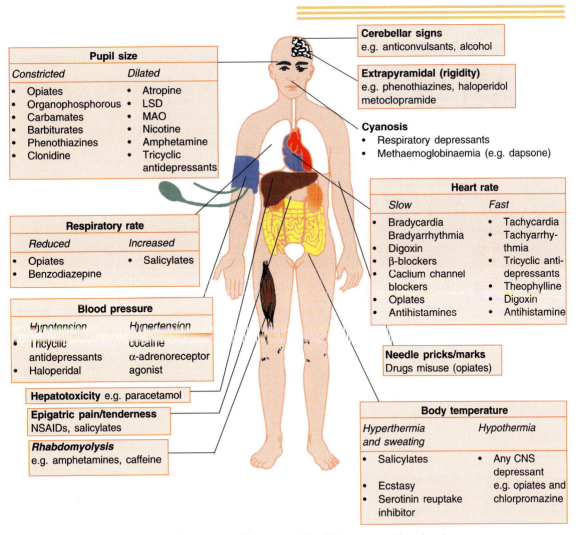

Fig. 75.1: Clinical manifestations (signs) in a case with poisoning

MANAGEMENT OF A CASE WITH POISONING

Any substance which produces adverse reactions/effects in a living organism is called *poison*. Acute poisoning is the common cause of morbidity and mortality throughout the world and is the most common cause of non-traumatic coma in young persons (< 35 years of age). Hospital-based data suggests that about 10% of all acute medical admissions are due to poisoning.

Types of Poisoning

1. *Self-poisoning:* It refers to the deliberate ingestion of an overdose substance/drug not meant for consumption. It is also called *suicidal or intentional poisoning*. Aluminium phosphide, OP compound poisoning are its examples.
2. *Accidental poisoning:* It occurs in children below 5 years of age, but can occur in adults, is either due to accidental exposure (inhalation of gases) or ingestion of fluid or substance from a wrongly labelled bottle, and also includes stings, bites or eating poisoned foods/plants (e.g. mushroom poisoning).
3. *Non-accidental poisoning:* Is a deliberate administration of a poison to a child.
4. *Homicidal poisoning:* Means to kill someone by poisoning.

Diagnosis

Although acute poisoning can mimic any acute illness, but the correct diagnosis is based on high degree of suspicion on history, is established on the physical examination, response to an antidote and clinical course.

History

Although accurate history is an important clinical weapon for diagnosis, but at times, is difficult to obtain from patients who are confused or obtunded and information obtained from the relatives and friends may not be dependable. The points to be noted on the history are given in Box 75.1.

> **Box 75.1: Important points on history-taking**
> - Time
> - Route of administration
> - Duration
> - Name and amount of the poison, chemical ingredients involved (summon the bottle/container/wrapper of poison to verify it)
>   The print code on the pills or lable may be used to identify the ingredients and potential toxicity of suspected poison by consulting a reference text, a computerised database, the manufacturer or a regional poisoning centre
> - Family, friends, police, pharmacists, physicians and employes should be asked regarding the habits, hobbies, behaviour, available medications and clinical grounds for suspicion of poisoning
> - Circumstances of exposure (location, surrounding, intent)
> - Symptomatology e.g. time of onset, nature and severity of symptoms
> - Time and type of first-aid given
> - Medical history for any acute illness
> - Psychiatric history
> - History of alcohol or drug overdose

Poisoning is likely to be missed if it is not suspected. The suspicious circumstances include:
1. Unexplained illness in a previously healthy person.
2. A history of underlying psychiatric illness such as depression.
3. Recent changes in health, economic status or social relationships.
4. Chemical exposure or illness following ingestion of food, drink or medication. The onset of illness in industrial workers or occupational workers may indicate chemical poisoning.
5. Patients falling ill immediately after landing from a foreign country or after arrest for criminal activity should be suspected of having an illicit drug concealed in body cavity (the GI tract).

Physical Examination

A search for the clothes, belongings and place of discovery may help to recover a suicidal note, or a container which may have the remaining tablets or chemical.

The physical examination should focus initially on the vital signs and cardiopulmonary and neurological status. Before proceeding for detailed clinical examination. First ensure A, B, C of cardiopulmonary resuscitation:
- The airway (A) is clear.
- The patient is breathing (B) properly and adequately.
- The circulation (C) is adequate and is not compromised. If the patient is alert and is hemodynamically stable, proceed to examination as follows:
    1. Level of consciousness: The Glassgow coma scale (given in chapter on coma) may be employed to assess the degree of unconsciousness though it has never been validated for use in poisoned patients.
    2. Look for respiratory effort and cyanosis, presence or absence of cough and gag reflex.
    3. Record pulse rate and blood pressure.
    4. Examination of eyes (for nystagmus, size of the pupil, and its reaction), abdomen (for bowel activity and bladder size) and skin (for burns, bullae, colour, warmth, moisture, pressure sores, puncture marks) to narrow down the diagnosis to a particular poison.
    5. Look for an evidence of trauma or physical illness.
    6. Temperature—measure with a low reading rectal thermometer.
    7. When history is unclear, all orifices should be examined for presence of chemical burns, and drug packets.
    8. The odour of breath or vomitus and the colour of the skin, nails or urine may give valuable informations for diagnosis.

The physical signs of the poisoning are given in the Figure 75.1 on front page. Diagnosis and differential diagnosis of the poisoning based on biochemical analysis is given in Box 75.2.

Laboratory Tests

In most patients, the diagnosis is made on the history and clinical signs alone. As these cases are medico-legal, hence, urine, serum and vomitus (or gastric lavage may be preserved for analysis especially where there is fatality. They may be useful to confirm or rule out suspected poisoning. Otherwise also, subsequent management of poisoned patients depends on the measurement of amount of toxin/poison and severity of the poisoning. Grading of severity is useful for clinical course and response to treatment.

In unconscious patients, a qualitative screen of the urine (e.g. urine immunofluorescence for drugs of misuse screening test) is an effective way to confirm recent use of drugs such as benzodiazepines, cocaine, opioids, ecstasy, and cannabis. Routine screens may not, however detect fentanyl derivatives, tramadol and other synthetic opioids. Occasionally measuring drugs of misuse and their metabolites in blood by gas chromatography-mass spectroscopy (GC-MS) may be required for medico-legal purposes. Personal communication with the laboratory is essential. A negative result on a screen may mean the poison is not detectable by the test used or its concentration is too low for detection at the time of sampling. In the latter situation, repeating the test at later time may give a positive result.

Response to Antidotes

The response to an antidote may be taken as a clue to diagnosis. Resolution of symptoms of hypoglycaemia with dextrose confirms hypoglycaemia. Resolution of altered mental status and abnormal vital signs within minutes of I.V. administration naloxone or flumazenil is virtually diagnostic of opiates and benzodiazepine poisoning respectively.

Box 75.2: Diagnosis and differential diagnosis based on laboratory assessment

Parameter	Differential diagnosis
Metabolic acidosis	Methanol, ethylene glycol, salicylate, carbon monoxide, ethanol poisoning.
An abnormally low anion gap	Bromide, iodine, lithium, nitrate, hypocalcaemia or hypermagnesaemia.
An Osmolal gap > 10 mmol/L (i.e. difference between measured serum osmolality and the calculated osmolality from serum Na+, glucose, urea)	Alcohol, glycol or ketone or an unmeasured electrolyte or sugar. It can be due to DKA or lactic acidosis from which poisoning has been differentiated.
Ketosis	Isopropyl alcohol and salicylate poisoning.
Hypoglycaemia	Poisoning by β-blockers, quinine, ethanol, OHA, and salicylates.
Hyperglycaemia	Poisoning by acetone, a beta-adrenergic agonist, a calcium channel blocker, iron or theophylline.
Hypokalaemia	Poisoning by barium, a beta-adrenergic agonist, a diuretic, theophylline
Hyperkalaemia	Poisoning with an α-adrenergic agonist, a beta blocker, digitalis, ACE inhibitors or fluoride.
Pulmonary oedema (ARDS) e.g. low PaO_2, low $PaCO_2$	Poisoning with carbon-monoxide, cyanide, an opoid, paraquat, salicylate or a sedative-hypnotic. Poisoning by inhaled gases, fumes or vapors (ammonia, metal oxides, mercury, phosphine (PH_3 due to aluminium phosphide poisoning).
Radio-opaque densities on abdominal X-rays	Ingestion of calcium salts, chloral hydrate, chlorinated hydrocarbon, heavy metals, illicit drug packets, iodinated compounds, K+ salts, psychotherapeutic agents, lithium, phenothiazines, salicylates or enteric coated tablets.
Bradycardia and AV block	Poisoning by antiarrhythmics, beta blockers, calcium channel blockers, cholinergic agents (carbonate and organophosphorus insecticide), digitalis, lithium or tricyclic-antidepressants.
QRS and QTc prolongation	Poisoning by antiarrhythmics, tricyclic antidepressants, heavy metals, lithium, local anaesthetic, meperidine and quinine and related antimalarial.
Tachyarrhythmias	Poisoning with digitalis, sympathomimetics, chloral hydrate, aliphatic or halogenated hydrocarbons and aluminium phosphide.

The prompt reversal of dystonia with I.V. benzotropine or diphenhydramine confirms drug-induced dystonia. *Vin rose urine colour* following a diagnostic use of desferoxamine confirms iron intoxication when measurements of serum iron and iron binding capacity test are not available immediately. Reversal of central and peripheral manifestations by physostigmine confirms anticholinergic poisoning.

Time Course of Events

It is also helpful in making a diagnosis of poisoning. Signs and symptoms developing acutely, peaking within several hours and subsequent resolution over hours or days in an otherwise healthy person suggest an acute poisoning.

Management

Principles

I. General management:
 - To support the vital functions (circulatory and respiratory).

II. Specific management:
 - To delay or prevent further absorption of poison.

- To enhance excretion of poison (through faeces or urine).
- To administer specific antidote, wherever applicable to prevent re-exposure.

Support of Vital Function

The supportive therapy may be needed to maintain physiological homeostasis until detoxification process is completed, and to prevent and treat secondary complications such as aspiration, bed sores, cerebral and pulmonary oedema, renal failure, rhabdomyolysis and generalised organ dysfunction due to prolonged hypoxia or shock.

A. Respiratory support:
- If respiratory depression is minimal, 60% O_2 via a mask may be sufficient. A nasopharyngeal or oropharyngeal airway should be inserted for constant monitoring for ventilation.
- Loss of gag or cough reflex is an indication for intubation (A gag reflex is assessed by positioning the patients on their side and making them gag using a sucker).
- Patients with severe excitation may also require intubation for airway protection.
- If ventilation remains inadequate, intermittent positive pressure ventilation (IPPV) should be instituted. Blood gas analysis is useful to confirm the need for IPPV.
- Hypoxaemia is common in unconscious patient, may go undetected after ingestion of poisoning (e.g. opiates, barbiturates etc.), hence, monitoring by oximetry or arterial blood gas analysis is mandatory for severely poisoned patients with depressed ventilation.
- Pulmonary arterial or capillary wedge pressure measurement is indicated in patients with pulmonary oedema to determine its nature. Drug-induced pulmonary oedema is usually noncardiogenic (normal or low capillary wedge pressure). A swan-ganz catheter may be put to measure the pressure and to monitor the fluid and diuretics therapy.
- Extracorporeal membrane oxygenation may be appropriate for severe but reversible respiratory failure.

B. Cardiovascular support:
- Hypotension (BP < 90 mmHg) is a common feature of drug overdosage, is caused by vasodilatation, hypovolaemia, myocardial depression, hypoxia etc. should be treated appropriately.
- Shocked patients (tachycardia, cold clammy skin, oliguria) should be managed accordingly.
- Arrhythmia are common. Find out the cause and treat it accordingly. Known arrhythmogenic factors such as hypoxia, acidosis and hypokalaemia should be corrected. Lidocaine and phenytoin are safe for drug-induced ventricular arrhythmias.
- Bradyarrhythmias due to beta blockers and calcium channel blockers may respond to glucagon and calcium respectively. Antibody (Fab antibody) to digoxin is indicated in digitalis-induced arrhythmias. Hypotension commonly accompanies bradyarrhythmia, should be managed simultaneously.

C. Care of unconscious patient (Read chapter on coma):
- In all cases, the patient should be nursed in the lateral position with lower leg straight and the upper leg flexed. In this position, risk of aspiration is minimized.
- Remove any obstructing object, vomitus or dentures. Maintain patent airway.
- Nursing care of mouth and measures to avoid pressure sore should be instituted.
- Unnecessary catheterization of bladder should be avoided. Condom drainage is best to avoid bed-wetting. Bladder in poisoned patients can be emptied by gentle suprapubic pressure.
- I.V. access and intravenous fluid to be started immediately and correct dehydration by I.V. fluids at least for 24 hours.

- Rest of the management is same as for any other unconscious patient including the monitoring of vital parameters (pulse, BP, temp, respiration, etc.).

D. Treatment of specific problems:
- *Convulsions/seizures:* These may occur in serious tricyclic antidepressants, antihistamine, phenothiazine and strychnine poisoning or may occur following drug withdrawal. Diazepam 10 mg I.V. is the standard treatment for fits of any cause. The patient should receive a loading dose of phenytoin (1g I.V. over 4 hours) followed by 100 mg 8 hourly if fits do not get immediately controlled with diazepam. Persistent fits must be controlled rapidly as they may otherwise result in hypoxia, brain damage and laryngeal trauma. The underlying cause should be corrected simultaneously.
- Hypothermia (rectal temperature (35°C) is a problem in elderly or in those poisoned with chlorpromazine or another neuroleptic. Hypothyroidism must be excluded. The patient should be covered with a space blanket and given intravenous and intragastric fluids at normal body temperature. Inspired gases should also be warmed to 37°C.
- Stress bleeding: Measures to prevent stress ulcers in poisoned patients include administration of antacids through ryle's tube or I.V. H_2 antagonists.
- Metabolic, renal and hepatic abnormalities; and secondary complications should be treated by standard measures.

Specific management: It depends on the route of exposure i.e. direct contact (eye, skin), ingestion (GI tract), inhalation (lungs and inoculation (blood). The steps of management are depicted in Figure 75.2

I. Steps to delay or prevent further absorption of poison

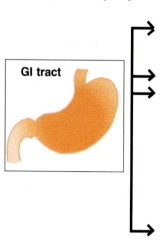

I. Decontamination of gastrointestinal tract

Gastric lavage: Only if a potentially life-threatening amount of toxic substance has been ingested within the last hour. Not to be used for acids, alkalis or petroleum distillates.

Induced emesis by syrup of ipecac.

Activated charcoal: 50 g can be given to an adult orally if a potentially toxic amount of poison has been ingested the last hour, but only if the toxin can be bound to charcoal. Multiple doses of charcoal are given (50 g every 4 hours) in poisoning by carbamazepine, dapsone, quinine and theophyline.

Catharsis: It is induced by cathartic salts (disodium phosphate, magnesium citrate, sodium sulphate) or saccharide (mannitol or sorbitol) to promote fecal excretion of poison. Contraindicated in corrosive poisoning and diarrhoea.

Whole bowel irrigation: Polyethylene glycol solution is given for potentially toxic ingestion of iron, lithium and theophylline and to clear packets of drugs from bodypackers

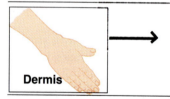

II. Decontamination of other sites

Removal of clothing/skin washing: Wash the skin with copious amounts of soap and water for chemical or pesticide exposures.

Contd.

Contd.

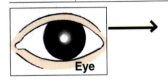

Irrigation of eyes:
- Wash eyes thoroughly for at least 15 minutes with normal saline or water.
- Remove particles from palpebral fissures. If pain persists, fluorescein drops and slit lamp examination for corneal damage are essential.

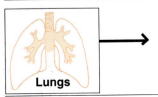

III. Exhalation of poison

Oxygen and bronchodilators: Give high-flow oxygen, e.g. 12 L/min. Nebulised β2-adrenoceptor agonists if patient has wheezing.

II. Steps to enhance poison excretion

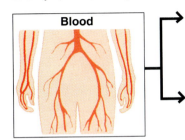

Urinary alkalinisation: Enhances elimination of salicylates and some pesticides, e.g. 2-4 D. Give 1 litre of 1.26% sodium bicarbonate I.V. over 3 hours. Check urine pH, remains between 7.5 and 8.5. Avoid use of large volumes i.e. forced diuresis, and watch for hypokalaemia.

Extracorporeal methods of elimination, e.g. haemodialysis or haemoperfusion: For serious poisoning with salicylates, theophylline, ethylene glycol, methanol, carbamazepine.

III. Neutralisation of poison by specific antidote
Antidotes counteract the effects of poisons by neutralising them (e.g. antigen-antibody reaction), by chelation (chemical binding) or by antagonising their physiological effects (activation of opposing nervous system activity, competitive inhibition). Antidotes can reduce both morbidity and mortality, but most antidotes are toxic too. The antidotes to various poisons are given in the box 75.3.

IV. Prevention of re-exposure
The method of poisoning prevention is depicted in Box 75.4.

Fig. 75.2: Steps of management in a patient with poisoning

Box 75.3: Commonly employed antidotes

Poison	Antidote
Paracetamol	N-acetylcysteine, methionine
Organophosporous and carbamates	Atropine (muscarine effects) pralidoxime (nicotinic effects)
Amanita phylloids	Benzylpenicillin
Calcium channel blockers	Calcium chloride/gluconate
Methanol and ethylene glycol	Ethanol
Iron	Desferroxamine
Opiates	Naloxone
Cyanide	Sodium nitrate, sodium thiosulphate
Anticholinergics	Physostigmine
Isoniazide	Pyridoxine
Lead, mercury, copper	BAL, calcium EDTA, D-pencillamine
Anticoagulants	Vitamin K
Beta blockers	Glucagon, adrenaline
Digitalis	Fab antibody

Box 75.4: Methods of poisoning prevention

Method	Mode of action
Addition of 'Bitrex' and other bittering agents to household products	• Prevents consumption of large quantities as it tastes bitter
Addition of antidote to the toxin e.g. combination tablets of methionine and paracetamol	• As antidote is incorporated, glutathione remains repleted and hepatocellular injury is prevented
Child-resistant containers	• Reduces chances of poisoning in children
Secure preservation (almirah, locked cupboard)	• Inaccessibility reduces chances of poisoning
Hazard warning signals	• Warning by label to potential toxicity, route of administration and protective measures
Education	• Warning on safe storage and handling of chemicals and drugs reduces poisoning incidence
Supervision	• Careful supervision reduces chances of poisoning in children
Legislation e.g. health and safety regulations	• Make a safe work place with safeguards in the use of dangerous chemicals

Chapter 76

Corrosive (Acid and Alkali) Poisoning

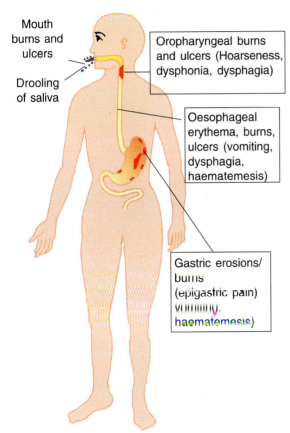

Fig. 76.1: Corrosive poisoning

These poisons corrode and destroy the local tissues commonly of mouth, pharynx and upper GI tract with which they immediately come in contact after ingestion (Fig. 76.1).

Mode of Action

Corrosive acids act locally and usually do not produce systemic effects. They produce coagulative necrosis by precipitation of tissue proteins which retards injury and limits the penetration into the tissue.

Types

- *Accidental:* It is common in children.
- *Suicidal:* It is common in adults.

Common Acid Poisons

- *Sulphuric acid:* It is present in toilet cleaner, battery acid, laboratory etc.
- *Hydrochloric acid:* It is present in toilet cleaner, soldering fluxes, laboratory etc.
- *Oxalic acid* (anti-rust).
- *Nitric acid* is used by goldsmiths, stone cleaners
- *Hydrofluoric acid* (present in toilet bowel cleaners, anti-rust compound and stone cleaners).

CORROSIVE ACID POISONING

Acute corrosive acid poisoning is common due to ingestion of an acid (sulphuric acid, HCl, nitric acid) present in many products of household use.

Clinical Features

The clinical manifestations depend on the concentration and quantity of acid consumed. The symptoms and signs are given Box 76.1.

Box 76.1: Symptoms and signs of corrosive acid poisoning

Site of injury	Symptoms	Signs
1. Mouth and oropharynx	• Pain in mouth, throat and drooling of saliva • Difficulty in speech (hoarseness or dysphonia) due to oedema of glottis • Choking and stridor • Constant cough, dyspnoea	• Oropharyngeal burns, ulcers, oedema, necrosis, discolouration of mouth • Deep mucosal burns may produce anaesthesia • Drooling of saliva over lips produces charring of skin over angles of mouth, chin and chest • In severe cases, the tongue is shapeless, a pulpy mass • Teeth may become chalky white and loose shine in severe poisoning (corrosion of teeth)
2. Oesophagus	• Painful swallowing, retrosternal pain, neck pain/tenderness • Haematemesis (vomiting with altered blood and mucus)	Oesophageal burns and ulcers. The mucosa is red and swollen
3. Stomach	• Epigastric pain, burning and tenderness • Vomiting. It is strongly acidic, will cause effervescence on coming in contact with earth and will stain clothes	Gastric burns
4. Respiratory tract (due to aspiration)	• Cough and dyspnoea • Hoarseness and dysphonia • Labored breathing	• Tracheitis and pneumonia • Pleural effusion may develop

In severe cases of acid poisoning following complications may occur:
1. **Hypotension and circulatory shock** due to vomiting and dehydration. The patient feels excessive thirst and tongue is dry. There is tachypnoea and tachycardia. There may be features of metabolic acidosis.
2. **Mediastinitis** due to rupture of oesophagus producing collection of air in the mediastinum (mediastinal emphysema). The mediastinal crunch (crunching sound on sternal compression) may be felt. There may be fever, increase in respiratory rate, constant cough and labored breathing.
3. **Stricture of oesophagus:** It develops on healing of acid burns in oesophagus producing oesophageal narrowing.

Investigations

1. *Routine laboratory tests:*
   - Complete hemogram, haematocrit.
   - Liver function tests.
   - Renal function tests (blood urea, serum creatinine).
   - Serum electrolytes.
2. *Arterial blood gas analysis.*
3. *Radiology:*
   - Chest X-ray. It may show diffuse mottling or ARDS like picture. In case of oesophageal perforation, air may be present in mediastinum (mediastinal emphysema).
   - Plain X-ray abdomen in case perforation is suspected.
4. *Endoscopy*: Laryngoscopy and upper GI endoscopy are done using a small-bore flexible

Corrosive (Acid and Alkali) Poisoning

endoscope as soon as the patient is hemodynamically stable and perforation is excluded. It documents the anatomical site and often severity of the injury (see Box 76.2).

Box 76.2: Fundoscopic classification of corrosive injury

Grade	Extent of injury
I	Oedema and hyperaemia only
IIa	Friability, erosions and superifical ulcerations
IIb	IIa (described above) *plus* discrete and deep ulcers
III	In addition to grade II changes, there are scattered areas of necrosis

Management

It depends on the extent of injury (Box 76.3).

A. *Immediate therapy*

1. *Fluid therapy:* Mild injury (grade I) can be managed with oral fluids. Moderate (grade II) injury requires I.V. fluids for 48 hours followed by small oral feeds of fluid. Severe injury initially may be treated by I.V. fluids, and may require feeding jejunostomy.
2. The important "Do's and "Don'ts" are given in Box 76.4.
3. *Post-resuscitation management:* Next step is to rule out an oesophageal and gastric perforation by:

Box 76.3: Extent of injury, management and complications

Endoscopic grading	Management	Complications
I	Oral fluids for 24-48 hours. Discharge the patient with advice of oral toilet with antiseptics and a soft diet	No complications
II (a and b)	• I.V. fluids for 24-48 hours, then start oral fluids • Begin with soft diet after 48 hours if patient can swallow	No complications
III	• In presence of dysphagia, nutritional supplementation intravenously or by a feeding jejunostomy • Antibiotics (a combination of an aminoglycoside and a cephalosporin) • Controversial use of steroids. A recent study in children has shown no benefit; while a meta-analysis published recently suggest beneficial effect of steroids • Resuscitate the patient for dehydration, shock etc.	Early perforation and GI haemorrhage

Box 76.4: Immediate "Do's" and "Don'ts" in corrosive acid poisoning

Don'ts
- Do not panic
- Make arrangements to transfer the patient to a hospital. Look at the oral cavity and remove any causatic granules and flakes gently
- Do not induce vomiting
- Do not put Ryle's tube as it may cause perforation of thinned mucosa of oesophagus or stomach. If still required, can be put only under endoscopic guidance

Do's
- Immediate liberal use of water or milk mixed with milk of magnesia, aluminium hydroxide and magnesium oxide to neutralise the acid. The best antidote is 5% magnesium oxide. Lime water, any vegetable oil or ghee, egg-white are other alternatives to neutralise the acid
- Correct hypotension with isotonic fluids and blood products. Suction of ice may reduce thirst
- If the patient has respiratory distress, do immediate tracheal intubation or tracheostomy
- Give oxygen
- Intravenous H_2 receptors blockers may be used for symptomatic relief and may help in early healing
- Use antibiotics if infection supervenes
- Relief of pain by morphine or pethidine
- Skin, oral and eye lesions may be irrigated with plenty of water

- Symptoms and signs.
- Chest X-ray and plain X-ray abdomen (film to be taken in erect position).

If there is no perforation, a cautious upper GI endoscopy by a small calibre flexible endoscope may be done by trained endoscopist. The endoscopy is safe and will delineate the injury and extent of mucosal damage. Depending on the classification of injury on endoscopy, proceed as given in Box 76.3.

In the event of perforation, thoracotomy and/or laparotomy is done at the earliest and oesophageal or gastric resection with appropriate bypass procedure may be required.

Long-term complications include oesophageal and gastric stenosis/stricture (Fig. 76.2) requiring endoscopic dilatation and corrective surgery.

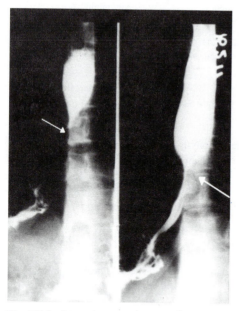

Fig. 76.2: Oesophageal stricture (↑) following corrosive (acid) poisoning

CORROSIVE ALKALI POISONING

Acute corrosive poisoning with alkali occurs due to ingestion of common household products containing alkali. Common alkaline products include industrial bleach, drain cleaners (sodium hydroxide), surface cleaners (ammonia, phosphates), laundry and dishwasher detergents (phosphates, carbonates), disk batteries, denture cleaners (borates, phosphates) and clinitest tablets (sodium hydroxide).

In India acids are more frequently implicated in poisoning than alkalis.

Mode of Action

Alkalis penetrate the tissues rapidly, produce corrosive effects by extracting water from the tissues causing tissue dehydration. They produce liquefactive necrosis of the tissues with which they come in contact with, therefore, there is higher risk of perforation of the oesophagus and stomach than acids do. Their action is bit slow but sustained one.

Types of Poisoning

- *Accidental ingestion.* It is common in children.
- *Suicidal.* It is common in adults especially females.

Clinical Features

1. Burning and severe pain extending from the mouth to the stomach due to corrosive alkaline injury, erythema, burns and ulceration. The pain radiates all over the abdomen.
2. Sudden caustic, soapy, nauseous taste in the mouth.
3. Vomiting soon follows which is strongly alkaline and contains frothy material with shreds of mucus and altered blood (haematemesis). The vomit will not effervescence when it comes in contact with the earth.
4. Dysphagia and dyspnoea may occur. Purging which is not seen in acidic poisoning is almost always present in alkali poisoning. There may be pain and tenesmus. Stools are mixed with blood and mucus.
5. Gastric and oesophageal perforation is common than acidic poisoning. It is a delayed sequelae. Complications include stricture of oesophagus or pylorus.

6. Alkali coming in contact with eyes cause oedema of conjunctivae, corneal ulceration and blindness.

Investigations

They are more or less same as discussed in acid poisoning.

Management

Management is same as that of acid poisoning because both produce corrosive injury to GI tract.
  i. Neutralization of alkali with weak acid should not be attempted as it may lead to further injury by liberating heat due to reaction with acids.
  ii. General supportive measures, treatment of shock, parenteral nutrition may be required.
  iii. The various Don'ts and Do's discussed in acid poisoning are also applicable here.
  iv. Glucocorticoids and silastic oesophageal stents have traditionally been used for alkali burns to prevent oesophageal stricture formation, but their efficacy is not proven. Animal studies suggest use of steroids. Prednisolone is used in the dose of 1-2 mg/kg every 4-6 hourly for at least 2 weeks.
  v. Prophylactic use of antibiotics is also recommended.
  vi. Oesophageal stricture or gastric outlet obstruction may require subsequent dilatation and bourginage or surgical reconstruction.

Chapter 77

Methylalcohol (Methanol) Poisoning

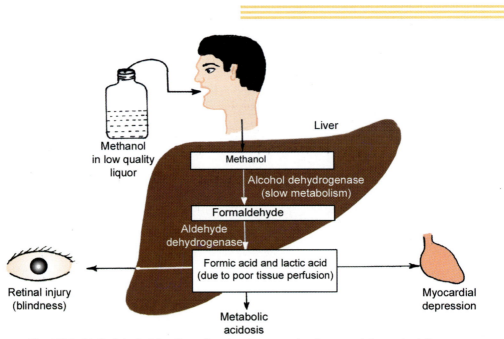

Fig. 77.1: Methylalcohol (methanol) poisoning—mechanisms and tissue toxicity

METHYLALCOHOL (METHANOL) POISONING

Methanol (methylalcohol) is used as a detergent, is a component of **varnishes, paint remo**vers, windshield washer solutions, copy-machine fluid, antifreeze solutions and **solvents. It is** also a denaturant used to make ethanol unfit for consumption.

Mode of Poisoning

Methanol poisoning occurs commonly due to accidental ingestion of cheap illicit liquor (hooch), may occur in isolation or in an epidemic proportion (*hooch tragedey*). People of lower socio-economic status are vulnerable to this poisoning.

Mechanisms of Action

After ingestion, it is rapidly absorbed and concentrated in the liver, GI tract, eyes and kidneys. Its level peaks within one to two hours of ingestion. Its binding is negligible. It is mainly metabolised in the liver (See Fig. 77.1) but upto 10% is excreted unchanged by the lungs and kidneys. In the liver, methanol is converted into formaldehyde and then into formic acid by the enzyme *alcohol dehydrogenase*. Both methanol and its metabolites are toxic, the latter causing more serious side-effects.

The half-life of elimination at low serum levels is 14-20 hours and at high serum level is 24-30 hours. Ethanol (ethylalcohol) competes with methanol for enzyme alcohol dehydrogenase for metabolism. Ethylalcohol has more affinity for this enzyme hence, has found place in its treatment by increasing the elimination half-life of methanol to 30-36 hours (In the absence of enzyme, methanol is not metabolised further).

The fatal oral dose of methanol is 30-240 ml (20-150 g), but 30 ml of a 40% solution can be fatal.

Clinical Features

The clinical features depend on the amount ingested. The time of onset of symptoms and signs after ingestion is variable and features are late in onset when ethanol is ingested concurrently. Hence, all patients of suspected methanol poisoning should be closely observed for an extended period of time before discharge.

The early manifestations are caused by methanol itself; while late features are produced by its toxic metabolities (formaldehyde and formic acid). The features are given in Box 77.1.

Diagnosis

The diagnosis is usually suggested by history of ingestion, ethanol-like intoxication, clinical features and an elevated serum osmolarity. It is confirmed by measurement of the serum methanol level (usually > 6 mmol/L or > 20 mg/dl). Later, the diagnosis is suggested by increased-anion gap, metabolic acidosis and elevated serum methanol and formate levels. Calculation of the osmolal gap and anion gap helps to assess the severity of intoxication because most centres do not have facility for methanol estimation.

$$\text{Serum methanol level (mg/dl)} = \text{Osmolal gap} \times 2.6$$

Investigation

1. ***Serum methanol level:*** More than 20 mg/dl levels are considered toxic; and more than 40 mg/dl indicate severe intoxication. A low or absent serum methanol level does not rule out serious intoxication in symptomatic patients because the whole methanol might have been metabolised to formic acid, hence, formate levels are elevated in such a situation.
2. ***Serum formate levels*** are elevated. Raised formate levels confirms the intoxication even if methanol levels are normal. Unfortunately, this investigation is not readily available.
3. ***Arterial blood gas analysis, serum osmolarity and anion gap*** must be done if there is suspicion of methanol poisoning. This helps to assess the severity also where methanol levels cannot be estimated.
4. ***Renal and liver function tests*** must be done if there is history of concurrent ethanol ingestion.
5. ***CT scan:*** CT scan of the brain may show bilateral putamen necrosis. A diagnosis of methanol poisoning can sometimes be made in retrospect on the basis of this finding.

Management

1. *Supportive measures*
    i. Removal of unabsorbed methanol by gastric aspiration and by administration of 50 g of activated charcoal to adsorb the poison. This measure is helpful if poisoning is < 4 hours duration.

Box 77.1: Symptoms and signs of methanol poisoning

Early	Late (after 24 hours)
1. At low concentration (> 20 mg/dl) • Nausea, vomiting and abdominal pain • Headache, vertigo, dizziness • Ethanol-like intoxication 2. At high concentration (> 40 mg/dl) • Alteration in consciousness • Convulsions • Coma • Metabolic acidosis • An increased osmolal gap (> 5 mOsm/L)	• Seizures • Severe metabolic acidosis • Increased osmolal gap (> 10 mOsm/L) • Visual disturbances e.g. clouding and diminished vision, dancing and flashing spots, fixed or dilated pupils, disc hyperaemia and blindness due to retinal injury • Coma • Severe intoxication may produce myocardial depression, bradycardia, shock etc. • Death may occur

ii. *Alkalinization of the urine* to enhance the elimination of formic acid.

iii. *Treatment of metabolic acidosis by sodium bicarbonate* A large amount of sodium bicarbonate may be needed. If blood pH is < 7.2 or serum HCO_3^- is < 15 mmol/L then I.V. $NaHCO_3$ is given after calculation as follows:

HCO_3^- = Body weight (Kg) × 0.4 × (difference between desired and measured bicarbonate level).

One half of the calculated deficit should be replaced within 4 hours for which 10-15 ampoules of 10 ml 7.5% $NaHCO_3$ are added to one litre glucose bottle and infused. Once the pH is > 7.2 or serum HCO_3^- level is > 18 mmol/L, no further bicarbonate administration is needed and patient is observed and monitored.

iv. *To correct volume deficit* by administration of fluids and parenteral nutrition supplementation with 10 to 25% dextrose to be given through a large vein via a cannula.

v. *Control of seizures* by I.V. diazepam (5-10 mg doses slowly at a rate of 1-2 mg/min) or I.V. phenytoin infusion in normal saline starting with a loading dose (18-20 mg/kg) followed by a maintenance dose of 100 mg 8 hourly.

2. **Specific measures**

   i. *Saturation of enzyme alcohol dehydrogenase by administration of ethanol:* Ethanol has stronger affinity for this enzyme and saturation of this enzyme by ethanol will prevent metabolism of methanol to toxic formaldehyde and formic acid metabolities. The indications of ethanol are:
   - When methanol measurement cannot be done but there is strong history and symptomatology to suggest the poisoning and osmolal gap is > 5 mOsm/L.
   - Presence of metabolic acidosis and osmolal gap is 5-10 mOsm/L.
   - Serum methanol level > 20 mg/dl.

   The dose of ethanol to be given to achieve its desired level of 100 mg/dl are depicted in Box 77.2. It is given in a loading dose followed by maintenance dose. Therapy should continue till methanol levels fall below 10 mg/dl and all signs of toxicity disappear.

   ii. *Supplement thiamine and folate.* Large doses of intravenous folate (50 mg or 1 mg/kg after every 4 hours) and thiamine 100 mg qid should be given. They enhance the metabolism of formic acid to CO_2 and H_2O.

   iii. *Haemodialysis:* It enhances the elimination of methanol and formic acid. Its indications are:

Box 77.2: Dosage of ethanol in methanol poisoning

Dose	Intravenous		Oral
	5%	10%	50%
Loading	15 ml/kg	7.5 ml/kg	1.5 ml/kg
Maintenance	2-3 (ml/kg/hr)	1 to 1.5 (ml/kg/hr)	0.2-0.3 (ml/kg/hr)
During dialysis	3-5 (ml/kg/hr)	1.5 to 2 (ml/kg/hr)	0.3 to 0.5 (ml/kg/hr)

- Serum methanol levels > 50 mg/dl (15 mmol/L).
- Suspected methanol poisoning with significant metabolic acidosis or osmolal gap > 10 mOsm/L.
- When clinical and metabolic abnormalities are resistant to preceding treatment.
iv. *A newer agent: 4-methylpyrazole (Fomepizole)* inhibits the enzyme alcohol dehydrogenase and thus prevents metabolism of methanol to its toxic metabolities. It is given as 10 mg/kg I.V. infusion over 1 hour before dialysis and repeated once or twice at 12 hours intervals. During dialysis, a dose of 1.5 mg/kg/hour is given. In fact, it is proposed as an alternative to ethanol as an initial therapy.

Treatment of methanol poisoning is summarised in Box 77.3.

Box 77.3: Summary of methanol poisoning treatment

Parameter	Supportive treatment	Ethanol therapy	Haemodialysis
Osmolal gap	< 5 mmol/L	5-10 mmol/L	> 10 mOsm/L
Methanol level	< 20 mg/dl	> 20 mg/dl	> 50 mg/dl

Chapter 78

Carbon Monoxide Poisoning

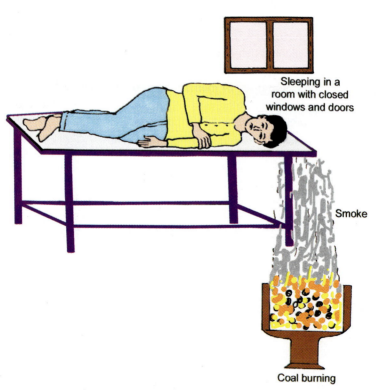

Fig. 78.1: Carbon monoxide poisoning

CARBON MONOXIDE POISONING

Carbon monoxide, a colourless, odourless and tasteless gas, is produced on combustion of any fuel gas in the absence of adequate oxygen and ventilation and may lead to domestic carbon monoxide poisoning. The most common source of carbon monoxide poisoning is smoke inhalation (Fig. 78.1). Other sources include heating systems in rooms that are not properly ventilated (e.g. gas, wood, kerosene heaters and stoves and brick ovens) and exhaust fumes of petrol engine.

Mechanism of Toxicity

Carbon monoxide readily combines with haemoglobin (has an affinity of 200-250 times than that of oxygen) to form carboxyhaemoglobin, prevents the formation of oxyhaemoglobin, thus, leads to decrease in oxygen carrying capacity of blood. It also shifts the oxygen dissociation curve to the left, further reducing the oxygen available to the tissues.

Carbon monoxide acts as a cellular poison, competes with oxygen for other haemato-proteins such as myoglobin, and enzymes (peroxidases, catalases and cytochromes). In the initial stage, it is transported to the tissues via plasma, and not via haemoglobin. Therefore, blood carboxyhemoglobin levels may be normal in early stages of poisoning.

Clinical Features

The clinical features of carbon monoxide poisoning are due to formation of carboxyhaemoglobin, the formation of which depends on the concentration, duration of exposure and activity of the person at the time of exposure. The clinical features depending on the level of toxicity are given in Box 78.1.

The subacute manifestations occurring within a few days of exposure include peripheral neuropathies, skin lesions (bullae, purpura), muscle necrosis (rhabdomyolysis, myoglobinuria) and renal damage (albuminuria, glycosuria).

Delayed manifestations which occur after 7-10 day of poisoning include headache, nausea, vomiting, aphasia, disorientation, gait abnormalities and incontinence.

Levels of carboxyhaemoglobin are not reliable indicators of severity of poisoning, therefore, mild, moderate and severe intoxication given in Box 78.1 is rough estimates of the levels.

Investigations

- Raised carboxyhaemoglobin level.
- Metabolic acidosis on blood gas analysis.
- Partial pressure of O_2 and calculated oxygen saturation by pulse oximeter may be normal as it cannot distinguish oxyhaemoglobin from carboxyhaemoglobin. Actual oxygen saturation is decreased.

Box 78.1: Symptoms and signs of carbon monoxide poisoning

Severity	Carboxyhaemoglobin	Symptoms and signs
Mild	< 25%	• Cherry-red or pink colour of skin • Dyspnoea on exertion, tachypnoea • Headache, lack of concentration, psychomotor retardation, fatigue, vertigo • Nausea, vomiting • Visual disturbances • Angina may be precipitated in patients with coronary artery disease
Moderate	25-50%	In addition to above, there may be confusion, seizures, collapse and cerebral oedema
Severe	> 50%	• Hypotension, slowing of pulse rate, respiratory depression, pulmonary oedema, coma • ECG abnormalities (ST-T changes, atrial fibrillation, ventricular ectopics and conduction defects). Angina may develop
Very severe	> 70%	• Rapidly fatal

Management

The main steps in the management of carbon monoxide poisoning are:

1. ***Supplement oxygen:*** The patient should be removed immediately from the source of exposure and 100% oxygen be administered. The half-life of carboxyhaemoglobin is 5 hours at room air which can be reduced to half by supplemental 100% O_2. Patients with mild symptoms require O_2 for just 4-6 hours to bring the carboxyhaemoglobin concentration to less than 5% which is safe.

2. ***Ventilatory support:*** Endotracheal intubation and mechanical ventilation with 100% oxygen are indicated in patients with coma, significant CNS dysfunction or cardiovascular instability.

3. ***ECG monitoring for cardiac arrhythmia:*** Patients with severe intoxication can develop hypotension, arrhythmias, ischaemic chest pain and CHF. The arrhythmias and hypotension should be treated appropriately.

4. ***Role of hyperbaric oxygen:*** The role of hyperbaric oxygen in the treatment of carbon monoxide poisoning is controversial but it is indicated in patients with coma, syncope and seizures and in patients with less severe symptoms and signs of CNS and CVS dysfunction that donot resolve with O_2 and supportive therapy. Hyperbaric oxygen therapy reduces the duration of toxicity and prevents the development of delayed sequelae.

Chapter 79

Copper Sulphate Poisoning

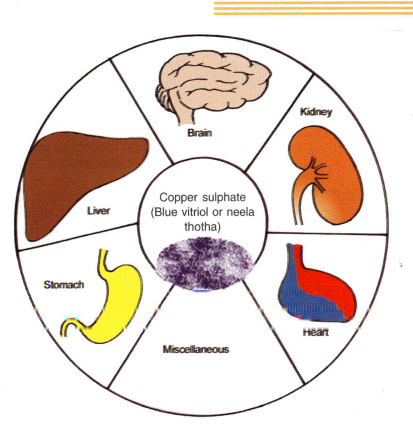

Fig. 79.1: Toxic effects of copper sulphate on various organ systems

COPPER SULPHATE POISONING

Copper as a metal is not poisonous but copper salts such as sulphate, carbonate and subacetate are poisonous in large amounts. Out of all salts, copper sulphate is usually encountered in poisoning due to its easy accessibility as *blue vitriol or neela thotha* which is a widely used compound. Accidental cases of poisoning outnumbers the suicidal cases but homicidal cases are rare. Copper sulphate is used in leather industry, ink-making industry and white washing. It is also added to impart a rich green colouration to preserved and tinned peas, vegetables and pickles, but the quantity used is so small to cause any toxic effect and the salt is rapidly converted to a harmless albuminate of copper. It is used in agriculture to control bacterial and fungal diseases and as an algaecide and herbicide. It is also used to kill slugs and snails in irrigation and municipal water treatment system.

Mode of Action

It is available as a dust, wetable powder or liquid concentrate. The lowest toxic ingested dose is 11 mg/kg.

It produces toxicity mainly by generating the free radicals (superoxide radicals) from molecular oxygen which disrupt the cellular membranes. It causes haemolysis by disrupting the RBC's membrane, denatures the haemoglobin and leads to formation of Heinz bodies. Even at low concentration, it interferes with cellular enzymes such as glucose-6 phosphate dehydrogenase, glutathione reductase and catalase (a free radical scavenger).

Clinical Features (Fig. 79.1)

After ingestion, it diffuses into the mucosal cells and then into blood producing systemic effects. It is largely caustic in nature. The toxicity is largely:

1. *Gastrointestinal:* Early symptoms pertain to its local effects on the GI tract. It produces burning pain in epigastrium, nausea, thirst, eructations and repeated violent vomiting and metallic taste. Vomiting reduces its toxic effects, but however, it may be retained in the stomach in an depressed consciousness state or in an unconscious victim. Vomitus is blue-green in colour and can be distinguished from bile by adding ammonium hydroxide to the vomitus, which turns deep blue (colour does not change with bile). Diarrhoea (rarely bloody), colic, ulceration and haemorrhagic gastritis can occur.
2. *Liver toxicity:* Jaundice may occur on 2nd to 5th day due to liver injury. Liver biopsy shows centrilobular necrosis with bile stasis.
3. *Renal toxicity:* It occurs on 3rd or 4th day of poisoning, manifests as proteinuria, haematuria (microscopic or macroscopic), oliguria and acute renal failure due to acute tubular necrosis. Diarrhoea, vomiting and dehydration promote renal toxicity.
4. *Neurological:* Manifestations include headache, muscle cramps and convulsions. In some cases, there may be complete paralysis of the limbs followed by drowsiness and coma.
5. *Cardiovascular manifestations:* They include headache, cold sweats, weak pulse, hypotension etc. Acute circulatory collapse develops as a complication due to consumption of a large dose and carries poor prognosis. It commonly occurs in those cases who do not have sufficient vomiting following ingestion leading to profound toxicity.
6. *Skin:* Copper sulphate is readily absorbed through the skin and can produce burning pain, itching and allergic dermatitis.
7. *Eye involvement:* Leads to conjunctivitis and keratitis.
8. *Others:* Diffuse myalgias, rhabdomyolysis, myoglobinuria, acute pancreatitis, acidosis, methemoglobinemia can occur. Death is due to shock or hepatorenal failure.

Chronic Copper Sulphate Poisoning

It occurs due to chronic exposure to copper sulphate, seen among miners due to inhalation of copper dust or fumes and also seen in welders. It may also occur following consumption of food contaminated with *vedigris* obtained from dirty copper vessels. Repeated ingestion of copper salts produces.
1. Haemolytic anaemia.
2. Metallic taste in mouth, nausea, vomiting, dyspepsia, abdominal pain and sometimes diarrhoea. Green and purple lining of the gums may be seen.
3. Impaired immune response.
4. Hepatic and renal damage.

Copper Sulphate Poisoning

5. Peripheral neuritis and atrophy of the muscles.
6. Conjunctivitis and corneal ulceration.
7. Skin, hair, urine and sweat become yellow-green.

Investigations

Copper sulphate produces intravascular haemolysis which is responsible for various complications. There is no correlation between haemolysis and serum copper levels. The various tests performed are:

1. ***Blood tests:*** There may be anaemia of normocytic normochromic type due to blood loss (haematemesis and malena) and haemolysis. Peripheral blood film may show small, crenated, fragmented RBCs and spherocytes. Reticulocytois is seen due to haemolysis.
2. ***Renal profile:*** Urine may show proteinuria, haematuria and haemoglobinuria. Blood urea and serum creatinine levels get elevated in presence of renal failure.
3. ***Liver function tests:*** Due to intravascular haemolysis, there may be unconjugated hyperbilirubinaemia. The enzymes are normal.
4. Hyperkalaemia may occur.

Management

1. ***General measures:***
    i. To remove the poison from the stomach by gastric lavage or nasogastric tube aspiration.
    ii. Stomach wash with 1% potassium ferrocyanide to form cupric ferrocyanide which is nonabsorbable and can be removed.
    iii. Administer white of egg or milk to form albuminate of copper which is insoluble and can be removed.
    iv. Catharsis by giving castor oil to promote excretion of unabsorbed copper sulphate through the intestine.
    v. I.V. fluids to maintain proper hydration. Blood transfusions may be needed for anaemia.
    vi. Symptomatic relief of gastric symptoms by antacids and H_2-antagonists.
2. ***Chelating agents:***
   Calcium EDTA, BAL and D-penicillamine are commonly employed chelating agents given in 5 days courses separated by 2-3 days of rest. The doses and side-effects of these drugs are given in Box 79.1.
3. ***Management of complications:***
   - Forced alkaline diuresis (50-100 mEq of $NaHCO_3$ in 100 ml of half saline) is indicated in case of intravascular haemolysis.
   - Circulatory support by adequate fluid replacement to prevent renal failure.
   - Peritoneal/haemodialysis if acute renal failure develops. The evidences also suggest that removal of copper by dialysis is also indicated in the early stages of poisoning when free copper is present in the circulation.
   - To prevent haemolysis, vit C, E and riboflavin can be given.

Box 79.1: Drugs and dosage of chelating agents in copper sulphate poisoning

Drug	Dosage	Side-effects
Calcium EDTA	15-25 mg/kg in 250-500 ml of 5% dextrose I.V. over a period of 1-2 hours twice a day for 5 days (Max dose is 50 mg/kg/day)	Raised intracranial pressure
BAL (Dimercaprol)	100 mg 8 hourly intramuscular for 2 days then 150 mg I.M. 12 hourly for 5 days	Nausea, vomiting, febrile reactions. Antihistamines given 30 minutes before the injection reduces these side-effects
Penicillamine	2 g/day orally in divided doses for one week	Skin rashes, fever, anaemia, agranulocytosis, proteinuria and nephrotic syndrome

Chapter 80

Epidemic Dropsy

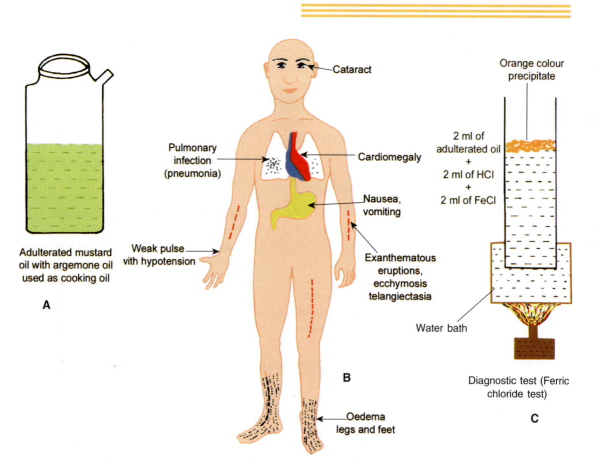

Fig. 80.1: Acute severe argemone oil poisoning (A) Adulterated mustard oil. (B) Clinical features. (C) Diagnostic test

EPIDEMIC DROPSY

Definition

It is defined as oedema (dropsy) occurring in epidemic form due to consumption of contaminated edible oil (mustard oil) with argemone oil—a toxic ingredient.

It is known to occur in epidemics in India, and recent epidemic of this poisoning has been reported from Delhi and the adjoining areas in 1990.

Mode of Poisoning

It is ingestional. Mustard oil is used as a cooking oil in certain parts of India especially West Bengal from where first epidemic broke. Mustard, sometimes gets contaminated with Mexican poppy (Argemone Mexicana) seeds (in India, it is known as sialkanta, Daurdy, Satyanashi, Brahmdandi or Pila datura). Consumption of this contaminated oil (Fig. 80.1A) leads to poisoning called *epidemic dropsy*. The toxic ingredients of argemone oil are *sanguinarine* and *disanguinarine*.

Mechanism of Action

The active ingredients present in argemone oil (sanguinarine and disanguinarine) are vasodilators, cause widespread vasodilatation in the deeper layer of skin, subcutaneous tissue, subperitoneal and sub-pericardial regions, and capillaries dilatation occurs also in viscera i.e. ovaries, uterus, liver, intestines and even (uvea and iris). There also occurs increased capillary permeability leading to exudation into subcutaneous tissue causing pitting oedema of legs and feet.

The extensive vascular dilatation combined with increased capillary permeability leads to hyperkinetic circulation, high cardiac output failure (collapsing pulse, wide pulse pressure) and progressive oedema. There occurs generalised anasarca similar to wet beri-beri.

> *Epidemic dropsy occurs due to widespread vasodilatation produced by active ingredients of argemone oil—a contaminant in edible oil.*

Clinical Features (Fig. 80.1B)

The most characteristic early feature is oedema of the extremities extending upwards and may become generalised. The extremities are warm and tender on pressure. There may be fever. Nausea and vomiting are also common, may even precede the onset of oedema. In addition, there may occur exanthematous eruptions on face, trunk and limbs. Telangiectatic and nodular eruptions may also be observed. Ecchymotic patches and bleeding has also been observed. There are signs of high cardiac output (warm extremities, bounding pulses, wide pulse pressure).

In severe cases, there is development of progressive cardiac failure leading to dyspnoea, tachypnoea, tachycardia and hypotension. The pulse is regular and bounding but in severe cases may become irregular and feeble. There is cardiomegaly and pericardial effusion may also be seen. There is significant degree of anaemia and patient may develop respiratory infections.

Diagnosis

It is based on:
  i. History of consumption of adulterated edible oil.
 ii. History of outbreak. Many persons of a family or a community or in an area may be involved.
iii. Clinical features.
 iv. Detection of argemone oil contamination in edible oil.

Tests Used to Detect Argemone Oil

1. *Nitric acid test (Fig. 80.2):* 5 ml of oil is shaken with an equal amount of nitric acid. On standing, the acid layer turns yellow, orange yellow or crimson depending on the amount of argemone oil. It is a sensitive test but not specific because of a high false positive rate, hence, if positive, must be confirmed by other tests.
2. *Ferric chloride test (Fig. 80.1C):* 2 ml of oil and 2 ml of concentrated HCl are mixed and heated in a water bath at 33–35°C for 2 minutes.

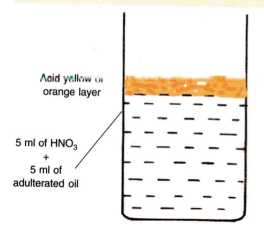

Fig. 80.2: The nitric acid test

Then add 8 ml of ethyl alcohol and mixture is heated in the water bath for 1 minute. Now 2 ml of ferric chloride solution is added and the tube is heated in the bath for further 10 minutes. The appearance of orange-red precipitate indicates presence of argemone oil.

3. **Paper chromatographic method:** It is most sensitive and specific method, can detect even low concentration of argemone oil adulteration upto 0.0001%.

Management

1. Removal or withdrawal of contaminated edible oil from the diet.
2. *Supportive treatment:* To relieve oedema and congestive heart failure if present, diuretics, digitalis and salt restriction are cornerstones of treatment.
3. The pulmonary infection may be treated by appropriate antibiotics.
4. Calcium, Vit C and Vit E have been used for restoration of damaged capillaries.
5. Steroids have been sometimes useful in severe cases.

Chapter 81

Organophosphates (Organophosphorus)

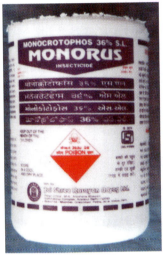

Fig. 81.1A: Monocrotophos—a common OP compound involved in poisoning

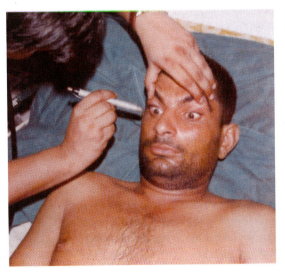

Fig. 81.1B: Looking for the signs of atropinisation during the treatment of OP poisoning. The signs of atropinisation include, mid-dilated pupils and clearing of pulmonary secretions (e.g. lungs become dry)

ORGANOPHOSPHATES

Definition

Organophosphorus compounds are widely used as agricultural, industrial and domestic insecticide. The poisoning may occur in isolation or in epidemics after ingestion of contaminated foodstuffs. Most of these compounds are available either as organophosphates (malathion, parathion, methyl-parathion, isomalathion, diazinon, dichlorvos, mipafox, tricholorophon and monocrotophos (Fig. 81.1A) etc. or carbamates (carbaryl, matacil etc.).

These compounds are available in powder form and are used as sprays. The formulations available contain 1-95% of an active ingredient so their toxicity varies widely.

Mode of Action (Fig. 81.2)

Organophosphorus compounds are potent inhibitors of acetylcholinesterase (AChE) and pseudo-cholinesterase (pseduo-ChE). In man, true ChE (AChE) in present in CNS and RBC's; while

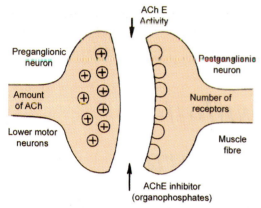

Fig. 81.2: Mechanism of action of AChE (acetyl cholinesterase) and its inhibitor at neuromuscular junction

pseudocholinesterase is present in liver, plasma and serum. The inhibition of these enzymes is due to irreversible binding of phosphate radical of organophosphates to active sites of enzymes. In case of carbamates this binding is reversible. The pharmacological and toxicological effects are due to accumulation of acetylcholine at synapses resulting in initial stimulation followed by paralysis of neurotransmission at cholinergic synapses. The cholinergic synapses are present in CNS, somatic nerves, autonomic ganglion, parasympathetic nerve endings and some sympathetic nerve endings like in sweat glands.

Absorption, Distribution, Metabolism and Excretion

Organophosphorus insecticides are absorbed through skin, lungs and gastrointestinal tract. The absorption through skin is slow but becomes rapid at high temperature (hot season) or in the presence of dermatitis. It is difficult to remove the poison from skin completely, hence, its absorption is prolonged.

The involvement of CNS shows that these compounds cross the blood brain barrier. Their distribution varies directly with water soluble partition characteristics. The knowledge of their distribution is important and useful for clinical picture and duration of poisoning. After half an hour of absorption, they are accumulated to highest degree in cervical brown fat and salivary glands; to a marked degree in liver, kidneys and adipose tissue; to fairly high degree in gastric and intestinal walls, thyroid, spleen, lungs and to lesser degree in CNS, muscles and bone marrow. After 4 to 5 hours, the concentration in adipose tissue and urine rises. The early relapse of poisoning indicates continued absorption; while late relapse is related to release from storage sites i.e. fat or adipose tissue.

Metabolism of organophosphorus compounds occurs particularly by oxidation, hydrolysis and by transfer of a portion of the molecule to glutathione, Hydrolysis by the enzymes is the only efficient method of its detoxification in mammals including man. After primary metabolic processes, they are excreted as phosphorus containing residues in the urine and faeces. There is no evidence of incorporation of residues into DNA, hence, no genetic damage occurs.

Acute Poisoning

Acute organoposphorus poisoning is second common cause of poisoning throughout India. The cases occur after skin exposure (uncommon) during mixing of powder with the solvent or while spraying (Fig. 81.1); after inhalation of fumes or vapours, after ingestion (most common) of compound itself or contaminated foodstuffs. About 70-80% of the poisoning is accidental and 20-25% cases are suicidal. The poisoning is more common in agricultural, industrial and domestic workers and chemists. No age is immune to this poisoning. In children it is mostly accidental and homicidal. The poisoning is more common in men than women (2:1). The severity of poisoning is highly variable. Majority of cases seem to belong to mild to moderate intoxication, hence accounting for low mortality (8-10%). Severe cases of poisoning occur after ingestion or inhalation. The signs and symptoms are due to muscarinic and nicotinic effects, appear within few minutes to few hours

Organophosphates (Organophosphorus)

Table 81.1: Clinical manifestations of acute severe organophosphorous poisoning

Organ/system	Signs and symptoms
A. Muscarinic effects	
GI Tract	Nausea, vomiting, diarrhoea, abdominal colic, involuntary defecation, increased peristalsis
Salivary glands	Excessive salivation
Eye (pupils, ciliary body and lacrimal gland)	lacrimation, blurring of vision, miosis, papilloedema
Respiratory (bronchial tree)	Bronchorrhoea, breathlessness, crackles, rales, pulmonary oedema, respiratory depression, suffocation
Heart	Bradycardia, cardiac arrhythmias, cardiac arrest, heart block of varying degree
Skin (sweat glands)	Hyperhidrosis
Nose	Rhinorrhoea
Urinary bladder	Involuntary urination and bed wetting
B. Nicotinic effects	
Striated muscles	Muscle twitchings, fasciculations, weakness, flaccid paralysis
Sympathetic ganglion	Pallor, tachycardia, elevation of BP
CNS manifestations	Giddiness, anxiety, restlessness, emotional lability, insomnia, nightmares, headache, tremors, apathy, withdrawal and depression, difficulty in concentration, drowsiness, confusion, slurred speech, ataxia, absence of reflexes, convulsions, cheyne-stokes breathing. Depression of cardiac and respiratory centres leading to fall of blood pressure, dyspnoea and cyanosis. Rarely acute Guillian-Barre syndrome reported.

(average 6-8 hours). The critical period is first 24 hours. The effects occur in varied combinations and also vary in time of onset, sequence and duration depending on the chemical, dose, duration and route of exposure. The classification of toxicity is based on clinical symptomatology (Table 81.1) and degree of inhibition of enzyme activity. In mild to moderate intoxication, the inhibition of the enzyme is significant to produce muscarinic and nicotinic effects but insignificant to produce respiratory depression, pulmonary oedema or cardiac arrhythmias.

Intermediate Type II Syndrome

These are usually neuropathic syndromes characterized by cranial nerves palsies and weakness of proximal limbs, neck and respiratory muscles. These syndromes usually develop 1-4 days after ingestion of pesticide with severe manifestations. The incidence reported in India is 15%. Recovery occurs within 4-10 days. Death is usually due to respiratory paralysis.

Diagnosis

Diagnosis is based on:
1. History and circumstances leading to exposure.
2. Presence of clinical manifestations (bronchoconstriction, pin-point pupils, fasciculations etc.).
3. Clinical and therapeutic response to atropine and oximes.
4. Confirmation of diagnosis by measurement of anticholinesterase enzyme in RBC's or plasma pseudocholinesterase enzyme.
5. Chemical analysis of body fluids (urine, blood, gastric lavage).

Management

All cases of poisoning should be sent to hospital as quickly as possible. Although symptoms may develop rapidly, delay in onset or steady increase in severity may be seen upto 24 hours after ingestion. The therapy may be graded according to severity of intoxication.
   a. **Latent poisoning:** (Serum ChE activity 50-90% of normal value). There are no clinical manifestations. The diagnosis is based on reduction in serum ChE activity by 10-20%. No treatment is required and observation for few hours is necessary. Prognosis is excellent.

b. *Mild poisoning* (serum ChE activity 20-50% of normal value). Treatment includes atropine 1-2 mg, I.V. and pralidoxime (PAM) 1g I.V. The prognosis is good.

c. *Moderate poisoning* (serum ChE activity 10-20% of normal value). Muscarinic and nicotinic effects are widespread without pulmonary oedema or respiratory paralysis. Atropine in doses of 1-2 mg, I.V. every 20-30 min is given till signs and symptoms of poisoning disappear or the signs of atropinization like mid-dilated pupils, clearing of rales and drying of pulmonary secretions appear. Pralidoxime 1g, I.V. stat is repeated if necessary. The treatment with atropine continues for 2-3 days with same dose but the interval between doses is increased.

d. *Severe poisoning* (serum ChE activity less than 10% normal value). The treatment modalities are as follows:

I. *Steps to remove the unabsorbed poison:* If insufficient amount of poison has been ingested, the unabsorbed poison should be removed and simultaneous steps taken to retard its absorption. The success of these measures depends on time since ingestion and speed of absorption of poison; steps to be taken are:

i. *Evacuation of stomach:*
- Induce emesis or do gastric lavage with lukewarm water or sodium chloride.
- Administer a slurry of activated charcoal (20 to 200 g with water or sorbitol) for adsorption of poison.
- Give catharsis with magnesium or sodium sulphate to enhance excretion in faeces.

ii. *Prevention of absorption from other sites*
- Wear protective gloves and remove the contaminated clothings.
- Meticulous washing of skin with alkaline soap or sodium bicarbonate solution is recommended.
- In the event of inhalation, extensive eye irrigation with water or saline should be given and patient removed to fresh air.

II. *Supportive measures:*
- Maintain open airway by oropharyngeal suction, endotracheal tube intubation.
- Maintain respiration by Ambu bag or mechanical means.
- Monitor blood gas analysis and respiratory rate.
- Administer intravenous fluids.
- Monitor pulse, blood pressure, urine output and ECG.
- Give antibiotics if necessary for pulmonary infection after culture and sensitivity.
- If convulsions are not controlled with atropine and PAM, give diphenylhydantoin.
- Sedate with diazepam, 5-10 mg, intramuscular.

III. *Administration of specific antidote:*

a. **Intermittent atropine therapy:** Atropine is given in the dose of 2-5 mg, I.V. in adults and 0.05 mg/kg I.V. slowly in the children every 5-10 min. till parasympathetic manifestations are controlled or early signs of atropinization appear (clearing of rales, drying of pulmonary secretions and mid-dilated pupils) (Fig. 81.1B). Tachycardia and pupillary dilatation are not good indicators of atropinization. The maintenance dose is given after the initial bolus at a continuous infusion at the rate of 0.02-0.08 mg/kg/hr, or intermittently as 1-2 mg with increase in the duration between doses; continued for 3-5 days and slowly withdrawn on 6th or 7th day. Sudden withdrawal may produce relapse or exaggeration of signs and symptoms.

b. *High dose continuous administration of atropine:* Some studies have shown that high doses of atropine (150 mg in 5% dextrose) drip over a period of 6 hours has been shown to be equally effective as intermittent therapy.

c. *Oximes (cholinesterase enzyme reactivators):* In adults pralidoxime (PAM) is given in doses of 1-2 g I.V. over 5-10 min or mixed in 250 ml of normal saline and infused over 30 min. The dose is repeated every 6-12 hours if muscle or diaphragmatic weakness or coma are not relieved. In severe poisoning PAM can be administered by continuous infusion (Adults: 500 mg/hr max. 12 g/24 hr; Children: 9-19 mg/kg/hr after an initial bolus). The titration should be based on clinical response. Oximes reactivate the ChE activity hence, are useful in severe cases of poisoning. PAM administration reduces the dose of atropine, hence, combination has been found to be very effective in treatment of moderate to severe early cases of poisoning. Oximes are not indicated in carbamate poisoning.

Chapter 82

Aluminium and Zinc Phosphide Poisoning

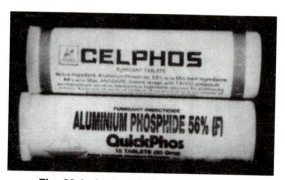

Fig. 82.1: Available packs of aluminium phosphide

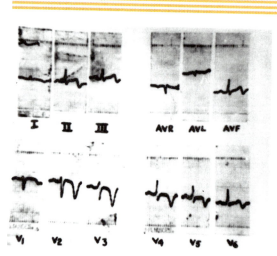

Fig. 82.3: ECG showing toxic myocarditis in a patient who presented with shock

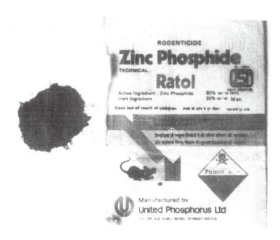

Fig. 82.2: Black-grey powder of zinc phosphide with 10 g packet

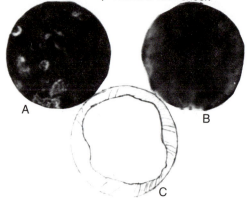

Fig. 82.4: Bedside positive silver nitrate paper test
A. Positive with gastric lavage B. Positive with breath
C. Normal control

ALUMINIUM PHOSPHIDE POISONING

Definition

Aluminium phosphide (AlP) is an ideal solid fumigant pesticide because of being efficacious, easy to use and low cost. It is available as tablets, (celphos, quickphos, alphose (Fig. 82.1), each weighing 3.0 g liberates 1.0 g of phosphine gas (PH_3). PH_3 being gaseous in nature diffuses uniformly throughout the stored grains, however, it does not affect the food value of grains. After fumigation, non-toxic residues left in the grains are phosphite and hypophosphite of aluminium. The poisoning involves younger generation and is mostly suicidal, occasionally accidental usually in children and rarely homicidal. It occurs in post-harvest season mostly in rural areas. The important factors for poisoning due to this agent is its easy availability in open market combined with easy accessibility at home especially that of farmers. Recently, cases of poisoning with exposed compound and its combined toxicity with alcohol have been reported. The zinc phosphide is used as rodenticide. It is a 10 g packet containing black coloured powder (Fig. 82.2).

Properties of Phosphine (PH_3)

Aluminium phosphide and zinc phosphide liberate toxic phosphine gas upon contact with water of HCl of stomach, which is responsible for its toxic effects. Each formulation of AlP contains 56% as active ingredient and 44% $(NH_4)_2 CO_3$.

$$AlP + 3H_2O \rightarrow Al(OH)_3 + PH_3 \uparrow \text{ (phosphine)}$$
$$AlP + 3HCl \rightarrow AlCl_3 + PH_3 \uparrow$$

Absorption, Distribution and Metabolism

Phosphine upon inhalation is freely absorbed by the lungs; the tablet when ingested releases phosphine rapidly which is absorbed through the gastrointestinal tract. A small amount of AlP is absorbed unchanged and deposited in the liver. The release of PH_3 from this unchanged absorbed AlP is slow which explains the extended toxicity of PH_3. After absorption, some phosphine is excreted through lungs and urine. Zinc phosphide is not water soluble but is lipid soluble, hence is slowly absorbed.

Mechanism of Action

Studies carried out on different animals showed non-competitive binding of cytochrome oxidase by phosphine leading to valency change of the heme iron and conformational change of prosthetic group. Later it was found that there is significant inhibition of catalase than cytochrome leading to accumulation of hydrogen peroxide (H_2O_2), an oxy-reactive species. Recent experimental studies showed extra-mitochondrial release of H_2O_2 and liberation of oxygen free radicals. Recently it has been claimed that inhibition of catalase and induction of SOD in humans lead to free radicals stress which brings out lipid peroxidation and protein denaturation of cell membrane leading to hypoxic cell damage. However, the exact mode of action is still unclear.

Acute Poisoning in Humans

AlP poisoning is either inhalational or ingestional while zinc phosphide is only ingestional. The clinical toxicity is more or less the same in both metal phosphide (AlP and Zn_3P_2) poisoning irrespective of the mode of poisoning except slight variation in initial symptoms. The signs and symptoms depend on the dose and severity of poisoning. Nausea and vomiting occur early in zinc phosphide poisoning.

Inhalation Toxicity

Mild exposure to PH_3 produces acute respiratory distress and irritation of mucous membrane. These may be associated with other symptoms such as dizziness, chest discomfort, nausea, vomiting, easy fatigue, headache etc. More severe toxicity produces ataxia, numbness and paraesthesia, tremors, diplopia, jaundice, muscular weakness, paralysis and muscular incoordination. Severe toxicity is

Poisonings

accompanied by shock, cardiac arrhythmia, congestive heart failure, ARDS, pulmonary oedema, convulsions and coma. Acute hepato-renal damage occurs much later. At a level of 400-600 ppm, it is lethal within half an hour.

Ingestional Toxicity

It could be mild or moderate to severe. It is common with both metal phosphides (AlP and Zn).

Mild Ingestional Toxicity

Marked systemic signs and symptoms do not occur except nausea, vomiting, headache, abdominal pain or discomfort. These symptoms are early and more prominent with zinc phosphide poisoning. These usually subside without any treatment except fluid replacement. The prognosis is good.

Moderate to Severe Poisoning

Systemic features appear early, are progressive and mostly fatal. Toxic dose of AlP in humans is 500 mg/70 kg. The time interval between ingestion and death reported is 1-106 hours (average 31 hours). The critical period of poisoning is first 24-36 hours. The systemic manifestations are given in Table 82.1.

Table 82.1: Systemic manifestations of moderately severe AlP or zinc phosphide poisoning in humans

System affected	Symptoms and signs
GI Tract	Nausea, vomiting, burning epigastrium, abdominal pain, diarrhoea and excessive thirst
CVS	Hypotension or shock, cardiac arrhythmias, myocardial ischemia, myocarditis, pericarditis, congestive heart failure
Respiratory	Cough, dyspnoea, crackles and rales, Type I and II respiratory failure
Hepatobiliary	Jaundice, hepatomegaly, raised transaminases
Renal	Oliguric and nonoliguric renal failure
CNS	Anxiety, fear, apprehension, restlessness, convulsions and terminally coma

Diagnosis

The diagnosis of AlP poisoning is based on (a) history of ingestion of AlP compound (b) clinical manifestations including shock (c) foul or decaying fish like smell (d) the ECG changes (Fig. 82.3) and metabolic acidosis. The confirmation is done either by qualitative silver nitrate impregnated paper test (Fig. 82.4) or by chemical analysis of blood or gastric fluid for phosphine.

Investigations

See Box 82.1.

Management

The main aim of management is to sustain life with appropriate resuscitative measures till PH_3 is excreted from body. Hence, early recognition and early institution of therapy are mandatory. The steps to reduce the mortality during first 24 hours include:

I. To delay absorption of phosphine through GI tract

a. Meticulous gastric lavage with $KMnO_4$ (1:1000) to be repeated twice or thrice so as to remove or oxidized unabsorbed poison.

Box 82.1: Investigations in metal (Al and Zn) phosphide poisoning

Investigation	Result
• Serum electrolytes.	Serum K^+ and Mg^{++} levels low
• Blood urea/creatinine	Normal, raised if ARF develops
• Blood gas analysis	Hypoxaemia, hypocarbia
• Serum HCO_3^- level and pH	Low, metabolic acidosis
• Serum cortisol	Low
• Blood phosphine levels (liquid gas chromatography)	High
• ECG	• Changes of myocarditis, arrhythmias
• Echocardiogram	• Global hypokinesia
• Chest X-ray	• Noncardiogenic pulmonary oedema may be present

b. A slurry of activated charcoal (50-100 g) to be given to adsorb PH_3.
c. Judicious use of antacid orally and H_2-blocker intravenously for symptomatic relief or gastrointestinal manifestations of PH_3.
d. Medicated liquid paraffin or magnesium sulphate may be given to accelerate its excretion through gut.

II. Steps to reduce organ toxicity

In the absence of an antidote and high affinity of PH_3 for enzyme systems, the organ toxicity develops rapidly. Heart is most vulnerable to PH_3 toxicity. Most of the organ toxicity is hypoxic and is due to oxidant injury produced by PH_3. Recently magnesium sulphate has been claimed to be an antioxidant and its use led to significant reduction in the mortality. Magnesium sulphate in addition to an antioxidant effect, is also useful as an antiarrhythmic and antihypoxic agent in this poisoning, hence, acts as a double-edged weapon for protection of the cells in the presence of hypoxia. A dose of 1 g of $MgSO_4$ I.V., stat is given followed by 1g every hour for next 3 hours and finally 1.0-1.5 g after every 4-6 hours for 3-5 days or till final outcome of these patients.

III. To enhance PH_3 excretion

Phosphine is stable and partially water soluble. It is excreted through breath and urine, therefore, adequate hydration and renal perfusion by low dose dopamine 1-3 µg/kg/min must be maintained. Diuretics are not useful in the presence of profound shock. However, if blood pressure is stable around 80 mmHg, then frusemide (20 mg I.V.) may be tried.

IV. Supportive measures

a. **Hypoxia:** It is managed by O_2 inhalation, patent airway by endotracheal intubation or assisted ventilation if necessary. Blood gas analysis should be monitored.

b. **Shock:** Intravenous fluids (4-5 L out of which 50% should be saline) should be given during first 3-6 hours guided by CVP, PCWP and monitoring of electrolytes. Blood pressure should be maintained above 70 mmHg. Low dose dopamine (1-3 µg/kg/min) combined with dobutamine (2.5-15 µg/kg/min) and intravenous hydrocortisone (200-400 mg after 4-6 hours) have been found effective. Steroids combat shock, reduce dose of dopamine and dobutamine, check the capillary leakage in the lungs (ARDS) and potentiate the responsiveness of shock to catecholamines and restore the low steroid levels.

c. **Arrhythmias:** Conventional antiarrhythmic drugs such as digoxin, xylocaine are ineffective. Atropine has not been found useful in bradyarrhythmia. Magnesium sulphate has been found effective in both bradyarrhythmias and tachyarrhythmia due to its membrane stabilising effect. Amiodarone has been tried with some success.

d. **Metabolic acidosis:** Moderate to severe metabolic acidosis is frequent in AlP poisoning. Intravenous sodium bicarbonate 50 m Eq may be given if arterial bicarbonate is < 15 mM/L, to be repeated to keep bicarbonate around 18-20 mmol. Dialysis can be carried out in case metabolic acidosis persists in haemodynamic stable patients.

e. **ARDS (Adult respiratory distress syndrome):** 100% O_2 is delivered by face masks or masks fitted with reserviour bag at moderate flow rate of 5-10 L to achieve PaO_2 of 60-70% with lowest inspired fraction of O_2 (FiO_2). Mechanical respiratory support and PEEP (positive end expiratory pressure) therapy are not recommended as patients remain in shocked state.

Table 82.2: Clinical features and electrocardiographic changes in 20 patients with zinc phosphide poisoning

1. **Clinical parameters**

Mean age (yrs)	26
Six ratio (F:M)	2:1
Amount ingested	7.5 g (5-20 g)
Mean duration of onset of symptoms (range)	30 min (20-40)
Interval between ingestion and hospitalisation	4.3 hours (1-8)
No. of cases with attempted suicide (%)	13 (65)
Accidental intoxication (%)	7 (35)

2. **Symptom and signs**

	No. of patient	%
• Profuse, black-coloured vomitus	20	100
• Restlessness, anxiety	20	100
• Palpitation, sweating	16	80
• Dyspnoea, tachypnoea	15	75
• Metabolic acidosis	12	60
• Shock (unrecordable BP and pulse)	8	40
• Hypotnesion (SBP < 90 mmHg)	3	15
• Pulmonary oedema	2	10
• Hepatomegaly (jaundice)	2	10

3. **ECG changes**

SVT or VT or ST segment change (ST↑ or ST↓)	2	10

Zinc Phosphide Poisoning—Diagnosis and Management

Zinc phosphide, a black coloured power, available by different names e.g. Ratol 10 g packet (Fig. 82.2), Fasco filed rat powder, kilrat, mouse con, Rometan etc. is used as rodenticide. The toxic effects are due to liberation of a toxic phosphine (PH_3) gas. The clinical picture is similar to aluminium phosphide poisoning with following exceptions:

1. It is a fat-soluble not water soluble, remains in the stomach for longer time, hence, local irritative symptoms such as nausea, vomiting, burning in epigastrium are early, more marked and more prolonged.
2. The poisoning is suicidal and ingestional only.

The clinical parameters, symptoms and signs, and ECG characteristic obsreved in a study are depicted in Table 82.2.

It is a lethal poison. Mortality is less than aluminium phosphide because of following factors:
- Not water soluble, hence, absorption is slow.
- Vomiting is early.
- Manifestations are less marked.

The treatment is supportive and symptomatic, is on the same lines as that of aluminium phosphide.

Chapter 83

Organochlorines

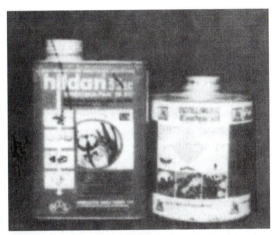

Fig. 83.1: Commonly used agents involved in organochlorine poisoning (endosulfan is available in tins)

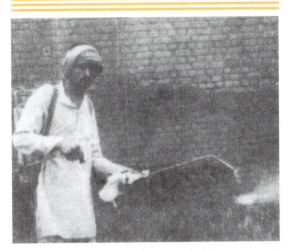

Fig. 83.2: Agriculture worker spraying the compound throughout the day, developed toxicity (mild) by ignoring preventive measures such as gloves were not worn. This patient developed seizures in the evening after 12 hours of exposure. The cause of poisoning was leaking spray nozzle and the plastic container carried on the back resulting in skin exposure

ORGANOCHLORINES

With advancement in agriculture production and widespread use of insecticides/pesticides in agriculture sector during the last 3 decades led to acute poisoning with these compounds. Poisoning with these compounds may be occupational (occupational workers) and partly due to their misuse accidentally (Fig. 83.1) or with suicidal intent. These types of mishaps are common in agricultural rural population and are attributed to illiteracy, ignorance, unemployment, mutual disputes and their ready availability in the home. In fact, this is one of the most common poisoning encountered throughout India and other developing countries where agriculture is the main profession.

Classification

The organochlorine compounds are classified into following 4 major groups depending on the biological activity and chemical composition.
1. ***Chlorinated ethane derivatives*** such as DDT and its analogs methoxychlor etc.

2. ***Hexachlorocyclohexane*** such as BHC (benzene hexachloride), lindane.
3. ***Cyclodiene derivatives*** such as chlordane, aldrin, dieldrin, endosulphan (Fig. 83.1) heptachlor.
4. ***Chlorinated camphenes*** such as toxaphene.

Organochlorines are synthetic compounds that are soluble in lipids and other solvents but not in water. Their main route of entry is through skin (during spray Fig. 83.2), GI tact (following ingestion) and lungs (following inhalations as aerosols). Their toxicity varies considerably and may be modified to a great extent by the toxicity of dissolving agent. The organochlorines are not much used now-a-days, hence, only few compounds are available in the market such as endosulphan and lindane (Fig. 83.1). They are safe and less toxic than organophosphorus compounds.

Mode of Action

The principal site of action is nervous system. They produce initial CNS stimulation followed by depression or paralysis.

Clinical Features

Acute toxicity follows after accidental or suicidal ingestion. Toxic dose is 10 mg/kg body weight. The initial symptoms are gastrointestinal (nausea and vomiting), which occur within 30 minutes to few hours followed by features of CNS stimulation such as hyperexcitability, headache, paraesthesias of lips and face, tremors and tonic-clonic seizures. Later, features of CNS depression such as paralysis, coma and respiratory failure may occur in severe cases leading to death.

Chronic toxicity due to repeated prolonged exposure in industrial workers occurs with neurological symptoms such as seizures (endosulphan) have been reported. Liver tumours, neuroblastoma in children and blood dysclasias have been also reported in workers after prolonged exposure.

Management

There is no specific antidote to this poisoning, hence, management is entirely symptomatic.
1. ***Removal of the compound:***
   - Repeated skin washings with soap and water to remove the poison from the surface of skin, if it is the route of poisoning.
   - Gastric lavage and induced vomiting: Gastric lavage with 2-4 L of plain water followed by administration of activated charcoal to adsorb the unabsorbed compound.
   - Induced catharsis may rapidly excrete the poison through GI tract.
2. ***Supportive treatment:***
   - Give respiratory support if there is respiratory failure.
   - Hyperactivity and convulsions may be controlled by diazepam (10 mg I.V. slowly). The dose can be repeated if necessary. Anticonvulsants are usually not needed.

Chapter 84

Plant Poison

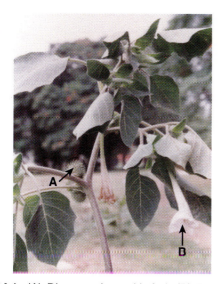

Fig. 84.1: (A) Dhatura plant with fruit (B) Dhatura flower indicated by arrows

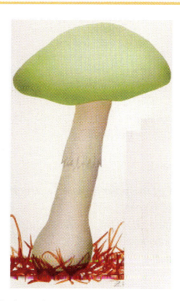

Fig. 04.2. Amanita phalloides (death cap-mushroom)

POISONING BY DHATURA AND OTHER RELATED PLANTS

Definition

It is poisoning produced by ingestion of fruits or seeds of a poisonous plant i.e. D. Stramonium (Jimpson seed), commonly called *dhatura plant*. It exists in two forms—white flowered and deep purple flowered plants. All parts of the plant are toxic but seeds and fruits are most toxic.

Other related plants include; atropia belladonna (deadly night-shade) and hyoscyamus niger.

Mechanisms of Toxicity

Ingestion of fruits or seeds of the plants produces toxic effects mainly due to anticholinergic properties. The active toxins in these plants are atropine and scopolamine, which block the acetylcholine receptors at post-ganglionic synapses of cholinergic nerve endings.

Clinical Features

Symptoms of toxicity appear immediately after ingestion usually within half an hour to one hour

Box 84.1: Clinical features of dhatura poisoning

Organ/System	Symptoms/Signs
Mouth	Dryness of mouth, tongue, mucous membranes and bitter taste.
GI tract	Burning pain in epigastrium, vomiting, difficulty in swallowing, distention and decreased bowel movements (constipation).
CVS	Tachycardia, hypertension initially followed by hypotension.
Urinary	Urinary retention, distended bladder
Eye	Dryness of eyes, red conjunctivae, dilated pupils.
CNS	Delirium, visual hallucinations, ataxia, disorientation, psychosis, extra-pyramidal features. In fatal cases, stupor, convulsions and coma supervene.
Skin	Dry flushed skin, hyperthermia.

which persist upto 24 to 48 hours. The clinical features are given in Box 84.1.

Management

1. *Removal of the poison from GI tract:*
   - Gastric lavage.
   - Activated charcoal administration to adsorb the unabsorbed poison.
2. *Symptomatic treatment:*
   - Urinary catheterization for retention of urine.
   - External cooling for hyperthermia.
   - Benzodiazepines (diazepam) for control of agitation.
3. *Role of physostigmine:* It is a cholinesterase inhibitor, appears to be useful on theoretical ground but its role is controversial. It may reverse coma, delirium and seizures. It has been found to precipitate cholinergic crisis, bradyarrhythmias and asystole.

Oleander Poisoning

Poisoning by yellow oleander (*cerebra thevetia* or *thevetia peruviana*) and white or pink oleander has been reported from south India. The kernels of the seeds of these plants are most toxic. These plants contain several glycosides which resemble digitoxin in action. These include peruvoside, ruvoside, thevetin A and B, gerebrin, thevetocin and oleandrin.

Clinical Features

They occur within 2-3 hours of ingestion. The toxic effects are due to toxic glycosides present in the seeds. The systemic effects are given in Box 84.2.

Box 84.2: Clinical features of oleander poisoning

System affected	Symptom and signs
GI tract	Nausea, vomiting, abdominal pain, diarrhoea
Pupils	Dilatation of pupils
CVS	Bradycardia, hypotension, AV blocks arrhythmias. The ECG shows ST-T changes, prolongation of PR-interval, AV dissociation, ventricular ectopics, VT and VF.
Liver	Jaundice
Renal	Renal failure, hyperkalaemia.
Nervous system	Tingling and numbness, restlessness

Management

1. *Gastric lavage and activated charcoal* to remove the poison from stomach.
2. *Fluid, electrolyte and acid-base balance:* Fluids should be given to correct dehydration and to prevent renal failure. Hyperkalaemia may require infusion of glucose with insulin. Acidosis may be corrected by sodium bicarbonate.
3. *Monitoring of the patients for cardiac rhythm*
   - Bradycardia and its related arrhythmia may be treated with atropine and transvenous pacing.
   - Lidocaine is effective against ventricular tachyarrhythmias.
4. *Role of digoxin-specific Fab-antibody:* It has been employed in life-threatening oleander poisoning with encouraging results.

MUSHROOMS POISONING

There are many poisonous mushrooms that can be confused with edible fungi and may be eaten by mistake. More than 95% of the fatalities due to mushroom ingestion are caused by the ingestion of *Amanita Phalloides* (the death-cap mushroom).

The mushroom *Amanita Phalloides* (Fig. 84.2) contains phallotoxins and amatoxins, which are thermostable toxins, interfere with cell metabolism. Amanita phalloides ("death cap") has an olive green cap, white gills and a skirt-like ring on the strip.

Clinical Features

In general, the sooner the symptoms occur, the less serious is the poisoning. There are three stages of the poisoning.

I. Initially nausea, vomiting, abdominal cramps, diarrhoea and profuse sweating appear within 2-3 hours of ingestion.

II. After 12 hours, patient complains of headache, dizziness and severe vomiting. This stage is marked by clinical improvement after volume replacement and lasts for 2-24 hours. During this stage, severe hepatocellular and renal damage becomes evident with rising blood urea, creatinine and liver enzymes.

III. The final stage (after 72 hours) is characterised by acute renal failure and massive hepatic necrosis with hypocalcaemia, sepsis and coma.

Diagnosis

It is made on:
- Clinical history of ingestion.
- Identification of the mushroom, if possible.
- Measurement of amatoxin in blood by radioimmunoassay.

Management

- Gastric lavage should be performed even in the late phases of poisoning because toxins have been demonstrated in duodenal aspirate as long as 36 hours of ingestion.
- Activated charcoal may be given to absorb the poison.
- Supportive treatment by I.V. fluids. The electrolytes, liver enzymes, blood urea, creatinine are to be monitored.
- Penicillin and silymarin inhibit uptake of amatoxin by liver cells, hence, have been associated with reduced mortality.
- The value of thioctic acid—a Kreb's cycle coenzyme is doubtful.

Chapter 85

Snake and Lizard Bites

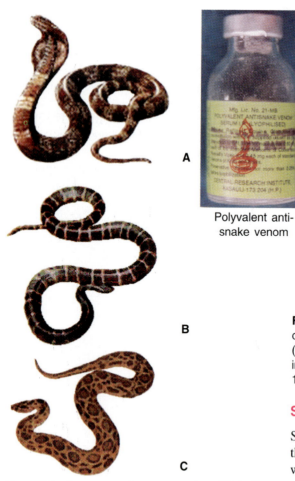

Fig. 85.1: Common poisonous snakes (A) Indian Cobra (Naja Naja) (B) Common krait and (C) Russell's viper

Polyvalent anti-snake venom

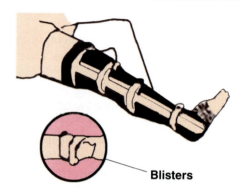

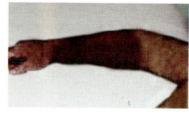

Fig. 85.2: Bite of cobra (Naja Naja). Note the swelling of the lower limb (common) and upper limb (uncommon) with local blistering and early signs of impending necrosis. By the side is a photograph of a 10 ml vial of lyophilised anti-snake venom

SNAKE BITE

Snake bite is a common problem in rural areas throughout the tropics including India. The field workers i.e. farmers, hunters, rice-pickers are particularly at risk. About 50 species of poisonous snakes are recognised but bites by few snakes are important clinically and create an emergency

Box 85.1: Common poisonous snakes and their identification

Types of snake	Identification
1. *Elapidae* (e.g. coral snake, cobras, Australian snake)	Coral snakes can be identified by red, yellow (or white) and black bands that completely encircle the body.
2. *Crotalidae* (pit vipers e.g. rattle snake and moccasins)	The heat sensing pits (foveal organs) are present between each eye and nostril. Rattle snakes produce sound by rattling the tail on the ground.
3. *Viperidae* (e.g. Russel's viper, European Adder)	They are characterised by their triangular heads, elliptical pupils, enlarged maxillary tongs and a single scale running over the full width of tail.
4. *Hydrophidae* (e.g. sea snakes)	They occur in coastal areas and bite in the presence of water.
5. *Colubridae* (e.g. mangrove snake)	

requiring prompt medical treatment. Poisonous species are given in Box 85.1 with their identification.

Cobra and kraits are found all over India, the Russell's vipers is more prevalent in the south and the saw-scaled viper is commonly found in the North and the West. Most bites are on the limbs because they are used by the person during his/her occupation.

Common snakes seen in India are: vipers (Russell's viper, scaled viper), cobra and the common krait (Fig. 85.1).

Immunological techniques have been developed for species identification of the snakes involved in the bites. An enzyme linked immunoassay (ELISA) can be used to identify a specific type of snake venom in a victim's blood, wound aspirate, or urine and this method has found place in clinical application throughout the world but is not used still in India.

Snake Venoms and Their Effects

Snake venom is a complex mixture of several chemical compounds such as enzymes, polypeptides, monoacids, amines, carbohydrate and lipids. They exert their effects in different ways:

- Elapidae neurotoxins produce neuromuscular paralysis by preventing the release of acetylcholine (ACh) or its action either pre-or post-synaptically. Death may occur due to respiratory paralysis.

- Viper venom produces coagulopathy at several points, Russell's viper venom activates coagulation factors such as factors V, IX, X, XIII, platelets and protein C. This effect causes fibrinolysis and DIC. It also contains a haemorrhagins that renders the vasculature leaky and produce local and systemic bleeding. Various proteolytic enzymes that cause tissue necrosis, also affect the coagulation pathway at various steps or impair organ function; myocardial depressant factors reduce the cardiac output. Saw-scaled vipers activate prothrombin, plasminogen and factor X and produce bleeding.

Sea snake venoms contain neurotoxins and myotoxin which result in muscle necrosis, myoglobinuria, hyperkalaemia and early acute renal failure.

Clinical Features

About one third of patients bitten by poisonous snake do not exhibit serious envenomation, because the amount of venom injected via a bite is highly variable and mainly depends on the length of the time since the snake had last bite and its aggression at the time of bite. However most of the patients present with features of apprehension and fear of intoxication, friends and relatives will frequently bring the snake with the patient for identification.

Local symptoms suggesting an effective bite include:

- Two clear-cut fang marks.
- Pain and swelling at the site of the bite.
- Painful regional lymph node enlargement
- Nausea, vomiting, headache, faintings and abdominal pain, may be due to over-reaction to the bite or earliest manifestations before envenomation, must be looked with highest degree of suspicion.

The clinical features of various snake bites are given in Table 85.1.

Investigations

Establish a physiological baseline profile for the following to monitor the progress and to act as a guide to the therapy.

1. *Coagulation profile:* It includes complete haemogram, bleeding time, clotting time, PTTK and fibrinogen degradation products (FDPs). Serial estimations may be done before antivenin therapy and after every 4 hours following antivenin because clotting defect produced by envenomation varies in duration and so is the restoration of the clotting time to normal due to antivenin therapy and resultant clearance of venom from the blood.

2. *Renal profile:* It includes urine examination, blood urea, serum creatinine to detect renal involvement as early as possible and to institute appropriate therapy.

Table 85.1: Clinical features of various snake bites

Elapid bite (Cobra and kraits)	Viper bite	Hydrophidae bite (sea snake)
Causative factor-neurotoxin	Causative factors—hemotoxin and haemorrhagins	Causative factors—myotoxin and neurotoxin
• Severe local reactions with blisters formation, and tissue necrosis appear within 1-2 hours. • Systemic effects: Neuroparalysis occurs within 6 hours but may be delayed upto 12 hours. The symptoms and signs are divided into preparalytic and paralytic syndromes. 1. *Pre-paralytic syndrome:* It includes vomiting, blurring of vision, drowsiness, heaviness of eyes and paraesthesias around the mouth. 2. *Paralytic syndrome:* It manifests with ophthalmoplegia, bilateral ptosis and spreads to involve muscles of palate, pharynx, tongue, jaw and limb paresis/paralysis. Finally, respiratory muscles may be involved producing generalised paralysis. Consciousness is maintained till respiratory depression. The syndrome is reversible either spontaneously or with antivenin over few days.	• Local swelling and oedema become obvious within few hours • Two clear-cut fang marks are seen Systemic effects: These result due to hypofibrinogenaemia, and consumptive coagulopathy. The symptoms and signs are: • Bleeding from the fang marks, blistering and necrosis become established within 24 hours • Bleeding may be obvious from the gums, nose, GI tract, urinary bladder. This is due to effect of haemorrhagins and DIC • Consequently to bleeding, hypovolaemia, shock and acute renal failure may develop • ECG changes and cardiac rhythm disturbances can occur • Panhypotuitarism can develop due to pituitary necrosis The features may reverse spontaneously or rapidly with specific antivenin therapy **GRADING OF VIPER BITES** (Table 84.2) Clinical features are as discussed above. Local swelling and necrosis are less marked. The preparalytic syndrome is more marked with rapid onset of paralysis	• Local tissue reactions are not seen • Paralytic features resemble that of elapid bite including respiratory muscle paralysis • Myotoxins produce rhabdomyolysis, myoglobinuria, and acute renal failure supervenes within 6-8 hours

Snake and Lizard Bites

3. *Arterial blood gas analysis:* It is done especially for elapid snake bite to detect impending respiratory failure and to plan the management.
4. *Routine EKG and X-ray chest* may be done to detect arrhythmias and cardiac involvement and/or respiratory infections.
5. *Creatine phosphokinase (CPK)* is greatly elevated in sea snake bite.
6. *ELISA* can be done rapidly and reliably at the bed side to identify a specific type of snake venom in a victim's blood, wound aspirate or urine. Venom levels by ELISA would give an estimate of the venom hours. This method has found clinical application throughout the world but unfortunately is not available in India.

Diagnosis

Diagnosis is based on:
1. **Reliable history of snake bite and identification of the killed snake:** Patients usually give a history of snake bite but this may be lacking in krait bite victims. Although *fang marks* are considered essential for fatal envenomation, but occasionally fatal envenomation can occur without *fang marks*. The development of severe local reactions with pain, swelling and necrosis is strongly suggestive of envenomation. In India, the killed snake is seldom brought for identification; immunodiagnostic methods are not developed and monovalent antivenom is not available. Hence, the identification of the snake is seldom done enthusiastically.
2. **Clinical features:** These have been discussed according to the snake bite (Table 85.1). Neuroparalytic features with or without local reactions occur due to cobra and kraits, respectively. Viper bites are characterised by local reactions, bleeding and DIC.
3. **Investigations:** They are useful to diagnosis of specific envenomation. Whole blood clotting time is a good bed side test that can be repeated frequently. If blood does not clot for 20 minutes at room temperature, it indicates systemic envenomation by viper bites. CPK is elevated in sea snake bite along with development of acute renal failure. Arterial blood gas analysis can identify the impending respiratory failure. Confirmation of the diagnosis is done by ELISA test for specific envenomation.

Complications

1. Extensive skin necrosis, gangrene, tetanus, secondary infection.
2. Shock, sepsis and organ system failure.
3. Acute adrenal insufficiency due to acute pituitary necrosis. Survivors develop the *Sheehan's syndrome*.
4. Cardiac arrhythmias, heart failure and hypotension.
5. Acute renal failure (acute tubular necrosis).
6. Respiratory failure.
7. Abortion in pregnant females.

Management

Aims of Treatment

- To retard the absorption of venom from the site of the bite.
- To neutralise the venom as quickly as possible.
- To prevent complications, tetanus, secondary infections.

  The management is divided into general and specific measures. General measures are directed against all types of snake bite, while specific are related to the toxicity observed and to the species involved.

Pre-Hospital (Field) Management— General Measures

It includes *"Don'ts"* and *"Do's"*:
A. *"Do's"* (to be done)
 i. All patients with suspected envenomation should be observed for upto 12 hours to rule out dry bite and to confirm envenomation.
 ii. *First Aid:*
  - Reassure the patient. Allay the anxiety and apprehension.

- Immobilise the bitten area to minimise the venom spread. An absorption delaying compression bandage preferably crepe bandage starting from the bite site extending upto the limbs prevents the lymphatic spread of the venom. Immobilise the limb by splinting during transportation.
- Tourniquet allowing a finger under it with difficulty should be tied if the bite has occurred within 2 hours, Tourniquet should not be released till antisnake venom has been given.

B. Important Don'ts (Rejected/Controversial Measures)
- Cruciate incision and suction.
- Local administration of antisnake venom
- Ice packs. It may cause ischaemia and tissue damage, hence, contraindicated.

Hospital Management

i. Once in the hospital, the victim should be monitored closely for vital signs, cardiac rhythm and oxygen saturation while a history is being recorded. A brief and thorough physical examination performed to evaluate presenting symptoms and signs.

ii. Gather informations regarding the event, approximate time of the bite, first-aid measures, previous episodes of bites and therapy received for that, known allergies and last date of tetanus immunization.

iii. The level of erythema/swelling in bitten extremity should be marked and the circumference measured at several locations and 10 cm proximally every 2-4 hours till swelling has stabilised.

iv. Large-bore intravenous access in two unaffected extremities should be obtained, or establish a **CVP line early** since these patients may develop sudden hypotension and may collapse.

v. Take blood for routine haemogram, clotting profile (BT, CT, PTTK, FDPs etc.) and for cross-matching and blood grouping. Perform urgent urinalysis for blood or myoglobin. In severe cases or in the face of significant comorbidity, arterial blood gas analysis, ECG and X-ray chest may also be got done.

vi. For relief of pain, use meperidine (pethidine) or any other analgesic. Aspirin should not be used as this may aggravate bleeding.

vii. Supportive therapy: Since snake venom contains clostridia, anaerobes and gram-negative organisms, patients should be given a combination of penicillin, metronidazole and aminoglycoside when local infection is very severe.

viii. All patients should receive tetanus immunoglobin/toxoid since the wound can act as a portal of entry.

ix. All vital signs (pulse, BP, respiration, urine output etc.) and laboratory parameters (coagulation profile, arterial blood gas analysis, renal and hepatic functions) should be monitored as hypotension, anaphylactic shock, renal failure and respiratory distress may all develop rapidly without any warning. Patient should be observed for atleast 24 hours for signs of systemic envenomation.

Specific Measures (Anti-Snake Venom—ASV)

Anti-snake venom is life-saving. Unfortunately monovalent antibodies (Fab antibodies now available in USA) for use and ELISA facility to diagnose specific snake venom are not available in India, therefore, polyvalent anti-snake venom (ASV) is used. Since this is an equine serum, reactions are common. However, the benefits of anti-venom are so great that the patients with a severe or progressive local reaction or clinical or biochemical features of systemic envenomation should receive it as quickly as possible depending on the grading of envenomation of different snake bite (Tables 85.2 and 85.3).

Adrenaline must be made available in the bedside emergency tray to manage anaphylaxis.

Snake and Lizard Bites

Table 85.2: Grading of vipers and allied bites and their respective management

Grading of bite	Clinical features	Management with ASV
I. (Mild)	Fang marks plus local swelling, paraesthesias	50 ml of ASV infused I.V.
II. (Moderate)	Fang marks plus local swelling limited to hands and/or feet. No systemic envenomation	100-150 ml of ASV infused I.V. in normal saline over 2 hours.
III. (Moderately severe)	Progression of the swelling beyond the site of the bite. Systemic reactions and laboratory changes present. History of bite by a toxic species or a large snake	150-200 ml of ASV as an infusion described above
IV. (Severe)	Pronounced and rapid progression of swelling, ecchymosis, severe systemic envenomation (signs and symptoms of toxicity plus abnormal laboratory parameters) and history of multiple bites by a large snake and/or highly toxic species	200 ml of ASV as an infusion in the manner described above. Repeated doses are necessary depending on the clotting time which is monitored

Caution: One must be sure of envenomation before antivenin therapy, as a dry bite which does not need treatment is not of uncommon occurrence.

Note:
- Repeat 50 ml doses every 4-6 hours for at least 48-72 hours. Studies have shown that clotting abnormalities may re-appear upto 72 hours after their apparent correction. This is attributed to delayed venom absorption from the site of the bite.
- Lophilized ASV is polyvalent, hence, is effective against bites of cobra, krait, Russell's viper and saw-scaled viper. lyphilised bowered ASV needs (pre-use reconstitution).
- Heparin worsens coagulopathy, hence, is not recommended.
- The ASV may be administered as long as 10 days to several weeks if signs of envenomation persist.
- Before starting antivenin therapy, enquiry must be made about any history of allergy and an intradermal sensitivity test performed by injecting 0.02 ml of saline diluted antiserum at a site distant from the bite. The injection site is then observed for at least 10 minutes for redness, pruritis or other adverse effects.

Table 85.3: Grading of elapid bites and its management

Grading of bite	Symptoms and signs	Management of ASV
IA.	No neuroparalytic features	For cobra bite. An initial high dose (200 ml) of
B.	Only local symptoms and signs	ASV is preferred. 100 ml may also be effective. Large doses are required for large snakes
II	Ophthalmoplegia and ptosis with or without local symptoms and signs	For krait bite, 100 ml of maintenance ASV may be required and should be given daily
III.	Grade II plus palatal, pharyngeal and limb paresis/paralysis	

Antihistamines and hydrocortisone must also be available to take care of immediate allergic reactions.

The hydrophides bites (sea snake bite) needs upto 1000 ml of monospecific antivenin initially for adequate neutralisation of venom.

Other Measures

1. *Neuroparalytic features* due to elapid bites (cobra bites only) may be treated with anticholinesterases. Edrophonium test positive patients should receive neostigmine 50-100 µg/kg every

4-6 hours or 25 µg/kg/hour infusion. Atropine sulphate 0.6 mg by infusion I.V. be given intermittently to relieve the side-effects of therapy.

2. **Treatment of hypotension and shock following viper bites (Russell's viper):** Early hypotension is due to pooling of blood in the pulmonary and splanchnic vascular bed, but later haemolysis and loss of intravascular volume contribute to it. Fluid resuscitation with normal saline or Ringer's lactate should be started immediately. If volume resuscitation fails to improve tissue perfusion, vasopressors (dobutamine, dopamine) may be administered. Intensive haemodynamic monitoring (CVP and/or pulmonary arterial pressures) can be helpful in such cases. Glucocorticosteroids may be useful to reverse adrenal insufficiency leading to shock. Diuretics may be used in case of fluid overload.

3. **Respiratory support:** Repeated pharyngeal suction, intubation and mechanical ventilation are important life-saving measures that should be used energetically. A rise in respiratory rate or fall in single breath count rather than arterial blood gas analysis should be the basis for mechanical ventilation. Where ventilators are not available, Ambu bags have been successfully employed for several hours.

4. **Renal failure:** Acute renal failure may be one of the gravest complication of viper bite, which is not reversed by ASV. Sea snake bite also produces rhabdomyolysis and acute renal failure due to myoglobinuria. Immediate and early treatment of ARF on usual lines with high doses of diuretics (frusemide) and/or dialysis should be instituted.

5. **Bleeding and DIC:** Blood loss, hypovolaemia and DIC should be corrected by fresh blood transfusion, or fresh frozen plasma and volume expansion. Heparin should not be used as discussed earlier.

6. **Treatment of compartmental syndromes:** If swelling in the bitten extremity causes subfacial oedema leading to impending tissue perfusion (muscle-compartment syndrome), surgical consulation may be sought to relieve it by possible fasciectomy while anti-snake venom continues. Compartmental syndromes are, however, rare after snake bites.

Prevention

1. *Primary*
   - Avoidance of contact with a snake by wearing protective knee length foot wear and thick gloves.
2. *Secondary*
   - Venoms toxoid: It is being used to immunise farmers in Japan. Elsewhere there has been progress with venoids to protect against the Russell's viper bite.
   - The production and modification of venom antigens by genetic engineering is an exciting new development in invention of snake venom vaccines.

LIZARD BITES

Bites from two venomous species of lizards (the gila monster, *Heloderma suspectum*) and the Mexican beaded lizard (*Heloderma horridum*) are encountered infrequently. The bites usually follow when attempts are made to capture or handle these creatures.

The venom contains proteases, phospholipases which are responsible for systemic effects.

Clinical Features

1. **Local symptoms and signs:** There is local pain, soft tissue oedema at the site of bite due to local venomous effects and mechanical trauma. Broken teeth may be embedded in the wound. Occasionally, local cyanosis and ecchymosis may develop.
2. **Systemic effects:** They include hypotension and shock, weakness, dizziness and diaphoresis.

Investigations

They are done to evaluate the venomous effects and to plan the treatment. These are:
- Complete blood count.
- Coagulation profile (BT, CT, platelet count, FDPs).

- Electrolytes estimation.
- Blood grouping and cross-matching.
- Urinalysis for renal involvement (blood, myoglobin).
- Electrocardiography (ECG).
- Soft tissue radiography of the bite to identify retained teeth.

Treatment

1. First aid measures for these bites are similar to snake bite (Read snake bite poisoning).
2. If the biting lizard is still attached to the victim, it should be detached by mechanical means (opening of its jaws).
3. Local pain is treated by analgesics (opiates).
4. The extremity should be splinted and elevated.
5. Cleansing and irrigation of the wound repeatedly.
6. Tetanus prophylaxis by immunoglobulin/toxoid.
7. If soft tissue radiography shows retained teeth, which should be removed by probing under local anaesthesia.
8. Supportive treatment: Fluids (intravenous normal saline or Ringer's lactate) should be given for hypotension and shock. Blood transfusions be given if bleeding occurs. Pain can be relieved by opiates and regional nerve blocks.
9. Antibiotics have no role.
10. No commercial antivenin exists. Mortality is low with supportive treatment.

Chapter 86

Scorpion Sting

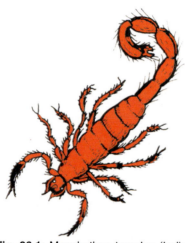

Fig. 86.1: Mesobuthus tamulus (Indian Red Scorpion)

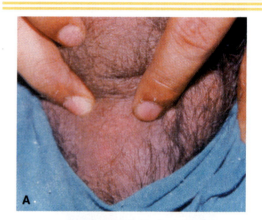

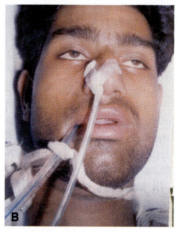

Fig. 86.2: Scorpion sting. **(A)** The site of bite is scrotum. Note the red scrotal area. It was tender. **(B)** The patient developed cholinergic (oculogyric crisis) and adrenergic crisis (blood pressure 180/130 mmHg) within 6 hours of the bite. Note: The patient recovered following treatment

SCORPION STING

Out of 1000 scorpion species known worldwide, only few are toxic to humans. In India, two species *mesobuthus tamulus* (Indian red scorpion) (Fig. 86.1) and *Palamnarus gravimanus* are of medical importance. Most of the cases of scorpion sting by mesobuthus tamulus have been reported from South India.

Farmers, farm workers, labourers, young children are at high risk. They are usually hit or stung while handling debris, paddy husk and harvesting grass without using protective measures (shoes) and scorpion stings human beings only when disturbed. Scorpions feed at night and remain hidden during the day in crevices or burrows or underwood, loose bark or logs of wood on the ground. They usually seek cool spots/places under building and often enter houses where they get entry into shoes, clothing or bedding or enter bathtubs and sinks in search of water.

Venom

Scorpion venom contains neurotoxins (polypeptides) that cause sodium channels to remain open and neurons to fire repetitively. The venom also contains enzymes (hyaluronidase) and serotonin which produce local reactions.

Clinical Features

1. ***Local symptoms and signs with or without systemic effects:*** These occur with stings by less poisonous scorpion or with scorpion with empty venom glands called *telson*. Pain, oedema and sweating appear at the sting site (Fig. 86.2). The pain may radiate along the involved dermatome and may be severe. The paraesthesia and hyperparaesthesia may be present, can be accentuated by tapping on the affected area (the tap test). These symptoms may subside within 24 hours without any systemic effects or may soon spread to other locations to produce systemic effects which are described below.

2. ***Systemic effects (Fig. 86.2B):*** Local effects may be followed by systemic effects due to spread of envenomation to other locations within few hours. Autonomic storm is the hallmark of poisoning by scorpion sting. It comprises:
   1. *Transient cholinergic manifestations:* These are:
      - Nausea and vomiting.
      - Profuse sweating all over the body.
      - Hypersalivation, lacrimation and rhinorrhoea.
      - Mydriasis (dilatation of pupils).
      - Priaprism (painful erection of penis).
      - Bradycardia, hypotension, bradyarrhythmias, ventricular premature beats with bigeminal pattern).

      These manifestations occur within few hours (4-5 hours) and subside within a day or two.
   2. *Transient adrenergic manifestations*
      - Puffy face, propped up eyes, oculogyric crisis, parasternal systolic lift, pansystolic or late systolic murmur due to papillary muscle dysfunction due to coronary vasospasm.
      - Cold extremities.
      - Perioral or generalised paraesthesias, muscle twitchings.
      - Patients can have hypertensive crisis (BP 200/140 mmHg) with sinus bradycardia (HR < 60/min).
      - Convulsions, transient hemiplegia, bilateral plantar extensor response can occur
      - At times acute pulmonary oedema.

3. ***Complications:*** Complications include tachycardia, arrhythmias, hypertension, hyperthermia, rhabdomyolysis and acidosis. Fatal respiratory arrest is common among young children and the elderly. Acute pancreatitis with severe pain abdomen has also been reported.

4. ***Late features:*** Asymptomatic hypotension (BP 70-90 mmHg) with bradycardia with warm extremities are seen in recovered patients (18-36 hours of hospitalization); are due to exhaustion of tissue catecholamines as a result of autonomic crisis, which persist for 3-5 days.

5. ***Electrocardiographic manifestations (Fig. 86.3):*** Tall tented T-waves, bradycardia, P-R prolongation, coronary sinus rhythm, VPCs in isolation or in runs can be observed.
   - Occasionally, ST segment elevation similar to acute MI may be observed due to vasospasm.
   - Conduction defects e.g. bundle branch block, fascicular block, complete heart block may appear transiently.

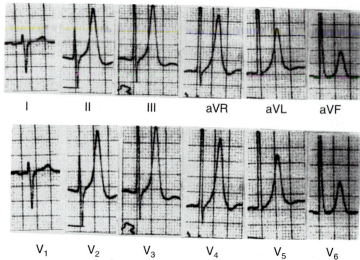

Fig. 86.2: Scorpion bite. The ECG shows tall tended T waves in leads I, II and V_2-V_6. This type of T wave change can occur in hyperkalaemia, CVA and early repolarisation syndrome

- Prolonged QTc with broad base, rounded top T waves are seen 24 hours of poisoning.

Investigations

They may reveal:
- Leucocytosis.
- Raised myocardial injury enzymes (CPK-MB).
- Low calcium and high potassium.
- Hyperglycaemia with reduction in serum insulin levels.

Management

1. **Pre-hospital or home management**
   - Identification of the offending scorpion aids in planning treatment.
   - Because most victims only experience local pain and discomfort, can be managed at home and asked to report to casualty and emergency department if signs of clinical envenomation i.e. cranial nerve or neuromuscular dysfunction develop.
   - Keep the patient calm and apply pressure dressings and cold packs to the sting site to reduce the absorption of the venom.
   - Pain can be relieved by local measures and by analgesics. Local anaesthesia can be given in case of intolerable pain which can be repeated. Oral diazepam is necessary to relieve anxiety.

2. **Hospital management**: Patient with cranial nerve or neuromuscular manifestations need immediate hospitalisation and aggressive support care and judicious use of antivenin to reduce mortality.
   i. *Correction of dehydration:* Dehydration resulting from vomiting, salivation, diaphoresis should be corrected by continuous oral rehydration solution. This helps to correct initial hypotension and shock. Parenteral crystalloid solutions or nasogastric feeding may be necessary in a confused agitated child. Electrolyte balance must also be corrected with fluid therapy.
   ii. *Scorpion antivenin*: Antivenin is available in India. Intravenous antivenin rapidly reverses cranial nerve dysfunction and muscular symptoms but does not affect local pain and paraesthesias. However, it does not prevent or protect the victim from

development of severe cardiovascular manifestations. Because of the risk of anaphylaxis or serum sickness following administration of goat serum combined with limited beneficial effects in experimental studies, recently it has been reported that scorpion antivenin is no better than placebo.

iii. *Supportive care:*
- *Control of restlessness and anxiety:* Although narcotics and sedatives can control restlessness and anxiety, these agents interfere with protective airway reflexes and should not be used in patients with neuromuscular symptoms unless endotracheal tube is inserted.
- *Control of hypertension/hypertensive crisis:* Various drugs like nifedipine, nitroprusside, hydralazine or prazosin have been used with success. Prazosin, a selective alpha-I adrenergic receptor blocker has found wide acceptance due to its pharmacological properties to antagonise the hemodynamic, hormonal and metabolic toxic effects of scorpion venom. Dose is 125-250 µg in children and 500 µg in adults, to be repeated 3-4 hourly until the signs of improvement appear.
- *Treatment of cardiac arrhythmia:* Bradycardia or bradyarrhythmias can be controlled with atropine. Runs of VPCs or VPCs with R on T phenomenon and VT respond to intravenous xylocaine and mexiletine. Intravenous amiodarone should be used with caution in patients with myocardial involvement and in presence of pulmonary oedema as it may further precipitate oedema.

5. **Other therapies:**
   - DIC, subdural haematoma may be treated with fresh blood transfusions.
   - Noncardiac pulmonary oedema or ARDS is rare with scorpion sting, may require tracheal intubation and oxygen administration.

Prevention

In scorpion-infested areas: shoes, clothing, bedding and towels should be shaken and inspected before being used. Removal of wood, stones, and debris from yards and composites help to remove the hiding sites for scorpion. Household spraying of insecticides can deplete their source of food.

Chapter 87

Sedative and Hypnotic Poisoning

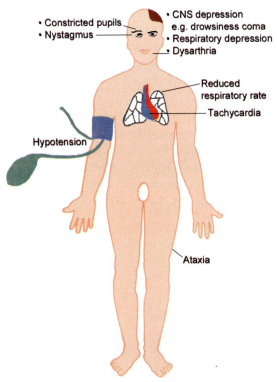

Fig. 87.1: Clinical manifestations of benzodiazepine poisoning

SEDATIVE AND HYPNOTIC POISONING

Sedative and hypnotic poisonings include:
- Benzodiazepines
- Non-benzodiazepines
- Barbiturates

1. Benzodiazepine Poisoning

Benzodiazepines are the commonly used sedatives and anxiolytic drugs in clinical practice. They are consumed in overdoses with suicidal intent. However, they are comparatively safe drugs even when taken in large doses. Mortality rates are low with this poisoning.

Mode of Action

Benzodiazepines potentiate the inhibitory effects of GABA on CNS neurones by binding to GABA receptors resulting in opening of chloride channels.

The drugs included in the group are given in Box 87.1.

Box 87.1: Commonly used benzodiazepines		
Long-acting	**Short-acting**	**Ultra-short acting**
• Chlordiazepoxide	• Alprazolam	• Estazolam
• Clonazepam	• Lorazepam	• Midazolam
• Diazepam	• Oxazepam	• Temazepam
• Flurazepam		• Triazolam
• Nitrazepam		
• Prazepam		
• Quazepam		

Clinical Features

All benzodiazepines are well absorbed and exhibit good protein binding (85-99%) and act as weak acids. They are metabolised in the liver and some

Sedative and Hypnotic Poisoning

have pharmacologically active metabolites. Metabolites are generally excreted in the urine along with the small amount of parent compound. Half life varies from 2 hours (short-acting agents) to 8 days (long acting drugs).

The toxic effects (Fig. 87.1) are evident within half an hour of an overdose and include:
- Weakness, hypotonia, hypotension.
- Ataxia, dysarthria.
- Constricted pupils.
- Drowsiness, respiratory depression and coma
- Pardoxical excitation may occur early in course of poisoning.

Diagnosis

It is based on:
1. Clinical history of intake and suggestive symptoms and signs.
2. Identification of metabolites in urine.
3. A response to *flumazenil* (an antidote) is a more sensitive diagnostic test.

Management

1. *Removal of unabsorbed drug* by repeated gastric lavage and administration of activated charcoal.
2. *Respiratory support:* Supplement oxygen, maintain the airway and intubate if there is altered sensorium and/or respiratory depression.
3. *Circulatory support:* Maintain circulation and monitor BP.
4. *Use of an antidote (flumazenil):* Flumazenil, a competitive benzodiazepine-receptor antagonist, can reverse CNS and respiratory depression. It is given in dose of 0.2 mg I.V. over 30 seconds followed by 0.3 mg at one minute and 0.5 mg at two minutes intervals until the desired effects are achieved or a total dose of 3 to 5 mg has been given. Patients must be monitored for relapse as flumazenil has short duration of action. Should relapse occur, the treatment can be repeated (at intervals of 20 minutes with a maximum dose of 3 mg/hour).

Failure to respond to flumazenil rules out benzodiazepine as the cause of poisoning. Flumazenil should not be used if mixed poisoning or tricyclic antidepressant poisoning is suspected.

Non-benzodiazepine Compound Poisoning

These compounds are taken alone or under the effect of alcohol:
1. *Buspirone:* It is a sedative, has less effect than diazepam. It interacts less with alcohol. Common manifestations of toxicity include: drowsiness, dysphoria, hypotension, bradycardia, paraesthesias, seizures, GI upset, dystonic reactions and priaprism. Treatment is by gastric lavage, activated charcoal administration and meticulous supportive care.
2. *Zolpidem:* Its effects are potentiated by consumption of alcohol. Common manifestations of toxicity include: nausea, vomiting, dizziness amnesia, drowsiness, respiratory and CNS depression. Supportive care, gastric lavage and activated charcoal are mainstay of treatment. Flumazenil has been found effective.
3. *Ecstacy (amphetamines):* Amphetamines or a neural 'designer' amphetamine (MDMA-3, 4 methylenedioxymethamphetamine, ectasy) are hallucinogenic in their effects. Effects occur within one hour of ingestion and last for 4-6 hours following doses upto 150 mg but upto 48 hours after ingestion of doses between 150-300 mg. Due to tolerance to these compounds, most users take the large doses.

The clinical features are given in Box 87.2.

Investigations

- Complete blood count.
- Renal and liver function tests.
- Blood glucose.
- Creatinine kinase (CK).
- ECG.
- Blood gas analysis.

Box 87.2: Clinical features of ecstasy/amphetamines

- Tachyarrhythmias e.g. supraventricular and ventricular
- Agitation or drowsiness are common
- Dehydration, hyponatraemia (dilutional)
- Nausea, muscle pain
- Hyper-reflexia, jaw clinching (trismus)
- Dilated pupils, blurred vision and visual halucinations
- Dry mouth, agitation

Note: Severe intoxication is characterised by convulsions, hypertension, coma and cardiac arrhythmias. A hyperthermic (5 HT like) syndrome may develop, characterised by rigidity, hyper-reflexia and hyperpyrexia leading to hypotension, metabolic acidosis, acute renal failure, DIC, hepatocellular necrosis, ARDS and cardiovascular collapse.

Management

1. Gastric lavage and activated charcoal administrations within one hour of ingestion are useful.
2. Patent airway must be secured before attempts are made to remove the poison from the stomach.
3. Intravenous fluids and electrolytes should be given to correct dehydration, hypotension and to prevent acute renal failure.
4. Monitor ECG, blood glucose, blood pressure and temperature.
5. The complications that are likely to be developed are given in Box 87.3 with appropriate treatment.

Barbiturate Poisoning

Barbiturates were the most frequently used antiepileptic drugs during seventies, hence, poisoning was common during that period. It has declined remarkably due to introduction of legislation by the Government of India to dispense the drug when prescription in triplicate is produced to the chemist. They are used as a sedative, hypnotic and as an antiepileptic.

Barbiturates are classified according to their duration of action as follows:
1. *Long-acting (6-12 hours)* e.g. phenobarbitone, barbital, pyrimidone.
2. *Intermediate-acting (3-6 hours)* e.g. amlobarbital, butabarbital.
3. *Short-acting (1-3 hours)* e.g. hexabarbital, secobarbital, pentobarbital.
4. *Ultra-short acting (< 30 minutes)* e.g. methohexital, thiopental.

Clinical Features

The initial features are mainly due to CNS depression followed by features of respiratory depression and hypotension.

1. *CNS depression:* Confusion, lethargy, depressed mental activity, decreased responsiveness to external stimuli, dilated pupils, depressed tendon reflexes and extensor plantar response are seen.

Box 87.3: Complications of ecstasy and their management

Complication	Management
• Hypertension	• Oral diazepam, nifedipine or doxazobin
• Hypertensive encephalopathy, infarction/stroke	I.V. nitrates or sodium nitroprusside
• Supraventricular tachycardia	I.V verapamil. Avoid β-blockers which cause hypertension due to unopposed alpha stimulation
• Amphetamine-induced angina	I.V. or sublingual nitrates. Avoid β-blockers
• Acute MI	• Avoid thrombolysis because MI is due to vasospasm • Nitrates
Hyperthermia	• Cool I.V. fluids, cold sponging • Dantrolene • Paralyse and ventilate the patient if above measures fail
Agitation or psychosis	• Oral diazepam. Avoid phenothiazines and haloperidol as they may precipitate convulsions

2. *Respiratory depression:* It causes Cheyne-Stoke's respiration, apnea, aspiration pneumonia and respiratory acidosis.
3. *Other features* include: hypotension, shock, hypothermia, acute renal failure and a characteristic bullous rash seen on pressure points like elbow or malleous after 2-3 days.

Investigations

A complete haemogram, renal and liver function tests, ECG, X-ray chest are routinely done in the poisoning. Serum barbiturate levels are mandatory to confirm the diagnosis, to judge its severity and to plan the treatment.

Management

1. *To remove the unabsorbed drug* from the stomach by gastric lavage, activated charcoal 50 g every 4 to 6 hours.
2. *To excrete the drug* through stool by catharsis.
3. *To enhance urinary excretion by forced alkaline diuresis in cycles.* It is useful for long-acting barbiturate poisoning.

Each cycle consists of 1000 ml of dextrose saline + 10 ml of KCl and 100 ml of NaHCO$_3$ followed by 1000 ml of 5% dextrose + 10 ml of KCl and 350 ml of mannitol in 60 kg adults. About 3-6 cycles are required depending on the severity. Urine output is to be measured, if it does not match with intake, a bolus dose of 40 mg frusemide may be given I.V. CVP line should be put and fluid balance maintained.

Complications of forced-alkaline diuresis include: circulatory overload, pulmonary oedema, electrolyte disturbance and mannitol, induced acute tubular necrosis.

4. *Removal of drug by extracorporeal means e.g. peritoneal or haemodialysis.* Haemodialysis is useful in poisoning due to long and short-acting barbiturates and haemoperfusion in short-acting one. The indications are given in Box 87.4.
5. *Respiratory support:* Maintain a patent airway. Intubate if assisted ventilation is required.
6. *Other measures:* Maintain electrolytes balance, temperature and BP.

Box 87.4: Indications of dialysis

1. Deep coma with areflexia, hypotension and respiratory depression.
2. Blood levels e.g. > 9 mg/dl of long acting and > 3.5 mg/dl for short-acting barbiturates.
3. Presence of renal failure and pulmonary oedema.

Part Ten

Internal Medicine

Systemic Anaphylaxis

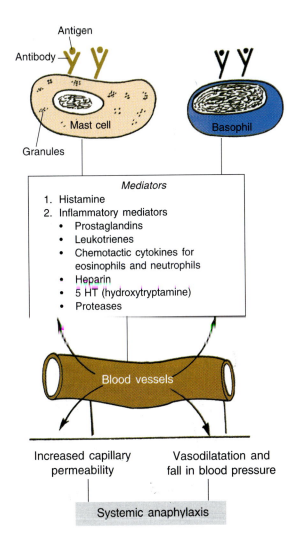

Fig. 88.1: Pathologenic mechanisms of anaphylaxis

ANAPHYLAXIS

Definition

Anaphylaxis is a systemic and life-threatening response of a sensitized human to an antigen, appears immediately within minutes of administration of specific antigen. It is characterized clinically by respiratory distress followed by vascular collapse or shock without antecedent respiratory difficulty. In fact, it is an antigen induced IgE-mediated immune reaction, occurs due to a variety of antigens.

Anaphylactoid reaction on the other hand occurs in an unsensitized person and is not IgE-mediated. Both anaphylaxis and anaphylactoid reactions produce similar symptoms and signs. Rarely, the life-threatening anaphylactoid reactions may occur during anaesthesia due to muscle relaxants such as alcuronium and pancuronium.

Exercise Induced Anaphylaxis

It is a unique form of allergy in which flushing sensation, a feeling of warmth and urticarial wheals develop in association with vigorous exercise. These symptoms do not occur with passive exercise or warming up.

Predisposing Factors

The patients having history of atopy, allergy and asthma are more prone to develop this reaction. This is due to release of histamine and other mediators (kinins) following the interaction of antigen with antibody (IgE) produced by B lymphocytes and bound to cell membranes of mast cell or circulating basophils leading to their degranulation (Fig. 88.1). The predisposing factors are given in Box 88.1.

Anaphylaxis may be caused by ingestion, inhalation or parenteral injection of an antigen that sensitizes the predisposed individuals.

> **Box 88.1: Predisposing factors for anaphylaxis**
> 1. **Drugs**
>   - Penicillin, cephalosporins amphotericin B
>   - Local anaesthetics e.g. procaine, lidocaine
>   - Vitamins e.g. thiamine, folic acid
>   - Contrast medium agents
>   - Occupational related agent e.g. ethylene oxide
>   - Antisera, dextran, albumin
>   - Cyclosporine
>   - Opiates
>   - NSAIDs and azo dyes
> 2. **Hymenopetra venoms**
>   - Hornets, wasp, honey bee, ants
> 3. **Heterologous proteins**
>   - Hormones e.g. insulin, vasopressin, paratharmone
>   - Enzymes e.g. trypsin, chymotrypsin, penicillinase
> 4. **Foods**
>   - Eggs, sea food, nuts, grains, beans
> 5. **Pollen extracts**
>   - Ragweed, grass, trees
> 6. **Nonpollen extracts**
>   - Dust mites, cot dander
> 7. **Idiopathic**
>   - Blood transfusion (immune complex mediated) e.g. whole blood, plasma and immunoglobulins.

Clinical Features

The symptoms and signs vary usually, appear immediately within few seconds to minutes after introduction of the antigen through injection but are late following ingestion and inhalation. These are:
1. **Respiratory manifestations:**
    i. *Acute bronchial obstruction:* There may be upper and lower airway obstruction leading to feeling of tightness in the chest with or without audible wheeze.
   ii. *Laryngeal oedema:* It is characterized by feeling of a 'lump' in the throat, hoarseness or stridor.
2. **Cutaneous manifestations:** A characteristic feature is urticarial eruptions (well-circumscribed cutaneous wheals with erythematous, raised serpiginous borders and branched centres) which are intensely itchy and may be localized or generalised. They seldom persist beyond 48 hours.

   A localized, nonpitting oedema, angioedema may also be present. It may be asymptomatic or may cause burning or tingling sensation.
3. **Cardiovascular manifestations:** Syncope, hypotension and tachycardia may occur before cardiovascular collapse.

   The associated ECG abnormalities with or without infarction may be noted in these patients, reflect either a primary cardiac event or can be due to critical reduction in blood volume.

Diagnosis

The diagnosis of anaphylaxis depends on:
   i. A reliable accurate history of administration of an antigen followed by acute onset of appropriate symptoms and signs.
  ii. Radioimmunoassay for defection of IgE antibodies. These assays require purified antigens.
 iii. Elevation of tryptase levels occurs due to mast cell activation, in an adverse systemic reaction, and are particularly informative with episodes of hypotension during general anaesthesia or when there has been a fatal outcome.

Management

Early diagnosis and early institution of treatment is mandatory since death may occur within minutes to hours after the first symptom. Ideally ABC of cardiopulmonary resuscitation should be achieved at the earliest in severe cases.

1. *Subcutaneous adrenaline (epinephrine):* Adrenaline (0.2 to 0.5 ml of 1:1000 dil), is given subcutaneously with repeat dose at 20 minutes interval. Mild to moderate symptoms can be controlled with single dose. If the patient does not improve with subcutaneous dosing, then 2-5 ml of epinephrine diluted in 1:10,000 may be given I.V. through an intravenous infusion line. In extreme cases or in whom I.V. line is not accessible, then adrenaline can be introduced via endotracheal route. In co-operative patients, nebulised epinephrine is effective.
2. *To retard the absorption of injected antigen:* If an antigenic material has been administered through an injection (insect stinger) into an extremity, its rate of absorption can be reduced by an application of a tourniquet proximal to injection site, administer 0.2 ml of 1:1000 epinephrine into the site, and remove without compression an insect stinger if insect bite is the cause of reaction.
3. *Intravenous glucagon:* 1 mg of glucagon I.V. over 5 minutes may be useful in epinehprine resistant cases.
4. *Volume expansion:* Volume expandors such as normal saline and vasopressor agents (e.g. dopamine) may restore vascular volume. Increased capillary leakage may require several litres of saline. About 90% patients respond to this therapy.
5. *Respiratory support:* Oxygen via a nasal catheter or IPP breathing of oxygen with 0.5 ml of isoproterenol diluted in 1:200 in saline may be helpful. Either endotracheal intubation or tracheostomy is mandatory for oxygen therapy in severe cases if progressive hypoxia develops.
6. *Other measures:* Parenteral antihistaminics and aminophylline are useful to control allergic symptoms and bronchospasm respectively. Steroids are not effective during an acute event but may alleviate the recurrence of bronchospasm, hypotension, and urticaria.

Prevention

1. If there is a definite history of past anaphylaxis with any known agent or procedure, even though mild, it is advisable to select another agent or procedure. A knowledge of cross-reactivity amongst the substances is crucial.
2. *A skin test* must be performed with allergenic extracts or when the nature of the past adverse reaction is unknown. Skin testing is of no value for non IgE-mediated reactions.
3. One should use special precautions while giving drugs to patients with history of hay fever, asthma and other allergic disorders.
4. Those who are known to be sensitive to insect bite should avoid visit to areas where such insects are likely to be present. Protective garments must be worn if they visit such areas, and they must be trained to inject adrenaline and antihistamine on the first symptom of anaphylactic reaction. Desensitization of such individuals may be necessary.
5. Venom immunotherapy to achieve venom specific IgG titres above 3.0 μg/ml in serum is recommended in persons having sting sensitivity. A 5 years treatment induces a state of resistance.

Heat Hyperpyrexia

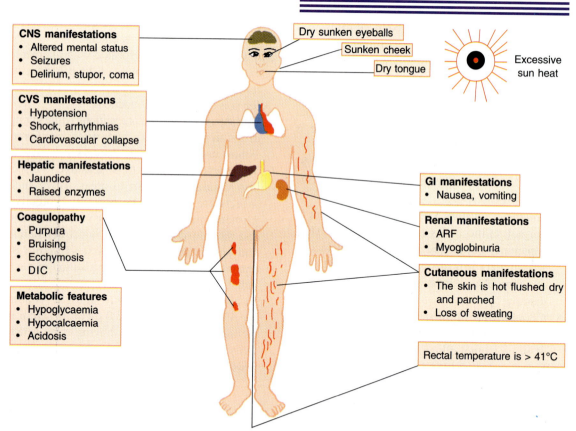

Fig. 89.1: Dry hot man due to heat stroke

Hyperpyrexia is defined as body temperature of greater than 40°C (106°F) and when it occurs due to exposure to high enviornmental temperature, then it is called *'heat hyperpyrexia'* or *"heat syndromes"*.

Acclimatisation is an effective protective mechanism against the effects of hot climate. It is an efficient mechanism accompanied by proper replacement of salt and water, helps to withstand heat stress. In acclimatised individuals, the concentration of sodium chloride in sweat is very low and this helps in the conservation of sodium chloride in hot climate. In contrast to this, unacclimatised individuals are predisposed to the effects of heat leading to *"heat hyperpyrexia or heat syndromes"*.

HEAT STROKE

Definition

It is a catastrophic condition which results from complete breakdown of thermoregulatory mechanism and is characterised by high grade fever usually > 41°C (> 106°F), loss of sweating and profound disturbance in consciousness.

> *Loss of sweating is the cardinal feature of heat stroke.*

Forms of Heat Stroke

1. *Exertional heat stroke:* It is a disorder of unacclimatized young persons particularly athletes, soldiers or labourers who perform strenuous work/task in hot and humid climate.
2. *Classical or nonexertional heat stroke:* It occurs among elderly, debilitated persons often in epidemic fashion during heat waves of hot season. The elderly bedridden, persons taking anticholinergics or anti-parkinsonian drugs or diuretics are most susceptibles.

Predisposing Factors

Many factors that can predispose to heat stroke are given in Box 89.1. It occurs in unacclimatised individuals in whom sweating is either absent or minimal.

Box 89.1: Predisposing factors for heat stroke	
• High environmental temperature	• Diabetes
	• Alcoholism
• Hot and humid condition/ atmosphere	• Dehydration or lack of water intake
• Old age	• Heavy exercise/work
• Debility	• Associated infection
• Obesity	• CVA

Clinical Features (Fig. 89.1)

All the body tissues are susceptable to heat injury. High temperature >41°C raises the BMR exuberantly and results in enzyme denaturation, protein coagulation and lipid liquefaction. Tissue injury depends on the absolute tissue temperature and duration of exposure. The systems involved are cardiovascular, CNS, renal and hepatic.

1. *Neurological manifestations:* Altered mental status, seizures, confusion, disorientation, stupor and coma may occur. Some patients who develop severe neurological features and survive may be left with permanent neurological complications i.e. cerebral (amnesia, dementia, hemiparesis), cerebellar (dysarthria, ataxia) and spinal cord (polyneuropathy).

2. *Cardiovascular manifestations:* Initially, the pulse is good volume and bounding, becomes weak and feeble due to development of shock, hypotension or cardiovascular collapse due to thermal myocardial injury and hypoxia. Cardiac arrhythmias and nonspecific ECG changes suggest myocardial damage and electrolyte disturbance. Death may occur due to circulatory collapse or sudden cardiac arrest.

3. *Renal manifestations:* Acute renal failure is common, occurs due to acute tubular necrosis as a result of ischaemia or myoglobinuria due to rhabdomyolysis (induced muscle necrosis by heat).

4. *Gastrointestinal manifestations:* Nausea, vomiting are common due to mucosal heat injury.

5. *Hepatic manifestations:* Liver necrosis may be due to direct heat injury resulting in jaundice. Elevations of bilirubin and SGPT are frequently encountered. Liver injury may result in late onset coagulopathy.

6. *Coagulopathy:* Direct injury to clotting factors results in early coagulopathy leading to petechiae and ecchymosis. Thrombocytopenia

can occur. Disseminated intravascular coagulation is seen only in severe cases.
7. *Cutaneous manifestations:* Metabolic acidosis occurs due to accumulation of lactic acid leading to acidotic breathing. Hypocalcaemia and hypokalaemia may occur. Sometimes hypoglycaemia may occur.

Management

Steps of management include:
1. **To reduce the temperature as quickly as possible by external means of heat dissipation (evaporative cooling):** Direct ice application with fanning to promote evaporation and heat loss is the most widely employed method and results in rapid cooling. Immersion in ice-cold water has been used. It is not only cumbersome but is associated with shivering and hypotension. Cooling effects should be stopped when core body temperature reaches to 38.5°C to prevent iaterogenic hypothermia. In severe cases, intravenous administration of cold fluid and iced gastric and peritoneal lavage or enema may be tried.
2. **Supportive care:**
   a. *A patent airway* should be established by endotracheal tube, if necessary. Adequate oxygenation is done by giving 100% oxygen. In comatosed patient with severe respiratory depression, assisted ventilation may be needed.
   b. *Fluid replacements* are usually small as compared to heat exhaustion. It consists of 1200-1500 ml of crystalloids, to be given under CVP monitoring in old persons. 50 ml of sodium bicarbonate is given to combat acidosis. Hypoglycaemia, if occurs may be treated appropriately.
   c. *Role of corticosteroids* is controversial, may be used to combat shock, cerebral oedema and adrenal insufficiency.
   d. *Urine output improves after external cooling and fluid replacement.* If urine output falls, mannitol 1.5 g/kg is given. Prolonged oliguria is an indication of dialysis.
   e. *Coagulopathy,* if develops may be treated with fresh blood transfusions or replacement of clotting factors.

HEAT EXHAUSTION

Definition

It is an another catastrophic condition of dysregulation of body temperature characterised by water and/or salt depletion due to profuse sweating. It is commoner than heat stroke.

Types

1. *Pure water depletion heat exhaustion:* It results from excessive sweating and inadequate water replacement by drinking. It occurs in acclimatised people (trained persons) because of increased ability to sweat. The patients with this type present with excessive thirst with signs of dehydration (feeble pulse, sunken eyeballs and cheeks, dry tongue etc.). As salt is not lost in sweat proportionately, therefore, there is rise in serum sodium and chloride with rise in osmolarity. Mental confusion, impaired sensorium, delirium, coma and death may occur. There is rise in body temperature (38°-40°C).
2. *Pure salt depletion heat exhaustion:* It is slow in onset, occurs in people working in hot and humid enviornment, especially in unacclimatised people (troops landed in hot climate) in whom salt loss in sweat is very high with replacement of water. The thirst is absent in this type. The skin is dry and inelastic. The symptoms pertain to dehydration and salt loss. These include fatigue, weakness, painful muscle cramps, nausea, vomiting and headache. Dehydration and hypotension develop subsequently. There is slight rise in body temperature. Confusion, delirium, coma supervene due to shock and cerebral oedema.

Rapid pulse, tachypnoea, raised temperature, signs of dehydration with profuse sweating are hallmark of heat-exhaustion irrespective of its type. Temperature is not as high as observed in heat stroke, is usually < 40°C.

3. *Combined type of heat exhaustion:* It is the most common type, presents with clinical picture of both pure types (a mixed picture).

Management

1. *Treatment irrespective of its types:* Shift the patient in a cool environment.
2. *Treatment of specific type*:
   i. *Pure water depletion type* needs judicious replacement of fluids. About 6-8 L of fluid should be given in first 24 hours and fluid therapy is continued until urine output is normal. The 5% dextrose is ideal when the patient does not take orally. Oral hydration with water may be needed in mild cases.
   ii. *Salt depletion type* needs replacement of fluid and salts by salted drinks orally (fruit drinks with 7 g of salt per litre, soups etc.). In unconscious patient, isotonic saline (2-4 liters) I.V. may be given within 24 hours and continued till urine output is normalised and sodium and chloride levels return to normal.
   iii. Monitor sodium and chloride.

MALIGNANT HYPERPYREXIA

Definition

It is an inherited abnormality of skeletal muscle sarcoplasmic reticulum that causes rapid increase in intracellular calcium levels in response to halothane or other inhalational anaesthetics or to succinylcholine.

Clinical Features

- Elevated temperature (hyperpyrexia).
- Muscle rigidity.
- Rhabdomyolysis.
- Acidosis.
- Cardiovascular instability i.e. tachycardia or rapid ventricular arrhythmias.

Treatment

- Cessation of anaesthesia.
- Administration of dantrolene to control rigidity. The recommended dose of dantrolene is 1 to 2.5 mg/kg of body weight given I.V. after every 6 hours for at least 24-48 hours or until oral dantrolene can be given, if needed.
- Procainamide should also be administered to patients with malignant hyperthermia (hyperpyrexia) because of likelihood of ventricular fibrillation in this syndrome.

Chapter 90

Hypothermia

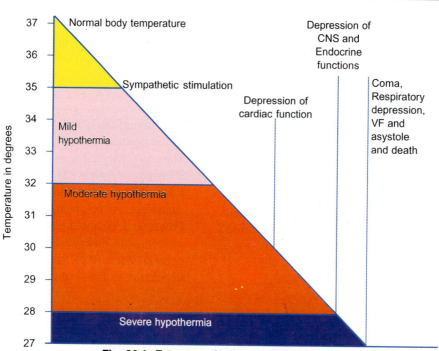

Fig. 90.1: Extremes of cold exposure

Definition

Hypothermia is defined as a core body temperature (rectal temperature) of 35°C or less. It is classified as *mild* (temp. between 35°C to 32°C), *moderate* (<32°C to 28°C) or *severe* (<28°C). This is depicted in Figure 90.1.

Pathogenesis

Hypothermia represents a loss of balance between heat production and the heat loss. Heat is generated in all the tissues and is lost by *radiation*, *evaporation*, *conduction* and *convection*. The balance between heat production and heat loss is regulated

Hypothermia

by the hypothalamus (preoptic and posterior region). Cold exposure activates the cold receptors in the skin and transmits the signal to hypothalamus via lateral spinothalamic tract. The hypothalamus (posterior region) activates the sympathetic nervous system to increase muscle tone and causes shivering. The shivering, in turn, increases the metabolic rate from normal level (40 to 60 kcal/h) to as high as 300 kcal/h. Shivering tries to conserve heat to overcome ambient temperature gradient, hence, is protective mechanism. Even at maximum metabolic rates, heat loss from the body can exceed heat production. As the body temperature drops to 30°C, metabolic process slows and shivering stops, thereby accelerating the development of hypothermia.

Causes

Extreme environmental conditions can cause hypothermia in healthy individuals. Most severe hypothermia occurs in persons with underlying medical conditions either due to excessive heat loss (environmental exposure) or inadequate heat production or both processes are involved (Table 90.1). It is hereby stressed that body temperature never falls below the environmental temperature.

1. *Iatrogenic hypothermia:* It can occur when semiconscious or unconscious patients are left uncovered in hospital room or during surgical procedures where large body surface areas are exposed to low temperature for long periods in the operating room.
2. *Intentional hypothermia* i.e. cold cardioplegia in cardiopulmonary bypass surgery.
3. *Accidental hypothermia:* Most environmental exposures are accidental. It can also occur due to interference with pathophysiologic events, anatomical disruptions and drugs. In the home enviornment in cold climates hypothermia occurs due to poor heating, clothing and poor nutrition, further contributed by drugs, illness, alcohol etc.

The outdoor hypothermia also involves climbers, skiers, arctic and anarctic travellers due to exposure to extreme low temperatures. Physical exhaustion and inadequate clothing are contributory.

Table 90.1: Causes of hypothermia

I. **Excessive heat loss**
   a. Environmental exposure
      - Accidental
      - Iatrogenic
   b. Increased continuous blood flow
      - Burn, psoriasis, toxic epidermal necrolysis.

II. **Inadequate heat production**
   a. Inadequate metabolism
      - Malnutrition and/or starvation
      - Hypothyroidism, adrenal insufficiency
      - Hepatic failure
      - Diabetic ketoacidosis and hypoglycaemia.
   b. Altered thermoregulation
      - Sepsis
      - Uraemia
      - Hypothalamic dysfunction, e.g. head trauma, stroke, tumour
      - Spinal cord injury—T_1 or above
      - *Shapiro's syndrome* (episodic spontaneous hypothermia with hyperhidrosis.
   c. Drug-induced
      - Barbiturates, phenothiazines, opiates, lithium, benzodiazepines
      - Alcohol.

Clinical Features

In mild hypothermia (core temp. 32-35°C), there is shivering and feeling of intense cold. The subject is alert and usually takes appropriate actions to rewarm e.g. huddling, extraclothing or exercise. There is tachycardia, increased cardiac output and peripheral vasoconstriction secondary to sympathetic stimulation. There may occur cold diuresis due to peripheral vasoconstriction leading to shunting of blood to central circulation.

In moderate hypothermia (core temp. 28-32°C), the ability to shiver is lost. Cardiac conduction is depressed. There is sinus bradycardia. Atrial fibrillation with slow ventricular conduction may occur. The EKG may show slow ventricular rate, T wave inversion and QT prolongation. At temperature of 28°C-30°C, **Osborne 'J' waves** (a positive upward deflection with J point elevation) appear at the junction of descending limb of R wave (QRS) with ST segment.

The neurological manifestations are diverse. At temperature of 32°, there is clouding of the consciousness with sluggish activity. As the temperature falls further (at 30°C), violent behaviour, confusion, disturbance of vision, ataxia, dysarthria may follow. Staggering, falling and faintings are common. Below 30°C to 28°C, there is depression of all the cerebral functions. Pulse and respiration become slow. There are slow pupillary as well as tendon reflexes.

In severe hypothermia (core temp. <28°C), there is loss of consciousness and patient becomes deeply comatosed at ≤ 25°C. As the coma increases, pupils become dilated and fixed, metabolic acidosis and pulmonary oedema leading to hypoxemia develop. The reflexes become lost and generalised rigidity simulating rigor mortis appears and patient may be mistaken as a dead man. Ventricular fibrillation and asystole may develop as temperature falls below 20°C and are the leading causes of death.

Investigations

Investigation may show:
1. Haemoconcentration (raised Hb and PCV).
2. Cold-induced granulocytopenia.
3. There may be evidence of hepatic and renal impairment (raised urea and creatinine).
4. Serum cortisol level may be low.
5. Coagulation profile may show depressed platelet function and DIC.
6. Arterial blood gas analysis may show hypoxaemia and metabolic acidosis.
7. Serum K^+ may be elevated.
8. X-ray chest and abdomen are important in patients with immersion hypothermia to see the evidence of aspiration.
9. EEG and evoked potentials. Evoked potentials show increase in latency and decrease in amplitude of visual, auditory and somatosensory potentials.

Severe hypothermia may be associated with isoelectric EEG which should not be taken as brain death and it is reversible.

10. ECG for Osborne 'J' waves and cardiac arrhythmias.

Management

The essence of therapeutic approach for these patients lies to bring the core body temperature slowly to normal while correcting metabolic abnormalities and treating cardiac arrhythmias. It is a medical emergency and requires energetic and immediate management. A common dictum quoted in the treatment of hypothermia is *"the person is not dead until it is warm and dead"* stresses the need of rewarming before a person is declared dead.

Steps of Management
1. Rewarming (active or passive, internal or external).
2. Supportive treatment for volume depletion, acid base disturbance, hypoxia and arrhythmias.
3. Treatment of underlying cause when patient becomes stable. Underlying hypothyroidism must be looked for, if present, must be treated. Avoid the precipitating factors.
4. Monitor temperature (core body), vital signs (pulse, BP, respiration, urine output), biochemical parameters (arterial blood gas, pH), ECG and electrolytes.

Rewarming

It is done to increase the body temperature by 0.5°C to 2°C/hr. Rewarming techniques can be active or passive, internal or external.

  i. *Passive external rewarming:* It is the easiest and safest method and should be done in each and every patient with mild hypothermia. It involves covering the patient with blankets and clothing in a warm environment to allow the endogenous heat production to correct the hypothermia. It is important to keep the head covered because upto 30% heat is lost from the head. A single layer of cotton blanket decreases the heat loss by 30%. Three layers of blankets reduce the heat loss by 50%.

ii. *Active external rewarming*: It involves direct application of heat sources (hot water bottles, heating blankets, heat lamps, submersion in a tank of hot water) to external body surfaces. This procedure may be hazardous as it may cause hypotension, or *"rewarming shock"* (associated with peripheral vasodilatation), paradoxical core acidosis and hyperkalaemia and can cause core temperature to drop even further (a phenomenon referred to as *"after drop"*). There is a risk of burn injury due to application of direct heat. Therefore, active rewarming should be done only on a young previously healthy person, with minimal pathophysiologic derangement. Direct heat to be applied only to the thorax if active rewarming is used.

Recently field treatment with insulating covers have been used with minimal loss of heat. It has also been observed that carbon fibre rewarming has resulted in a rapid rise in core temperature. Convection warmers have been used in operation theatres for management of peri-operative hypothermia.

iii. *Active internal rewarming*: The simplest method is airway rewarming in which the patient inspires humidified oxygen heated to 42°C via face mask or endotracheal tube and this technique raises the core temperature by 1 to 2°C/hr.

Warmed intravenous fluid and lavage of the stomach, bladder or colon with warmed fluids have a limited warming effects, may not be of much help when rapid rewarming is needed. Heated peritoneal and pleural lavage induce rapid rewarming (2-4°C/h), should be used only in moderate to severe hypothermia with cardiovascular instability or when external rewarming is ineffective.

The most efficient rewarming technique is extracorporeal blood warming by haemodialysis or cardiopulmonary bypass. Both methods require continuous removal of blood that is circulated and warmed externally before being reinfused. These methods are used for rapid rewarming in severe hypothermia when other methods are ineffective.

Supportive Measures

1. *Correction of volume depletion:* Warmed normal saline or 5% dextrose saline may be given intravenously. Lactate Ringer's solution should be avoided.
2. *Physical manipulation of the patient* should be minimized. Central venous line, nasogastric tube and endotracheal tube should be inserted carefully because of likelihood of cardiac arrhythmias.
3. *Treatment of acidosis:* It does not require any treatment except rewarming.
4. *Treatment of sepsis*: If it is a possibility then treat it with appropriate antibiotics. Broad-spectrum antibiotics are employed before a culture or sensitivity report is received.
5. *Correction of hypokalaemia*: Rewarming alone corrects hypokalaemia.
6. *Correction of hyperglycaemia:* Rewarming often corrects hyperglycaemia, if persists after rewarming a small dose of insulin may be used.

Monitoring

1. Monitoring of temperature by rectal thermometer designed to measure the lower body temperature.
2. Continuous cardiac monitoring is required for detection of arrhythmias. Atrial arrhythmias are common and reverse with rewarming alone. Ventricular arrhythmias are usually refractory to drugs and to defibrillation. Bretylium tosylate (5 µg/kg I.V.) is the agent of choice.

When cardiac arrest is present, active internal rewarming and cardiopulmonary resuscitation (CPR) should be initiated simultaneously.

Treatment of underlying cause

Treatment or removal of underlying cause/precipitating cause once the patient becomes stabilised after rewarming. A careful search should be made for any underlying cause or precipitating cause, and should be corrected or treated. Alcohol should be avoided in future.

Chapter 91

High Altitude Related Emergencies

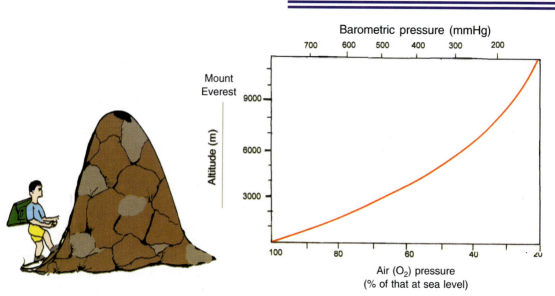

Fig. 91.1: Diagram showing the decrease in oxygen and barometric pressure with increasing heights

HIGH ALTITUDE RELATED ACUTE DISORDERS

High altitude environment is different than the environment at ground level. It is characterised by hypobaric hypoxia, low temperatures and increased radiation (ultraviolet and ionising) and most of high altitude disorders are attributed to hypoxia.

Altitudes above 2700 m is defined as *high altitude*. Most low-landers on reaching these heights develop biophysiological changes related to acclimatization to these heights. Failure of acclimatization or acute effects of these biophysiological changes lead to diseases found at these heights. Altitude above 5500 m is termed as *extreme altitude*. At extreme altitude, permanent adaptation or acclimatization of man does not occur.

Physiological Changes to High Altitude

1. *Hyperventilation:* It is mediated via peripheral chemoreceptors due to hypoxia and is the earliest change that occurs on ascent to high altitude.

2. *Hyperventilation is followed by hypocapnia* that leads to respiratory alkalosis which is compensated by renal bicarbonate excretion.
3. *Hypoxia* leads to pulmonary vasoconstriction.
4. *Secondary polycythaemia* occurs as a response to hypoxia, is mediated through erythropoietin production. Although it is a physiological response and increases O_2 carrying capacity of blood but leads to an increase in blood viscosity which can be deleterious specially at extreme heights. It may lead to venous thrombosis and may predispose to pulmonary embolism.
5. *There is decrease in partial pressure of oxygen and barometric pressure with increasing heights* (Fig. 91.1). At 5000 m height, the partial pressure of O_2 is reduced to 50%. The oxygen saturation falls with increase in altitude. Below 2500 m, the reduction in O_2 saturation is small and no symptoms other than exertional dyspnoea appear. All syndromes of high altitude appear at heights > 2700 m.
6. *Other changes* include: increase in sympathetic tone, and long-term changes of increase in capillary density and intracellular oxidative enzymes.

Classification

Depending on the onset of manifestations, high altitude disorders may be classified into *acute*, *subacute* and *chronic* (see Table 91.1). Here only acute disorders will be discussed. Most of the high altitude illnesses occur in travellers and mountaineers.

ACUTE MOUNTAIN SICKNESS

It is a benign and reversible condition, occurs in travellers ascending to altitude of 3000 m (40-50%).

Hypoxia, stimulation of renin-angiotensin-aldosterone and ADH release resulting in fluid retention are the underlying pathogenic mechanisms. Hypoxia leads to cerebral vasodilation with increased blood flow. Fluid retention leads to oedema.

Clinical Features

The symptoms develop within 6 to 24 hours of an ascent and vary in severity from trivial to incapacitating (uncommon). Headache is the predominant presenting symptom which is generally frontal, throbbing, aggravated by exertion and is more severe in the morning. It is due to cerebral vasodilatation induced by hypoxia.

In more severe cases, headache is associated with malaise, anorexia, giddiness, insomnia, nausea and vomiting. Ataxia and peripheral oedema may be present.

In minority of cases, more serious sequelae such as high-altitude pulmonary oedema (HAPO) and high-altitude cerebral oedema (HACO) may also occur.

Table 91.1: Classification of high altitude disorders

1. *Acute*
   - Benign form e.g., acute mountain sickness
   - Malignant forms
     — High altitude pulmonary oedema
     — High altitude cerebral oedema
2. *Subacute*
   - Subacute infantile or adult mountain sickness
3. *Chronic*
   - Chronic mountain sickness
4. *Others*
   - High altitude pulmonary arterial hypertension
   - High altitude retinopathy
   - Thrombotic episodes
   - Gastrointestinal problems

Management and Prophylaxis

1. In mild cases, rest and an analgesic are just adequate. Symptoms resolve after 12-48 hours at a stable altitude but may recur with further ascent.
2. Persistent symptoms or severe form of illness respond to acetazolamide in the dose of 250 mg 8 hourly for 2-3 days. Acetazolamide is a carbonic anhydrase inhibitor, hence response to it indicate alkalosis as the probable cause of these symptoms. Dexamethasone (8 mg stat) followed by 4 mg 6 to 8 hourly may be useful if symptoms persist.

3. Patients with severe form need to be monitored closely for evidence of HAPO as minority of cases may develop it.
4. Acclimatizing by ascending gradually is the best prophylaxis.

HIGH-ALTITUDE PULMONARY OEDEMA (HAPO)

Definition

High altitude pulmonary oedema is a serious condition that occurs rarely due to exposure to high altitude in association with severe physical exertion in unacclimatized yet otherwise healthy young persons.

Predisposing Factors

Rapidity of ascent, young age (< 25 years), heavy exertion and the presence of mountain sickness are common precipitating events.

An incidence of 1-4% at altitude of 4000 m has been reported. It is more common in highlanders who re-enter high altitude after a short sojourn to low altitudes. Recent data shows that acclimatized high-altitude natives also develop this syndrome on return to high altitude after a brief stay at lower altitude.

Pathophysiology

The mechanism for high-altitude pulmonary oedema is obscure. It is an example of noncardiogenic pre-arteriolar high-altitude pulmonary oedema characterised by increase in cardiac output and pulmonary arterial pressure while pulmonary capillary wedge pressure and left atrial pressures are normal. There is increased capillary permeability of alveolar capillary membrane due to mismatch perfusion (areas of over and under perfusion lead to stress failure) induced by hypoxia. Higher incidence of HAPO in re-entrants to high altitude indicates larger hypoxic pulmonary response to ascent to further heights after brief stay at lower altitudes.

Clinical Features

The *clinical manifestations* usually start with symptoms suggestive of acute mountain sickness followed by dry mouth and breathlessness. The cough later on becomes productive with frothy mucoid expectoration which may be blood-stained (haemoptysis). The chest pain or discomfort may also occur.

On examination, patient looks ill, tachypnoea and tachycardia are present. BP is normal. There may be mild to moderate pyrexia. Central cyanosis occurs late. Optic fundi may show retinal haemorrhage in 10-15% of cases. Presence of papilloedema indicates associated cerebral oedema. There are signs of noncardiogenic pulmonary oedema, i.e. medium to coarse crepitations are heard on both lung fields.

Investigations

There may be leucocytosis. X-ray chest shows bilateral or unilateral diffuse haze due to alveolar oedema mostly involving the midzones and lower zones of the lungs. The cardiac size is normal. The pulmonary artery is dilated and prominent. ECG shows right axis deviation and sinus tachycardia. There may be 'T' wave inversion in right-sided chest leads. Arterial blood gas analysis may show hypoxaemia with hypocapnia or normocapnia.

Management

Unless recognized and treated rapidly, this may lead to cardiorespiratory failure, collapse and death.

Steps of Treatment

1. **Descent to lower altitude:** It should take place as early as possible.
2. **Reversal of hypoxia by oxygen:** Oxygen should be administered at high flow rates with a face mask, if possible. In mild to moderate cases, this is sufficient.
3. **Role of Gamow bag:** A portable pressure bag can be used in patients where descent to lower

altitude is not feasible; usage of this bag can effectively reduce the altitude by about 1800 m for the patient inside.

4. **Diuretics** have a limited role, can be used only in severe cases not responding satisfactorily to O_2. Frusemide (20-40 mg) may be given intravenously.
5. **Morphine** and **bronchodilators** are not indicated.
6. **Antibiotics** may be used if there is an evidence of infection (purulent sputum, fever, leucocytosis).
7. **Oral or sublingual nifedipine** can be given to reduce pulmonary arterial pressure and subsequently to relieve oedema.
8. **Nitric oxide (15 ppm) combined with oxygen** has been shown to have excellent beneficial effect.
9. **Role of steroids** is controversial.

The mortality rate in untreated or inadequately treated patients is as high as 50%. When treated early the mortality is less than 10%.

High Altitude Cerebral Oedema (HACO)

It is the least common high altitude associated disorder but is a serious and potentially fatal condition like HAPO, and most of times is associated with acute mountain sickness and HAPO.

The pathophysiology is similar to acute mountain sickness and HAPO. Worsening hypoxaemia leading to severe cerebral vasodilatation combined with increased capillary permeability contribute to it. Brain in fatal cases may show flattening and widening of gyri, narrowing of sulci and punctate haemorrhage in white matter. Dural venous sinus thrombosis is often seen.

Clinical Features

It occurs at moderate height of 3500-4000 m in sensitive individuals.

It usually follows acute mountain sickness and HAPO, hence, their features are usually present. In addition, patients present with rapidly progressive cerebral symptoms such as hallucinations or behavioral change, confusion, blurring of vision, dizziness, vomiting and ataxia. Speech is often slurred. Alteration in consciousness is a characteristic feature; coma appears in severe cases. Focal neurological signs (hemiparesis), abnormal plantar response can also occur. The optic fundi may show retinal haemorrhage and papilloedema.

Management

1. **Rapid descent to lower altitude** and **oxygen therapy** are mainstay of treatment.
2. **Decongestive therapy:** High dose parenteral steroids, mannitol and diuretics have been used successfully as decongestive therapy, but their efficacy is difficult to judge as these treatment are usually given in field conditions.

Chapter 92

Electrical and Lightning Injuries

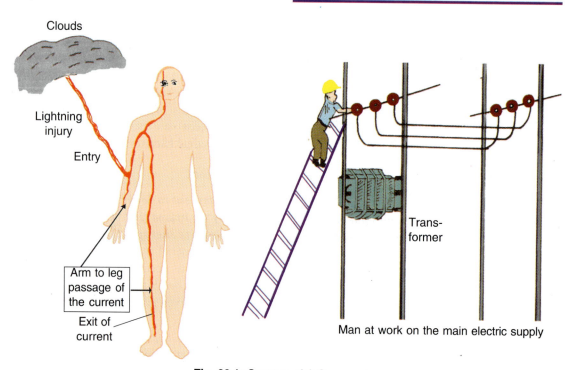

Fig. 92.1: Sources of A.C. current

ELECTRICAL AND LIGHTNING INJURIES

Definition

Injuries inflicted by an electrical current when coming in contact with live wires or electrical gadgets are called *electrical injuries*. The severity and distribution of electrical injury depends on:

i. *Type of current (direct or alternating):* At low voltage, alternate current (supplied for household use) is more dangerous than direct current (DC). At higher voltages, both alternate current (AC) and direct current (DC) are equally dangerous or lethal.

ii. *Amount and voltage of current:* High voltage current produces violent muscular contractions and may throw the patient away from the source of current but even a small contact may be lethal. On the other hand, a low voltage current causes spasms in the muscles and person may remain in contact with the source causing extensive injuries or death.

iii. *Resistance offered by the body:* Human body is a bad conductor of electricity, but wet perspiring soft skin makes it more vulnerable by lowering its resistance. If resistance offered by the body is high, then local tissue destruction results only; while at low resistance, systemic effects on the heart and brain appear.

iv. *Pathway of the current:* Whenever current flows through a conductor, heat is generated and skin being the most resistant tissue of the body gets the most heat at the point of entry as well as at exit. The two danger zones for electrical injury are brain and the heart where immediate effects of heating become evident.

v. *Duration of current:* The prolonged the contact, the more serious is the effect.

Lightning injury is direct current of short duration and most of the current flashes over the outer surface of the body (Fig. 92.1). Lightning injuries are similar to electrical injuries in all aspects. The passage of lightning electricity from arm to arm or arm to leg is most likely to involve the spinal cord. It may cause immediate effect by heating the nervous system, while delayed spinal cord syndrome is due to secondary vascular occlusion. About 30% victims seriously injured by lightning die, while 70% may have permanent sequelae.

Clinical Features

The AC current being more dangerous than DC can cause immediate death due to ventricular fibrillation and respiratory arrest. The clinical features can be divided into immediate and remote or late effects. They are given in Box 92.1.

Management

1. *Basic measures:* The victim should be freed from the current at once after switching off the mains. A dry pole or a stick of wood, leather belt or rubber should be used during separation. If there is fire, it should be extinguished with sand only. Do not use water or other liquids.

2. *Cardiopulmonary resuscitation:* Immediate cardiopulmonary resuscitation may be lifesaving, hence, should be started at once. Breathing and circulation should be supported in an unconscious patient using mouth to mouth respiration and external cardiac compression. Airway should be maintained. Ventricular fibrillation should be treated with defibrillation. All patients with cardiac arrhythmias should be monitored in intensive care unit for 48 hours.

Box 92.1: Clinical features of electrical/lightning injuries

1. *Immediate:* They usually appear within few hours and may affect the various systems as follows:
   i. Local heat effects:
      - Local burns at the point of entry and exit.
      - Sinking of hair, blisters, fissures, charring, ecchymosis and lacerations.
      - Deep extensive tissue damage (rhabdomyolysis), oedema with compression and focal neuropathies or plexus lesions.
   ii. Features due to fall
      - Fracture, dislocation, head injury.
   iii. Systemic features
      - Cardiovascular e.g. shock, ventricular fibrillation and cardiac arrest.
      - Respiratory e.g. hypoxia and asphyxia.
      - Neurological e.g. consciousness may be lost with electrical injury either from syncope or from immediate concussion or cerebral oedema. Other features include visual disturbance, headache, amnesia, speech disturbance, tingling and muscular contractions, convulsions, motor paralysis and stroke. Temporary tinnitus and deafness may be experienced.
      - Renal e.g. acute renal failure.

2. *Remote or late effects:* They are usually permanent.
   - Neurological e.g. seizures, myelopathy, neuropathy, causalgias, motor neurone disease like features, tetanus.
   - Visual: Cataract is an occasional late sequel to the electrical flash and may appear as late as 2 years of injury.

Artificial respiratory support with an oxygen supply should be started. Assisted ventilation may be used, if required.
3. ***Other measures:***
    i. *Treatment of shock:* Intravenous fluids should be given in cases with deep extensive burns and tissue damage leading to shock. Usual fluid used is Ringer's lactate 0.5 ml/kg/h. Fluid and electrolyte balance is maintained to prevent acute renal failure.
    ii. *Tetanus:* Tetanus toxoid should be given. Penicillin and other broad spectrum antibiotics are used as clostridia may infect the tissue.
    iii. *Treatment of burn and local tissue damage:* High voltage injury with deep tissue damage may require surgical exploration, debridement of necrotic tissue. Amputation may be needed with extensive damage.
    iv. *Acute renal failure:* It may occur due to shock or *rhabdomyolysis* leading to myoglobinuria. Adequate hydration and in some cases, hemodialysis may be required to maintain renal functions.

Chapter 93

Drowning and Near Drowning

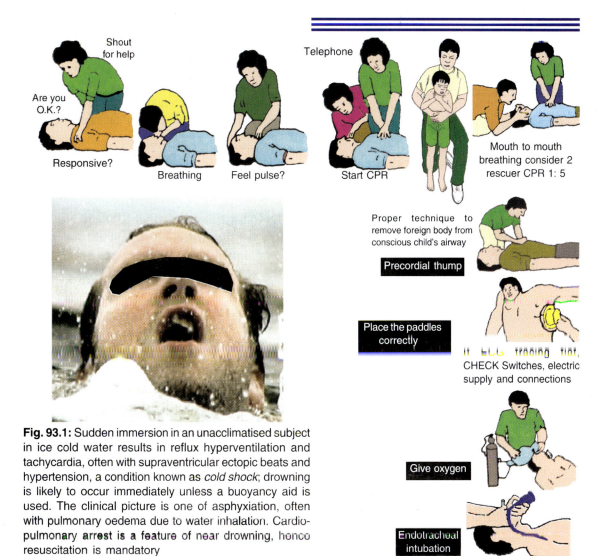

Fig. 93.1: Sudden immersion in an unacclimatised subject in ice cold water results in reflux hyperventilation and tachycardia, often with supraventricular ectopic beats and hypertension, a condition known as *cold shock*; drowning is likely to occur immediately unless a buoyancy aid is used. The clinical picture is one of asphyxiation, often with pulmonary oedema due to water inhalation. Cardiopulmonary arrest is a feature of near drowning, hence resuscitation is mandatory

Definition

It is an unexpected tragedy in which a previous healthy person dies or is exposed to severe cerebral hypoxia (asphyxiation) and suffers permanent brain damage.

Near drowning: It refers to a condition from which a person is rescued alive.

Dry drowning: Drowning without aspiration of water into the lungs is called *dry drowning.* It occurs in 10% of cases. Apnoea is the cause of hypoxaemia. Death follows intense laryngospasm.

Wet drowning: It refers to entry of water into the lungs. It occurs in 90% cases. Ventilation-perfusion mismatch is the cause of hypoxaemia.

Pathophysiology (Fig. 93.1)

1. Consequent to submersion, breath holding occurs for a variable period till the accumulating CO_2 stimulates the respiratory centre sufficiently enough to force an inspiration which results in aspiration of water into the lungs (wet drowning). In about 10% of cases, death may occur due to asphyxia without any entry of water into the lungs (dry drowning). Apnoea is the cause of hypoxaemia and laryngospasm is the cause of asphyxia and death.
2. About 90% of drowning victims aspirate the water into the lungs. Fresh water aspiration alters the surface tension properties of the alveolar surfactants and makes the alveoli unstable which causes a decreased ventilation-perfusion ratio with hypoxaemia and development of diffuse pulmonary oedema. Hypertonic sea water pulls extra amount of fluid from plasma into the lungs with the result alveoli become fluid-filled with normal perfusion. This event also causes right to left shunting with venous admixture in the lungs. With both types of water, pulmonary oedema occurs.
3. Fresh water in the alveoli is hypotonic, and is rapidly absorbed, impairs alveolar surfactant function and leads to alveolar collapse which promotes intrapulmonary right to left shunting (pulmonary venous admixture).
4. About 85% of patients of near-drowning aspirate 22 ml/kg of water or less which does not significantly affect blood volume or serum electrolytes concentration. When a large amount of fresh water is aspirated, it causes haemodilution, acute hypervolaemia and severe haemolysis, but this development has been reported rarely. With rapid redistribution of water and development of pulmonary oedema, even fresh water victims frequently demonstrate hypovolaemia by the time they reach the hospital.
5. Aspiration of grossly contaminated water may lead to severe pulmonary infection.
6. Occasionally, death may occur due to injury to head or cervical spine, as in the case of divers.

> *Hypoxaemia, and metabolic acidosis are mainly responsible for abnormal cardiovascular and renal functions.*

Causes

Drowning is particularly common in children. Drowning may be a secondary event during swimming, may occur due to unrelated factors such as sudden occurrence of an epileptic fit or a stroke or myocardial infarction. The initiating event is usually unknown. The causes of drowning in various age groups are given in Box 93.1.

Box 93.1: Causes of drowning according to age

1. *Infants or young children*
   - Domestic bath
   - Garden pools
2. *Adolescents*
   - Swimming pool
   - Rivers
   - Other bathing sites
3. *Adults*
   - Water sports, boating, fishing etc.
   - Occupational
4. *Older persons*
   - Domestic baths

Clinical Features

Those who are rescued alive (near drowning), are often unconscious and not breathing. Hypoxaemia, hypocarbia and metabolic acidosis are invariable features. The oral cavity may contain a foreign body which may be inhaled and lead to respiratory obstruction and asphyxia.

Some recover spontaneous ventilation and consciousness rapidly. There may be features of acute lung injury such as tachypnoea, tachycardia, cyanosis and pulmonary oedema (ARDS). The acute lung injury recovers within 48-72 hours unless complicated by infection.

Early complications include:
- Dehydration.
- Gastric distension.
- Hypotension.
- Haemoptysis.
- Cardiac arrhythmias.
- Hypothermia (submersion in cold water). It may be protective and recovery have been reported after prolonged immersion in cold water in children.

It must be remembered that survival may be possible after submersion for a period of upto 30 minutes in very cold water without brain damage. The outcome depends on duration of immersion, intensity of acidosis, presence of cardiac arrest and time-delay before resuscitation.

Management

Regardless of the conditions surrounding a drowning or near drowning, following steps of treatment (Fig. 93.2) must be adhere to:

1. Retrieve or remove the victim from the water and stabilise his/her head and neck if trauma is being suspected.
2. ABC (**A**irway, **B**reathing and **C**irculation) of cardiopulmonary resuscitation (CPR) must be instituted immediately, even in the water if this does not danger the rescuer.

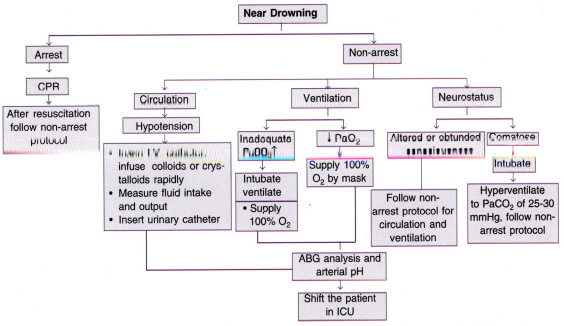

Fig. 93.2: Algorithm for a near drowned victim to be followed in order of priorities—Guidelines only; assume victim had normal arterial blood gas values (ABGs) before near drowning

3. If the patient is unconscious, clean the oral cavity off debris or any foreign body and protect the airway as needed for endotracheal intubation and ventilatory support if required subsequently.
4. Establish an intravenous access as early as possible.
5. Provide supplemental oxygygen and ventilatory support to overcome hypoxaemia until the blood gas analysis proves it is no longer required.
6. Monitor cardiac rhythm by ECG as soon as possible.
7. Monitor body temperature and restore it to normal.
8. If spontaneous breathing patient has persistent respiratory insufficiency, continuous positive airway (CPAP) breathing is useful in maintaining arterial oxygenation.
9. If patient has cardiovascular instability, evaluate cardiac output and effective circulatory volume by invasive monitoring, and measure serum electrolytes.
10. Evaluate renal function and cerebral status as indicated.

Note: The American Heart Association as well as special committee of Institute of Medicine (1994) have recommended that an abdominal thrust should not be used routinely in victims of submersion because of two reasons:
1. It may lead to regurgitation of gastric contents into the lungs or aspiration of the vomitus.
2. It may further delay ventilatory and circulatory resuscitation.

Therefore, abdominal thrust should only be used when the airway is obstructed with a foreign body or when victim fails to respond to mouth-to-mouth breathing.

Glucocorticoid therapy, prophylactic antibiotic therapy and monitoring of intracranial pressure are no longer recommended.

Chapter 94

Hanging and Strangulation

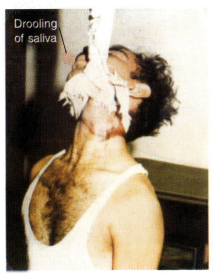

Fig. 94.1: Hanging

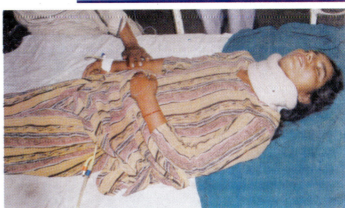

Fig. 94.2: Dislocation of cervical spine due to hanging for which neck collar has been applied

Definition

Hanging is a form of asphyxia produced by suspension of the body by a ligature around the neck which constricts the neck by the weight of the body (Fig. 94.1). In hanging, the ligature runs from the front above the thyroid cartilage symmetrically upwards on both sides of the neck to the back (occipital region).

A ligature mark around the neck is diagnostic of hanging.

In partial hanging, the bodies are partially suspended; the toes or feet touching the ground or are in a sitting, kneeling, lying down prone or any other position. The weight of the head acts as constricting force instead of the body.

Strangulation: Strangulation is also a form of asphyxia similar to hanging caused by constriction of the neck by a ligature without suspending the body. The ligature is U-shaped pulled by the manual force around the front and back of neck and person stands behind the body. Strangulation can be attempted using both hands around the neck called *throttling*.

Ligature used: The ligature used include a rope, metallic chains, wire, leather strap or belt, bed sheet, scarf, dhoti, sari, turban etc. It must be remembered that these cases are medicolegal cases, hence, every physician is duty bound to complete the medicolegal formalities including medicolegal report (MLR). A doctor who examines the patient first of all should note the following:

1. Ligature used.
2. Ligature mark on the neck. One should note whether it corresponds to the material used for hanging.
3. One should ascertain the length and texture of the ligature and to verify whether it was sufficient to hang the victim.
4. Before removing the ligature; one should ascertain, the width, nature and composition, mode of application and type of the knot used during hanging.

    Sometimes, the rope may break and becomes detached and the victim will be found lying on the ground with a ligature around the neck.
5. A suicidal note may be present at the site of hanging if it is suicidal hanging. The note should be procured and handed over to the police.

Clinical Features

The symptoms and their pathogenesis are described in the Table 94.1.

Table 94.1 symptoms of hanging and strangulation	
Causes/mechanisms	*Symptoms*
1. **Stretching of neck** by constricting force	• The neck is elongated and head is turned to the side opposite to knot. • Pain in the neck due to fracture or dislocation of cervical vertebrae (Fig. 94.2).
2. **Cerebral anoxia** due to constriction of carotid arteries. Asphyxia develops rapidly due to sudden compression of wind-pipe	• Face is pale. There is loss of power and sensory disturbances such as flashes of light, ringing and hissing noises in the ears, mental confusion, disturbance in consciousness and convulsion. Death may occur rapidly as patient can do nothing to help himself or herself.
3. **Venous congestion** due to constriction of jugular veins and rise in venous pressure in the head	• Congestion of head and neck. When the constricting force is great, then face becomes puffy, oedmatous, congested and cyanotic. • The eyes are wide open, bulging and suffused. The pupils are dilated. • The tongue is swollen, protruding and often bruised. • Patechial haemorrhages are common in the skin of eyelids, conjunctivae, face, forehead. • Bloody froth may escape from the mouth and nostrils. Bleeding may occur from the nose and ears. • The hands are clenched. • The genital organs may be congested and there may be discharge of urine, faeces and semen. *These asphyxial signs may be absent if death occurs quickly.*
• Stimulation of cervical sympathetic by the ligation knot. It may occur sometimes	• The pupil is dilated and the eye on the same side may remain open. It indicates antemortem hanging (*le facie sympatheique*).
• Increased salivation due to stimulation of salivary glands by the ligature	Drooling of saliva from the angle of the month when the head is dropping forward.

Diagnosis

It is based on:
  i. Ligation mark running around the neck i.e. obliquely in hanging and transverse in strangulation.
 ii. Presence of abrasions, ecchymosis and redness around the ligation mark.
iii. Dribbling or drooling of saliva from the angle of the mouth.
 iv. Ecchymoses of larynx or epiglossitis.
  v. Symptoms and signs of asphyxia.

Management

  I. **Pre-hospital management:**
     When you witness a victim:
     - Cut the ligature and remove it. Keep the ligature for inspection of forensic expert.
     - Make the patient to lie flat with cervical spine supported.
     - Loosen all his/her clothes and allows him/her to breath fresh air.
     - If the patient is unresponsive, call for help and activate emergency medical services (phone and call for van).
     - Start ABC of cardiopulmonary resuscitation.
 II. **Treatment in the hospital:**
     - O_2 inhalation.
     - Procure I.V. line and start glucose drip
     - Endotracheal intubation and breathing by ambu bag if there is or has been respiratory arrest
     - Removal of secretions by intermittent suction.
     - Continue rescue breathing.
     - Complete the medicolegal formalities.
     - Use anticonvulsants for control of convulsions. If convulsions not controlled by anticonvulsants, use midazolam, assisted ventilation and neuromuscular blockade.
     - Use mannitol or I.V. steroids to reduce raised intracranial tension though its benefit is debatable.
     - Take the emergency X-ray of the cervical spine and seek orthopedic consultation for any cervical injury. If necessary, a cervical collar may be used to support the cervical spine.
III. **Treatment in Respiratory Intensive Care Unit (RICU)**
     - If there is respiratory difficulty or arrest or anoxic encephalopathy, shift the patient to RICU for respiratory support.
     - Respiratory stimulants may be used.

Causes of Death

- Asphyxia.
- Venous congestion and raised cerebral venous pressure.
- Combined asphyxia and venous congestion.
- Reflex vagal inhibition.
- Fracture or dislocation of cervical vertebrae.

Complications

- Aspiration pneumonia.
- Pulmonary oedema.
- Infections.
- Oedema of larynx.
- Hypoxic encephalopathy. Cerebral infarction.
- Brain abscess.

Sequelae/After Effects

- Hemiplegia.
- Epileptiform convulsions.
- Amnesia (loss of memory).
- Dementia.
- Cervical cellulitis.
- Retropharyngeal abscess.
- Parotitis.
- Persistent coma.
- Cerebellar ataxia, myoclonus.
- Korsakoff's amnesic state.
- Choreoathetosis.

Part Eleven

Acid-base and Electrolyte Disturbance

Chapter 95

Acid-base Disturbance

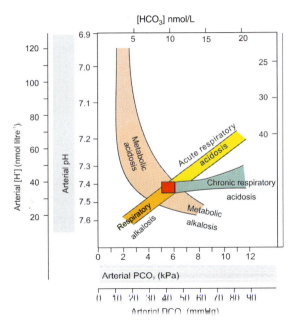

Fig. 95.1: The Flenley acid-base nomogram. This was derived from a large number of observations in patients with 'pure' respiratory or metabolic disturbances. The bands show the 95% confidence limits respresenting the individual varieties of acid-base disturbance. The rectangular area shows the approximate limits of arterial pH and PCO_2 in normal individuals. When the point obtained by plotting (H^+) against $PaCO_2$ does not fall within one of the labelled bands, compensation is incomplete or a mixed disorder is present

Definition

The acid-base is maintained within a narrow range. Acid-base disturbance occurs when disease process causes disruption of normal homeostatic mechanisms or when the acid or alkali burden presented exceeds the adaptive capacity of these mechanisms (Fig. 95.1).

The ability to manage acid-base disturbance is essential for the treatment of critically ill patients. Therefore, it is essential to understand its pathogenesis and pathophysiology to arrive at correct conclusion and to intervene timely for their correction so as to avoid life-threatening disturbance.

Terminology Used

An *acid* is a chemical substance that can release or donate (H^+) ion in solution; while a *base* is a substance that would accept this (H^+) ion concentration.

Hydrogen ion concentration has traditionally been expressed as pH, the negative logarithm of (H^+). The normal pH is maintained within a narrow range by means of a precise balance between acid production and excretion but this may contribute to complacency about the real magnitude of changes in (H^+) ion (See Box 95.1).

- Normal arterial pH varies from 7.36 to 7.42. It is maintained by intracellular and extracellular buffers; and by renal and respiratory regulatory mechanisms.

Acid-base and Electrolyte Disturbance

Box 95.1: Relationship between H⁺ and pH

pH	(H⁺) ion nmol/L	Calculation of H⁺ concentration
6.9	126	In the pH range of 7.25 to 7.55, do the following steps:
7.0	100	
7.1	79	• Drop 7 and the decimal point
7.2	63	• Substract the value obtained from 80 will be the result of H⁺ ion in nmol/L
7.3	50	
7.4	40	For example, if 7.25 is pH, then by deleting 7 and decimal, one gets 25 which is substracted from 80, results in 55 nmol/L which is H⁺ ion concentration
7.5	32	
7.6	25	

- Intracellular pH varies from 6.40 to 7.35.
- pH is negative (–) log of hydrogen ion concentration (H⁺).
- $PaCO_2$ = 40.0 ± 4.0 mmHg (35-45 mmHg).
- HCO_3^- = 24 ± 2 mEq/L (20-30 mEq/L).

Central to understanding of acid-base disturbance is the carbonic acid-bicarbonate buffer pairing. This is expressed in the *Henderson-Hasselbatch equation*:

$$(H^+) = 181 \times PaCO_2/HCO_3^-$$

(Here 181 is the dissociation coefficient of carbonic acid in the presence of carbonic anhydrase).

From this equation, it is clear that acidaemia is directly related the ratio between CO_2 tension and plasma bicarbonate concentration in blood. In the equation, *carbonic acid-bicarbonate* acts as a buffer which means that the combination can react with any strong acid or base added to the system and thereby minimising alterations in the pH. Thus, sodium bicarbonate combines with acid (inorganic or organic) and forms the sodium salt of that acid while carbonic acid splits into H_2O and CO_2 which is eliminated by the lungs

$$HCl + NaHCO_3 \rightarrow NaCl + H_2CO_3$$
$$H_2CO_3 \rightarrow CO_2 + H_2O$$

Primary Acid-base Disorders

They are discribed in Figure 95.2.

Acidosis: It is a condition in which hydrogen ion concentration rises, or would rise in the absence of compensatory mechanisms.

Alkalosis: It is a just reverse of acidosis.

Respiratory: The term respiratory is used when the primary disturbance is in the CO_2 tension because main excretion of CO_2 is through lungs.

Metabolic: The term metabolic is used when the primary disturbance is in plasma HCO_3^- concentration.

Base deficit: It is the difference between the actual plasma bicarbonate and the normal value. Base

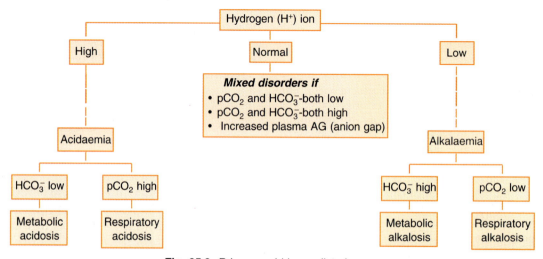

Fig. 95.2: Primary acid-base disturbance

deficit is seen in metabolic acidosis; while base excess occurs in metabolic alkalosis.

Plasma anion gap (AG) = $Na^+ - (Cl^- + HCO_3^-)$

It is the difference between unmeasured anions and unmeasured cations:

= 12 ± 3 mEq/L provided the level of albumin is 4.0 g/dl; for every decline of albumin by 1.0 g/dl, substract 4 from the normal value for the AG.

Regulation of Acid-base Balance

The mechanisms include:
- Chemical buffering system
- Regulation of $PaCO_2$ by neurorespiratory control (e.g. respiratory system).
- Handling of HCO_3 by the kidneys.

Under normal conditions, a steady state of $PaCO_2$ is maintained at 40 mmHg by a balanced state of CO_2 production and excretion. Hypercapnia means underexcretion of CO_2 resulting in its retention, occurs as a result of hypoventilation rather than excess CO_2 production. Similarly hypocapnia (overexcretion of CO_2) results from hyperventilation. Increase or decrease in $PaCO_2$ represents dearrangements of neural respiratory control or due to compensatory changes in response to primary alterations in the plasma HCO_3^-.

Primary changes in $PaCO_2$ can cause acidosis or alkalosis as discussed above, depending on whether $PaCO_2$ is above (respiratory acidosis) or below (respiratory alkalosis) the normal value of 40 mmHg. Primary alteration in $PaCO_2$ evokes a similar buffering and renal adaptation. A primary change in the plasma bicarbonate as a result of metabolic or renal factors results in compensatory changes in ventilation that blunt the changes in blood pH that would occur otherwise. Such respiratory alterations are referred to as *secondary or compensatory changes* since they occur in response to primary metabolic change.

In acid-base disturbance, primary change is either in regulation of $PaCO_2$ due to defective neural respiratory control or due to primary alteration of bicarbonate (HCO_3^-.)

Basic Principles

Carbohydrate and fat metabolism: Complete combustion of carbohydrate and fat in the liver and muscles produces CO_2 which forms carbonic acid if respiratory function is normal. Therefore, respiratory acidosis results due to decreased removal of CO_2; and respiratory alkalosis due to increased removal of CO_2.

Incomplete combustion of these metabolic fuels results in the formation of organic acids such as lactic acid, hydroxybutyric acid, acetoacetic acid and the fatty acids. If the production of these acids exceeds the metabolising capacity of the liver, will result in lactic acidosis and diabetic ketoacidosis.

Aminoacid metabolism: Metabolism of aminoacids produces HCO_3^- and NH_4^+ ions. These may combine in liver to form urea resulting in no net acid or base production provided CO_2 is removed by respiration normally.

Alternatively: If NH_4^- is excreted in the urine but HCO_3^- remains within the body, this will result in alkali retention which is equivalent to H^+ excretion. NH_4^+ excretion in the tubular diseases cause systemic acidosis.

Sulphuric acid, hydrochloric acid and phosphoric acid produced from metabolism of amino acids are known as "fixed acids" which cannot be metabolised further to CO_2 hence are not removed by respiration. They are removed as sulphate, chloride or phosphate and as H^+ ion by renal excretion. Absorption of ingested acids and alkali results in acidosis and alkalosis respectively.

Renal handling of H^+: Secretion of H^+ ion into distal tubule is dependent on an aldosterone-sensitive pump which exchanges Na^+ for H^+ or K^+.

Excretion of hydrogen ions is, therefore, dependent on the delivery of sodium to the distal tubule:
 i. Increased sodium delivery to the distal tubules induced by diuretics and hyperaldosteronism results in increased excretion of H^+ and K^+ leading to alkalosis and hypokalaemia.

ii. Decreased sodium delivery due to hypovolaemia or hypoaldosteronism, cause acidosis and hyperkalaemia.

By the same mechanisms, increased K^+ delivery leads to acidosis and alkalosis.

Renal handling of HCO_3^- (Fig. 95.3): The kidneys regulate plasma HCO_3^- by three processes; (i) *reabsorption of filtered HCO_3^-, (ii) formation of titratable acid, and* (iii) *excretion of NH_4^+ in the urine.* The kidneys filters approximately of 4000 mmol of HCO_3^- per day. To reabsorb this load of HCO_3^-, the renal tubules must secrete an equal amount (4000 mmol) of H^+ ions. About 80-90% of HCO_3^- is reabsorbed from the proximal tubules and remainder from the distal tubule; the latter secrete protons to defend systemic pH. The quantity of secreted protons is represented in the urine as titratable acid and NH_4. In metabolic acidosis, kidneys increase NH_4^+ production and excretion. NH_4^+ production and excretion are impaired in chronic renal failure, hyperkalaemia and renal tubular acidosis.

Diagnosis of Acid-base Disorders

1. Clinical history and investigations should be taken into consideration to reach at a proper diagnosis.
2. In complicated cases, the acid-base normogram (Fig. 95.1) is invaluable. The H^+ and $PaCO_2$ are measured in arterial blood as well as the bicarbonate. Care should be taken to obtain the arterial blood sample for gases without using excessive heparin. In the blood gas analysis, pH and $PaCO_2$ are measured, and the HCO_3^- is calculated from *Henderson-Hasselbatch equation*. The calculated value should be compared with measured HCO_3^-. If the values for calculated and measured HCO_3 differ by more than 10% (> 2.2 mmol/L) and the patient is afebrile, a laboratory error in the pH, $PaCO_2$ or HCO_3^- should be suspected. Repeat these measurements as one does not want to make a decision based on an error.

$$H^+ = PaCO_2 \times 24/HCO_3^-$$

3. If the values from a patient lie in one of the bands in the normogram (Fig. 95.1), it is likely that only one abnormality is present. If H^+ is high (pH is low) but the $PaCO_2$ is normal, the intercept lies between two bands; the patient has respiratory dysfunction leading to failure of CO_2 elimination, but this is partly compensated for by metabolic acidosis, stimulating respiration and CO_2 removal (this is the most common acid-base mixed abnormality in clinical practice).

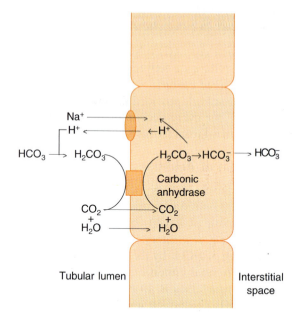

Fig. 95.3: Reabsorption of sodium bicarbonate in the renal proximal tubule. Bicarbonate is reclaimed by secretion of H^+ into the lumen in exchange for Na^+. This results in formation of H_2CO_3 which is then broken down into CO_2 and H_2O. These are absorbed and converted back to H_2CO_3, which now dissociates into H^+ ion and HCO_3^-. The net result is reabsorption of Na^+ and HCO_3^-. This process is dependent on carbonic anhydrase within cells and the luminal surface cells balance is a complex

4. The most common causes of acid-base abnormalities should always be kept in mind while probing the history for clues about aetiology. For example, established chronic renal failure is expected to cause a metabolic acidosis and chronic vomiting frequently causes metabolic; alkalosis and patients with chronic obstructive pulmonary disease or a sedative drug overdose often display a respiratory acidosis. The drug history is important as thiazide diuretics may cause hypokalaemia with metabolic akalosis. The carbonic anhydrase inhibitor, acetazolamide can result in metabolic acidosis.
5. Blood for electrolytes should be simultaneously drawn with arterial blood gases. Metabolic acidosis leads to hyperkalaemia as a result of cellular shifts in which H$^+$ is exchanged with K$^+$ or Na$^+$. Diabetic ketoacidosis, lactic acidosis, diarrhoea and renal tubular acidosis are often associated with potassium depletion.

Types of Disturbance

1. *Simple acid-base disturbance:* These are most common, include metabolic (alkalosis or acidosis) or respiratory (alkalosis or acidosis). Each primary acid base disorder is characterised by a specific physiological response which returns the plasma (H$^+$) and pH towards normal but not into normal range except in respiratory alkalosis.
2. *Mixed acid-base disturbance:* Absence of the predicted physiological response indicates the mixed acid-base disorder i.e. more than one acid-base disturbance.

Predicted Physiological Responses

Primary respiratory disturbances (primary change in PaCO$_2$) involve secondary metabolic responses (secondary change in HCO$_3^-$) and primary metabolic disturbances elicit predictable respiratory responses. Physiological compensation in various acid-base disturbances is given in the Table 95.1.

Table 95.1: Predicted physiological responses in simple acid-base disorders

Disorder	Response
Metabolic acidosis:	PaCO$_2$ will decrease (↓) by 1.25 mmHg per mmol/L fall (↓) in HCO$_3^-$
Metabolic alkalosis:	PaCO$_2$ will increase (↑) by 0.75 mmHg per mmol/L rise (↑) in HCO$_3^-$
Respiratory acidosis:	
• Acute:	HCO$_3^-$ will rise (↑) by 1 mmol/L per 10 mmHg rise (↑) in PaCO$_2$
• Chronic:	HCO$_3^-$ will rise (↑) by 4 mmol/L per 10 mmHg rise (↑) in PaCO$_2$
Respiratory alkalosis:	
• Acute:	HCO$_3^-$ will decrease (↓) by 2 mmol/L per 10 mmHg fall (↓) in PaCO$_2$
• Chronic:	HCO$_3^-$ will decrease (↓) by 4 mmHg per 10 mmHg fall (↓) in PaCO$_2$

Note: The rise and fall is from the normal values of bicarbonate 25 mmol/L and PaCO$_2$ of 40 mmHg

METABOLIC ACIDOSIS

Metabolic acidosis is characterised by:
- Reduction in plasma HCO$_3^-$.
- Rise in (H$^+$) ion and fall in pH.
- PaCO$_2$ is reduced secondarily by hyperventilation. Metabolic acidosis can be detected by finding a high plasma anion gap (AG) > 15 mEq/L even without a pH or HCO$_3^-$ change called—*high anion gap metabolic acidosis.*

Aetiology

The physiological disturbances that give rise to metabolic acidosis include either an addition of exogenous acids or there is failure of acid excretion leading to high anion-gap acidosis.

On the other hand, metabolic acidosis that results due to loss of HCO$_3$ results in normal anion gap.

The disturbances leading to metabolic acidosis are given in Box 95.2. In most situations, metabolic acidosis is accompanied by sodium and water depletion.

The causes of metabolic acidosis are classified into increased anion gap acidosis and normal anion gap acidosis (Table 95.2).

Acid-base and Electrolyte Disturbance

> **Box 95.2: Disturbances associated with metabolic acidosis**
> - Overproduction of acids other than H_2CO_3 by disordered metabolism.
> - Addition of exogenous acid (ingestion of acids).
> - Failure to excrete acids other than H_2CO_3 at a rate equal to their generation.
> - Loss of bicarbonate in the urine or through GI tract

The first step is to identify whether acidosis is due to retention of HCl or to another acid. This is achieved by calculating the anion gap. The calculation of anion gap is simple as follows:

- The normal cations in plasma are Na^+, K^+, Ca^{++} and Mg^{++}.
- The normal anions in plasma are Cl^- and HCO_3^-, negative charges present on albumin, phosphate, sulphate, lactate and other organic acids.
- The sum of the positive and negative charges are equal.
- Measurement of Na^+, K^+, Cl^- and HCO_3^- are usually easily available.

Anion gap = (unmeasured anions)–(unmeasured cations). The normal anion gap is 8 to 14 mmol/L.

Table 95.2: Differential diagnosis of metabolic acidosis

Mechanisms	Conditions	Accumulating acid
I. High anion gap metabolic acidosis		
i. Addition of excessive acids to extracellular fluid		
a. Organic acids	Ketoacidosis e.g. diabetes, alcoholism and starvation	• Acetoacetic • β-hydroxybutyric
	Lactic acidosis	Lactic acid
b. Poisoning	• Methanol poisoning	Formic
	• Ethylene glycol posioning	Glycolic and oxalic
	• Salicylate poisoning	Salicylic and lactic
ii. Failure to excrete acid at a normal rate		
• Decreased GFR and inadequate renal NH_4 production	Acute on chronic renal failure	Sulphuric, phosphoric and hydrochloric
II. Normal anion gap metabolic acidosis		
i. Loss of bicarbonate		
• In urine	• Proximal renal tubular defect	Hydrochloric
	• Acetazolamide	Hydrochloric
	• Hyperparathyroidism	
	• Tubular damage due to drugs heavy metals	
• From gastrointestinal tract	• Diarrhoea, fistulae, ileostomy and ureterosigmoidostomy	Hydrochloric
ii. Failure to excrete acid at normal rate		
• Failure of the distal tubular H^+ secretory system	Distal renal tubular acidosis	Hydrochloric

Acid-base Disturbance

Clinical tip: A useful mnemonic for causes of a raised anion gap recalls Kussmaul:

- K for ketosis (diabetes, alcoholism, malnutrition)
- U for uraemia
- SS for salicylate poisoning
- M for methanol poisoning
- A for ethylene (formerly spelt as aethylene glycol poisoning)
- U for uraemia
- L for lactic acidosis.

Box 95.3: Causes of lactic acidosis

Type A: Conditions associated with tissue hypoxia	Type B: Impaired mitochondrial function
• Shock due to any cause (septic shock is the most common)	• Diabetes mellitus
• Respiratory failure	• Hepatic failure
• Carbon monoxide and cyanide poisoning	• Severe infection
• Severe anaemia	• Drugs (metformin, isoniazid, salicylates)
	• Toxins (ethanol, methanol)
	• Congenital enzyme defects

Renal Tubular Acidosis (RTA)

It includes a group of conditions characterised by hypercholeraemic metabolic acidosis. Any condition affecting tubular function can lead to RTA. Three variants are described:

1. *Proximal hypokalaemic RTA (former type II)* is caused by failure of sodium bicarbonate reabsorption in the proximal tubule. It is characterised by acidosis, hypokalaemia, an inability to lower the pH of urine below 5.5 despite systemic acidosis and bicarbonate loss in urine.
2. *Distal hypokalaemic RTA (former type I)* is due to failure of H^+ excretion in the tubule. It is characterised by acidosis, hypokalaemia, inability to lower urinary pH less than 5.5 despite systemic acidosis and low urinary ammonium production.
3. *Distal hyperkalaemic RTA (fromer type IV)* is caused by defective hydrogen ion secretion. There is hyporeninaemia and hypoaldosteronism. It is characterised by hyperkalaemia, acidosis in a patient with mild chronic renal insufficiency usually caused by tubulointerstial disease.

One of the most common types of metabolic acidosis is lactic acidosis in which lactic acid production from pyruvate in the muscle, skin, brain and RBCs exceeds its removal by the liver and kidneys. The causes of lactic acidosis (type A and B) are given in Box 95.3.

Clinical Features of Metabolic Acidosis

1. *Respiratory manifestations:* Severe metabolic acidosis usually manifests with stimulation of respiration leading to hyperventilation (Kussmaul's respiration), respiratory distress and air hunger.
2. *Cardiovascular features:* Severe acidosis may lead to mycardial depression resulting in reduced cardiac output, fatigue and hypotension. Cardiac arrhythmias may occur.
3. *Cerebral features:* There may be confusion, drowsiness and fits.
4. *Miscellaneous features:* Insulin resistance, hyperkalaemia and increased protein catabolism.
5. *Features of underlying disorder:* In many cases, features of underlying disorder and presence of sodium and water depletion may dominate.

Management

1. The underlying cause of acidosis should be identified whenever possible. Organic acidosis such as ketoacidosis may be treated with insulin and lactic acidosis may be treated by managing the shock with fluids.
2. Poisoning and metabolic acidosis due to fixed acid accumulation require treatment for their elimination through kidneys (alkaline forced diuresis) or by dialysis or haemofiltration.
3. *Alkali therapy:* The role of sodium bicarbonate is controversial. Risk of $NaHCO_3$ therapy include hypervolaemia and hypertension due to excessive sodium load and overshoot alkalosis in recovery period. Therefore, $NaHCO_3$ is not used in moderate acidosis but it may be used in acute severe acidaemia (pH < 7.1) to improve cardiac function and lactate utilisation. The

blood (H^+) and HCO_3 as well as anion gap should be monitored closely.
4. In chronic renal failure, oral sodium bicarbonate supplement may be required on a long-term basis.

METABOLIC ALKALOSIS

It is characterised by:
- Increase in plasma bicarbonate ($HCO_3 > 25$ mmol/L).
- pH > 7.40.

It is less common than metabolic acidosis. It is usually a response to an HCl, KCl and NaCl deficit. In health, when plasma (HCO_3^-) rises above normal, urinary excretion of (HCO_3^-) increases rapidly. It is therefore very unusual to observe metabolic alkalosis in the presence of normal renal function.

Aetiology and Pathogenic Mechanisms

A number of factors stimulate bicarbonate reabsorption and hydrogen ion secretion because of altered renal function see Box 95.4.

Box 95.4: Conditions which sustain metabolic alkalosis

1. Strong stimulus to reabsorb sodium (i.e. hypovolaemia) particularly in the presence of low plasma chloride
2. Increased (H^+) ion secretion by renal tubules
   - Increased delivery of Na^+ to distal tubule (e.g. loop diuretics)
   - High $PaCO_2$ due to chronic respiratory failure
   - Potassium depletion
   - Excess mineralocorticoids

There are important relationship between tubular handling of Na^+, K^+ and (H^+) ions. In the distal tubule where there is final composition of urine, reabsorption of Na^+ generates an electromechanical gradient which derives both K^+ and (H^+) ions from the tubular cells into the lumen (Fig. 95.3). Thus, if kidneys are avidly retaining sodium due to any cause (aldosterone and other mineralocorticoids), it cannot retain K^+ and (H^+) ion. If the intracellular K^+ concentration is already low because of K^+ depletion, there is obligatory rise in secretion of H^+ ions.

Sodium is reabsorbed from nephron either with chloride or with bicarbonate. If chloride is deficient, then there is preferential reabsorption of bicarbonate which will worsen the alkalosis and will prevent the additional excretion of bicarbonate by the distal tubule which is necessary to correct an established metabolic alkalosis.

The causes of metabolic alkalosis are given in the Table 95.3.

Table 95.3: Common causes of metabolic alkalosis

1. ***Administration of exogenous alkali (HCO_3^- load)***
   - Acute alkali administration
   - Milk-alkali syndrome
2. ***Loss of Na^+, Cl^-, H^+ and water (extracellular fluid depletion)***
   - Vomiting or gastric aspiration
   - Congenital chlorodiarrhoea
   - Diuretics (thiazides, frusemide, bumetanide)
   - Oedematous state (effective ECF is reduced)
3. ***Expansion of ECF (extracellular fluid), hypertension, K^+ deficiency and mineralocorticoid excess***
   - High renin: e.g. renal artery stenosis, accelerated hypertension.
   - Low renin: e.g. primary aldosteronism, Cushing's syndrome, Bartter's syndrome, adrenal enzyme defect.
   - Others: e.g administration of liquorice, carbenoxolone

The classical pardigm sustaining metabolic alklosis due to vomiting and administration of diuretics is presented in the Figure 95.4.

Clinical Features

Patients of metabolic alkalosis may be asymptomatic or may complain of symptoms related to volume depletion or hypokalaemia.
1. *Symptoms due to volume contraction/depletion:*
   - Weakness, muscle cramps and postural dizziness.
2. *Symptoms due to hypokalaemia:*
   - Polyuria, polydipsia and muscle weakness.
3. *Symptoms of cerebral dysfunction:*
   - Altered mental status, apathy, confusion and drowsiness.

Acid-base Disturbance

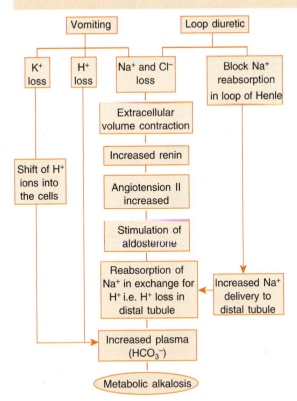

Fig. 95.4: Schematic representation of pathogenesis of metabolic alkalosis. Metabolic alkalosis may be due to vomiting or loss of gastric contents or to use of diuretics

4. *Acute alkalosis:* Acute severe alkalosis may cause:
   - Respiratory depression.
   - Cardiac arrhythmias (supraventricular or ventricular).
   - Tetany due to lowered ionised calcium (Trousseau's sign positive).
5. *Severy long-standing alkalosis may be associated with:*
   - Reduced renal function and uraemia.

Management

1. Mild to moderate alkalosis may not require any treatment.
2. *Correction of underlying stimulus for HCO_3^- generation:* If primary hyperaldosteronism is present, its correction will reverse alkalosis. The (H^+) loss by the stomach can be prevented by H_2 blockers. Stop the loop diuretics if patient is taking.
3. *To remove the factors that sustain HCO_3^- reabsorption:* In patients without renal disease, restoration of ECF (extracellular fluid) volume and the plasma chloride and K^+ concentration will remove the stimulus to renal (H^+) secretion and allow renal excretion of excess bicarbonate.

   In patients who have lost gastric contents e.g. in pyloric outlet obstruction, should be replaced with isotonic (0.9%) NaCl solution (3-6 litres/day) and sufficient KCl to restore K^+ deficit (40-60 mmol/day).

   Patients who are on continuous gastric aspiration should also have the volume of aspirate replaced by I.V. infusion of an equal amount of isotonic saline solution containing KCl (20 mmol/L).

   Alkalosis associated with K^+ deficiency is corrected by stopping the diuretics (potassium losing) and administration of sufficient KCl to restore body K^+ to normal.
4. *Treatment of saline-resistant cases:* Unusual cases, termed saline-resistant are associated with marked K^+ deficits (> 1000 mmol), Mg^{++} deficiency, Bartter's syndrome, or primary hypermineralocorticoid states. Therapy in these cases must be directed toward the underlying pathophysiological problem.
5. *Treatment of severe alkalosis:* If associated conditions preclude infusion of saline or alkalosis is severe (pH > 7.55), HCO_3^- loss can be accelerated by use of acetazolamide (250-500 mg orally or I.V.). Dilute HCl (0.1 N) or NH_4Cl may be used as acidifying agent.

   If renal function is impaired, haemodialysis against dialysate low in (HCO_3^-) and high in (Cl^-) can be effective.

RESPIRATORY ACIDOSIS

Respiratory acidosis results when the effective alveolar ventilation fails to keep pace with the rate of CO_2 production. As a result, there is retention

Acid-base and Electrolyte Disturbance

of CO_2 leading to rise in $PaCO_2$ and H^+ ion, and HCO_3^- (See the Fig. 95.1 on front page).

Predicted Physiological Response

1. In acute respiratory acidosis, the plasma HCO_3^- will rise by 1 nmol/L with 10 mm rise in $PaCO_2$.
2. In chronic respiratory acidosis, the plasma HCO_3^- will rise by 4 nmol/L with 10 mmHg rise in $PaCO_2$.

The kidneys respond by increased H^+ secretion so that urine becomes acidic and bicarbonate is added to the blood. The distinction between respiratory acidosis and metabolic alkalosis can be made by the fact that (H^+) ion is characteristically raised in respiratory acidosis and reduced in metabolic alkalosis. A chronically raised $PaCO_2$ is compensated by renal retention of HCO_3 and the (H^+) ion returns to normal. A constant arterial HCO_3 concentration then usually become established within 5 days. This represents primary respiratory acidosis with compensatory metabolic alkalosis.

Causes

Respiratory acidosis results due to severe pulmonary disease, respiratory muscle fatigue, or abnormalites in ventilatory control (depression of medullary respiratory centre) and is due to the increase in $PaCO_2$. The causes are enumerated in the Table 95.4.

Clinical Features

The clinical features vary according to severity and duration of the respiratory acidosis, the underlying disease, and whether there is accompanying hypoxaemia.

1. A rapid rise in $PaCO_2$ (acute hypercapnia) may cause anxiety, dyspnoea, confusion, psychosis and hallucinations and may progress to coma—called acute hypercapnic encephalopathy.

	Table 95.4: Causes of respiratory acidosis (acute and chronic)	
	Acute	*Chronic*
1. Depression of respiratory centre in medulla i.e. ventilatory control	• Drugs e.g. opiates, anaesthetics, sedatives • Cardiac arrest • Stroke • Central sleep apnoea • Infection	• Extreme obesity (PickWickian syndrome) • CNS lesion (rare)
2. Diseases of chest wall and respiratory muscles	• Myasthenic crisis • Guillain-Barre syndrome • Severe hypokalaemia • Drugs e.g. aminoglycosides, organophosphorous compound, curare, succinylcholine • Peroidic paralysis	• Poliomyelitis • Multiple sclerosis • Amyotrophic lateral sclerosis • Diaphragmatic paralysis • Scoliosis • Myxoedema
3. Airway obstruction	• Asthma • Aspiration of foreign body or vomitus • Obstructive apnoea • Laryngospasm	• Thymoma • Tonsillar hypertrophy • Paralysis of vocal cords • Aortic aneurysm
4. Disorders of lung parenchyma	• Severe asthma or pneumonia • Acute exacerbation of chronic lung disease • Pneumothorax • ARDS • Acute cardiogenic pulmonary oedema	• COPD • Pulmonary emphysema • Interstitial fibrosis
5. Mechanical ventilation	• Improperly adjusted and not supervised	• Large increase in alveolar dead space

2. Lesser and slowly rising $PaCO_2$ (chronic hypercapnia) leads to sleep disturbances, loss of memory, daytime somnolence, personality changes, impairment of coordination and motor disturbances such as flapping tremors and myoclonic jerks. Headache and signs of raised intracranial pressure including papilloma may occur.
3. Cardiovascular effects of respiratory acidosis include increased cardiac output, normal or increased BP, warm skin, bounding pulse and diaphoresis.

Investigations

1. Arterial blood gas analysis shows rise in $PaCO_2$ and H^+ ion with fall in blood pH.
2. Pulmonary function tests include spirometry, diffusion capacity for carbon monoxide, lung volumes and arterial $PaCO_2$ and O_2 saturation. These tests help to determine if respiratory acidosis is due to lung disease.
3. Non-pulmonary causes need appropriate tests for assessment of chest wall, pleura and neuromuscular functions.
4. Measurement of haematocrit in each and every case.

Management

1. *Acute respiratory acidosis:* It can be life-threatening and measures to reverse the underlying cause should be undertaken simultaneously with restoration of adequate alveolar ventilation. These are:
   - Prompt removal of underlying cause.
   - Establish patent airway.
   - Administer O_2 carefully which should be titrated in patients of COPD with CO_2 retention. O_2 can be given at 6 L/min if PaO_2 is less than 65 mmHg.
   - Improvement of pulmonary functions by using bronchodilators, clearing of bronchial secretions, treatment of infection and avoiding fluid overload.
   - When patient is in coma, or has extreme hypercapnoea ($PaCO_2 > 80$ mmHg) or severe acidosis (pH < 7.1) tracheal intubation with assisted ventilation may be needed.
2. *Chronic respiratory acidosis:* It is frequently difficult to correct as one can rarely remove the underlying cause. Measures taken are aimed at improving lung functions such as cessation of smoking, use of O_2, bronchodilators, glucocorticoids, diuretics and controlling infection. Excessive O_2 and sedatives are to be avoided. Acute exacerbation of chronic hypercapnia may need mechanical ventilation.

RESPIRATORY ALKALOSIS

Respiratory alkalosis occurs when alveolar hyperventilation results in excessive loss of CO_2 (fall in $PaCO_2$) and fall in H^+ ion and rise in pH.

Predicted physiological response (See the Table 95.1)
1. In acute respiratory alkalosis, HCO_3^- will fall by 2 mmol/L with 10 mm fall in $PaCO_2$.
2. In chronic respiratory alkalosis, HCO_3^- will fall by 4 mmol/L with 10 mmHg fall in $PaCO_2$.

Causes

The causes are given in Box 95.5.

> **Box 95.5: Common causes of respiratory alkalosis**
>
> 1. Hypoxia due to acute attack of bronchial asthma, pulmonary oedema, pulmonary embolism and acute circulatory failure. Chronic hypoxia occur in cyanotic heart disease, high altitude and pulmonary fibrosis.
> 2. CNS disorders (e.g. CVA, brain tumour, encephalitis).
> 3. Pregnancy.
> 4. Gram-negative septicaemia or endotoxaemia.
> 5. Hepatic failure.
> 6. Drugs e.g. salicylate poisoning.
> 7. Anxiety induced hyperventilation.
> 8. Pain.
> 9. Excessive mechanical ventilation.

Clinical Feature

They are due to hyperventilation and hypoxaemia. Paraesthesias, circumoral numbness, chest wall tightness or pain, light-headedness, dizziness, inability to take an adequate breath and rarely tetany or convulsions may occur. In digitalised patients, cardiac arrhythmias and cardiac arrest may occur.

Investigations

1. Arterial blood gas analysis demonstrates an acute or chronic respiratory alkalosis, often with hypocapnia in the range of 15 to 30 mmHg and no hypoxaemia. Arterial pH is high.
2. The plasma (K^+) is often reduced and the (Cl^-) increased. In acute hyperventilation syndrome, ionised calcium level may be reduced.
3. In chronic respiratory acidosis and alkalosis, the kidneys return H^+ towards normal by transiently increasing or decreasing the rate of NH_4 excretion and thereby increasing the plasma HCO_3^- in chronic respiratory acidosis or decreasing the plasma HCO_3^- in chronic respiratory alkalosis.

Management

When diagnosis of respiratory alkalosis is made, its cause should be investigated. The diagnosis of hyperventilation syndrome (common cause) is made by exclusion. In difficult cases, it may be important to rule out other conditions such as pulmonary embolism, coronary artery disease and hyperthyroidism.

The treatment of respiratory alkalosis is directed towards the alleviation of the underlying cause. If respiratory alkalosis complicates ventilator management, changes in dead space, tidal volume, and frequency can minimize the hypocapnia. In chronic respiratory alkalosis, measures to treat respiratory alkalosis itself are generally not required.

In patients with anxiety-hyperventilation syndrome, reassurance of the patient or sedation, or rebreathing into a closed system (a paperbag) during symptomatic attacks and attention to underlying psychological stress may be beneficial. Antidepressants are not recommended. Beta blockers may ameliorate the anxiety induced hyperadrenergic state.

In severe alkalaemia, along with the treatment of primary disorder, skeletal muscle paralysis and assisted mechanical ventilation may be required.

Hypokalaemia, a common accompaniment must be corrected.

MIXED ACID-BASE DISORDERS

Definitions

Mixed acid-base disorders are defined as independently coexisting disorders, not merely compensated responses, are often seen in critically ill patients in critical care units. The diagnosis of mixed disorder should be considered in the clinical context. The causes of mixed acid-base disorders are given in the Table 95.5.

Table 95.5: Common causes of mixed acid-base disorders

1. *Metabolic acidosis and respiratory acidosis (common)*
   - Cardiopulmonary arrest
   - Severe pulmonary oedema
   - Sedative and salicylate poisoning
   - Pulmonary disease with renal failure or sepsis
2. *Metabolic acidosis with respiratory alkalosis*
   - Salicylate overdose
   - Recent alcoholic binge
   - Combined hepatic and renal insufficiency
3. *Metabolic alkalosis with respiratory alkalosis*
   - Chronic respiratory disease with diuretic therapy, steroid therapy, severe vomiting, reduction of hypercapnia by ventilation
4. *Metabolic acidosis and metabolic alkalosis*
   - Severe vomiting in patients with underlying renal failure, diabetic ketoacidosis and alcoholic ketoacidosis

Mixed respiratory and metabolic acidosis or mixed respiratory and metabolic alkalosis can lead to dangerous extremes of pH. A patient first of all may have simple acid-base disturbance due to underlying cause, develops second acid-base disorder as a result of complication. For example a patient with diabetic ketoacidosis (metabolic acidosis) may develop a respiratory problem leading to respiratory acidosis or alkalosis.

When metabolic acidosis and metabolic alkalosis coexist in the same patient, the pH may be normal or near normal. When the pH is normal, an elevated anion gap denotes the presence of a metabolic acidosis. A diabetic patient with ketoacidosis may develop metabolic acidosis due to renal dysfunction.

Management

Management involves the treatments described above for each element of the disturbance.

Chapter 96

Disorders of Sodium Balance

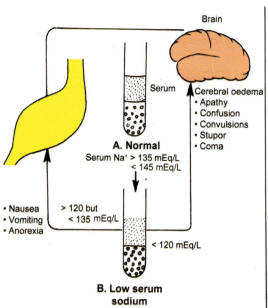

Fig. 96.1: Clinical effects of hyponatraemia (A) Normal, (B) Low sodium concentration

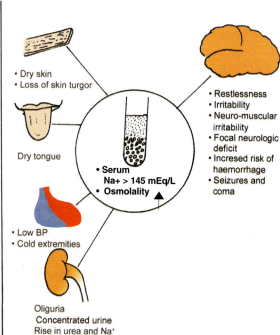

Fig. 96.2: Clinical features of hypernatraemia

The electrolyte disturbances involve sodium, potassium, calcium and magnesium. The electrolyte abnormalities are commonly encountered clinically in a wide spectrum of diseases especially in a critically ill patients and contribute to increased mortality due to the underlying disease. The electrolyte disturbance is the common reversible factor in an irreversible disease process. The diagnosis of these disorders is based on clinical suspicion in an underlying disorder and confirmation is done by estimation in serum.

Basic Physiology of Sodium and Water

Water is the most abundant constituent of the body, comprising 60% of the body weight (42 L water) in a 70 kg man and 50% in women. The difference

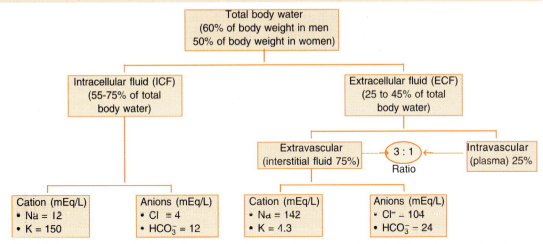

Fig. 96.3: Distribution of total body water and major cations and anions in different compartments.

in two sexes is due to relative proportions of adipose tissue. The distribution of water in two major compartments i.e. extracellular (extracellular fluid-ECF) and intracellular (intracellular fluid-ICF) is given in the Figure 96.3. The ECF is further subdivided into intravascular (plasma water) and extravascular (interstitial spaces) in a ratio of 1:3.

In a healthy person:
- Serum sodium varies from 136 to 145 mEq/L (Fig. 96.1).
- Serum potassium varies from 3.5 to 5.5 mEq/L.
- Serum osmolality ($2 \times Na^+$ plus K^+ in mEq + blood sugar and urea in mg ÷ by 18) varies from 280-295 mOsm/kg

HYPONATRAEMIA

Definition

A plasma Na^+ concentration less than 135 mEq/L usually reflects a hypotonic state called *hyponatraemia*.

Abnormalities of plasma sodium concentration and hyponatraemia are almost always due to disturbance in water metabolism.

Pseudohyponatraemia: Plasma is 93% water, the remaining 7% consists of plasma proteins and lipids. Since Na^+ is dissolved in plasma water (aqueous phase), increasing the non-aqueous phase artificially (increasing proteins and lipids) will lower the Na^+ concentration measured per liter of water. This is called *spurious* or *pseudohyponatraemia*. The plasma osmolality remains normal. The Na^+ ion concentration measured by Na^+-sensitive glass electrode remains normal. This type of hyponatraemia is of little significance, needs evaluation of the underlying cause such as hyperproteinaemia and hyperlipidaemia.

The causes of pseudohyponatraemia are:
- Hyperlipidaemia and hyperproteinaemia.
- Post-transurethral resection of prostate/bladder tumour.
- Hyperglycaemia.
- I.V. mannitol.

Isotonic or hypotonic or dilutional hyponatraemia may complicate transurethral resection of the prostate or bladder because large volumes of iso-osmotic (mannitol) or hypo-osmotic (sorbitol or glycine) bladder irrigation solution can be absorbed resulting in dilutional hyponatraemia. The metabolism of absorbed sorbitol or glycine to CO_2 and water may lead to hypotonicity of the accumulated fluid and solutes are not rapidly excreted.

Hypertonic hyponatraemia: It is characterised by increased plasma osmolality, is seen in hyperglycaemia and intravenous administration of mannitol. This is due to the fact that, during uncontrolled or poorly controlled diabetes, the glucose being an effective osmole draws water from the muscle cells resulting in hyponatraemia. Plasma Na^+ concentration falls by 1.4 mmol/L for every 100 mg/dl rise in plasma glucose.

Causes

The causes of hyponatraemia are given in the Table 96.1 along with clinical features and respective treatment.

In general, hypotonic hyponatraemia is due to either a primary water gain (and secondary Na^+ loss) or a primary Na^+ loss (and secondary water gain). Hyponatraemia associated with hypovolaemic shock is due to contraction of the ECF volume stimulating *thirst* and ADH secretion. The increased water ingestion and impaired renal excretion result in hyponatraemia.

Hyponatraemia is commonly due to a decrease in the diluting capacity of the kidneys. The diuretic-induced hyponatraemia is always due to *thiazide* diuretics because they lead to Na^+ and K^+ depletion leading to ADH-stimulated water retention. This is uncommon with loop diuretics because they impair only the maximal urinary concentration capacity which limits the ADH-mediated water retention.

Hyponatraemia associated with oedematous states (e.g. congestive heart failure, nephrotic syndrome, cirrhosis of liver, hypoproteinaemic states) is due to expansion of extracellular fluid and retention of Na^+ (See the Table 96.1). All these disorders lead to contraction of effective blood volume leading to excessive thirst and ADH stimulation.

Hyponatraemia due to syndrome of inappropriate antidiuretic hormone (ADH) secretion (SIADH) is the most common cause of normovolaemic hyponatraemia and is commonly due to the nonphysiologic or inappropriate release of ADH from the posterior pituitary or an ectopic source. Renal free water excretion is impaired while the regulation of Na^+ balance is unaffected.

Hormonal excess or deficiency such as Addison's disease and hypothyroidism may lead to hyponatraemia and should not be confused with SIADH. This is due to primary water gain (via ADH) secondary to Na^+ loss due to adrenal insufficiency.

Finally, hyponatraemia may occur in the absence of ADH or renal failure. This is due to inability of the kidneys to excrete the dietary waterload.

In primary (psychogenic) polydipsia compulsive water drinking may overwhelm the normally large renal excretory capacity of 12 L/d. These patients usually have underlying psychiatric illnesses and may be taking medications such as phenothiazines which cause dry mouth due to their anticholinergic effect and lead to excessive thirst.

Beer potomania is an another example of such hyponatraemia because beer drinkers have a poor dietary intake of proteins and electrolytes and consume large amounts of beer which may exceed the excretory capacity of the kidneys resulting in hyponatraemia.

Clinical Features (Fig. 96.1)

Symptoms and signs depend on the rate of change and severity of hyponatraemia. At plasma sodium level above 120 mmol/L (mEq/L), gastrointestinal manifestations (nausea, vomiting, anorexia) are common and neurological manifestations uncommon. At plasma Na^+ level below 120 mmol/L, neurological manifestations (apathy, lethargy, confusion, absent reflexes, seizures, stupor and coma) will occur in addition to GI manifestations if the onset is acute or a rapidly developing hyponatraemia. This is due to osmotic water shift leading to increased intracellular fluid volume specifically the brain cells swelling or cerebral oedema. Children and young menstruant females who develop acute hyponatraemia due to injudicious postoperative hypotonic fluid management are at a greater risk of death or permanent neurological deficit. Over-aggressive treatment has been associated with "*acute central pontine myelinolysis* which leads to permanent neurological impairment and carries a high mortality. This is

Disorders of Sodium Balance

Table 96.1: Pattern of hyponatraemia; its causes, clinical features and management

Disturbance	Causes	Clinical manifestations	Management
1. Body water ↓ • Total body ↓↓ sodium	*i. Extra-renal* • Vomiting • Diarrhoea • Burns • Sweating • Pancreatitis *ii. Renal-oses* • Excess of diuretics • Osmotic diuresis (e.g. hyperglycaemia, tubulointerstitial (disease) • Salt-wasting nephropathy • Hypoaldosteronism *iii. Cerebral salt wasting*	i. Low jugular/central venous pressure. ii. Features of ECF depletion • Thirst • Concentrated urine • Dizziness, weakness, oliguria, postural hypotension • Apathy, confusion • Tachycardia • Cold extremities • Reduced skin turgor	• Volume replacement with isotonic saline—normal saline • If severe, use colloid initially • Avoid excess water intake
2. • Body water ↑ • Total body Sodium: Normal	• Psychogenic water drinking • Iatrogenic water excess i.e. I.V. dextrose solutions, absorption of hypotonic bladder irrigation fluid-called pseudohyponatraemia • SIADH (dilutional hyponatraemia)	• Normal JVP • No signs of ECF depletion or excess	• Water restriction (e.g. 500 ml/day) • Severe cases may require hypertonic saline with extreme care and expert advice
3. • Body water ↑ • Total body ↑ sodium	Oedematous states such as: • CHF • Nephrotic syndrome • Liver cell failure • Renal failure	• There is pitting oedema of face, extremities • JVP is raised in CHF and renal failure • Other features of cardiac, renal and liver disease	• Diuretic therapy • Salt restriction

seen in overcorrection of chronic hyponatraemia than acute. Older male patients, and particularly alcoholics are at risk.

Investigations

1. *Plasma osmolality:* Most patients with hyponatraemia have low plasma osmolality. If plasma osmolality is normal with hyponatraemia, then pseudohyponatraemia must be ruled out.
2. *Urine osmolality:* Urine osmolality and specific gravity of less than 100 mOsm/kg and 1.003, respectively occurs in patients with primary polydipsia. If this is not low, then ADH release due to pain, nausea, drugs or physiological response to haemodynamic stimuli may be suspected or it may be SIADH.
3. *Urine Na^+ concentration:* Volume depletion (hypovolaemia) with normal renal functions results in a urine concentration of Na^+ less than 20 mmol/L because Na^+ is reabsorbed from the tubules. The finding of a urine Na^+ concentration greater than 20 mmol/L indicates a salt-wasting nephropathy, diuretic therapy, hypoaldosteronism or occasionally vomiting.
4. *Serum sodium levels:* Low levels less than 135 mEq/L indicate hyponatraemia irrespective of its cause.

SYNDROME OF INAPPROPRIATE SECRETION OF ADH (SIADH)

Definition

It is characterised by a defect in osmoregulation of ADH (vasopressin) from posterior pituitary. Normally, water overload, hyponatraemia and a low plasma osmolality would suppress ADH and produce a very dilute urine, but in this syndrome, all these factors cannot suppress ADH, hence, there is inappropriate or persistent secretion of ADH either from posterior pituitary, or there is ectopic production of ADH by a tumour. The presence of ADH leads to inappropriate concentration of the urine (urine osmolality above that of plasma) and retention of water (i.e. there is normovolemia).

Table 96.2: Causes of inappropriate secretion of ADH (SIADH)

1. *CNS disorders*
   - Meningitis
   - Encephalitis
   - Brain abscess
   - Brain tumour
   - Delirium tremens, psychosis
   - CVA
   - Hydrocephalus
   - Head trauma
   - Guillain-Barre syndrome
2. *Pulmonary disorders*
   - Pneumonias (viral or bacterial)
   - Lung abscess
   - Tuberculosis
   - Cystic fibrosis
3. *Neoplasm*
   - Carcinoma of bronchus (small cell), pancreas, duodenum, urinary tract, lymphoma, thymoma and mesothelioma
4. *Drug-induced*
   i. *Hypoglycaemics* e.g. Chlorpropamide, tolbutamide
   ii. *Antidepressants* e.g. Amitriptyline, fluoxetine
   iii. *Major tranquillisers,* e.g. Haloperidol, fluphenazine
   iv. *Anti-epileptics* e.g. Carbamazepine
   v. *Chemotherapeutic drugs* e.g. Cyclophosphamide, vincristine, vinblastine
   vi. *Thiazide diuretics* e.g. Hydrochlorthiazide
   vii. *Opiates* e.g. Morphine
   viii. *NSAIDs*
5. *Miscellaneous*
   - Pain
   - Severe nausea
   - Postoperative period

Serum urea concentration is often low because of dilution by retention of water.

Causes

The causes of SIADH are listed in the Table 96.2.

Clinical Features

They are same as discussed under hyponatraemia.

Diagnosis

The diagnosis is based on the fact that the patients with SIADH have normovolaemia with hyponatraemia and there is no evidence of cardiac, renal, hepatic and endocrinal cause to explain impaired water excretion. The diagnostic criteria are depicted in Box 96.1 and an approach to diagnosis is illustrated in Figure 96.3

Disorders of Sodium Balance

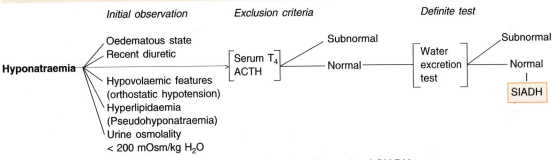

Fig. 96.3: An approach to the diagnosis of SIADH

Box 96.1: Diagnostic criteria for SIADH

1. Essential
- Plasma osmolality low i.e. less than 270 mOsm/kg H_2O (normal is > 280 mOsm/kg)
- Plasma urea low i.e. 2.3 mmol/L (normal 4-6 mmol/L)
- Uric acid level is low
- Plasma sodium low i.e. about 124 mmol/L (normal 135-145 mmol/L)
- Urine osmolality is higher than plasma i.e. about 430 mOsm/kg (should be < 150 mOsm/kg in face of low plasma osmolality)
- Elevated urinary sodium excretion > 20 mEq/L
- Clinical normovolaemia
- Absence of endocrinal (thyroid, adrenal), renal, hepatic and cardiac failure

2. Supplemental
- *Abnormal water load test.* Patient is unable to excrete at least 90% of a 20 ml/kg water load in 4 hours and/or failure to dilute urine osmolality to < 100 mOsm/kg
- Plasma vasopressin (ADH) levels are elevated inappropriate to the plasma osmolality
- Improvement of plasma Na^+ levels with fluid restriction

Management

1. Restriction of fluid intake to 800 to 1000 ml/day. Since this fluid intake is always less than urinary output plus insensible fluid loss, a negative water balance ensues that results in gradual daily reduction in weight, a progressive rise in serum Na^+ concentration and osmolality, and symptomatic improvement. Fluid restriction to be continued until serum Na^+ exceeds 135 mmol/L.

2. The underlying cause should be corrected wherever possible. Fluid restriction to be continued until the cause is corrected.

Plasma osmolality, serum Na^+ and body weight should be monitored daily or frequently until serum Na^+ exceeds 135 mmol/L.

3. If water restriction is poorly tolerated or ineffective, demeclocycline—a potent inhibitor of ADH, may be given in doses of 900-1200 mg/day. Patient receiving demeclocycline should be followed carefully to detect any evidence of renal failure, bacterial superinfection, or excessive drug-induced water loss.

4. When syndrome is very severe, hypertonic saline (300 ml of 3% or 5% sodium chloride) should be infused intravenously over 3-4 hours. To avoid the possibility of inducing pontine myelinolysis, the serum sodium concentration should not be raised too rapidly. Frusemide may be used along with to reduce the chances of congestive heart failure state.

HYPERNATRAEMIA

Definition

Hypernatraemia is defined as plasma sodium concentration greater than 145 mEq/L. Hypernatraemia in fact is hyperosmolar state because Na^+ is a major effective ECF osmole and a major determinant of osmolality.

Acid-base and Electrolyte Disturbance

Table 96.3: Causes and management of hypernatraemia

Disturbance	Total body sodium	Causes	Urinary finding	Management
1. Pure water losses (normovolaemic hypernatraemia)	Normal	1. *Extra-renal losses* • Skin (sweating, fever) • Respiratory (tachypnoea)	Hypertonic urine	• To restore water dificit by water replacement
		2. *Renal losses* • Diabetes insipidus (central, nephrogenic)	Hypo or ISO or Hypertonic urine	
2. Sodium and water deficit (hypovolaemic hypernatraemia	Low	1. *Extra-renal losses* • GI tract (diarrhoea) • Skin (burns, sweating)	Hypertonic urine (urine $Na^+ < 10$ mEq/L	• Replace Na^+ deficit by hypotonic saline
		2. *Ranal losses* • Osmotic diuresis (glycosuria, urea, mannitol) • Postobstructive diuresis	Iso or hypotonic urine (urine $Na^+ > 20$ mEq/L)	
3. Addition of Na^+ (Hypervolaemic hypernatraemia)	Increased	• Primary hyper aldosteronism • Cushing's syndrome • Excessive saline administration	Isotonic or hypertonic urine	Diuretics and water replacement

Hypernatraemia may be due to primary Na^+ gain or water deficit. The two physiological responses to hypernatraemia are increased water intake stimulated by thirst and excretion of concentrated urine reflecting ADH secretion in response to an increased osmolality.

Causes

In practice, hypernatraemia results either due to decreased water intake or increased water loss or both. It commonly occurs in elderly patients with intercurrent illnesses. Since water is distributed between ICF (intracellular fluid) and the ECF (extracellular fluid) in a ratio of 2:1, a given amount of solute-free water loss will result in a two-hold greater reduction in ICF compartment than ECF comparment.

These causes are given in the Table 96.3.

Clinical Features (Fig. 96.2)

The clinical manifestations are as a result of hypertonicity which shifts water out of the cells leading to contraction of ICF volume. A decreased brain cell volume results in CNS features and increases the chances of brain haemorrhage. The symptoms and signs are:

1. **Symptoms and sign of CNS involvement:**
   - Altered mental status, restlessness, lethargy, weakness.
   - Neuromuscular irritability e.g. muscular twitchings, hyper-reflexia, tremulousness, ataxia.
   - Focal neurological deficits.
   - Occasionally seizures and coma.
   - Polyuria and excessive thirst.
2. **Symptoms and signs of volume depletion:**
   - Severe thirst.
   - Dryness of tongue, loss of skin turgor.
   - Tachycardia, hyopotension.
   - Oliguria, concentrated urine, raised urea and Na^+.
3. **Vascular consequences:** There are increased chances of intracerebral and subarachnoid haemorrhage leading to irreversible neurological sequalae.

Management

The treatment of hypernatraemia depends on two important determinants—ECF volume status and rate of development of hypernatraemia (Table 96.3).

1. *Hypovolaemic hypernatraemia:* The main aim is to restore ECF volume by isotonic saline infusion; and plasma osmolality is corrected by half-saline or 5% dextrose.
2. *Hypervolaemic hypernatraemia:* Diuretics and water replacement is needed (See Table 96.3). In the presence of renal insufficiency, dialysis may be required.
3. *Normovolaemic hypernatraemia:* It is treated by water replacement either orally or parenterally with 5% dextrose.

Calculation of water replacement is as follows:

$$\text{Desired total body water} = \frac{\text{Actual plasma Na}^+}{\text{Desired plasma Na}^+} \times \text{Actual total body water}$$

$$\text{Water replacement} = \text{Desired total body water} - \text{Actual total body water}$$

4. *Treatment of diabetes insipidus:* Read textbook of medicine.

Chapter 97

Acute Disturbance of Potassium Balance (Dyskalaemia)

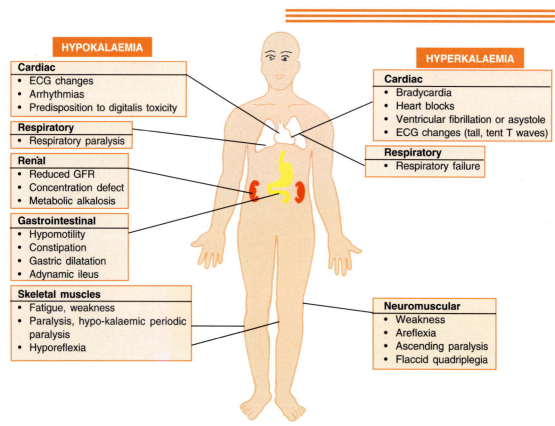

Fig. 97.1: Clinical manifestations of potassium disturbance

ACUTE POTASSIUM IMBALANCE (DYSKALAEMIAS)

The total body potassium is 3500 mEq. Potassium is the major intracellular cation. Only 2% is found in the extracellular fluid (ECF). The ratio of intracellular to extracellular potassium concentration is 38:1, and changes in the normal potassium concentration have an important influence on the neuromuscular transmission and resting membrane potentials, most significantly in the heart (Fig. 97.1).

Acute Disturbance of Potassium Balance (Dyskalaemia)

Regulation of Potassium Balance
(Fig. 97.2)

The two mechanisms are:
1. *Distribution of potassium between intracellular and extracellular fluid.*
2. *Excretion of K^+ by the kidneys mainly and to some extent in the stool and sweat.*

Potassium is pumped into cells in exchange for sodium by Na^+/K^+ ATPase, in a ratio of 3 sodium to 2 potassium ions. This creates a negative intracellular voltage. The intracellular K^+ concentration remains constant at around 150 mmol/L because of passive leakage from cells through non-selective K^+ channels. Certain drugs i.e. β adrenergic agonists and insulin shift the K^+ from extracellular compartment into the cells through Na^+/K^+ ATPase stimulation, hence, are useful for treatment of hyperkalaemia.

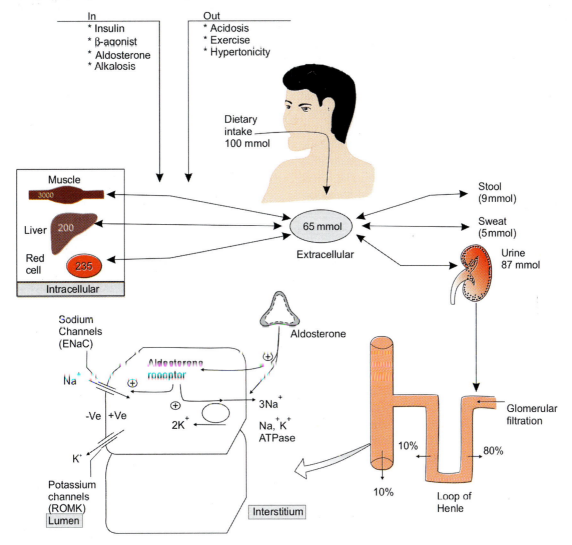

Fig. 97.2: Total body potassium distribution, renal K^+ handling and secretion of K^+ by distal tubular mechanism. The tubular cell illustrated is the principal cell of the cortical collecting duct

Acidosis, exercise, digoxin and hypertonicity have reverse effect i.e. they shift K^+ out of the cells into extracellular compartment by inhibiting the Na/K^+ ATPase mechanism. Hyperkalaemia is commonly seen in metabolic acidosis. The plasma potassium is therefore most vulnerable to factors influencing the shift of K^+ between extracellular and intracellular compartments.

3. *Potassium excretion:* Most of the dietary K^+ is excreted through kidneys. In the kidneys, about 90% of filtered K^+ is reabsorbed actively in the proximal tubule and thick ascending limb. About 10% escapes the reabsorption which is sufficient to maintain K^+ balance in the presence of normal renal function. This is the reason that hyperkalaemia does not occur in the presence of normal GFR. However, if GFR is reduced, then active secretion of K^+ by the distal tubule is necessary to avoid progressive accumulation of K^+ and eventual hyperkalaemia. The active secretion of potassium is mediated by aldosterone, which stimulates Na^+/K^+ ATPase and opens luminal sodium and potassium channels to facilitate sodium reabsorption and potassium secretion. In health, plasma levels of aldosterone rises parallel to increase in plasma potassium. The other stimulus to aldosterone is angiotensin II, thus, any factor which inhibits angiotensin production will blunt the hormonal and renal response to rising potassium level. This is the reason of hyperkalaemia due to ACE inhibitor therapy, NSAIDs therapy (inhibit prostaglandin-mediated renin release) and beta blockers (inhibit renin release). Drugs which block the action of aldosterone (e.g. spironolactone, amiloride) also cause hyperkalaemia particularly in the presence of renal failure.

HYPOKALAEMIA

Definition

It is defined as serum potassium level less than 3.5 mEq/L. It is a common and serious problem in sick hospitalised patients especially on diuretics.

Aetiopathogenesis

Hypokalaemia may result from:
  i. Decreased net intake.
  ii. Shift into the cells and/or.
  iii. Increased net loss.

Diminished dietary intake:
It cannot be a sole cause of hypokalaemia because urinary excretion can effectively be decreased to less than 15 mmol/L as a result of net K^+ reabsorption in the distal tubule. Secondly, the amount of K^+ in the diet almost always exceeds that excreted in the urine. However, it is made clear that decreased dietary intake can exacerbate the potassium depletion secondary to increased loss through the gastrointestinal tract and kidneys. An usual cause of decreased intake is ingestion of clay (geophagia) which binds dietary K^+ and iron. It was customary among African-Americans.

Movement of potassium into the cell:
The intracellular shift of K^+ into the cells may transiently decrease the K^+ concentration without altering total body K^+ content. Metabolic alkalosis leads to hypokalaemia. Uncontrolled hyperglycaemia may lead to K^+ depletion by osmotic diuresis; while treatment of diabetic ketoacidosis with insulin results in hypokalaemia due to intracellular shift of K^+ under the effect of insulin. Stress induced catecholamines release and use of beta-adrenergic agonists also promote cellular uptake of K^+ (Fig. 97.2). Anabolic states can result in hypokalaemia by this mechanism. Massive transfusion with thawed washed RBCs, may cause hypokalaemia as flattened RBCs loose half of their K^+ content during storage. This is called *iatrogenic hypokalaemia. Spurious hypokalaemia (pseudohypokalaemia)* is seen with leucocytosis (count > 50,000/mm^3).

Increases net loss
Excessive sweating causes loss of K^+ through skin. Hyperaldosteronism enhances K^+ excretion in the urine. Profuse diarrhoea, WDHA syndrome, laxative abuse cause loss of K^+ through the stool. Most cases of chronic hypokalaemia are due to

renal K⁺ wasting. Increased renin and aldosterone levels lead to renal K⁺ wasting and hypokalaemia. Primary hyperaldosteronism (Conn's syndrome) or adrenocortical hyperplasia, and renin-secreting tumours of juxtaglomerular apparatus (Bartter's syndrome), renal cell carcinoma, Ovarian and Wilm's tumour may produce hypokalaemia due to hyper-reninaemia.

Renal K⁺ wasting with suppressed renin and aldosterone level is seen in Liddle' syndrome (an autosomal dominant disease).

The causes of hypokalaemia are given in the Table 97.1.

Clinical Features

The clinical manifestations vary from patient to patient even with same degree of hypokalaemia, and their severity depends on the degree of hypokalaemia. Symptoms seldom occur unless serum K⁺ concentration falls below 3 mEq/L. Paralytic ileus and cardiac arrhythmias are usually seen in hypokalaemia with serum K⁺ level < 2.5 mEq/L. The clinical manifestations are as a result of more negative resting membrane potential of various cells. The clinical features are enumerated in the Box 97.1 and Figure 97.1.

Diagnosis and Differential Diagnosis

An approach to differential diagnosis is depicted in Figure 97.4. The diagnosis of hypokalaemia depends on:

i. History of decreased K⁺ intake and K⁺ loss (medications, vomiting and diarrhoea).
ii. Physical examination e.g. hypertension, diabetes.
iii. Laboratory tests
  - Urinary K⁺ and chloride.
  - Plasma and urine osmolarity.
  - Acid-base status.
iv. Exclusion of spurious hypokalaemia. Spurious hypokalaemia (pseudohypokalaemia) seen with leucocytosis (> 50,000/mm³) and

Table 97.1: Causes of hypokalaemia

1. **Reduced intake**
   - Inadequate dietary intake
   - Starvation
   - Clay ingestion
   - Potassium free I.V. fluids
2. **Shift of K⁺ into the cells**
   - Metabolic alkalosis
   - Insulin effect
   - β-adrenergic agonists and alpha-adrenergic antagonists
   - Anabolic state
   - Others such as hypothermia, hypokalaemic periodic paralysis, pseudohypokalaemia, barium toxicity
3. **Increased loss**
   a. *Losses from gastrointestinal tract*
   - Vomiting and diarrhoea
   - Aspiration of upper GI contents
   - Fistulae
   - Villous adenoma of colon
   - Ureterosigmoid anastomosis
   - Laxative abuse
   b. *Losses from the kidneys*
   - Defective proximal reabsorption of K⁺
     – Recovery phase of ATN (diuretic phase)
     – Following relief of urinary tract obstruction
     – Proximal renal tubular acidosis (RTA)
     – Drug induced tubular damage e.g. amphotericin
   - High urine flow rates and Na⁺ delivery to distal nephrons
     – Loop and thiazide diuretics
     – Uncontrolled diabetes (osmotic diuresis)
     – Bartter's syndrome
     – Gitelman's syndrome
   - *Mineralocorticoid receptors stimulation*
     – Primary hyperaldosteronism (Conn's syndrome)
     – Secondary aldosteronism e.g. ECF depletion, renal artery stenosis, accelerated hypertension, liver cirrhosis, cardiac failure and nephrotic syndrome
     – Cushing's syndrome or steroids therapy
     – Carbenoxolone, liquorice use.

redistribution of K⁺ seen in certain clinical settings must be excluded before evaluating K⁺ deficit/depletion.

Box 97.1: Clinical features of hypokalaemia

1. **Cardiac**
   - *The EKG abnormalities (Fig. 97.3)*
     - Appearance of U wave
     - Prolongation of QTc interval
     - Flattening of T wave/inversion
     - ST segment depression
     - Prolongation of P-R interval
     - Widening of QRS
   - *Arrhythmias*
     - Atrial and ventricular ectopics
     - Ventricular tachycardia, torsades de pointes, ventricular fibrillation
   - *Predisposition* to digitalis toxicity and digitalis-induced arrhythmias
2. **Neuromuscular**
   - *Gastrointestinal*
     - Hypomotility
     - Constipation
     - Adynamic ileus
   - *Genitourinary*
     - Dilatation of bladder
   - *Striated muscle*
     - Fatigue, weakness
     - Rhabdomyolysis
     - Paralysis-hypokalaemic periodic paralysis
     - Hyporeflexia
   - *Respiratory*
     - Respiratory paralysis
3. **Renal**
   - Decrease in GFR
   - Concentration defect
   - Metabolic alkalosis
4. **Endocrine**
   - Decrease in aldosterone
   - Decrease in insulin

Management

Aims and objectives
- To correct the K^+ deficit.
- To minimise ongoing losses.

1. **Correction of potassium deficit:** It is safer to correct hypokalaemia via oral route with exception of periodic paralysis. The degree of potassium depletion does not correlate well with plasma K^+ concentration, therefore, while correcting the potassium deficit and assessing the response to treatment, plasma K^+ concentration should be monitored frequently. Potassium chloride is usually the preparation of choice for hypokalaemia with metabolic alkalosis. Potassium bicarbonate (gluconate, citrate, acetate are metabolised to HCO_3) tends to alkalinize, hence, is more appropriate for hypokalaemia associated with metabolic acidosis. In diabetic ketoacidosis, potassium phosphate is the ideal salt. However, KCl can be used in any of the conditions. Ulcers in the small bowel are reported with enteric coated KCl tablets.

Patients with severe hypokalaemia or those unable to take any thing by mouth require intravenous replacement therapy with KCl. For intravenous therapy, the maximum concentration should not exceed 60 mEq/L and rate of infusion should not exceed 20 mEq/hour. In emergency situation, in patients with paralysis, digitalis intoxication or hepatic coma, K^+ can be infused rapidly (< 40 mEq/hour) with EKG monitoring in ICU.

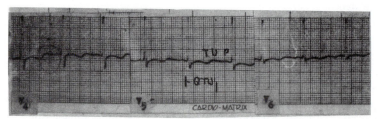

Fig. 97.3: Hypokalaemia. Note prominent U wave, prolonged QTU interval, ST segment depression and T wave inversion

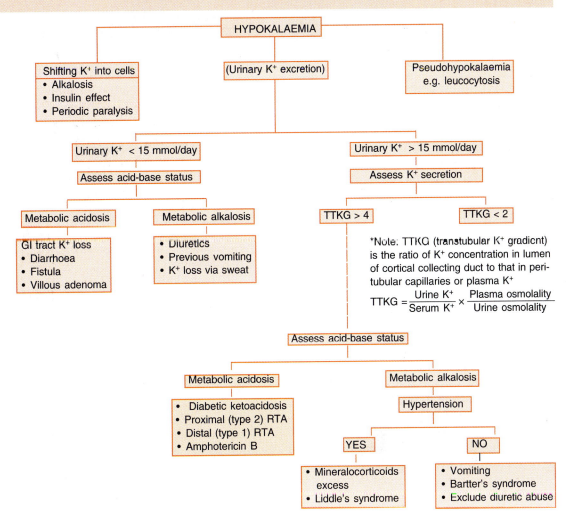

Fig. 97.4: A clinical approach to diagnosis of hypokalaemia

Fluids with K⁺ concentration > 40 mEq/L should be administered through a large vein to avoid phlebitis

Note: KCl should be mixed in normal saline since dextrose solutions may initially exacerbate hypokalaemia under the effect of insulin.

Hypomagnesaemia and hypokalaemia occur concomitantly in most of the conditions responsible for hypokalaemia. Magnesium deficiency is the most overlooked electrolyte abnormality in the intensive care setting. Tissue magnesium deficit is an important cause of refractory hypokalaemia. Lack of response to potassium replacement suggests the need for magnesium replacement even in the presence of normal Mg^{++} level. It is very difficult to administer large quantities of magnesium orally because magnesium salts produce diarrhoea. With repletion of magnesium losses, the renal potassium wasting resolves.

In addition to potassium salts, supplementation therapy with potassium-sparing diuretics (spironolactone, triamterene, amiloride) may be helpful.

2. **To minimise ongoing losses:** If there is an identifiable and correctable cause of K^+ loss, then it should be rectified to stop or minimise ongoing losses.

HYPERKALAEMIA

Definition

Serum potassium concentration more than 5.5 mEq/L is called *hyperkalaemia*. It occurs as a result of either K^+ release from the cells or decrease renal loss.

Potassium adaptation: The rapid K^+ excretion in response to increased dietary consumption is called *potassium adaptation*. This is the reason that increased K^+ intake is rarely the sole cause of hyperkalaemia.

Iatrogenic hyperkalaemia: May result from over enthusiastic parenteral K^+ replacement or in patients with renal insufficiency.

Pseudohyperkalaemia or spurious hyperkalaemia: An artificially elevated K^+ concentration due to K^+ movement out of cells immediately prior to or following venepuncture is called *pseudohyperkalaemia*. The various contributing factors are:
- Prolonged use of a tourniquet with or without repeated fist clenching.
- Haemolysis.
- Marked leucocytosis or thrombocytosis. The clot formation results in release of K^+ from the cells.

Pseudohyperkalaemia should be suspected in an otherwise asymptomatic patient with no obvious underlying cause. If proper venepuncture technique is used and plasma K^+ instead of serum if measured will be found to be normal.

Causes

The causes of hyperkalaemia are listed in the Table 97.2. In diabetic ketoacidosis, hyperkalaemia is

---

Table 97.2: Causes of hyperkalaemia

1. **Increased K^+ intake**
   - Overzealous intravenous K^+ replacement
   - High K^+ containing foods or drugs
2. **Release of intracellular K^+ following cell death**
   - Bleeding into GI tract, soft tissues or body cavities with lysis of RBCs
   - Intravascular haemolysis
   - Rhabdomyolysis or tissue damage by crush injuries
   - Tissue necrosis due to ischaemia/hypoxia
   - Catabolic states e.g. fasting
3. **Shift of K^+ out of cells (extracellular shift)**
   - Metabolic acidosis
   - Hypoinsulinaemia (diabetic ketoacidosis)
   - Drugs e.g. beta blockers, digoxin (in toxic doses)
   - Hypoaldosteronism and hyporeninaemia
   - Hypertonicity of ECF
   - Strenuous exercise
   - Tissue hypoxia
   - Hyperkalaemic periodic paralysis
4. **Impaired renal excretion of K^+**
   a. Reduction in GFR
      - Acute renal failure
      - Chronic renal failure (GFR < 15 ml/min)
      - Urinary tract obstruction
   b. Reducted renal blood flow
      - Hypovolaemia
      - Circulatory failure
   c. Impaired tubular secretion of K^+
      i. Primary hypoaldosteronism
         - Adrenal insufficiency (Addison's disease)
         - Adrenal enzyme deficiency
      ii. Secondary hypoaldosteronism
         - Hyporeninaemia
         - ACE inhibitors
         - NSAIDs
         - Gordon's syndrome
         - Beta blockers
         - Cyclosporin
         - Heparin
      iii. Resistance to aldosterone
         - Pseudohypoaldosteronism
         - Tubulointerstitial disease
         - Transplanted kidneys
         - Amyloidosis
         - Sickle-cell disease
         - Drugs (e.g. K^+ sparing diuretics, trimethoprim, pentamidine)
5. **Spurious hyperkalaemia (pseudohyperkalaemia)**
   - Tissue damage during venepuncture
   - Incorrect blood sampling and improper handling
   - Haemolysis
   - Marked leucocytosis or thrombocytosis

relatively common because of metabolic acidosis (extracellular shift of K⁺), hypoinsulinaemia and hypovolaemia (impaired K⁺ excretion) despite an overall K⁺ deficit accumulating during the preceding period of osmotic diuresis. With treatment, hyperkalaemia rapidly resolves and may be followed by significant hypokalaemia.

Spurious hyperkalaemia is caused by release of K⁺ *in vitro* from abnormal or damaged cells such as abnormal WBCs in leukaemia, haemolysis and incorrect blood sample collection or poorly handled blood specimens that have been left for too long at room temperature before separation and analysis.

Chronic hyperkalaemia is virtually associated with decreased renal K⁺ excretion due to either impaired secretion or diminished distal solute delivery.

Clinical Features

Since the resting membrane potential is related to the ratio of the ICF to ECF potassium concentration, hence, hyperkalaemia prolongs depolarization of the cell membrane. Prolonged depolarisation impairs membrane excitability leading to neuromuscular and cardiac manifestations. Clinical features usually appear when serum K⁺ is 6.5 mEq/L. The manifestations include:

1. **Neuromuscular manifestations:** They include tingling, paraesthesias, weakness, areflexia, ascending paralysis and respiratory paralysis.
2. **Cardiac manifestations:** There may be bradycardia which may progress to complete heart block, ventricular fibrillation or asystole.

The ECG manifestaions correlate well with rise in plasma K⁺ level. There may be tall, tented T waves (Fig. 97.5), ST segment depression, first degree AV block, and QRS widening. Finally, a biphasic *sine wave* (representing fusion of widened QRS and T waves) develop signalling imminent ventricular standstill which is a terminal event in hyperkalaemia.

Management

Aims and objectives:
1. To counteract cardiac toxicity.
2. To shift K⁺ into the cells.
3. To remove the excessive K⁺ burden from the body.

Therapeutic approach to hyperkalaemia depends on the clinical setting, the ECG changes and serum potassium levels. Aggressive anti-hyperkalaemic therapy should be immediately initiated if serum potassium concentration exceeds 6.5 mEq/L or at any level of hyperkalaemia if EKG abnormalities except tall tented T waves are present which include absent P wave, widened QRS or a ventricular arrhythmia. Potentially fatal hyperkalaemia rarely occurs unless K⁺ level exceeds 7.5 mEq/L. It is wise to overtreat this disorder rather than under-treatment. The therapeutic measures employed are depicted in the Box 97.2. They are:

1. **To counteract cardiac toxicity:** Administration of calcium gluconate decreases membrane excitability thus antagonises the effects of

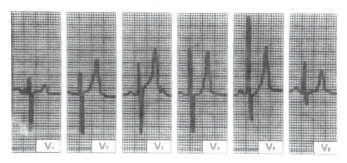

Fig. 97.5: Hyperkalaemia: Note tall tented T waves

Box 97.2: Therapies for acute hyperkalaemia

Treatment	Mechanism of action	Onset of action	Duration of action
1. Calcium gluconate (10-30 ml of 10% solution I.V.)	Antagonises membrane effect, counteracts cardiac toxicity	Few minutes	30-60 minutes
2. Glucose 50 g i.e. 500 ml of 10% dextrose with 10 units of regular insulin infusion	Shifts the potassium into the cells	15-30 minutes	4-6 hours
3. Nebulised salbutamol or albuterol (10-20 mg as nebulised aerosol)	— Same as above —	15 minutes	2 hours
4. Sodium bicarbonate (44-132 mEq I.V.)	Shifts K^+ into the cells	30 minutes	4 hours
5. Cation-exchange resin (sodium polystyrene sulphonate) • Oral 40 g in 20 ml of 70% sorbitol to avoid constipation • Enema (50-100 g)	There is removal of K^+ by exchange of Na^+	120 minutes 60 minutes	4-6 hours
6. Dialysis • Haemodialysis • Peritoneal dialysis	Removal of K^+ from circulation	Few minutes after start	—

hyperkalaemia on cardiac conduction and has an immediate onset of action. In the setting of hypotension or cardiac arrest, calcium chloride should be preferred because it releases calcium ions into circulation immediately without requiring prior hepatic deconjugation of the parent compound.

Calcium is useful to conteract the effects of hyperkalaemia on heart by increasing the threshold potential and thereby exerting an anti-arrhythmic action.

2. **To promote intracellular shift of K^+:** Insulin causes K^+ to shift into cells by mechanisms already discussed, and lowers the serum K^+ levels. Although glucose alone will stimulate insulin release from normal β-cells of pancrease but for a more rapid response, exogenous insulin is administered with glucose (glucose neutralised drip) to prevent hypoglycaemia. A commonly recommended combination is 10 to 20 IU of insulin with 25 to 50 g of glucose.

Alkali therapy with I.V. $NaHCO_3$ can also shift the K^+ into the cells. This is safest when administered as an isotonic solution of 3 ampoules per litre (134 mmol/L $NaHCO_3$). Alkali therapy is reserved for severe hyperkalaemia associated with metabolic acidosis.

Calcium gluconate and $NaHCO_3$ should not be mixed as they can precipitate from a solution.

3. **Removal of the excessive potassium burden from the body:** Excessive potassium burden can be removed by diuretics (loop and thiazide diuretics).

A cation-exchange resin promotes the exchange of Na^+ for K^+ in the gastrointestinal tract and lowers K^+ concentration by 0.5 to 1.0 mmol/L within 1 to 2 hours and last for 4-6 hours. The cation-exchange resin is used in sodium phase (sodium polystyrene sulphonate) either orally or by enema.

Definite therapy for hyperkalaemia is removal of K^+ by haemodialysis. This should be reserved for patients with renal failure and those with life-threatening hyperkalaemia unresponsive to other measures.

4. **Treat the underlying cause of hyperkalaemia**, if found. This may involve dietary modification, correction of metabolic acidosis, volume expansion etc.

Part Twelve

Skin Emergencies

Chapter 98

Acute Urticaria and Angioedema

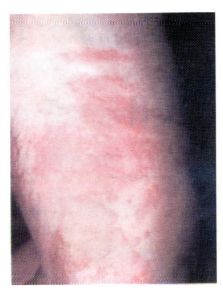

Fig. 98.1A: Acute urticaria: Following exposure to a drug

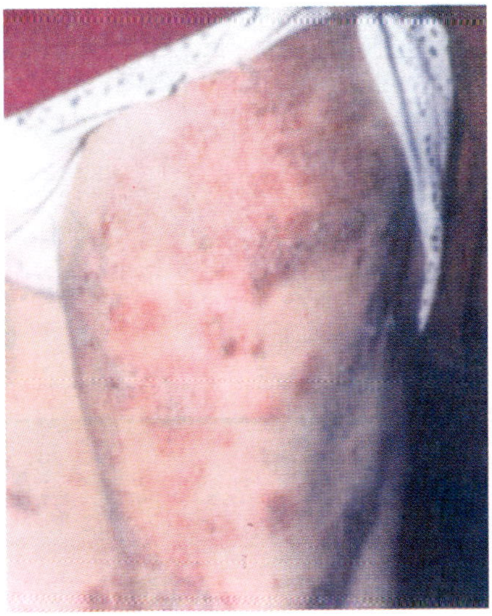

Fig. 98.1B: Papular urticaria: Papular urticaria following an insect bite

ACUTE URTICARIA AND ANGIOEDEMA

Definition

Acute urticaria is defined as transient urticarial (hives) pruritic lesions consisting of a central wheal surrounded by an erythematous halo lasting for less than 2 months (Fig. 98.1). Urticaria is due to dilatation of dermal vessels whereas *angioedema* (Fig. 98.2) results due to dermal oedema as well as subcutaneous oedema. Angioedema occurs alone or in combination with urticaria (e.g. urticarial vasculitis and physical urticaria).

Causes

Acute urticaria has a wide variety of allergic aetiologies (see Box 98.1), but it is difficult to ascertain its cause in emergency situations. However, cause is not needed in the management of urticaria. A significant number of patients have no identifiable cause.

Clinical Picture

The patient usually presents with pruritis and circumscribed, raised, erythematous lesion

522 Skin Emergencies

> **Box 98.1: Common causes of acute urticaria and angioedema**
>
> **Immune-mediated**
> - Atopy
> - Physical urticaria (e.g. dermatographism, solar, cold and cholinergic urticaria caused by sweating)
> - Antigen sensitivity e.g. pollens, foods (milk and its products, egg, nuts, chocolate and shellfish), drugs, helminths
> - Hereditary angioedema
> - Serum sickness
> - Blood transfusion reactions
> - Necrotising vasculitis
> - Hepatitis B infection
>
> **Non-immune causes**
> 1. *Mast cell releasing agents*
>   - Mastocytosis
>   - Food additives e.g. tartrazine
>   - Opiates, radiocontrast media, antibiotics
> 2. *Prostaglandin inhibitors*
>   - Aspirin
>   - NSAIDs
>   - Azo dyes
>   - Benzoates.

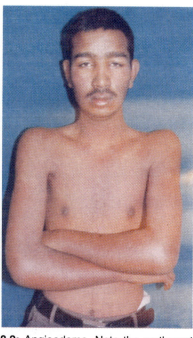

Fig. 98.2: Angioedema. Note the erythematous skin with oedema around the eyelids, face and subcutaneous tissue

(wheals). They are raised because of dermal oedema which may extend deep into the tissue resulting in subcutaneous swelling called angioedema. Hence, urticaria and angioedema may occur in any location together or individually. The sites of involvement include: The eyelids (Fig. 98.1), lips, tongue, larynx and GI tract as well as subcutaneous tissue.

The wheals (lesions) appear suddenly and do not last longer than 48 hours but may continue to occur for indefinite periods. Several attacks may be associated with laryngeal oedema, diarrhoea, abdominal pain, vomiting, dizziness, syncope, hypotension or shock and bronchospasm—called anaphylactic syndrome. Laryngeal involvement may be potentially fatal if not treated urgently.

In children urticaria may be associated with fever or pain abdomen (worm infestation).

Investigations

- TLC and DLC may show eosinophilia.
- IgG levels are raised and complement levels are low in immune mediated urticaria.
- Cryoglobulins and cold haemolysins may be detected in cold urticaria.
- Stool examination for worm infestations.
- LE cells, hepatitis B surface antigens for systemic causes of purpura.

Treatment

1. Patient should avoid triggering factor.
2. **Antihistamines** are the mainstay of treatment in acute urticaria. In adequate doses, antihistamines alone are sufficient to control the symptoms and corticosteroids are not needed. Similarly parenteral antihistamines are usually not indicated.
   - A **sedative H_1 antihistamine** is preferred at night such as long-acting chlorpheniramine maleate (8-12 mg) or bromopheniramine 12-

24 mg or hydroxyzine HCl 10-50 mg.
- **Non-sedative H_1 antihistamines** such as terfenadine (60 mg bid) or astemizole (10 mg daily) or Loratidine (10 mg/day) or cetrizine (10 mg daily) are useful for daytime use.
- **Hydroxyzine HCl or cyproheptadine HCl** have wider spectrum of action than routine H_1 receptor-blocking agents. Angioedema will often rash and better with these agents.
- **Combination treatment:** Antihistaminics (H_1 blockers) may be used in combination with H_2 receptors blockers (ranitidine, famotidine).
- **Corticosteroids** are indicated orally or parenterally only when the antihistamines fail to control the symptoms.
- **Subcutaneous adrenaline** (1:1000 dil) is used for anaphylaxis to control the laryngeal oedema and hypotension, can be repeated safely after 15-20 minutes if there is no tachycardia. Other measures such as tracheostomy, infusion of saline, dopamine and I.V. steroids may be employed as already discussed in the management of anaphylactic shock.

Most patients with acute urticaria recover completely from the acute attack and may remain well throughout their lives.

Chapter 99

Erythroderma and Exfoliative Dermatitis

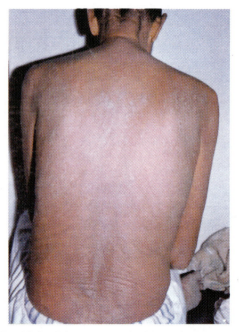

Fig. 99.1: Erythroderma (exfoliative dermatitis)

Definition

Erythroderma is a nonspecific inflammatory condition characterised by redness of the skin surface involving more than 90% of the body surface. There may be associated scaling, erosions, pustules as well as shedding of hair and nails.

Table 99.1: Causes of erythroderma

1. **Primary cutaneous disorders**
   - Psoriasis
   - Dermatitis (atopic, stasis, contact, seborrhagic)
   - Pityriasis rubra pilaris.
2. **Drugs** e.g. sulphonamides, salicylates, penicillins, hydantoin, thioacetazone, gold, allopurinol, captopril carbamazepine.
3. **Systemic diseases**
   - Cutaneous T cell lymphoma.
   - Lymphoma.
4. **Idiopathic.**

Aetiology

Males are more commonly affected (2-3 times) than females. The causes are given in the Table 99.1.

Clinical Features

Erythroderma developing in primary eczema or dermatitis, underlying malignancy and following drug intake is often sudden. The cutaneous inflammation is seen as erythema (redness) and scaling within few days. The scalp and body hair may fall along with nails in erythroderma of few weeks duration, secondary changes such as erosions and pustules may be associated.

Drug induced erythroderma (exfoliative dermatitis) often begins as morbilliform eruption or it may arise as diffuse erythema. Fever and eosinophilia often accompany the eruption and occasionally there is an associated interstitial nephritis.

Potential systemic manifestations include fever, chills, hypothermia, reactive lymphadenopathy, peripheral oedema, hypoalbuminaemia and high output cardiac failure.

Investigations

- TLC and DLC for leucocytosis, eosinophilia.
- ESR may be raised.
- Urea and electrolytes may be monitored.

Complications

- Disturbance of temperature regulation due to diffuse involvement of skin leading to hypothermia.
- High output cardiac failure due to vasodilatation.
- Dehydration due to water loss and there may be dyselectrolytemia.

Treatment/Management

- Hospitalization and bed rest.
- Nutritional supplements e.g. high protein intake, multivitamins and mineral.
- Stop the drug if it is the underlying cause.
- Check and treat secondary infections with appropriate antibiotics.
- Physiological saline compresses for 30 minutes 4 times a day is helpful in removing the scales, debris and bacteria.
- Emollients (liquid paraffin) after short lukewarm bath is helpful. Sedative antihistamines may be used to control pruritis, sometimes, low potency steroid creams or ointments may be used except in psoriatic erythroderma.
- Treat appropriately the complications such as high output state, hypoalbuminaemia, hypothermia and water and electrolyte imbalance.
- Specific treatment for psoriasis or malignancy may be instituted if it is the underlying cause.

Chapter 100

Pemphigus

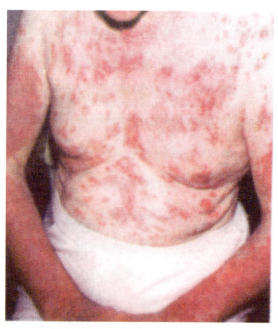

Fig. 100.1: Bullous pemphigus

PEMPHIGUS

Definition

Pemphigus is the most common autoimmune blistering (bullous) disorder involving the skin and the mucous membrane.

Types

Histologically, there is acantholysis and cell separation and intradermal blister formation. Depending on the cleavage level within epidermis and different clinical patterns, two forms are recognized, each with a variant.
1. Pemphigus vulgaris and its variant pemphigus vegetans.
2. Pemphigus foliaceous and its variant pemphigus erythematosus.

Aetiology

The IgG class of autoantibodies directed against intracellular cement substance of the epidermal keratinocytes identified as desmogleins lead to formation of clefts (acantholysis and cell separation) in the epidermis. Similar antibodies have also been demonstrated in patients with burns, bullous pemphigoid and penicillin-induced eruptions. Pemphigus like eruptions can be produced by some drugs e.g. captopril, d-penicillamine and rifampicin. Rarely pemphigus may be associated with thymoma, myasthenia gravis, SLE, carcinoma and lymphoproliferative diseases.

Clinical Features

1. **Pemphigus vulgaris:** It is very common disease in India, involves younger persons in the age groups of 20-40 years.
   It presents commonly with oral erosions followed by skin lesions such as generalized flaccid blisters (vesicles) or bullae usually on normal looking skin, that quickly rupture to leave large denuded areas which crust and

continue to spread without further blistering at the same area.

The **sites of oral lesion** are buccal and palatine mucosae. The lesions are painful, tender and heal slowly. Other uncommon sites are conjunctivae, pharangeal, laryngeal and anorectal mucosae. The sites of blisters are scalp, face, axillae and groin.

Nikolsky's sign is positive which means tangential pressure (sliding pressure) on the unaffected skin may cause separation of the epidermal layers and denudation of the skin.

Asboe—Hansen's sign indicates bulla spreading or blisters spreading by lateral and perpendicular pressure applied on intact blisters.

Pemphigus vegetans: It is a variant of pemphigus vulgaris, is a much milder form of the disease which may begin either as vesicles or blisters that eventually develop hypertrophic granulation or vegetative granulation. Oral lesions may occur. Inter triginous involvement is common. The initial moist vegetative lesions turn dry later on.

Pemphigus foliaceous: It is a less common disease and lesions are superficial blisters and erosions that appear on the face, neck and upper trunk. Oral lesions are rarely seen. The course of the disease is more or less similar to pemphigus vulgaris.

Pemphigus erythematosus. It is a variant of pemphigus foliaceous. Erythematous, scaly, hyperkeratotic dry plaques (lesions) are seen in butterfly distribution over the face starting from the nose spreading over the cheeks. Oral mucosa is rarely involved. Though it resembles SLE but systemic involvement never occurs.

Diagnosis and Investigations

The diagnosis is made by:
1. **Tzanck smear:** The blister is ruptured and the base is scrapped with the scalpel and smear is made on a glass slide. Staining with Giemsa reveals acantholytic cells with large dense nuclei and a rim of cytoplasm.
2. **Skin biopsy from a fresh blister and its histopathology:** Histopathology shows intradermal cleft which is subcorneal in pemphigus foliaceous and its variant but is suprabasal in pemphigus vulgaris and its variant. Acantholytic cells are seen in clefts. In pemphigus vegetans, hyperkeratosis, acanthosis and intradermal eosinophilic abscesses are seen.
3. **Immunofluorescence:** Direct immunofluorescence reveals deposition of IgG in the intercellular space of both involved and uninvolved skin. Less commonly IgM and IgA may be found. Indirect immunofluorescence shows IgG antibodies which corresponds with the severity of the disease.
4. **ELISA:** Recently ELISA tests that can detect IgG auto antibodies to desmoglein-1 and 3 have been developed that will help for rapid diagnosis.

Treatment

- General supportive measures include compresses with $KMNO_4$ or simply with soap and water.
- Maintain fluid and electrolyte balance.
- Treatment of infection by antibiotics.
- **Immunosuppression:** Systemic steroids (prednisolone 1-2 mg/kg/day orally) along with cytotoxic agents like cyclophosphamide or azathioprine (1 mg/kg/day) are the main drugs used in the treatment of pemphigus. Cyclophosphamide pulse therapy or cyclophosphamide plus steroid pulse therapy have been employed for severe cases and have been beneficial.
- Topical or intralesional steroids help the mild cases. Topical $AgNO_3$ (0.5%) may be used to promote healing.

Chapter 101

Skin Infections

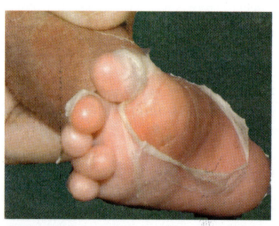

Fig. 101.1: Staphylococcal scalded skin syndrome (SSSS). Note the peeling of the skin preceded by redness and tenderness in an infant. The skin lesions are similar to toxic epidermal necrolysis

SKIN INFECTIONS

Skin infection is very common in clinical practice. Every physician shall see some form of cutaneous infection in his day-to-day practice. It is stressed here, that sometimes, the serious and/or potentially serious skin infection may pose an emergency situation, therefore, it is imperative for the physician to know the site of their localisation, degree of involvement and presence of toxaemia/septicaemia. The following skin infections may pose as an emergency.

1. **Staphylococcal Scalded Skin Syndrome (SSSS—Fig. 101.1):** It is a severe form of skin disease produced by exotoxins elaborated by *S. aureus* of phase group 2. It affects infants and young children, is characterised by diffuse/extensive erythema and fever, followed by widespread flaccid bullae formation and exfoliation. The raw areas are extremely tender but not purulent. There is significant fluid and electrolyte loss. Secondary infection is common. The entire illness resolves within 10 days. It can be, however, fatal in 2-3% cases due to hypovolaemia and sepsis.

Treatment

1. Local care of denuded skin.
2. Replacement of fluids and electrolyte to correct hypovolaemia and electrolyte imbalance. The electrolytes should be monitored.
3. **Antibiotics:** The antistaphylococcal antibiotics are most useful. Parenteral cloxacillin is the treatment of choice.

Toxic Shock Syndrome (TSS)

It is an acute life-threatening intoxication or endotoxaemia produced by toxin-producing strains of *S. aureus*. It is characterised by fever, hypotension, rash, multiorgan dysfunction (at least 3 organs must be involved) and desquamation during the early convalescent period. The disease was recognised with a large outbreak in menstruating women because menstruation is the most common setting for TSS but non-menstruation cases also occur frequently (50%). It affects both sexes and all ages. It is common in menstruating women using tampons.

> *The toxins responsible for TSS include toxic shock syndrome toxin I (TSST-1), pynogenic exotoxin C and endotoxin F.*

The syndrome in non-menstrual cases complicate skin lesions of many types including burns, insect bites, varicella lesions and surgical wounds. Postoperative disease develops hours to days following a surgical procedure.

Clinical Features

- Patient is toxic and ill-looking. There is tachypnoea and tachycardia.
- General symptoms e.g. nausea, vomiting, abdominal pain, diarrhoea, muscular pains and headache.
- Features of hypotension e.g. dizziness, vertigo, low urinary output and perspiration.
- **Rash:** The macular erythematous rash develops over first 2 days of illness. It is usually generalised. There may be conjunctival suffusion, periorbital oedema.
- **In menstruating women**, there may be purulent vaginal discharge and vaginal mucosa is red.
- A strawberry tongue develops in 50% cases.
- There is involvement of multiple organs e.g. brain, kidneys, lungs, liver, GI tract etc. Mental status is clear.

Investigations

- TLC, DLC may show neutrophilic leucocytosis.
- There may be anaemia, thrombocytopenia.
- Urine may show pyuria, haematuria, proteinuria.
- There may be hypoalbuminaemia, raised blood urea and creatinine.
- Raised SGOT and SGPT levels.
- There may be hypocalcaemia and hypophosphatemia.
- Creatinine phosphokinase (CK) levels are elevated.
- Blood cultures are usually negative.

Treatment

- Decontamination of the site of toxin production e.g. removal of tampons and debridement of surgical wounds.
- Correction of fluids and electrolyte balance. Liberal administration of fluids including saline should be used to resuscitate shock. Pressure agents e.g. dobutamine may be used to resuscitate shock unresponsive to fluids. The dose of dobutamine is same as described in management of peripheral circulatory failure. (Read as emergency chapter 71).
- Electrolytes particularly hypocalcaemia and hypomagnesaemia may be corrected and maintained.
- **Antibiotics:** Semisynthetic penicillins (nafcillin, oxacillin) or vancomycin are the drugs of choice. In serious infection, clindamyin 900 mg I.V. 8 hourly alone or with vancomycin have been used.
- Infusion of neutralizing antibody to TSST-1 (immunoglobulin) as a single dose of 400 mg/kg generates a protective level of antibody.

Complications

- Multiple organ failure due to hypoperfusion.
- Massive oedema due to hypoalbuminaemia.
- Adult respiratory distress syndrome.

Chapter 102

Stevens-Johnson Syndrome

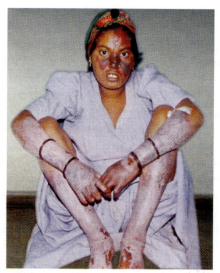

Fig. 102.1: Stevens-Johnson syndrome

Definition

The Stevens-Johnson syndrome describes a severe erythema multiforme (erythematous maculopapular lesions) with a widespread bullous disease associated with oral and genital ulceration and marked constitutional symptoms.

Causes

1. **Infections:**
   - Viral e.g. herpes simplex.
   - Mycoplasma.
   - Yersinia, tuberculosis, histoplasmosis.
2. **Drugs:**
   - Sulphonamide.
   - Codein.
   - Thiacetazone.
   - Carbamazepine.
   - Phenytoin.
   - Phenobarbitone.
3. **Connective tissue disease**—a rare precipitating factor.
4. **Topical applications.**

Clinical Features

1. *Constitutional symptoms:* The onset is acute with mild fever, sore throat, malaise and prostration.
2. *Skin lesions:* Extensive bullous eruption of the skin and mucous membranes. The skin lesions are distributed symmetrically on the dorsum of hands, feet, the forearms, legs, face and neck. Total percent of body surface area detachment is less than 10% which differentiates it from another potentially fatal condition called toxic epidermal necrolysis where > 30% of the body area shows detachment of skin.
3. *Systemic manifestations* include iritis, urethritis, gastritis, arthritis and haemorrhages e.g. haemoptysis. There may be difficulty in respiration. Dehydration occurs due to fluid and sodium loss. Hypotension can occur.

Treatment

The disease has usually a spontaneous resolution subsiding within few weeks. Stevens-Johnson syndrome can be recalcitrant and can be fatal.

The emergency measures include:

1. **Immediate:**
   - Removal of the cause e.g. infection, drug etc. All drugs the patient was taking must be stopped immediately. If that is not possible, substitute them with chemically unrelated drug.
   - Symptomatic treatment with antihistamines and calamine lotion. The antihistamines can be used intravenously. Calamine lotion is used locally.

2. **Specific emergency treatment**
   - Maintenance of a patent airway.
   - Good nutrition supplementation.
   - Proper fluid and electrolyte administration to correct hypovolaemia and electrolyte disturbance. BP and electrolytes should be monitored.
   - Prevention of secondary skin infection of skin lesion by appropriate antibiotic therapy.
   - Care of mouth and eyes.
   - Good nursing care.
   - **Systemic corticosteroids:** A short course of steroids (prednisolone 60-80 mg daily then gradually tapered off) may be used to overcome acute phase and to relieve constitutional symptoms.

Index

A

Abdominal pain (Read biliary colic)
Abscess
    amoebic 75-77
Absolute neutrophil count 321
ACE inhibitors
    AMI 132
    heart failure 147
Acetylcysteine 19, 83
Acid-base disturbance 489-501
    primary 490
    types 493
Acute disseminated encephalomyelitis (ADEM) 270
Acute mountain sickness 473
Acute muscarinic effects 429
Acute ST-elevation myocardial infarction 127-133
Acute pulmonary oedema 153
Acute respiratory distress syndrome (ARDS) 16-19
    causes of 17
    differential diagnosis 18
    management 18
    radiological features 18
Acute tubular necrosis 392
Acute urticaria and angioedema 521
    causes 521
    clinical Picture 521
    treatment 522
Acrocyanosis 316
Acyclovir 268
Addison's disease 369
Adrenaline 358
Adrenal insufficiency 368-371
    causes 369
    clinical features 369
    treatment 370

Advanced cardiac life support (ACLS)
    cardiac arrest 193
    diuretics therapy 405
    electric shock 376
    implanted cardioverter defibrillator (ICD) 196
    lightning 476
Agranulocytosis 319-322
Albumin serum 81
Albuminocytological dissociation 280
Aldosteronism
    hypoaldosteronism 516
    primary 516
    secondary 516
Allopurinol 334
Alteplase 130
Aluminium phosphide poisoning 432-436
    ARDS in 434, 435
    arrhythmias in 435
    magnesium sulphate in 435
    manifestations of 434
    shock 435
    treatment 434-435
Amaurosis fugax 238
Aminophylline 15, 158
Ambulance 159, 160
Amphetamines 455
Amphotericin-B 322
Amrinone 138, 151
Anaphylaxis 461-463
    anaphylactic reactions 461
    anaphylactoid reactions 461
    exercise induced 461
Antilymphocyte globulin 326
Amylase
    serum 72

Angina
    β blockers in 179
    clinical presentation 178
    management 179
    printzmetal 189
    unstable 177, 188
Angiodysplasias 64, 67
Angioedema 462, 521
Angiography 63, 66
    UGI bleed 61
    LGI bleed 65
Anoproctoscopy 66
Anion gap 491
Anticholinergics 56, 234
Anticoagulants 26
    heparin 26, 131, 179
    oral 179
Antihistaminics 56, 63, 233
Antiphospholipid syndrome 369
Antiplatelet therapy
    CVA 244
Antipsychotic drugs 212
Anti-rabies vaccine 103
Aortic aneurysm 188
Aortic dissection 136, 188
Aortic regurgitation
    acute 135
Aplastic anaemia 323-327
    causes 321
    clinical features 324
    management 325
Aplastic crisis 298
Arginine vasopressin (AVP) 506
Artemether 123
Artesunate 123
Ascending venography 24
Asphyxia 34
Aspirin 129, 243
Assisted ventilation
    in ARDS 19

Atrial fibrillation 162, 362
Atrial flutter 164
Atrial natriuretic peptide 398
Atrial tachycardia 162
Atropinisation 430
AV nodal reentry 161
   accessory pathway 160
   antidromic tachycardia 162
   circus movement tachycardia 159
   orthodromic AVRT 161

B

Barium examination
   enema 66
   UGI 63
Basic life support (BLS) 193, 194
Benign paroxysmal vertigo 233
Benzodiazepines 454
Beta blockers
   acute coronary syndrome 177
   heart failure 147
   AMI 132
Biliary colic 85-87
   causes 86
   ERCP 86
   pain 86
   treatment 87
Bisphosphonates 381
Bites
   lizard 448
   snake 442
Bone marrow examination 325
Bone marrow transplantation
   aplastic anaemia 310
   leukaemias 328
Brain abscess 257
Bretylium 166
Bronchial asthma
   acute severe 12-15
   assisted ventilation 15
   beta-2 agonists 15
   corticosteroids in 15
   ipratropium bromide in 15
Bronchiectasis 4
Broncho-alveolar lavage 18
Budd Chiari syndrome 80

C

CABG 180
   acute coronary syndrome 177

Calcitonin 382
Calcium
   gluconate 378, 518
   serum levels 376
Calcium channel blockers
   acute coronary syndrome 177
   in ATN 359
   myocardial infarction 127
   vertigo 230
Caloric test 231
Captopril 201
Carbon-monoxide poisoning 418-420
Cardiac arrest 191-196
Cardiac enzymes 128
   CPK-MB 189, 190
Cardiac output 142
Cardiac pacing
   AV blocks 170-172
   heart failure 147
   SA block 170
Cardiac tachyarrhythmias 159-168
Cardiac tamponade 182-186
   causes 183
   clinical features 183
   management 185
   pericardial effusion 183
Cardiogenic shock 134-139
   definition 135
   echocardiography in 136
   management 136-139
Cardiomyopathy
   dilated 155, 192
   hypertrophic 192
Cardioversion 162
Carvedilol 152
Catatonia 214
Cavernous sinus thrombosis 287
Central pontine myelinolysis 504
Central venous pressure (CVP) 143
Cerebral infarction 237
Cerebral edema
   acute high altitude 475
   acute, in hyponatremia 502
   acute hepatic encephalopathy 83
Cerebral malaria 121-124
   acute pulmonary oedema in 124
   clinical features 122
   therapy 113
Cerebral vasospasm 249
Cerebral venous
   sinus thrombosis 286

Charcot's triad 86
Chelating agents 423
Chest pain 187-190
   angina, prinzmetal 189
   angina, stable 188
   angina, unstable 188
   causes 188
   myocardial infarction 190
Charcoal
   activated 406
   for poisoning/drug overdosage 407
Choking 35
Cholangitis
   acute biliary colic 85-87
   causes of 86
   clinical features 86
   investigations 86
   obstructive 86
Cholecystitis
   acute 85
Cholera 112-114
   clinical features 113
   diagnosis 113
   management 113
   prevention 114
   vaccine 114
Chronic bronchitis
   acute exacerbation 40
Chvostek's sign 377
CPK-MB 178, 179
Clostridium tetani 106
Colchicine 305
Colloids 145
Colon cut off sign 72
Colonoscopy 66
Coma 213-218
Coma vigil 214
Complete heart block 171
   acute myocardial infarction 127
Compresison devices in DVT 27
Congestive heart failure 147-152
Continuous positive airway pressure (CPAP) 19
Conus medullaris lesion 276
Copper sulphate poisoning 421-423
Cord compression 274-279
   AVM 279
   causes 274

clinical features 274
infective 276, 274
management 278
neoplastic 278, 279
Coronary angiography 181
Coronary artery disease
clinical manifestations 170
Coronary syndrome 177-181
β-blockers 181
clinical presentation 178
Corrosive injury to GIT 409-413
endoscopic classification 410
management 411
prevention 411
Cortisol, plasma 369
Crohn's disease 66
Cryoprecipitate 317
Cullen's sign 70
Cyclosporine 326, 335
Cytokines 315

D

Dantrolene 467
DC shock 162
DDAVP 312
D-dimer ELISA test 23-24, 317
Decontamination
gut 406
skin 406
Decortication 50
Deep vein thrombosis
pulmonary embolism 20-28
prevention of stroke 243
Defibrillation 194
Dehydration 59, 113, 118
assessment of 113
Delirium 207-212
causes 209
clinical features 209
delirium tremens 212
substance induced and substance withdrawal 210
Dementia 211
Demyelinating disease 280
Demylination disorders 270
Dengue fever 96-98
bleeding manifestations 96
clinical features 96
dengue hemorrhagic fever 97
dengue shock syndrome 97

differential diagnosis 98
management 97
Desmopressin 312
Devic's disease 271
Dhatura poisoning 439
Diabetes insipidus 509
Diabetic ketoacidosis 345-351
cerebral oedema in 347
clinical features 346
insulin therapy, in 348
laboratory picture of 347
treatment of 348
Dialysis
indications in ARF 398
modes 397
peritoneal 397
Diarrhoea 57-60
causes 58
large bowel 58
samll bowel 58
Diazepam
tetanus 108
seizures 254
Diazoxide 200, 204
Digital subtraction angiogrpahy (DSA) 241
Digitalis
digoxin 150
heart failure 147
Dimercaprol 423
Disseminated intravascular coagulopathy 314-318
acute 315
causes of 315
chronic 316
heparin therapy in 317
in leukaremia 329
treatment of 317
Dizziness 230
faintness 230
psychiatric 228
Dobutamine
cardiogenic shock 135
Donor reactions
cause of 339
clinical features 339-340
prevention 341
Donors
aphresis 341
autologous 355

Dopamine 138
renal-dose 396
D-penicillamine 423
Drainage of liver abscess 78
Droperidol 212
Drowning 479-482
near drowning 480
dry drowning 480
wet drowning 480
Duodenal ulcer 61
Dysentery 119-120
amoebic 120
bacillary 120

E

Echocardiography
in pericardial effusion 184
cardiogenic shock 135
Electrical alternans 184, 185
Electrocoagulation 63
Electroenephalogram (EEG) 217, 252
Electroconvulsive therapy (ECT) 212
Electrocution 476-478
and acute renal failure 475
electrical burns 478
shock 478
tetanus 478
Electrolyte disturbance 489-518
Electromechanical dissociation (EMD) 191
Electrophysiological studies
in GB syndrome 282
pulmonary 20-28
Emphysema 31
Empyema 45-50
clinical features 46
management 48
open drainage 50
pneumonia 45
Encephalitis 265-278
acute 265
arboviral 265
causes of 265
clinical features 266
diagnostic approach 266
herpes simplex 265
Japanese B 266
lymphocytic choreomeningitis virus 266

management of 267
mumps 266
Encephalopathy
    enteric 101
    hepatic 79-84
    hypertensive 197
Endoscopy
    endoscopic haemostasis 64
    UGI 62
Epidemic dropsy 424-426
    clinical features 425
    diagnosis 425
    management 426
Epinephrine
    in anaphylaxis 462
    in cardiac arrest 191
ERCP 73
Ergotamine 224
Erythroderma and exfoliative dermatitis 524
    clinical Features 524
    management 525
    treatment 525
Esmolol 163, 200
Etidronate 382
Evoked potential 271

F

Fibrinogen degradation products 316
Fibrinolysis 314
Fludrocortisone 229, 370
Flumazenil 83
Food poisoning 58, 115-118
Forced alkaline diuresis 423
Foreign body airway obstruction 35
Fosphenytoin 253
Fresh frozen plasma 317
Fursemide 151, 158, 204

G

Gas gangrene 110-111
Gastric
    lavage 406
    ulcer 61
Glomerulonephritis, acute 386
Glucagon 358, 463
Glucocorticoid deficiency 370

Glucose-insulin-potassium (GIK) 132
Graft versus host disease 335
Granulocyte-Macrophage colony stimulating factors 322, 327
Grey Turner's signs 70
Guillain-Barrè syndrome
    classification 281
    clinical features 281
    diagnostic criteria 283
    intravenous immune globulin (IVIg) 284
    plasmaphreiss in 284
Gum hypertrophy 329

H

Haemetemesis 62
Haematochezia 57
Haemolytic crisis 298
Haemolytic uremic syndrome 307
Haemoperfusion 407
Haemophilia 308-13
    clinical features 310
    management 311
    physiotherapy 313
Haemodialysis 390, 397
    in drug intoxications 457
    in hyperkalemia 518
    in poisoning 407
Haemoptysis 3-6
    angiography 5
    left ventricular failure 153
    management 5
    pseudo-haemoptysis 3
    recurrent 4
    role of bronchoscopy 5
Haemopump 139
Haemolytic disease of the new born 337
Haemostatic support 317
Haloperidol 212
Hampton's hump 22
Hanging and Strangulation 483
    cerebral anoxia 484
    sequelae 485
    stretching of neck 484
    venous congestion 484
Headache 219-224
    causes 20

cluster 21
    management 224
    subarachnoid hemorrhage 246
Heart blocks 171-174
Heart failure 147-152
    causes 148
    clinical features 148
    definition 147
    diagnosis 149
    echo 150
Heat
    exhaustion 466
    stroke 465
Heimlich's manoeuvre 38
Hepatic encephalopathy 79-84
    acute 79
    causes 80
    chronic 83
    clinical features 80
    complications 83
    grades 80
    management 81
Hepatic failure
    features 80
Herniation syndromes
    central 291
    uncus's transtentorial 292
Histaminergic drugs 234
Hooch 414
Horner's syndrome 240
Hydralazine 204
Hydrocephalus
    chronic 249
Hydrophobia 102
Hypercalcemia 379-382
    causes of 379
    clinical features 380
    treatment 381
Hypercapnia
    respiratory failure 40
Hyperkalaemia 516-18
    acute 516
    calcium salts, in 517
    causes 516
    chronic 517
    clinical features 517
    management 517
    nebulized albuterol, in 518
Hypernatremia 507
    causes 508

Index

euvolemic 508
hypervolemic 508
hypovolemic 508
management 509
Hyperosmolar hyperglycemic
   clinical features 353
   etiology 352
   investigations 335
   management 354
   nonketotic coma 352-355
Hypertension
   accelerated 198
   malignant 201
Hypertensive
   emergencies 199
   encephalopathy 198
   renal emergencies 199
   pregnancy related states 200
   urgency 198
Hyperthermia 464-467
   malignant 467
   therapeutic effects 467
   treatment of 467
Hyperventilation 472
Hypoaldosteronism 516
Hypocalcaemia 375-378
   causes of 376
   clinical features 376
Hypoglycaemia 356-360
   causes 357
   clinical features 358
   management 359
   reactive 357
   spontaneous 357
   tests for 359
   unawareness 358
Hypokalaemia 512-16
   causes 513
   differential diagnosis 513
   management 514
   manifestations 514
   refractory 515
Hypomagnesemia 515
Hyponatremia 503
   adrenal insufficiency 370
   causes 504
   neuropsychiatric manifestations
      of 504
   and SIADH 506
Hypoparathyroidism 376

Hypotension
   postural and syncope 229
   orthostatic 232
Hypothermia 468-471
   accidental 469
   intentional 469
Hypothyroidism 365
Hypoventilation 40
Hypoxemia 40, 43
Hypoxia 473

I

Idioventricular rhythm 172
Immunophenotyping 330
Impedances plethysmography 24
Implantable cardioverter defibrillator 196
Inferior vena caval filter 28
Inflammatory bowel disease 66
Intercostal tube drainage (ICTD) 32, 48
International normalisation ratio (INR) 25
Interstitial nephritis, acute 381
Interventricular septum
   rupture of 139
Intraaortic balloon pump (IABP) 138
Intracranial pressure
   increased in 291
   monitoring 289
   reduction 292
Intravenous pyelography 395
Ipratropium bromide 15

K

Keith-Wegener retinopathy 198
Ketoacidosis
   alcoholic 348
   diabetic 345
Ketosis
   starvation 348
Kussmaul's breathing 347
Kussmaul's sign 184, 185

L

Labetolol 202
Labyrinthitis 232

Laser photocoagulation 63
Leukemia 328-335
   acute lymphoblastic 329
   acute myeloid 329
   acute promyelocytic 331
   clinical features 329
   evaluation of 329
   French-American-British (FAB)
      classifcation 330
   leukemic blasts, ALL 330
   subleukemia 328
   treatment 332
Leukemia cutis 329
LGI Bleed 65-67
   angiography 66
   causes of 65
   clinical features of 65
   treatment 67
Lidocaine 160, 166
Lipase serum 71
Liver abscess 75-78
Lizard bites 448
Lock jaw 107
Lorazepam 109, 212
Loss of consciousness (coma) 213-218
   causes 214
   management 217
Lugol's iodine 364
Lung resection 50

M

Magnesium
   acute myocardial infarction 127
   ventricular tachycardia 167
Malaria, severe 122
Mallory Weiss tear 54, 64
Mannitol 82
Meckle's diverticulum 65
Megaloblastic crisis 299
Melana 61, 65
Meniere's disease 234
Meningitis 255-264
   antibiotic in 257
   aseptic 260
   bacterial 255
   benign recurrent lymphocytic 260-261
   clinical features 256
   treatment 257

tubercular 261
viral 260
Metabolic acidosis 493-496
  causes 495
Metabolic alkalosis 496
  causes 496
Methemoglobinemia 71
Methyl alcohol poisoning 414-417
  CT scan picture in 415
  ethyl alcohol in 416
  metabolic acidosis 416
  serum methanol level 415
  serum osmolol gap 415
  treatment 417
Methylprednisolone 272
Metronidazole 77
Microangiopathic hemolytic anemia 314
Midazolam 109
Migraine 222
  acute 224
  provoking factors 222
  vertigo 234
Miller Fisher syndrome 281
Milrinone 138
Mitral regurgitation 135
  acute 135
Multiple-organ dysfunciton syndrome (MODS) 91
Myelitis
  demylinating 270
  postinfections 270
Myelopathy
  compressive 274
  non-traumatic 278
  traumatic 278
Myocardial infarction 127-133
  clinical features 128
  diagnosis 128
  management 128
  secondary prophylaxis 132
Myocarditis 9
Myoglobin, serum 179
Myxedema coma 365-367
  clinical features 365
  hypothermia 366
  investigations 366
  management 366
  precipitating factors 365

N

Neomercazole 364
Nephritic syndrome 385-389
  causes 386
  clinical features 386
  dialysis 389
  management 387
  plasmapheresis 389
Neuromyelitis optica 270
Neurolabrynthitis 233
Neuroleptic 234
Neutropenia 319-322
  causes 320
  cyclic 321
  drug induced 320
  treatment 321
Nicardipine 200
Nitrates 129
  nitroglycerine 129, 179
Non-benzodiazepine sedative compounds 455
Non-invasive positive pressure ventilation in COPD 42-43
Norepinephrine 138
NSAIDs 54, 62
Nystagmus 231

O

Obstructive uropathy 392
Oculocephalic reflex 217
Oesophageal varices 61, 64
Oliguria 386
Open lung biopsy 9
Ophthalmoplegia 373
Oral rehydration solutions 59, 114
Organochlorines 437-438
Organophosphorous compounds 407
  poisoning 428
    grading of poisoning 429
Osborne "J" waves 469
Osmolality, serum 506-507
  urine 506
Oxygen therapy 11, 19
  hyperbaric 420

P

Pacemaker 170
Palla's sign 22
Pamidronate 382
Pancrea divisum 70
Pancreatic necrosis 69
Pancreatitis 68-74
  abscess 69
  acute 68
  ascites 69
  causes of 70
  clinical features 70
  drugs causing 70
  imaging 71
  management of 72-73
  necrotising 73
  pseudocyst 69, 71
  severe 69
Panhypopituritarism 373
Papillary muscle dysfunction 158
Paraplegia 274
  acute 274
  causes of 274
  signs and symptoms 275
  spinal shcok 276
Parapneumonic effusion 45
Parathyroid hormone 375
Pemphigus 526
  clinical Features 526
  ELISA 527
  erythematosus 527
  foliaceous 527
  Hansen's sign 527
  Nikolsky's sign 527
  treatment 527
  types 526
  vegetans 527
Percutaneous
  transluminal coronary angioplasty (PTCA) 131, 181
Pericardiectomy 186
Pericardiocentesis 186
Pericarditis 183
Phenobarbitone 253
Phenothiazine 56
Phenytoin 253
Phosphine (PH_3) 433
  blood levels 434
  inhalation of 433
    manifestations 434

Pituitary
  adenomas 372
  apoplexy 372
Plant poisoning 439-441
  dhatura 439
  mushroom 441
Plasmapheresis
  in nephritic syndrome 388
  in thrombotic thrombocytopenic purpura 306
Platelet
  concentrates 317
  dysfunction 397
  transfusions 305
Pleural effusion 45
  pancreatitis 54
  peel 49
Pleurodhesis 33
Plicamycin 382
Pneumatic compression devices 27
Pneumocystis carini
  pneumonia 8
  pneumothorax in 30
Pneumomediastinum 410
Pneumonia 7-11
  aetiology 9
  antibiotic therapy 10
  atypical presentation 8
  bronchyscopy 9
  management 10
  severity 9
  typical 8
Pneumothorax 29-33
  interstitial lung diseases 30
  pneumocystis carini pneumonia 30
  primary spontaenous 30
  secondary sponatenous 30
  tension 31
  traumatic 29
Poisoning 401-408
  accidental 402
  acute 402
  barbiturate 456
  benzodiazepines 454
  homicidal 402
  oleander 440
  mushroom 441
  sedative hypnotic 454-457
  self 402
  zinc phosphide 436

Polyneuritis, acute inflammatory demyelinating 280-285
Polyvalent anti-snake venom 446
Positive end expiratory pressure (PEEP) 19
Postural syncope 229
Potassium, serum 512, 516
Potassium channel openers 181
Pralidoxime (PAM) 431
Presyncope 225
Procainamide 159, 162
Promethazine 56
Propofol 253
Propranolol 364
Propylthiouracil 364
Pseudoaneurysm 139
Pseudo-haemoptysis 3
Pseudohyponatremia 503
Psychosis 210
Pulmonary angiogrpahy 5, 24
Pulmonary artery 141
Pulmonary edema 153-158
  acute 153
  clinical features 155
  high altitude 473
  in mitral stenosis 155
  non-cardiogenic 16
  re-expansion 33
Pulmonary embolism 20-28
  diagnosis 25
  ECHO in 26
  management 26
  probability 24
  prophylaxis 27
Pulsus paradoxus 185
Purpura
  Henoch-Schonlein (HSP) 307
  thrombocytopenic 301-305
  thrombotic thrombocytopenic (TTP) 206-308
Physostigmine 440

Q

Quinine 123

R

Rabies 102-105
  clinical features 102-103
  immunization
    acute 102

antirabies serum 103
  passive 103
  immunoglobulin (HRIG) 103
  incubation period 103
  management 102
  paralytic 103
  treatment 103
Raised intracranial pressure 289-292
  clinical features 290
  idiopathic 291
  management 292
Ranson's criteria 74
Reflux oesophagitis 61
Rehydration 113
Renal failure
  acute 390-398
    causes of 391
  biopsy 395
  post renal 391
    causes 391
  prerenal 391
    causes 391
Renal vein thrombosis 393
Respiratory acidosis 497
  causes of 498
Respiratory failure 39-44
  classification 40
  clinical features 41
  definition 329
  management 41-43
  type I 40
  type II 40
Reticulocytosis 296
Revascularisation 128, 133
  myocardial infarction 128
Rewarming
  active external 471
  passive external 470
Rhabdomyolysis 477
Rib resection 50
Risus sardonicus 106
Rose spots 100

S

Salbutamol 15
Scorpion sting 450-453
Seizures
  complex partial status 252
  nonconvulsive status 252

540 Emergency Medicine

Sepsis 91-95
  causes of 92
  clinical features 92-93
  definitions 91
  diagnosis 92
  management 93-95
  predisposing factors 92
  shock 91
Sequestration crisis 300
Sheehan's syndrome 369
Shock
  acute circulatory failure 142
  AMI 127
  cardiogenic 134
  septic 91
SIADH 506
  causes of SIADH 506
  demeclocycline in 506
  diagnostic criteria 506
  management 507
Signal-averaged ECG 228
Silent chest 13
Silver nitrate paper test 432
Sinus node dysfunction 170
Skin infections 528
  clinical Features 529
  treatment 528, 529
Snake bite 442
  elapid bite 444
  hydrophidae bites 444
  management 445
  viper bite 444
Snakes
  cardiotoxic 444
  hemotoxic 444
  myotoxic 444
  neurotoxic 444
Sodium, serum 502
  nitroprusside 202
Somatostatin
  octreotide 64
Spinal cord compression 273-279
  causes of 274
  clinical features 274
  localisation of lesion 276
  management 278
Staphylococci
Status asthmaticus 12

Status epilepticus 251-254
  classification 252
Stevens-Johnson syndrome 530
  causes 530
  clinical Features 530
  treatment 531
Sting-scorpion 450
Stokes-Adam attacks 174-176
Streptokinase 129
Stress ulceration 64
Stroke 235-245
  acute ischemic 235
  aetiology 237
  ischemic 237
  ischemic penumbra in 236
  neuroprotective 243
  lacunar stroke 237
  management 242
  prevention of 245
  rehabilitation 245
  types of 237
Subarachnoid hemorrhage 246-250
  causes of 247
  complications 249
    imaging 249
  management 249
  symptoms of 247
Sudden cardiac death (SCD) 191-196
  causes 192
  cardiomyopathy 192
  coronary artery disease 192
  left ventricular dysfunction 192
  management 193
  survival 191
Sumatriptan 224
Supraventricular tachyarrhythmias 161
Swan Ganz catheterization 135, 141
Syncope 225-229
  carotid sinus 229
  differential diagnosis of 229
  Holter 228
  micturition 226
  neurocardiogenic 227
  postural 229
  vasodepressor 226
  vasovagal 229
Syndrome of inappropriate AVP secretion 506

T

Temperature
  core 469
  monitoring 471
  skin surface 464
Tetanus 106-109
  cephalic 107
  clinical features 107
  complications 109
  immunization 109
    active 109
  incubation period 107
  local 107
  management 108
  neonatal 107
Tetanus immune globulin (TIG) 108
Tetanus toxoid 109
Tetany 376
Thoracentesis 47
Thoracoscopy 50
Thrombin time 316
Thrombocytopenia 301-305
Thrombolysis 26, 129
  in AMI 130
  intrapleural 50
  pulmonary embolism 20
Thromboplastin 26
Thumpversion 166
Thyroid storm 361-364
  apathetic 362
  beta-blockers 364
  clinical features 362
  factitious 362
  Grave's disease 362
  management 363
  precipitating factors 362
TIA 236
Toxic-shock syndrome 376, 528
tPA 130
Transfusion reactions, acute 339
Transient global amnesia 238
Transjugular intrahepatic
  portosystemis shunt 64
Transplantation 82
  hepatic 79
Transtracheal aspiration 9
Transverse sinus thrombosis 287

Index

Traveller's diarrhea 58
Trismus 108
Troponins 178
Trousseau's
   sign 377
Tubercular, meningitis 261
Tumor lysis syndrome 334
Typhoid carrier 99
Typhoid 99-101
   clinical features 100
   complications 100
   management 101
   state 101

U

UGI bleeding 61-64
   balloon tamponade 64
   endoscopy 63
   in peptic ulcer 63
Ulcerative colitis 66
Upright tilt testing 227

Urine
   low ouput 386
   specific gravity 394
Urokinase 123

V

V/Q mismatch 40
   scan 24
Valporate 254
Vasopressin 64
Vasovagal syncope 229
Ventricular fibrillation 166, 168
   causes 168
Ventricular tachycardia 165-167
   diagnosis 164
   sustained VT 165
   treatment 161
Vertebrobasilar
   infarction 240
Vertigo 230-234
   acute 230

BPPV 233
   causes 230
   central 233
   management of 233
Vestibular rehabilitation 234
Vestibulo ocular reflex 217
Vibrio cholerae 112
Vomiting 53-56
   causes 54
   clinical evaluaiton 54
   drug therpay 55

W

Waterhouse-Friederichsen syndrome 369
Westermark's sign 22
Widal test 100
Wilson's disease 80

Z

Zollinger Ellison syndrome 54
Zolpidem 455